D1476797

DIAGNOSTIC CYTOLOGY and HEMATOLOGY

of the Dog and Cat

DIAGNOSTIC CYTOLOGY and HEMATOLOGY
of the Dog and Cat

Third Edition

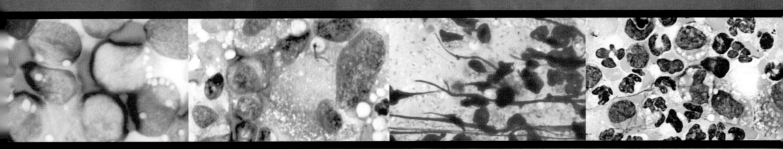

Rick L. Cowell, DVM, MS, MRCVS, DACVP
Clinical Pathologist
IDEXX Laboratories, Inc.
Stillwater, Oklahoma

Ronald D. Tyler, DVM, PhD, DACVP, DABT
Harlingen, Texas

James H. Meinkoth, DVM, PhD, DACVP
Professor
Department of Veterinary Pathobiology
Center for Veterinary Health Sciences
Oklahoma State University
Stillwater, Oklahoma

Dennis B. DeNicola, DVM, PhD, DACVP
Clinical Pathologist
Chief Veterinary Educator
IDEXX Laboratories, Inc.
Westbrook, Maine

With 1,032 illustrations

MOSBY

ELSEVIER

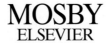

11830 Westline Industrial Drive
St. Louis, Missouri 63146

DIAGNOSTIC CYTOLOGY AND HEMATOLOGY
OF THE DOG AND CAT, THIRD EDITION

ISBN: 978-0-323-03422-7

Copyright © 2008, 1999, 1989 by Mosby, Inc., an affiliate of Elsevier Inc.

Library of Congress Control Number: 2007928088

Vice President and Publisher: Linda Duncan
Senior Acquisitions Editor: Anthony Winkel
Developmental Editor: Maureen Slaten
Publishing Services Manager: Pat Joiner-Myers
Senior Project Manager: Gena Magouirk
Design Direction: Margaret Reid

Printed in Canada

Last digit is the print number: 9 8 7 6 5 4 3 2 1

Contributors

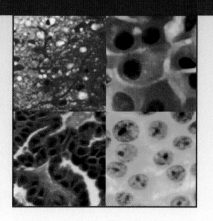

Robin W. Allison, DVM, PhD, DACVP
Associate Professor
Department of Veterinary Pathobiology
Center for Veterinary Health Sciences
Oklahoma State University
Stillwater, Oklahoma
Subcutaneous Glandular Tissue: Mammary, Salivary,
*   Thyroid, and Parathyroid*
Vaginal Cytology

Claire B. Andreasen, DVM, PhD, DACVP, MS
Professor and Chair
Department of Veterinary Pathology
College of Veterinary Medicine
Iowa State University
Ames, Iowa
Nasal Exudates and Masses

Christian Bédard, DMV, IPSAV, DACVP, MSc
Assistant Professor
College of Veterinary Medicine
Université de Montréal
Saint-Hyacinthe, Montréal (Québec), Canada
Cerebrospinal Fluid Analysis

Deborah C. Bernreuter, DVM, MS
Clinical Pathologist
IDEXX Laboratories, Inc.
Irvine, California
The Oropharynx and Tonsils

Dori L. Borjesson, DVM, PhD, DACVP
Associate Professor
Department of Pathology, Microbiology,
   and Immunology
School of Veterinary Medicine
University of California–Davis
Davis, California
The Pancreas

Rick L. Cowell, DVM, MS, MRCVS, DACVP
Clinical Pathologist
IDEXX Laboratories, Inc.
Stillwater, Oklahoma
Sample Collection and Preparation
Cell Types and Criteria of Malignancy
Selected Infectious Agents
Cutaneous and Subcutaneous Lesions
The External Ear Canal
Effusions: Abdominal, Thoracic, and Pericardial
Transtracheal and Bronchoalveolar Washes
The Lung and Intrathoracic Structures
The Kidneys
The Bone Marrow

Mitchell A. Crystal, DVM, DACVIM
Chief of Medicine
North Florida Veterinary Specialists
Consultant, Vet Med Fax and Associates
Jacksonville, Florida
Cerebrospinal Fluid Analysis

Dennis B. DeNicola, DVM, PhD, DACVP
Clinical Pathologist
Chief Veterinary Educator
IDEXX Laboratories, Inc.
Westbrook, Maine
Selected Infectious Agents
Round Cells
The Lung and Intrathoracic Structures

Michel Desnoyers, DVM, PhD, DACVP
Professor
College of Veterinary Medicine
Université de Montréal
Saint-Hyacinthe, Montréal (Québec), Canada
Cerebrospinal Fluid Analysis

Kate English, BSc, BVetMed, DipRCPath, MRCVS
Lecturer, Veterinary Clinical Pathology
Department of Pathology and Infectious Diseases
The Royal Veterinary College
North Mymms
Hatfield, Hertfordshire, United Kingdom
Transtracheal and Bronchoalveolar Washes

Patty J. Ewing, DVM, DACVP, MS
Director, Clinical Laboratory
Department of Pathology
Angell Animal Medical Center
Boston, Massachusetts
The Kidneys

Peter J. Fernandes, DVM, DACVP
Clinical Pathologist
IDEXX Veterinary Services, Inc.
Altadena, California
Synovial Fluid Analysis

Susan E. Fielder, DVM, MS
Resident
Department of Veterinary Pathobiology
Center for Veterinary Health Sciences
Oklahoma State University
Stillwater, Oklahoma
The Musculoskeletal System

T.W. French, DVM, DACVP
Associate Professor
Population Medicine and Diagnostic Sciences
College of Veterinary Medicine
Cornell University
Ithaca, New York
The Liver

Carol B. Grindem, DVM, PhD, DACVP
Professor, Clinical Pathology
Department of Population Health and Pathobiology
College of Veterinary Medicine
North Carolina State University
Raleigh, North Carolina
The Bone Marrow

Kenneth S. Latimer, DVM, PhD, DACVP
Professor
Department of Veterinary Pathology
College of Veterinary Medicine
University of Georgia
Athens, Georgia
Nasal Exudates and Masses
The Gastrointestinal Tract

Peter S. MacWilliams, DVM, PhD, DACVP
Professor, Clinical Pathology
Department of Pathobiological Sciences
School of Veterinary Medicine
University of Wisconsin–Madison
Madison, Wisconsin
The Spleen

Jeanne M. Maddux, DVM, PhD, DACVP
Aurora Animal Clinic
Fairbanks, Alaska
Subcutaneous Glandular Tissue: Mammary, Salivary, Thyroid, and Parathyroid

Edward A. Mahaffey, DVM, PhD, DACVP
Watkinsville, Georgia
The Musculoskeletal System

James H. Meinkoth, DVM, PhD, DACVP
Professor
Department of Veterinary Pathobiology
Center for Veterinary Health Sciences
Oklahoma State University
Stillwater, Oklahoma
Sample Collection and Preparation
Cell Types and Criteria of Malignancy
Selected Infectious Agents
Cutaneous and Subcutaneous Lesions
Cerebrospinal Fluid Analysis
Effusions: Abdominal, Thoracic, and Pericardial
Transtracheal and Bronchoalveolar Washes
The Lung and Intrathoracic Structures
The Kidneys

Joanne B. Messick, VMD, PhD, DACVP
Associate Professor, Veterinary Clinical Pathology
Comparative Pathobiology
School of Veterinary Medicine
Purdue University
West Lafayette, Indiana
The Lymph Nodes

Dennis J. Meyer, DMV, DACVIM, DACVP
Executive Director, Navigator Services
Charles River Preclinical Services
Reno, Nevada
The Liver

Rebecca J. Morton, DVM, PhD, DACVM
Associate Professor
Department of Pathobiology
Center for Veterinary Health Sciences
Oklahoma State University
Stillwater, Oklahoma
Sample Collection and Preparation

Patricia N. Olson, DVM, PhD, DACT
CEO
Morris Animal Foundation
Inglewood, Colorado
Vaginal Cytology

Penny K. Patten, DVM, DACVP
Resident
Department of Veterinary Pathobiology
Center for Veterinary Health Sciences
Oklahoma State University
Stillwater, Oklahoma
The External Ear Canal

Keith W. Prasse, DVM, PhD, DACVP
Professor and Dean Emeritus
College of Veterinary Medicine
University of Georgia
Athens, Georgia
The Eyes and Associated Structures

Pauline M. Rakich, DVM, PhD, DACVP
Athens Diagnostic Laboratory
College of Veterinary Medicine
University of Georgia
Athens, Georgia
Nasal Exudates and Masses
The Gastrointestinal Tract

Theresa E. Rizzi, DVM, DACVP
Instructor, Clinical Pathology
Department of Veterinary Pathobiology
Center for Veterinary Health Sciences
Oklahoma State University
Stillwater, Oklahoma
Effusions: Abdominal, Thoracic, and Pericardial

Tracy Stokol, PhD, DACVP, BVSc
Assistant Professor
Population Medicine and Diagnostic Sciences
College of Veterinary Medicine
Cornell University
Ithaca, New York
The Liver

Mary Anna Thrall, DVM, DACVP, MS
Professor
Department of Microbiology, Immunology
  and Pathology
College of Veterinary Medicine and Biomedical Sciences
Colorado State University
Fort Collins, Colorado
Vaginal Cytology

Ronald D. Tyler, DVM, PhD, DACVP, DABT
Harlingen, Texas
Sample Collection and Preparation
Cell Types and Criteria of Malignancy
Selected Infectious Agents
Cutaneous and Subcutaneous Lesions
The External Ear Canal
Effusions: Abdominal, Thoracic, and Pericardial
Transtracheal and Bronchoalveolar Washes
The Lung and Intrathoracic Structures
The Kidneys
The Bone Marrow

Dana Walker, DVM, PhD, DACVP
Principle Pathologist and Site Director
Clinical Pathology Department
Bristol-Myers Squibb
Syracuse, New York
Peripheral Blood Smears

Julie L. Webb, DVM
Resident
Department of Pathology
College of Veterinary Medicine
University of Georgia
Athens, Georgia
The Gastrointestinal Tract

Karen M. Young, VMD, PhD
Clinical Professor
Department of Pathobiological Sciences
School of Veterinary Medicine
University of Wisconsin–Madison
Madison, Wisconsin
The Eyes and Associated Structures

Joseph G. Zinkl, DVM, PhD, DACVP
Professor Emeritus
Department of Pathology, Microbiology,
  and Immunology
School of Veterinary Medicine
University of California–Davis
Davis, California
Examination of the Urinary Sediment
The Male Reproductive Tract: Prostate, Testes, and Semen

Preface

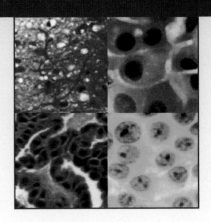

Cytologic evaluation of blood, fluid, and tissue specimens is an especially valuable diagnostic aid in veterinary medicine. Reliable, confident interpretation of carefully obtained, well-preserved, representative cellular samples is essential for accurate diagnosis, prognosis, and treatment. *Diagnostic Cytology and Hematology of the Dog and Cat, Third Edition* is a comprehensive yet practical reference designed to help the reader develop and enhance the necessary clinical laboratory and interpretive skills for a wide variety of pathologic conditions seen in everyday practice, along with those less frequently encountered.

The goal of this reference text is to provide small-animal veterinary clinicians and cytology students with the knowledge and skills required to apply cytodiagnostic techniques to sample collection, preparation, microscopic assessment, and interpretation. It is intended to be a familiar and trusted bench-top reference and guide alongside the microscope. The numerous tables and flowcharts that accompany the text assist the reader in the correlation of cytologic findings with clinical signs and history, physical examination, diagnostic imaging, and other clinical laboratory findings to achieve the most accurate and specific diagnosis possible, while being rapid and efficient.

Written in a logical, highly visual manner, we believe we have provided a resource that will establish and maintain a secure clinical foundation for the technical as well as interpretive aspects of cytological diagnostic screening. The straightforward text is organized for quick information retrieval. Over 1000 high-resolution, full-color photomicrographs illustrate pertinent features of lesions, aid in the differentiation of normal cells from abnormal cells, and demonstrate the variability of patterns seen in certain conditions. Helpful and easy-to-follow algorithms and tables are distributed throughout the text to facilitate rapid and efficient progression through the diagnostic process. Because inappropriate sample collection and poor slide preparation are often the major impediments to sample quality, we have included valuable preparation tips to guide the clinician through the initial workup and around the common pitfalls to the best diagnosis. This not only facilitates accurate on-site diagnosis but also permits the practitioner to confidently submit diagnostic-quality samples to a cytopathologist for interpretation.

This edition maintains the practical diagnostic approach of its predecessors, and four new chapters—*Cell Types and Criteria of Malignancy, Selected Infectious Agents, Round Cells,* and *The Pancreas*—have been added to broaden the text's scope for greater usefulness.

In addition, chapters from the previous edition have been substantially updated to include recently recognized conditions, new terminology, and new procedures. Three chapters in particular—*Effusions: Abdominal, Thoracic, and Pericardial; The Lung and Intrathoracic Structures;* and *The Gastrointestinal Tract*—offer more expanded coverage and have been reorganized to integrate relevant information for better understanding.

The authors hope that you will truly find this one of the most used references in your clinical library. We also believe that, with the knowledge and skills you glean from use of this resource, you will reduce your clinical time and frustrations and, most importantly, improve the quality of care you deliver to your patients and their people.

Rick L. Cowell
Ronald D. Tyler
James H. Meinkoth
Dennis B. DeNicola

Acknowledgements

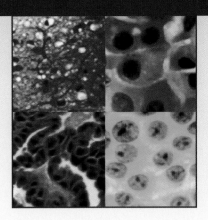

We thank our families for their support and understanding. Many other people deserve acknowledgement and sincere thanks also. These include Elsevier's excellent editors and staff and the many veterinary pathologists at IDEXX laboratories who sent slides or pictures for use in the text, especially Drs. Dean Cornwell, Desiree Lipscomb, Tammy Johnson, Debbie Bernreuter, and Pete Fernandes.

It was an honor and privilege to work with each of the authors. They are exceptional veterinarians, scientists, and teachers. We thank them for sharing their time, talent, and expertise, and we thank their families for sharing them. Finally, we would like to thank IDEXX Laboratories for generously supporting veterinary education and this book in particular.

Rick L. Cowell
Ronald D. Tyler
James H. Meinkoth
Dennis B. DeNicola

Contents

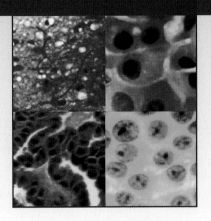

Sample Collection and Preparation

J.H. Meinkoth, R.L. Cowell, R.D. Tyler, and R.J. Morton

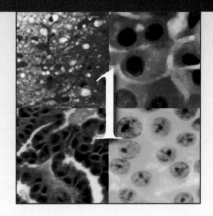

CHAPTER

The role of cytology as a diagnostic tool in veterinary medicine continues to expand. Cytology is a reliable method of obtaining a tissue diagnosis in a minimally invasive way. As clinicians have increased their use of this diagnostic methodology and cytopathologists have become more experienced with a wider variety of lesions, the variety of tissues sampled, the spectrum of disease processes identified by cytology, and the reliability and precision of the diagnoses for lesions of many tissues have increased. The widespread availability of ultrasonography has greatly enhanced the ability to accurately sample focal lesions deep within body cavities. Cytology and histopathology will remain complementary diagnostic procedures, reflecting a trade-off between the lower degree of invasiveness of sample collection with cytology and the increased amount of information available from the ability to evaluate tissue architecture with histopathology.

Other than the experience of the cytopathologist evaluating the samples, one of the major factors determining the diagnostic value of cytologic specimens is the quality of the sample. The diagnostic yield of cytology is noticeably higher in the hands of clinicians who have a great deal of experience with obtaining cytologic specimens. With histologic specimens, once the tissue sample is collected and placed in an appropriate amount of formalin, laboratory technicians handle the remainder of sample preparation. With cytology, the clinician is faced with the responsibility of not only collecting an adequately representative specimen, but also preparing the slides that are to be examined and, often, staining of the slides as well. Because the cells to be examined are not grossly visible during sample collection and slide preparation, it is often difficult to tell whether an adequate specimen has been obtained at the time of the sampling procedure.

Collection and preparation of cytologic specimens is definitely a skill gained only through experience and refinement of technique based on the results obtained. Many clinicians (and owners) are understandably frustrated when a sample submitted is determined to be nondiagnostic. Fortunately, an understanding of some basic principles of sample collection and familiarity with some of the more common pitfalls related to cytologic sample preparation (often learned by hard experience) can eliminate many nondiagnostic results.[1-5] Finally, knowing which samples have a high probability of yielding diagnostic information and which samples do not is important in determining when to use cytology and in preparing the owner for the results that are likely to be obtained.

METHODS OF SAMPLE COLLECTION

There are several methods of collecting samples for cytologic analysis. The indications for each are outlined in Table 1-1.

Fine-Needle Biopsy

Fine-needle biopsy (FNB) can be performed using a standard syringe and needle with or without aspiration (described later). This is probably the best overall method for sampling any mass or proliferative lesion, as well as for sampling any subcutaneous glandular organ, such as lymph node, mammary gland, or salivary gland.[4] FNB is also best suited for minimally invasive sampling of internal organs or masses. FNB allows collection of cells from deep within the lesion, avoiding surface contamination with cells and organisms that often plague impression smears, swabs, or scrapings.

Selection of Syringe and Needle: FNBs are collected with a 22- to 25-ga needle and a 3- to 20-ml syringe. The softer the tissue, the smaller the needle and syringe used. It is seldom necessary to use a needle larger than 22-ga for aspiration, even for firm tissues. When needles larger than 22-ga are used, tissue cores tend to be aspirated, resulting in a poor yield of free cells. Also, larger needles tend to cause greater blood contamination.

The size of syringe used is influenced by the consistency of the tissue being aspirated. Softer tissues, such as lymph nodes, often can be aspirated with a 3-ml syringe. Firm tissues, such as fibromas and squamous-cell carcinomas, require a larger syringe to maintain adequate negative pressure (suction) for collection of a sufficient number of cells. A 12-ml syringe is a good choice if the texture of the tissue is unknown.

TABLE 1-1

Indications for Various Methods of Sample Collection

Collection Method	Indications for Uses	Comments
Fine-needle biopsy (aspiration or nonaspiration method)	Masses (surface or internal) Lymph nodes Internal organs Fluid collection	Best method for minimally invasive sampling of internal organs/masses Best method for cutaneous/subcutaneous masses because it avoids surface contamination
Impression smear	Exudative cutaneous lesions Preparation of cytology samples from biopsy specimens	Most useful for identification of infectious organisms May yield only surface cells and contamination (problem with ulcerated tumors) With biopsy specimens, it is imperative to blot excess blood from sample Impression smears of biopsy specimens must be made before exposure of biopsy sample to formalin
Scraping	Used with flat cutaneous lesions that are not amenable to fine-needle biopsy Preparation of cytology samples from poorly exfoliative biopsy specimens	With dry cutaneous lesions (e.g., ringworm), it is important to scrape sufficiently to obtain some blood/serum to help cells stick to slide
Swab	Vaginal smears Fistulous tracts	Generally used only when anatomic location not amenable to collection by other means With fistulous tracts, most useful in classifying type of inflammatory response and identifying infectious organisms

Preparation of the Site for Aspiration: If microbiologic tests are to be performed on a portion of the sample collected, or a body cavity (peritoneal and thoracic cavities, joints, etc.) is to be penetrated, the area of aspiration is surgically prepped. Otherwise, skin preparation is essentially that required for a vaccination or venipuncture. An alcohol swab can be used to clean the area. If the samples are being collected using ultrasound guidance, it is important to avoid the use of ultrasound gel, substituting alcohol as a contact agent instead. Ultrasound gel stains pink with commonly used cytology stains. Even a small amount of ultrasound gel picked up as a contaminant when the needle passes through the skin is enough to completely obscure the cells and render a slide nondiagnostic.

Aspiration Procedure: With the standard aspiration method of FNB, the mass is stabilized with one hand while the needle, with syringe attached, is introduced into the center of the mass (Figure 1-1). Strong negative pressure is applied by withdrawing the plunger to about threefourths the volume of the syringe (Figure 1-2). If the mass is sufficiently large and the patient sufficiently restrained, negative pressure can be maintained while the needle is moved back and forth repeatedly, passing through about two thirds of the diameter of the mass. With large masses, the needle can be redirected to several areas within the mass to increase the amount of tissue sampled. Alternatively, several different areas of the mass can be sampled with separate collection attempts. Care should be taken to not

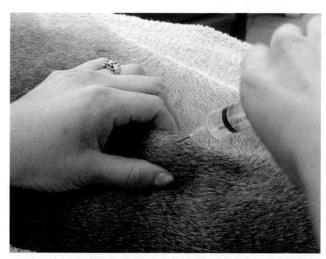

Figure 1-1 Aspiration technique of FNB. The mass is stabilized with one hand while the needle is introduced into the center of the mass. The hand holding the syringe is used to pull back on the plunger, creating negative pressure. *(Courtesy Oklahoma State University teaching files.)*

allow the needle to exit the mass while negative pressure is being applied because this can result in either aspiration of the sample into the barrel of the syringe (where it may not be retrievable) or contamination of the sample with tissue surrounding the mass.

The negative pressure should not be applied for more than a few seconds in any one area. Often, there will be

A   **B**   **C**

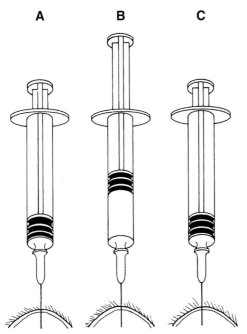

Figure 1-2 Fine-needle aspiration from a solid mass. After the needle is within the mass **(A)**, negative pressure is placed on the syringe by rapidly withdrawing the plunger **(B)**, usually one half to three fourths the volume of the syringe barrel. The needle is redirected several times while negative pressure is maintained, if this can be accomplished without the needle's point leaving the mass. Before the needle is removed from the mass, the plunger is released, relieving negative pressure on the syringe **(C)**.

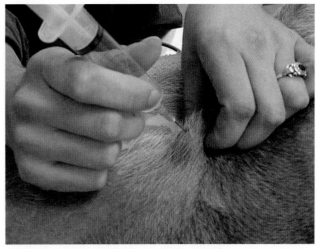

Figure 1-3 Nonaspiration technique of FNB. The syringe is held at or near the needle hub with the thumb and forefinger. Note that the syringe is prefilled with air. The free hand is used to stabilize the mass. This technique allows greater control over movement of the needle. *(Courtesy Oklahoma State University teaching files.)*

no material visible in the syringe or in the hub of the needle even though an adequate sample has been obtained. With excessive force or prolonged application of negative pressure, disruption of blood vessels will eventually occur and the sample will be contaminated with peripheral blood, diluting the tissue cells and rendering the sample nondiagnostic.

After several areas are sampled, the negative pressure is released and the needle is removed from the mass and skin. The needle is removed from the syringe and air is drawn into the syringe. The needle is replaced onto the syringe and some of the tissue in the barrel and hub of the needle is expelled onto the middle of a glass microscope slide by rapidly depressing the plunger. When possible, several preparations should be made, as described later in this chapter ("Preparation of Slides").

Nonaspiration Procedure (Capillary Technique, Stab Technique): Many people prefer to collect FNB without the application of negative pressure, and this technique can yield samples of equal or better quality than those obtained with the standard aspiration technique.[4,5] The non-aspiration technique works well for most masses, especially those that are highly vascular.[1,4] This technique is similar to the standard fine needle aspiration biopsy technique, except no negative pressure is applied during collection. The procedure is performed using a small-gauge needle on a 5- to 12-ml syringe. The barrel of the syringe is filled with air

prior to the collection attempt to allow rapid expulsion of material onto a glass slide. The syringe is grasped at or near the needle hub with the thumb and forefinger (much like holding a dart) to allow for maximal control (Figure 1-3). The mass to be aspirated is stabilized with a free hand, and the needle is inserted into the mass. The needle is rapidly moved back and forth in a stabbing motion, trying to stay along the same tract. This allows cells to be collected by cutting and tissue pressure. Care must be taken to keep the needle tip within the mass to prevent contamination with surrounding tissue. The needle is then withdrawn and the material in the needle is rapidly expelled onto a clean glass slide, and a smear is made using one of the techniques listed later in this chapter (see "Preparation of Slides"). Having the syringe pre-filled with air allows the sample to be expelled onto a slide more quickly, thereby helping to avoid desiccation (drying out) of the collected cells and coagulation of the sample. Generally, material sufficient for only one smear is collected. If possible, it is optimal to perform multiple collection attempts at various sites within the mass to increase the chance of obtaining diagnostic material and to ensure a representative sampling of the lesion.

Collection Tip
Make and submit multiple slides—This is one of the most important things that can be done to increase the diagnostic yield. Small-gauge needles are used for collecting cytologic specimens and the procedure is usually relatively painless. It takes less time to perform several collection attempts and prepare multiple slides when the animal is first presented than to repeat a procedure after finding the slide(s) to be nondiagnostic, often after the animal has already been discharged from the hospital. This is particularly important if sedation/anesthesia is required for collection. It is optimal to stain and briefly examine one or two slides to ensure that they are adequately cellular while the patient is still in the hospital (or before animal is recovered, if anesthesia/sedation is required).

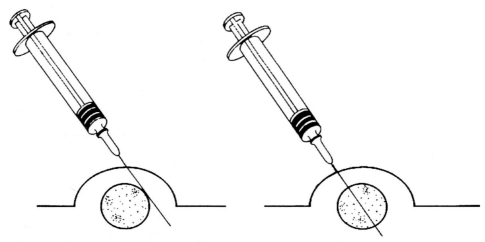

Figure 1-4 Geographic miss. Sometimes the needle is not in the area containing representative tissue of the lesion during sample collection. This is common in obese animals where the lesion may be surrounded by abundant subcutaneous fat. *(Courtesy Oklahoma State University teaching files.)*

If the slides stained are not cellular, additional collection attempts can be performed immediately.

There are many reasons why any one slide may be nondiagnostic. The slide may not have any diagnostic cells because the needle missed the lesion during collection (geographic miss) (Figure 1-4) or may have been in a nonrepresentative portion of the lesion (e.g., an area of inflammation or necrosis within a neoplasm (Figure 1-5). In addition, some lesions simply do not exfoliate cells well. Even if adequate cells were collected, many times the cells do not spread out well and the slides are too thick to evaluate (especially common with lymph node aspirates) or all of the cells are ruptured during smear preparation (Figure 1-6). Even in the hands of clinicians who are highly experienced in sample collection, it is not unusual to evaluate multiple slides from a single lesion and have all but one of the slides be nondiagnostic for one reason or another.

If possible, a minimum of four to five slides, representing collection attempts from several sites within the lesion, should be submitted from any lesion. If some of the samples appear to be excessively thick or if little to no material is apparent on the slides, make additional slides. With multiple slides the odds are better that at least one of them will be of diagnostic quality.

If multiple masses are sampled, always use a new needle and syringe with each mass. If this is not done, slides from one mass may be contaminated with cells left in the needle from previous collection attempts.

Collection Tip
Avoid blood dilution—Blood contamination (hemodilution) is another common cause of nondiagnostic slides. FNB with aspiration will collect the tissue of least resistance. If blood vessels within the lesion have been ruptured, the tissue of least resistance will be peripheral blood. Once significant blood contamination has occurred, it is difficult to salvage the sample. Additional collection attempts using a clean syringe and needle should be performed.

The two major causes of blood contamination are the use of too large a needle (<22-ga) and prolonged aspiration.

Larger-bore needles do not usually collect more cells, but are more likely to rupture small blood vessels. As said before, material is often not visible in the syringe during sample collection, despite adequate numbers of cells being present within the needle. Any time material is visible in the hub of the needle, the collection procedure should be stopped and slides made immediately.

Some lesions are highly vascular, making it difficult to avoid blood contamination, even with good collection technique. In these cases, use of a nonaspiration technique may result in less blood contamination and more tissue cells for evaluation.

Collection Tip
Don't be timid—Other reasons for poor cellularity of a sample are inadequate negative pressure (aspiration technique) and slow or shallow needle passages (nonaspiration technique). Needle passages should be quick and of sufficient length (although the size of the mass may limit the length of the needle pass).

Impression Smears

Impression smears can be made from ulcerated or exudative superficial lesions (Figure 1-7) or tissue samples collected at surgery or necropsy. Impression smears from superficial lesions often yield only inflammatory cells even if the inflammation is a secondary process; neoplastic cells may not exfoliate in exudates or impression smears of ulcerated masses. If possible, FNB of tissue under the ulcerated/exudative area should be collected in addition to the impression smears. Inserting the needle at a nonulcerated area will help reduce contamination during collection. Impression smears of exudates or ulcers are most beneficial for determining if bacterial or fungal organisms are present. Keep in mind that bacteria may reflect only a secondary bacterial infection.

Ulcers should be imprinted before they are cleaned. The lesion should then be cleaned with a saline-moistened surgical sponge and reimprinted or scraped.

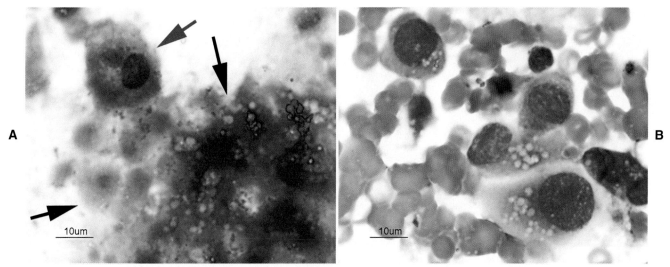

Figure 1-5   Samples collected from a prostatic carcinoma with areas of necrosis. **A,** Most slides were from aspirates of necrotic areas and contain predominantly necrotic cellular debris *(black arrows)*. A single partially intact cell is present *(blue arrow)*. These slides would be nondiagnostic. **B,** One of the aspiration attempts sampled a nonnecrotic area and the resulting slides contained numerous intact cells allowing a diagnosis to be made. This demonstrates the importance of sampling multiple sites of a mass. *(Courtesy Oklahoma State University teaching files.)*

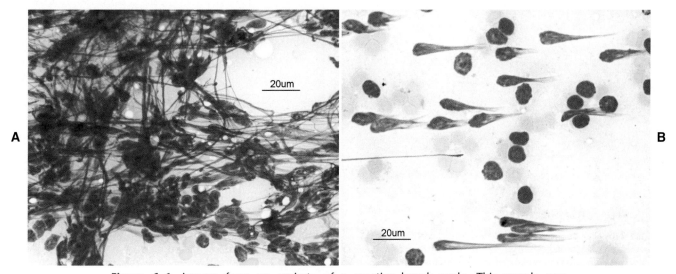

Figure 1-6   Images from an aspirate of a reactive lymph node. This sample was nondiagnostic because all of the cells have been ruptured due to excessive downward pressure being applied during sample preparation. **A,** The linear streaks of material represent nuclear chromatin of ruptured cells. **B,** Ruptured cells often appear to have "comet tails" all going the same direction. *(Courtesy Oklahoma State University teaching files.)*

To collect impression smears from tissues collected during surgery or necropsy, the tissue should first be cut so that there is a fresh surface for imprinting (Figure 1-8). Next, the excess blood and tissue fluid should be removed from the surface of the lesion being imprinted by blotting with a clean absorbent material (Figure 1-9). Excessive blood and tissue fluids inhibit tissue cells from adhering to the glass slide, producing a poorly cellular preparation. Also, excessive fluid inhibits cells from spreading and assuming the size and shape they usually have in air-dried smears. After excess blood and tissue fluids have been blotted from the surface of the lesion, the surface of the

lesion is touched (pressed) against the middle of a clean glass microscope slide and lifted directly up (Figure 1-10). This should be repeated several times so that several tissue imprints are present on the slide. If the excess blood has been adequately removed, the tissue will stick somewhat to the slide and will appear to peel off the slide, if removed slowly. Properly made slides will have slightly opaque areas at the areas of the impressions but should not have excessively thick areas of blood (Figure 1-11).

No further smearing of the material is necessary. Do not slide the tissue around on the glass surface because this causes cells to rupture. When possible, several slides

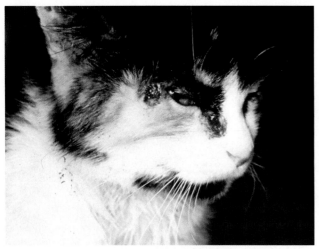

Figure 1-7   Ulcerative, exudative lesions on the face of a cat. This lesion is well suited for impression smears. Slides from these lesions revealed inflammatory cells and many *Sporothrix* organisms. *(Courtesy Oklahoma State University teaching files.)*

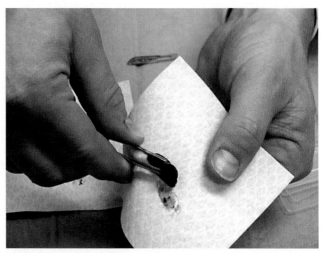

Figure 1-9   The surface of the tissue is blotted several times against an absorbent material to remove excess blood and tissue fluid. This is extremely important to avoid slides that contain only peripheral blood. *(Courtesy Oklahoma State University teaching files.)*

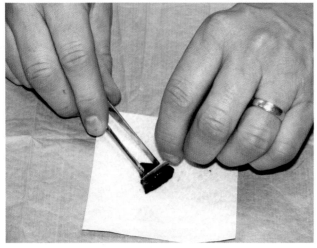

Figure 1-8   Impression smear of tissue removed at surgery. The tissue is trimmed so that there is a fresh surface for making the impression smear. If normal tissue surrounding a mass has been excised, it is important to be sure that the tissue is cut through the area of interest. *(Courtesy Oklahoma State University teaching files.)*

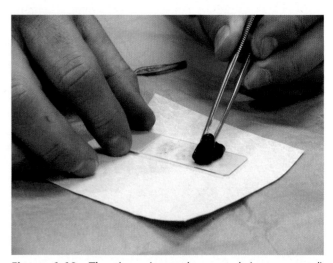

Figure 1-10   The tissue is gently pressed (not smeared) several times against the surface of a clean glass slide. *(Courtesy Oklahoma State University teaching files.)*

should be imprinted so that a few can be retained in case special stains are necessary. After making sufficient impression smears, the tissue used should be placed in an appropriate amount of formalin so that it may be submitted for histologic evaluation if necessary.

Scrapings

Scrapings can be made from external lesions or tissue obtained from surgery or necropsy. Generally, scrapings will result in more cellular slides than will impression smears; however, like impression smears, scrapings may contain mostly surface contamination or inflammation if made from the surface of ulcerated cutaneous lesions. Generally,

scrapings are not as valuable for diagnosing neoplasia as slides made from FNB. Scrapings are valuable in collecting samples from cutaneous lesions that are flat and dry and thus not amenable to FNB or impression and from samples collected at surgery or necropsy (Figure 1-12).[4] Two examples of lesions in which scrapings are beneficial are feline eosinophilic granuloma complex lesions and dermatophytosis. Scrapings are prepared by holding a scalpel blade perpendicular to the lesion's blotted surface and pulling the blade toward oneself several times. When scraping dry, nonulcerated lesions, such as dermatophyte lesions, scrapings should be sufficiently deep to cause exudation of serum/blood. This proteinaceous fluid will help the cells (and hairs when looking for dermatophytes) collected to adhere to the slide and prevent them from being washed off during staining. The material collected

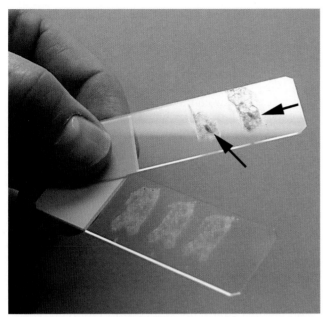

Figure 1-11 The resulting slides from an impression smear. The slide on the bottom is properly made and has several slightly opaque areas where the tissue has been touched to the slide indicating cells have probably been transferred to the slide. The slide on top has excessive peripheral blood *(arrows)* indicating that the tissue was not properly blotted against absorbent material prior to making the impression smear. This slide will likely contain only peripheral blood, or if cells are present, they may not be well spread out. *(Courtesy Oklahoma State University teaching files.)*

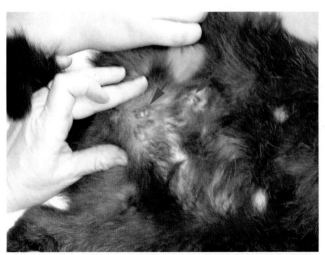

Figure 1-12 Multiple plaque-like and raised lesions on the ventrum of a cat with eosinophilic granuloma lesions. The lesions were not thick enough to obtain good aspirates but yielded diagnostic cells via scraping. The ulcerated lesions are those that have already been scraped *(arrows)*. Scraping to the point of obtaining a small amount of blood/serum helps the cells adhere to the slides and also increases the chance of bypassing surface contamination and obtaining representative cells. *(Courtesy Oklahoma State University teaching files.)*

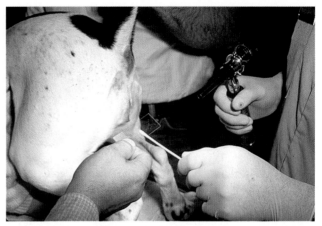

Figure 1-13 Preparation of a vaginal swab from a dog. The swab containing the sample is gently rolled along the slide. Sliding or smearing the swab across the slide will result in excessive rupturing of the cells. *(Courtesy Oklahoma State University teaching files.)*

on the blade is transferred to the middle of a glass microscope slide and spread either by smearing gently with the scalpel blade or by one of the techniques described later for preparation of smears from aspirates of solid masses.

Swabs

Generally, swabs are used only when other collection methods are not practical, such as when obtaining samples from the vagina or external ear, or within fistulous tracts. Swabs from the external ear canal and fistulous tracts are most useful for identifying infectious organisms. Swabs are collected from the site using a sterile cotton swab. If the lesion is moist, the cotton swab need not be moistened. However, if the lesion is not very moist, moistening with sterile saline is suggested. Moistening the swab helps minimize disruption of the cells that might occur during collection and sample preparation. Use of lubricant gels (such as K-Y Jelly) should be avoided when collecting swabs because they can coat the sample and interfere with staining of the cells, rendering the slide uninterpretable. Once the sample has been collected, the swab is gently rolled across the surface of a clean glass slide. It is important to not swipe the swab across the slide because this will often result in rupture of all the cells (Figure 1-13).

PREPARATION OF SLIDES: SOLID TISSUE ASPIRATES

Slide-Over-Slide Smears ("Squash Preps")

When used properly, this is generally the best method for preparing slides from FNB or scrapings of solid tissue lesions. The goal is to prepare a thin film in which the cells are spread out into a single layer, without rupturing the cells. The material collected from the FNB procedure is expelled near one end (~½ inch) of a clean glass slide (sample slide). A second glass slide (spreader slide) is placed on top of, and perpendicular to, the slide containing the sample directly over the specimen (Figure 1-14). The specimen will usually spread out between the two slides due to the weight of the spreader slide alone. If the sample is thick or granular and does not spread out well, light momentary downward pressure may be applied to the spreader slide and then released.[4] The spreader slide is then lightly drawn out across the length of the bottom slide, spreading the sample (Figure 1-15). Despite the name *squash prep*, it is important that no downward pressure is applied to the spreader slide while smearing the sample because this usually results in rupturing the majority of the cells.

When done correctly, this technique does a good job of spreading out the cells, even those in clusters, so that cellular detail can be adequately evaluated. The main disadvantage of this method, particularly in inexperienced hands, is excessive cell rupturing. Lymphoid cells are particularly

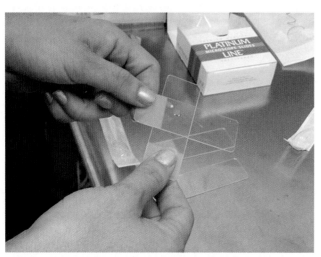

Figure 1-14 Squash preparation. Once the sample has been placed on a clean glass slide, a second slide is place on top of the sample and will be used to spread out the sample. It is important that no downward pressure be applied with the top slide during spreading of the sample. *(Courtesy Oklahoma State University teaching files.)*

fragile and will often rupture if even moderate pressure is used when preparing slides with this technique.

Blood Smear Technique

With many samples, especially lymph node aspirates, the material expelled from the syringe onto the slide will have enough tissue fluid and/or blood that the sample can be smeared out as if making a blood smear (Figure 1-16).[4] This technique will result in less cell rupturing, especially with fragile cell populations, and generally produces thin smears with intact cells that are well spread out.

As with the slide-over-slide technique, the sample is expelled from the syringe near one end of the sample slide. The long edge of the spreader slide is placed onto the flat surface of the sample slide in front of the sample. The spreader slide is tilted to a 45-degree angle with respect to the sample slide and pulled backward about a third of the way into the aspirated material. The spreader slide is then smoothly and rapidly slid forward, as if making a blood smear. The smear should end in a feathered edge at least ½ inch from the opposite end of the spreader slide. This is important because many automated slide stainers do not stain the entire slide, but leave an unstained area approximately ¼ to ½ inch thick on either end of the slide. Cells in these areas will not be stained and therefore cannot be evaluated. Even when using dip-staining methods that stain the entire slide, material at the very edges of a slide may be impossible to view on some microscopes. If the sample smear extends all the way to the edge of a slide, additional slides should be made, and a smaller amount of sample should be put on the slide.

"Starfish" Preps

Another technique for spreading aspirates is to drag the aspirate peripherally in several directions with the point of a syringe needle, producing a starfish shape (Figures 1-17 and 1-18). This technique tends not to damage fragile cells, but allows a thick layer of tissue fluid to remain

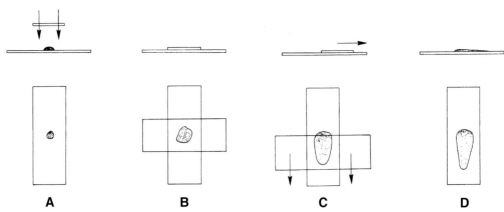

A   **B**   **C**   **D**

Figure 1-15 Squash preparation. **A,** A portion of the aspirate is expelled onto a glass microscope slide and another slide is placed over the sample. **B,** This spreads the sample. If the sample does not spread well, gentle digital pressure can be applied to the top slide. Care must be taken not to place excessive pressure on the slide, causing the cells to rupture. **C,** The slides are smoothly slid apart. **D,** This usually produces well-spread smears but may result in excessive cell rupture.

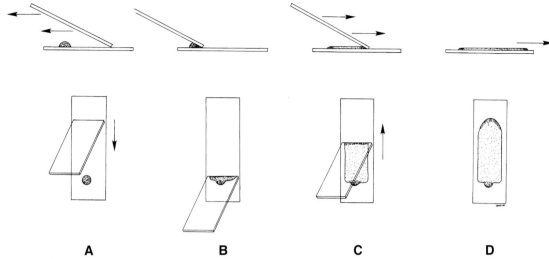

A   **B**   **C**   **D**

Figure 1-16 Blood smear technique. **A,** A drop of fluid sample is placed on a glass microscope slide close to one end, then another slide is slid backward to contact the front of the drop. **B,** When the drop is contacted, it rapidly spreads along the juncture between the two slides. The spreader slide is then smoothly and rapidly slid forward the length of the slide, producing a smear with a feathered edge (**C and D**).

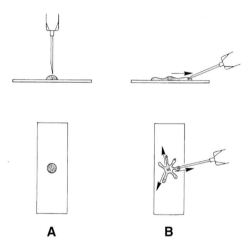

A   **B**

Figure 1-17 Needle spread or "starfish" preparation. **A,** A portion of the aspirate is expelled onto a glass microscope slide. **B,** The tip of a needle is placed in the aspirate and moved peripherally, pulling a trail of the sample with it. This procedure is repeated in several directions, resulting in a preparation with multiple projections.

around the cells. Sometimes, the thick layer of fluid prevents the cells from spreading well and interferes with evaluation of cell detail. Usually some acceptable areas are present, however.

Preparation Tip

Don't let the sample dry/clot—If the sample clots or dries out on the slide before smears can be made, the cells may not spread out sufficiently to be evaluated. Also, the cells will often be distorted or not stain well because they are incorporated in a clot. One common mistake is for people to spray the sample from the needle onto the slide from a long distance. This results in the sample being spread out in many small drops over the slide, much like a shotgun

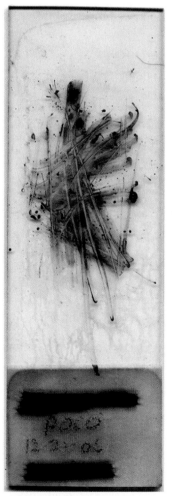

Figure 1-18 Slide prepared using starfish or needle spread technique depicted in Figure 1-17. Blue streaks indicating cellular areas are seen where the needle was dragged repeatedly across the slide and through the sample. *(Courtesy Oklahoma State University teaching files.)*

blast (Figure 1-19). The problem is that these small drops tend to dry before the operator has time to make a smear. When viewed under the microscope, small clusters of poorly spread-out cells (Figure 1-20) are seen, and it is usually impossible to adequately visualize the morphology of the cells. When transferring the sample to the slide, the edge of the needle should be held very close to the slide and the sample should be sprayed in one drop if possible. The sample should then be immediately smeared using one of the techniques described previously. If sufficient sample is obtained to put on more than one slide, it is important to make all smears quickly before the sample dries. When using the nonaspiration technique, pre-filling the syringe with air will shorten the time between sample collection and smear preparation and will reduce the likelihood of the sample clotting before smears can be made.

Preparation Tip

Avoid making too thick a smear—Smears that are too thick will not have cells adequately spread out, making the cells impossible to evaluate. Samples that yield thick smears are those that are contaminated with excessive amounts of peripheral blood or samples collected from tissues that easily exfoliate large numbers of cells (e.g., lymph node aspirates). Ideally, only a small drop of sample should be applied to a slide (about the size of drop used in making a blood smear). If a large amount of sample is applied to a single smear, the smear generally ends up being too thick. If the sample extends all the way to the far end of the slide, the smear will probably be too thick.

Generally, the amount of sample being applied to the slide can be controlled when the material is expelled from the syringe. If too large a drop is applied to a slide, a thin smear can still be obtained by using the blood smear technique. The spreader slide is drawn back just to the point that it barely contacts the sample, which will begin to spread across the surface of the spreader slide by capillary action, and then is rapidly smeared forward. Alternatively, the spreader slide can be placed flat on top of the sample, as when preparing a slide-over-slide technique. Then the spreader slide is lifted up and used to transfer a portion of the sample to another clean glass slide, on which a smear can be made. This technique can be repeated more than once if needed, and finally the remaining material on the initial sample slide is smeared out. In this way, several thin smears can be made from one large drop of sample.

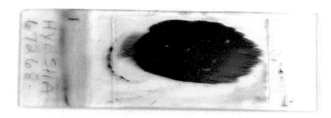

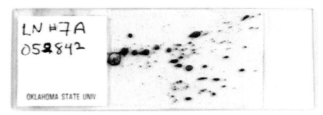

Figure 1-19 Example of a poorly smeared sample. The slide on top is well made. However, the bottom slide shows what happens when a sample is sprayed onto the slide from a distance resulting in a shotgun blast–like arrangement of small drops. These drops dry quickly and then cannot be spread out. *(Courtesy Oklahoma State University teaching files.)*

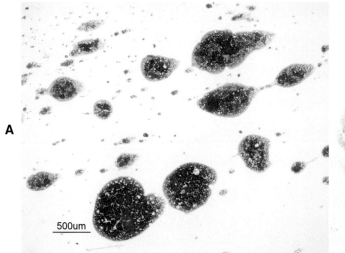

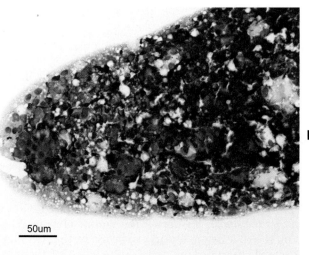

Figure 1-20 Photomicrograph of slide shown on the bottom of Figure 1-19. **A,** Low-magnification image shows that the cells are all present in thick drops where the sample landed and that they were not spread out before the sample dried. **B,** Higher-magnification image of one of the drops shows that the individual cells cannot be seen, resulting in a nondiagnostic sample. *(Courtesy Oklahoma State University teaching files.)*

PREPARATION OF SLIDES: FLUID SAMPLES

A fluid sample can be obtained when sampling body cavities (e.g., thoracocentesis, joint tap), performing washings (e.g., transtracheal wash), or when aspirating a cystic lesion (e.g., benign cyst, cystic tumor, sialocele). Proper handling of fluid samples is essential to obtaining diagnostic information. The two main considerations are preserving cell morphology during transit of the sample and preparing smears that are sufficiently cellular to allow for adequate evaluation.

Any fluid sample on which cytologic evaluation is going to be performed should be placed in an appropriate amount of ethylene-tetra-acetic acid (EDTA). EDTA will prevent coagulation of the sample (which can alter cell counts obtained from the specimen) and help preserve cell morphology during transport to the laboratory. This is especially important if the sample will be mailed. Usually, but not always, EDTA will adequately preserve cell morphology overnight and possibly longer. Refrigeration of the sample will prolong the length of time that readable smears can be made from the sample. If culture of the fluid is anticipated, a portion of the sample should be placed separately into an appropriate transport media or other sterile tube. It is important that a sufficient amount of sample fluid be added to the EDTA tube. EDTA has a very high refractive index and if only a small amount of sample is added to a large EDTA tube, the total protein estimation determined by a refractometer will be artifactually elevated.

Even when fluid samples are placed in EDTA tubes and refrigerated or kept cool with ice packs, cells will undergo aging changes and eventually become too degenerate to evaluate. Depending on the cellularity, type of cells present, and physical composition of the fluid (i.e., protein concentration), significant morphologic changes may occur within 24 hours. The best way to preserve cell morphology is to send premade, air-dried smears. Once smears are made, cell morphology will be preserved for several days, even without fixation of the slides. If possible, premade smears should always be made and sent along with the fluid sample itself. Glass slides should never be placed in the refrigerator because condensation forming on the slide can result in lysis of the cells.

Fluid samples can vary from virtually acellular (cerebrospinal fluid) to extremely cellular (septic exudate). Depending on the nature of the sample, different techniques can be used to produce slides of adequate cellularity. Smears can be prepared directly from fresh, well-mixed fluid or from the sediment of a centrifuged sample using blood smear (direct smears) (see Figure 1-16), line smear (Figures 1-21 and 1-22), and squash prep (see Figure 1-15) techniques. Table 1-2 outlines the samples to be prepared and submitted from fluid samples based on the characteristics of the specimen.

The blood smear technique (direct smear) usually produces well-spread smears of sufficient cellularity from homogenous fluids containing ≥5000 cells/µl but often produces smears of insufficient cellularity from fluids containing <5000 cells/µl. The line smear technique can be used to concentrate fluids of low cellularity but often does not sufficiently spread cells from highly cellular fluids. In general, translucent fluids are of low to moderate cellularity, whereas opaque fluids are usually highly cellular. Therefore, translucent fluids often require concentration,

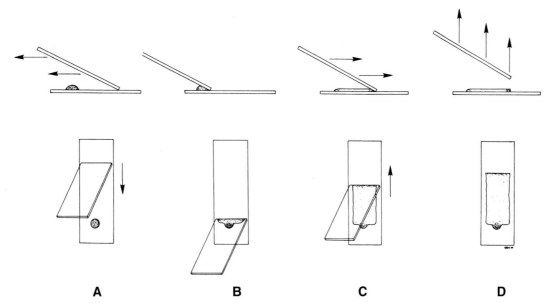

Figure 1-21   Line smear concentration technique. **A,** A drop of fluid sample is placed onto a glass microscope slide close to one end, and another slide is slid backward to contact the front of the drop. **B,** When the drop is contacted, it rapidly spreads along the juncture between the two slides. **C,** The spreader slide is then slid forward smoothly and rapidly. **D,** After the spreader slide has been advanced about two thirds to three fourths of the distance required to make a smear with a feathered edge, the spreader slide is raised directly upward. This produces a smear with a line of concentrated cells at its end, instead of a feathered edge.

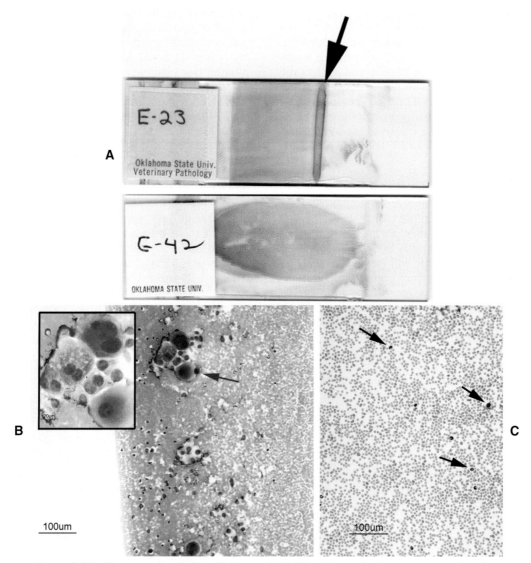

Figure 1-22 Line smear made from fluid sample. **A,** The slide on the bottom was made using a standard blood smear technique. Toward the right, the sample forms a typical feathered edge. The slide on the top was made using a line smear technique. Toward the right, the smear ends abruptly, forming a thick line with a higher concentration of large nucleated cells *(arrow).* **B** and **C,** Images taken from the line smear of a fluid sample. The main portion of the smear (**C,** *right*) is of low cellularity, consisting mostly of blood but with low numbers of nucleated cells *(black arrows).* These relatively small cells are neutrophils and macrophages. At the line edge (**B,** *left*), there are increased numbers of nucleated cells, especially clusters of large neoplastic epithelial cells. Inset shows higher magnification of cell cluster indicated by the red arrow. **(A** *courtesy Oklahoma State University teaching files.)*

either by centrifugation or by the line smear technique. When possible, concentration by centrifugation is preferred. The squash prep technique often spreads viscous samples (e.g., transtracheal wash [TTW]) and samples with flecks of particulate material better than the blood smear and line smear techniques.

To prepare a smear by the blood smear technique, place a small drop of the fluid on a glass slide about ½ inch from the end. Slide another slide backward at a 30- to 40-degree angle until it contacts the drop. When the fluid flows sideways along the crease between the slides,

quickly and smoothly slide the second slide forward until the fluid has all drained away from the second slide. This makes a smear with a feathered edge.

To concentrate fluids by centrifugation, the fluid is centrifuged for 5 minutes at 165 to 360 G. This is achieved by operating a centrifuge with a radial arm length of 14.6 cm (the arm length of most urine centrifuges) at 1000 to 1500 rpm. After centrifugation, the supernatant is separated from the sediment and analyzed for total protein concentration. The sediment is resuspended in a few drops of supernatant by gently thumping the side of the tube.

TABLE 1-2

Methods of Preparing Cytology Slides from Fluid Samples

Types/Characteristics of Fluid	Samples to Prepare/Submit
Peripheral blood for cytology	Make several air-dried direct smears (blood smear method)
	Submit remainder in EDTA
Clear, transparent fluids (e.g., abdominal fluid)	Make 1-2 direct smears (can be used to estimate cellularity) and line smears
	Centrifuge a portion of the sample and make smears from sediment
	Submit a portion of fluid in EDTA
	Submit a portion of fluid in sterile container if culture is desired
Turbid/opaque fluids	Make 1-2 direct smears
	Submit a portion of the fluid in EDTA
	Submit a portion of the fluid in sterile container if culture is desired
Clear fluid with flecks or mucous strands (e.g., transtracheal wash fluid, bone marrow samples in EDTA)	Make several direct smears from fluid
	Make "squash preps" (slide-over-slide preps) of particles/mucous strands removed from the fluid using either a pipette, needle, or capillary tube
	Submit a portion of the fluid in EDTA
	Submit a portion of the fluid in sterile container if culture is desired

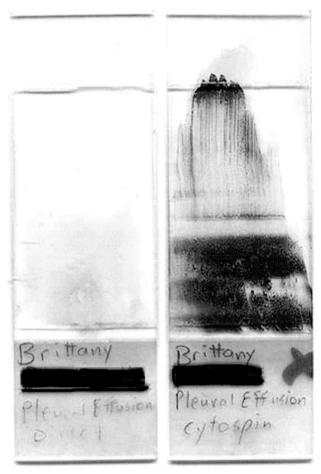

Figure 1-23 Direct smear *(left)* and concentrated smear made from sediment *(right)* of pleural effusion from a dog. The dark color on the concentrated smear is the result of markedly increased cellularity. *(Courtesy Oklahoma State University teaching files.)*

A drop of the resuspended sediment is placed on a slide and a smear is made by the blood smear or squash prep technique (Figure 1-23). Sediment concentrated slides can produce highly cellular smears even from fluids of low cellularity and help identify cells present in low numbers (Figure 1-24). When possible, several smears should be made by each technique. When slides are made from the sediment of a fluid sample, it is not possible to estimate the cellularity of the sample from the slides, so it is imperative to retain a portion of sample for cell counts, which are important for determining the mechanism of fluid accumulation.

When the fluid cannot be concentrated by centrifugation or the centrifuged sample is of low cellularity, the line smear technique (see Figure 1-21) can be used to concentrate cells in the smear. A drop of fluid is placed on a clean glass slide and the blood smear technique is used, except the spreading slide is stopped and raised directly upward about three fourths of the way through the smear. This will result in a line containing a much higher concentration of cells than the rest of the slide (see Figure 1-22). Unfortunately, the cells that are present in the line may not be well spread out, making evaluation difficult.

Collection Tip

Fluid from solid lesions—Sometimes fluid is obtained when sampling a mass or other proliferative lesion. When this occurs, as much fluid as possible should be drained from the lesion and handled as described previously. The lesion should then be reevaluated. If a solid tissue component still remains, that component should be sampled by FNB using either the aspiration or non-aspiration technique. Many times, cystic neoplasia will not exfoliate overtly neoplastic cells into the cystic fluid. The material obtained from direct FNB may have a completely different cell population than that present in the fluid itself.

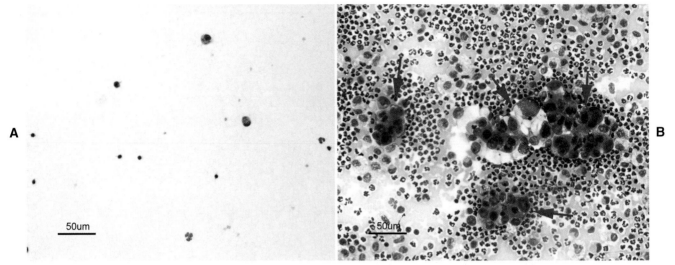

Figure 1-24 Photomicrographs taken from slides shown in Figure 1-23. **A,** Low-magnification image taken from direct smear of pleural fluid shows relatively sparse cellularity consisting mostly of nondegenerate neutrophils and macrophages. This image is representative of the slide. **B,** Low-magnification image taken from the concentrated sediment preparation of the same fluid sample. The slide is highly cellular. In addition to the neutrophils and macrophages seen on the direct smear, clusters of neoplastic epithelial cells *(arrows)* are easily found.

STAINING CYTOLOGIC PREPARATIONS

To Stain or Not to Stain?

If you intend to send the slides to a laboratory for evaluation, it is not necessary to stain the slides or do any special fixation at all. Air-dried smears will hold up quite well over the length of time necessary for transport to an outside laboratory. In fact, if the slides are to be submitted for analysis, unstained slides are preferable. This will allow the cytologist to stain the smears with the type of stain he or she is used to viewing. However, it is usually advisable to stain at least one slide to ensure that an adequately cellular sample was obtained before paying for interpretation of the smears.

Types of Stain

Several types of stains have been used for cytologic preparations.[6] The two general types most commonly used are the Romanowsky-type stains (Wright's stain, Giemsa stain, Diff-Quik) and Papanicolaou stain and its derivatives, such as Sano's trichrome. Papanicolaou stains and their derivatives require the specimen to be wet-fixed, (i.e., the smear must be fixed before the cells have dried). Usually this is achieved by spraying the smear with a cytologic fixative or placing it in ethanol immediately after preparation. Such procedures are not necessary, and are actually undesirable, if the samples are to be stained with Romanowsky-type stains. Papanicolaou-type stains give excellent nuclear detail and are routinely used in human cytopathology.[6] However, these stains require multiple staining steps, do not stain many organisms or cell cytoplasm well, and are not practical for use in most clinics. They are rarely used in veterinary cytology, even in large commercial laboratories. The remainder of this chapter (and text) deals with Romanowsky-type stains.

Romanowsky-type stains are inexpensive, readily available to the practicing veterinarian, and easy to prepare, maintain and use. They stain organisms and the cytoplasm of cells excellently. Though nuclear and nucleolar detail cannot be perceived as well with Romanowsky-type stains as with Papanicolaou-type stains, nuclear and nucleolar detail are sufficient for differentiating neoplasia and inflammation and for evaluating neoplastic cells for cytologic evidence of malignant potential (criteria of malignancy). Smears to be stained with Romanowsky-type stains are first air-dried. Air-drying partially preserves (fixes) the cells and causes them to adhere to the slide so that they do not fall off during the staining procedure.

There are many commercially available Romanowsky-type stains, including Diff-Quik, DipStat, and other quick Wright's stains. Most, if not all, Romanowsky stains are acceptable for staining cytologic preparations. Diff-Quik does not undergo the metachromatic reaction. As a result, granules of some mast cells do not stain. When mast-cell granules do not stain, the mast cells may be misclassified as macrophages or plasma cells. This can lead to confusion in examination of some mast-cell tumors. The variation between different Romanowsky-type stains should not cause a problem once the evaluator has become familiar with the stain he or she uses routinely.

Each stain usually has its own unique recommended staining procedure. These procedures should be followed in general but adapted to the type and thickness of smear being stained and to the evaluator's preference. The thinner the smear and the lower the total protein concentration of the fluid, the less time needed in the stain. The thicker the smear and the greater the total protein concentration of the fluid, the more time needed in the stain. As a result, fluid smears with low protein and low cellularity, such as some abdominal fluid samples, may stain better using half or less of the recommended time. Thick smears, such as smears of neoplastic lymph nodes, may need to be stained twice the recommended time or longer. Each person tends to have a different technique that he or she prefers. By trying variations in the recommended time intervals for stains, the evaluator can establish which times produce the preferred staining characteristics.

Poor staining quality is a common problem for a variety of reasons. It can be confusing to the novice when trying to examine is or her own slides because the cells may appear completely unrecognizable. Most staining problems can be avoided by the following precautions:[4]

- Use only new, clean slides. Attempts to re-use slides are usually doomed to failure. Even if they are cleaned and dried, the samples often do no spread out well or do not stain properly because the surface properties of the glass have been altered.
- Use fresh, well-filtered (if periodic filtering is required) stains. Over time with repeated use, stains will "fatigue," form excessive precipitate, or may become contaminated with organisms or cell debris from previous slides.
- Make sure that the slides are completely air-dried before staining. This is particularly important when examining blood smears. Some water will remain even after slides appear grossly to have dried. Slides should be air-dried for 5 to 10 minutes or dried briefly with a hair dryer prior to staining.
- Do not touch the surface of the slide or smear at any time. Likewise, make sure the slide is not contaminated with ultrasound gel or other lubricant gels (e.g., K-Y).

Table 1-3 gives some problems that can occur with Romanowsky-type stains and some proposed solutions to these problems. One of the most commonly encountered problems is simply understaining the slides. Slides are often understained when they are highly cellular or stained with old stains. With well-stained smears, the nucleus of most cells should be a dark purple and there should be clear demarcation of the nucleus and cytoplasm (see Chapter 2). When slides are understained, cells and nuclei may appear pink, it may be difficult to distinguish the boundary between the nucleus and the cytoplasm, or the cells may just appear excessively faded or "muted." It may be difficult for the beginning cytologist to recognize understaining if he or she is not familiar with what the cells should look like. However, most cytology preparations will contain some neutrophils or other peripheral blood cells whose morphology is more likely to be familiar to the observer. These cells can be used as an internal control for staining quality. It is important to remember that if the slides appear understained, they can simply be placed in the stains for an additional period of time. However, restaining should optimally be done before immersion oil is placed on the slides.

SUBMISSION OF SAMPLES TO THE LABORATORY

If the clinician is not going to evaluate the slides in-house, the final step in processing of cytologic samples is ensuring that they arrive at the laboratory intact. Many well made, potentially diagnostic slides have met their doom at the hands of various postal services. Thin cardboard slide mailers (Figure 1-25) do not offer adequate protection for slides being mailed to outside laboratories and often result in broken, unreadable slides. Rigid plastic or Styrofoam mailers (Figure 1-26) are suitable for mailing slides and generally prevent breakage. If these are not available, slides should be wrapped in protective material (i.e., paper towel) and mailed in a small, sturdy box. Alternatively, slides can be placed in a large plastic pill bottle and then placed in a mailing envelope.

If samples of body fluids are submitted along with slides, small EDTA tubes will fit inside standard Styrofoam slide mailers or can be placed inside a larger cardboard box. Most overnight mailing services require that body fluids be double-sealed and placed in specially designed plastic envelopes, which they provide.

Slides mailed to an outside laboratory should be labeled with patient and owner name and the location from which the sample was collected. Microscope slides used for cytology (or hematology) should have frosted or colored edges that can be written on with a pencil. It is difficult to permanently label slides without frosted edges and this can lead to samples being mixed up. The ink from most marking pens (even so-called permanent markers) is soluble in cytologic stains and fixatives and will wash off during the staining procedure, leaving the slides unidentified. In contrast, pencil markings on frosted slides will not erase during staining. Many nonfrosted slides arrive at labs with patient identification written on small pieces of white bandage tapes affixed to the edge of the slide. With many types of automatic slide stainers, these labels must be removed before the slides can be stained, again leading to potential misidentification of the sample.

As a final note, unstained cytology slides should never be mailed with, or even stored near, samples in formalin. Formalin fumes will penetrate most any packaging, even biopsy samples in plastic jars with screw top lids that are sealed in plastic zip-top bags. Formalin fumes partially fix the cells on air-dried smears and markedly interfere with subsequent staining (Figure 1-27), often making the slides totally uninterpretable.

SUBMISSION OF SAMPLES FOR CULTURE

Although this text deals primarily with cytologic evaluation of samples, with many samples (particularly fluids) submitted for cytology, culture is also indicated. Culture results are strongly influenced by sample collection, preparation, and transport. The following procedures are suggested to optimize success in culturing lesions and fluids:

- Call the laboratory before collecting the sample.
- Collect the sample as aseptically as possible.
- Submit fresh samples for culture.
- Use proper methods for collection and transport of the sample.
- Use a timely transportation service.

Call the Laboratory before Collecting the Sample

Techniques, media, days when cultures are read or subcultures are performed, and so forth, often vary from laboratory to laboratory. By contacting the laboratory to which

TABLE 1-3

Some Possible Solutions to Problems Seen with Common Romanowsky-Type Stains

Problem	Solution
Excessive blue staining (red blood cells may be blue-green)	
Prolonged stain contact	Decrease staining time
Inadequate wash	Wash longer
Specimen too thick	Make thinner smears if possible
Stain, diluent, buffer, or wash water too alkaline	Check with pH paper and correct pH
Exposure to formalin vapors	Store and ship cytologic preps separate from formalin containers
Wet fixation in ethanol or formalin	Air-dry smears before fixation
Delayed fixation	Fix smears sooner if possible
Surface of the slide was alkaline	Use new slides
Excessive pink staining	
Insufficient staining time	Increase staining time
Prolonged washing	Decrease duration of wash
Stain or diluent too acidic	Check with pH paper and correct pH; fresh methanol may be needed
Excessive time in red stain solution	Decrease time in red solution
Inadequate time in blue stain solution	Increase time in blue stain solution
Mounting coverslip before preparation is dry	Allow preparation to dry completely before mounting coverslip
Weak staining	
Insufficient contact with one or more of the stain solutions	Increase staining time
Fatigued (old) stains	Change stains
Another slide covered specimen during staining	Keep slides separate
Uneven staining	
Variation of pH in different areas of slide surface (may be due to slide surface being touched or slide being poorly cleaned)	Use new slides and avoid touching them before and after preparation
Water allowed to stand on some areas of the slide after staining and washing	Tilt slides close to vertical to drain water from the surface, or dry with a fan
Inadequate mixing of stain and buffer	Mix stain and buffer thoroughly
Precipitate on preparation	
Inadequate stain filtration	Filter or change the stain(s)
Inadequate washing of slide after staining	Rinse slides well after staining
Dirty slides used	Use clean new slides
Stain solution dries during staining	Use sufficient stain, and do not leave it on slide too long
Miscellaneous	
Overstained preparations	Destain with 95% methanol and restain; Diff-Quik–stained smears may have to be destained in the red Diff-Quik stain solution to remove the blue color; however, this damages the red stain solution
Refractile artifact red blood cells with Diff-Quik stain (usually due to moisture in fixative)	Change the fixative

the sample will be submitted, such things as optimal sample type, transport medium, day of the week to submit the sample, and the like can be discussed. Also, some laboratories furnish culture supplies. Expensive and/or quickly outdated supplies, such as blood culture tubes, may be ordered from the laboratory as needed. Early communication with the laboratory also allows the laboratory to prepare for the sample and ensure that any special media required are available.

Collect Samples as Aseptically as Possible

All samples should be collected as aseptically as possible. Even samples collected from lesions that naturally are exposed to secondary contamination, such as cutaneous ulcers, should be protected from further contamination. When samples are collected from more than one lesion, care should be taken not to cross-contaminate the samples. Finding the same organism in several different lesions is strong evidence that the organism is involved in development of the lesions. Therefore, cross-contamination of samples from different lesions can lead to misinterpretation of culture results. When fluids are collected, anticoagulant and serum tubes should not be assumed to be sterile. Serum tubes generally are identified as *sterile* or *nonsterile* on the label of the tube. Also, EDTA, because of its effect on bacterial cell walls, can be bacteriostatic or bactericidal and should be avoided.

Submit Fresh Samples

Samples should be submitted as soon after collection as possible. Fluid aspiration, resection of lesions to be cultured, exploratory surgeries during which culture is

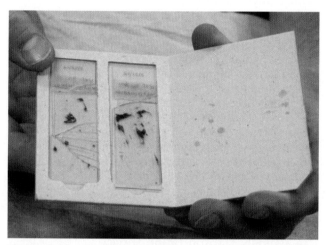

Figure 1-25 Cardboard containers do not offer sufficient protection for mailing slides. If the slides are not put in additional protective packaging, they often become broken in transit. *(Courtesy Oklahoma State University teaching files.)*

anticipated, and other procedures that may produce samples to be cultured should be scheduled to allow immediate transportation of samples to the laboratory. During transport, samples should be kept cool but not frozen.

Use Proper Methods for Collection and Transport of Samples

Tissue and fluid samples usually are more rewarding than swab samples for isolation of a causative agent. Individual tissue samples submitted for culture should be about 4 cm^2 or larger. Whirl-Pak bags, which are sterile and sealable, are excellent for submitting samples for culture. If the interior of the tissue is to be cultured by the laboratory, clean and sealable plastic bags are sufficient. To avoid cross-contamination, all tissues should be packaged separately. To prevent drying during transport, small biopsies, such as punch biopsies of skin lesions, should be placed in a transport system with maintenance medium. Avoid shipping biopsies in sterile saline because this may result in falsely negative culture results.

Fluid samples (i.e., urine, milk, joint fluid, thoracic fluid, abdominal fluid, abscess aspirates) to be cultured should be placed in containers that are sterile and leakproof, such as sterile Vacutainer tubes, small Whirl-Pak bags, or sterile disposable syringes.

For collection of samples for which swabs must be used (epithelial surfaces, fistulous tracts), the swabs should be placed in a maintenance medium that allows preservation with little to no replication of microbes so that the quantity and quality of the microbial flora of the swab remain as intact as possible. A variety of transport tubes containing maintenance media are commercially available for optimal transport of swabs for isolating bacteria, chlamydia, or viruses (Culturette, Transwab, Transtube, and CultureSwab). The bacterial media systems usually support a wide variety of bacteria for up to 72 hours at

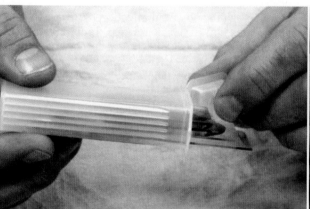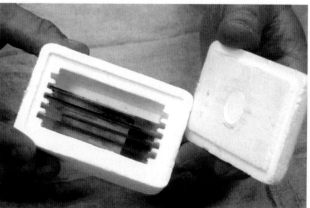

Figure 1-26 Rigid plastic **(A)** and Styrofoam mailers **(B)**, shown here, do a good job of protecting slides for mailing. Slides in these types of containers can usually be put directly in mailing envelopes with no additional protective packaging. *(Courtesy Oklahoma State University teaching files.)*

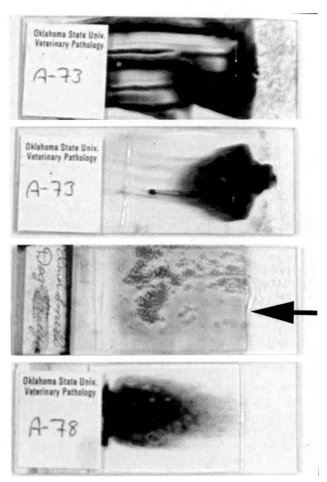

Figure 1-27 Effect of formalin fumes on unstained cytology slides. The slide second from the bottom *(arrow)* was mailed with a biopsy sample in formalin. After staining, the slide has a characteristic color that is different from the other slides that were not exposed to formalin. This partial fixation alters the staining of the cells and often makes it impossible to interpret the sample.

20° to 25°C. Swabs without media can dry out during transport, resulting in false-negative results, whereas swabs submitted in broth culture medium often are overgrown by contaminants. Separate swabs should be submitted if additional cultures for fungi and/or viruses are desired.

Samples for anaerobic culturing require special handling and transport. The main objective is to limit, as much as possible, the exposure of the sample to oxygen and, thus, to air. Swabs are the least desirable means for specimen collection for anaerobes because of the difficulty of limiting the exposure of the sample to air. Fluids for anaerobic culturing should be collected in syringes, with air excluded. The needle is then plugged with a sterile rubber stopper or bent double to prevent intake of air and transported immediately to the laboratory for culture. If samples for anaerobic culturing cannot reach the laboratory within 2 hours, the sample must be placed into some type of anaerobic transport system. Several

commercial systems are now available for transporting all types of specimens for anaerobic culture. Port-A-Cul Systems contain a prereduced transport medium in a soft agar with reducing agents to maintain anaerobiosis and offer vials for fluid specimens, jars for small tissues and swabs, and tubes for swabs. Also available are self-contained, gas-generating systems that provide their own anaerobic atmosphere once the sample is placed in the container and the system sealed. Such systems are available for swabs (Anaerobic Culturette, Becton Dickinson Microbiology Systems) and as sealable plastic bags (Bio-Bag, Gas-Pak Pouch). The bags can be used for transporting large tissue specimens, fluids contained within syringes, and aerobic swab systems for anaerobic culturing.

In general, samples submitted for fungal culture should be collected and transported in the same manner as samples for bacterial culture, with the exception of dermatophyte cultures.

Scrapings and hair plucked from the periphery of suspected dermatophyte lesions should be submitted in clean containers that remain dry during transit. Bacterial overgrowth of dermatophyte cultures is a common problem and can be eliminated by disinfecting suspect dermatophyte lesions with alcohol prior to obtaining samples. Vacutainer tubes and similar tightly sealable containers are to be avoided because condensate tends to form within them, allowing overgrowth of contaminants. Clean paper envelopes are suitable specimen containers. For transport, the envelope should be packaged within a more durable wrapper. Swabs are the least preferred samples for fungal cultures and should never be used for dermatophyte isolation attempts.

Use a Timely Transportation Service

Care in collection of samples can be for naught if the samples are not received in the laboratory in a timely manner, which generally means 48 hours or less. Most microbiology laboratories deal with various carriers on a daily basis and can advise what carrier to use. Packaging specimens to guard against breakage and leakage not only protects against specimen loss but also protects package handlers against potential infection. Be aware that special requirements must be taken when shipping biohazardous materials, including some clinical specimens. If in doubt regarding how to package specimens for transport, contact the microbiology laboratory to which the specimens will be sent.

References

1. Meyer DJ: The acquisition and management of cytology specimens. In Raskin RE, Meyer DJ (eds): *Atlas of Canine and Feline Cytology*. Philadelphia, Saunders, 2001, pp 1-17.
2. Lumsden JH, Baker R: Cytopathology techniques and interpretation. In Baker R, Lumsden JH (eds): *Color Atlas of Cytology of the Dog and Cat*. St. Louis, Mosby, 2000, pp 7-20.
3. Menard M, Papageorges M: Fine-needle biopsies: How to increase diagnostic yield. *Comp Cont Ed Pract Vet* 19: 738-740, 1997.

4. Tyler RD, Cowell RL, Baldwin CJ, et al: Introduction. In Cowell RL, Tyler RD, Meinkoth JH (eds): *Diagnostic Cytology and Hematology of the Dog and Cat*, ed 2. St. Louis, Mosby, 1999, pp 1-19.

5. DeMay, RM: *The Art and Science of Cytopathology*. Chicago, ASCP, 1996, pp 464-483.

6. Jörundsson E, Lumsden JH, Jacobs RM: Rapid staining techniques in cytopathology: A review and comparison of modified protocols for hematoxylin and eosin, Papanicolaou and Romanowsky stains. *Vet Clin Path* 28:100-108, 1999.

Cell Types and Criteria of Malignancy

J.H. Meinkoth, R.L. Cowell, and R.D. Tyler

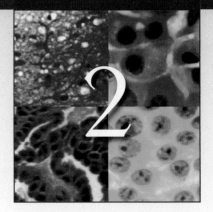

CHAPTER

Examining cytologic preparations often presents a potentially confusing array of different cell types, as well as a potentially endless variety of cell debris and contaminants as well. With experience, most of the common lesions are recognized quickly. For the beginner, or even the experienced cytologist, when confronted with a lesion or sample site not previously encountered, it is helpful to keep in mind certain fundamental questions that need to be considered when evaluating a sample. An orderly approach to examining slides and answering certain questions that can be answered based on cytology will reduce the chances of missing important information or misdiagnosing/over-diagnosing the sample. Cells can usually be classified into one of a few basic categories, based on common features shared by different cells in that category. Recognizing the common features of the different basic cell types sometimes makes it possible to classify cells that are at first not obviously recognized.

ARE SUFFICIENT NUMBERS OF WELL-STAINED, WELL-PRESERVED, INTACT CELLS PRESENT TO EVALUATE?

A basic premise of cytology is that interpretations are generally based on whole populations of cells, not on low numbers of individual cells. Any one cell or few cells from a lesion may show features that are atypical or unusual. This is especially true if cells are coming from a tissue in which the cells are not well preserved or exposed to injurious stimuli. Cells coming from inflammatory reactions or areas of tissue repair often show cellular atypia that is the result of dysplasia. In addition to atypia seen with inflammation and tissue repair, cells that undergo aging changes may be difficult to interpret. Cells present in fluid samples (e.g., thoracocentesis, abdominocentesis) may undergo morphologic changes over time if slides are not made immediately upon collection. These changes can range from subtle alterations such as cellular or nuclear swelling and altered staining characteristics to overt pyknosis or lysis. Even if slides are prepared immediately upon collection, cells may have undergone in-vivo aging. Cells from the fluid portion of cystic lesions, such as some mammary tumors, or cells that have been in prolonged contact with urine, such as urine sediment preparations or urethral/bladder samples collected by traumatic catheterization, often have significant artifacts that must not be misinterpreted as criteria of malignancy.

Interpretations based on inadequately cellular specimens may not contain a representative sample of the lesion giving a false impression of normalcy or, even worse, may result in a false impression of neoplasia that is not really present. Although there is no easily defined limit to the question, "How many cells are enough?", slides should have numerous cells per field across a large portion of the slide. When a large lesion is being evaluated, several smears of good cellularity collected from different areas of the lesion should be evaluated to assess any variability that may be present within different parts of the lesion. Large neoplasms may have areas of inflammation or necrosis that will yield markedly different cell populations than adjacent areas.

The cellularity of the smear is often evident the moment the slides are stained. A slide containing high numbers of nucleated cells is visibly blue after staining. Slides that are perfectly clear after staining probably have low numbers of nucleated cells, although there may still be sufficient cells present for a diagnosis. Therefore, cellularity must be confirmed by looking at the slide under the microscope. Even for practitioners who do not have the time or desire to evaluate cytology preparations themselves, it is beneficial to stain one or two smears and determine that an adequately cellular specimen is being sent off for evaluation.

When examined microscopically, the slides should first be scanned using low power (10× to 20×) to assess the cellularity of the slide and find the area(s) containing the highest number of well-stained, well-spread-out, intact cells for evaluation (Figure 2-1). Cells are often unevenly distributed across the slides, especially with impression smears or aspirates of solid tissue lesions. Even with slides made from fluid samples, large cells may all be pulled out to the feathered edge, where they can be easily overlooked if the whole slide is not scanned first (Figure 2-2).

After locating the cellular areas of the slides, it is important to determine whether the cells are sufficiently spread out for evaluation, intact and well stained. This

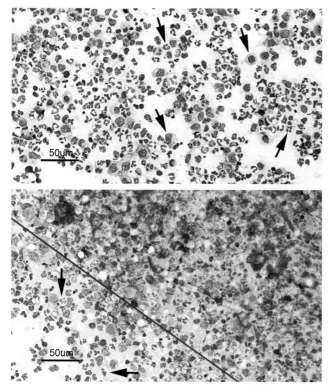

Figure 2-1 Low-power image of different areas of a slide. The top image shows an area that although highly cellular, is well spread out and the cells are well stained. Although cell detail is difficult to evaluate at this magnification, it is possible to see the characteristic nuclear shape of some well-spread-out neutrophils and to differentiate the nucleus and cytoplasm of mononuclear cells *(arrows)*. The lower image shows another area from the same slide where the cells are not well spread out and thus have not stained well. Most of the area above and to the right of the red line is too thick to evaluate. A few well-spread-out cells are seen in the lower left *(arrows)*.

can usually also be done on low power (10× to 20×), which will allow a greater portion of the slide to be evaluated in a short time. Inexperienced cytologists often frustrate, themselves by spending an inordinate amount of time trying to identify cells that cannot be interpreted because they are not spread out, are poorly stained, or are ruptured. Intact, well-stained, well-spread cells should have a clearly evident demarcation between the nucleus and cytoplasm (Figure 2-3). The nucleus may be irregularly shaped (particularly in neoplastic cells), but the nuclear outline should be smooth and distinct. A fuzzy appearance around the outline of the nucleus generally indicates that the cell has been minimally traumatized during sample collection and/or preparation. More significant cell trauma can result in the nucleus appearing fragmented or full of holes (see Figure 2-3). Severely traumatized cells will often appear as strands of light pink nuclear chromatin (Figure 2-4). Some traumatized/ruptured cells will be present in virtually any cytologic specimen. The sample is usually still interpretable if the majority of the cells are intact; however, the traumatized cells are typically not evaluated, particularly when determining criteria of malignancy,

because ruptured nuclei may appear enlarged and nucleoli may appear more prominent. If the majority of the cells are traumatized/ruptured, additional samples usually need to be collected.

Cells that are not well spread out often stain diffusely dark and it is difficult to distinguish the line of demarcation and color distinction between the cytoplasm and nucleus (Figure 2-5). Also, poor staining (even in well-spread-out cells) can result in a less distinct demarcation between nucleus and cytoplasm.

Nucleoli will often be more prominent than usual in understained cells, and this can result in a false impression of malignancy if this artifact is not recognized. The nuclei of well-stained cells are usually a dark purple color, generally more intensely and deeply stained than the surrounding cytoplasm. There will be some variation in the intensity and pattern of nuclear staining between cell types. If you are unsure whether light staining of nuclei is a characteristic of the cell or the result of understaining, it may be helpful to evaluate the staining of more familiar cells, if any are present. Usually, some neutrophils will be present as the result of peripheral blood contamination or inflammation within the lesion and make a good reference to evaluate how well cells are stained (and spread out).

In most specimens, there will be significant variation in cellularity, degree of cell spreading and, hence, staining quality from area to area on the slide. This is particularly true of very cellular specimens (i.e., lymph node aspirates), which may have areas that are of diagnostic quality even if the majority of the slide is thick and understained. Diligent scanning of the slides on low power is necessary to find these areas before attempting to evaluate the cells at higher magnification. If the entire slide is found to be understained, restaining the slide before immersion oil is added may improved the staining quality and result in a diagnostic sample.

ARE ALL OF THE CELLS ON THE SMEAR INFLAMMATORY CELLS?

A good initial decision, particularly for the beginning cytologist, is to determine if the smear is composed entirely of inflammatory cells. In most general practices, inflammatory lesions are probably more commonly sampled than neoplastic lesions. Also, most clinicians initially feel more comfortable recognizing inflammatory cells because they are more familiar with the morphology of these cells, having viewed them many times in peripheral blood smears. Many clinicians choose to screen their cytology specimens, interpreting inflammatory lesions in-house while submitting those composed of tissue cells for outside evaluation. Although inflammatory cells in tissues often look the same as they do in peripheral blood, some may appear different because of morphologic changes induced by being present in a focus of inflammation or simply because they are not well spread out. It is important to remember that one may not be able to identify every cell present on a slide (or even on any given field), and that the interpretation is based on the entire cell population present. If a lesion is found to be composed entirely of

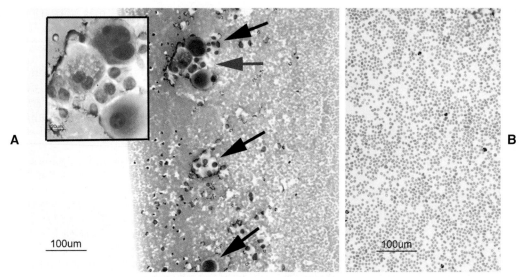

Figure 2-2 Images from a slide made from hemorrhagic pleural effusion showing uneven distribution of cells on the slide. **A,** Numerous large clusters of cells *(arrows)* have all been pulled out to the edge of the smear. Some of these show marked atypia allowing for a diagnosis of neoplastic effusion (carcinoma). Inset shows higher magnification of atypical cell cluster indicated by the red arrow. **B,** The majority of the smear contained predominantly erythrocytes with a few small nuclei (neutrophils and macrophages) visible. Scanning on low power quickly allowed the atypical cells to be found at the edge of the smear. These could have easily been overlooked if the observer started out at high magnification in the body of the smear.

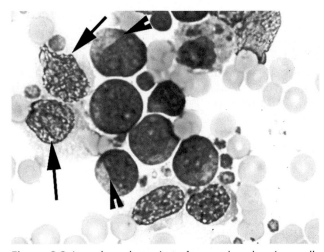

Figure 2-3 Lymph node aspirate from a dog showing well-spread-out cells. A clear distinction can be seen between the nucleus and the cytoplasm *(arrowheads).* Several traumatized cells are also present. Note that their nuclear chromatin appears excessively fragmented *(arrows).*

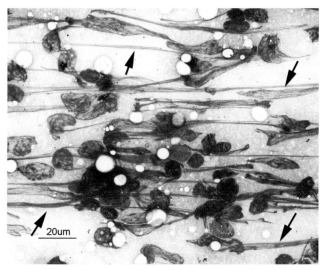

Figure 2-4 Severely traumatized cells. The streaks of material *(arrows)* represent smeared-out nuclear chromatin from ruptured cells.

inflammatory cells, the relative percentages of the various types of inflammatory cells should be noted, because this may provide clues as to the etiology of the inflammation. Finally, a search for infectious agents should be conducted. A discussion of the various inflammatory patterns and morphology of common infectious agents will be covered more completely in Chapters 3 and 5 of this text. The basic types of inflammatory cells and their morphologic variations are later in this chapter.

Neutrophils

Neutrophils are commonly found in cytologic specimens. Their morphology is often similar to that observed in peripheral blood smears (Figure 2-6). Normal neutrophil nuclei stain dark purple and contain one to multiple distinct segments or lobes. The neutrophil cytoplasm is typically clear. Neutrophils are phagocytic cells and typically are the cells that phagocytize pathogenic bacteria, if present (see Figure 2-6). Neutrophils contain intracytoplasmic granules. However, the neutrophil granules in most domestic

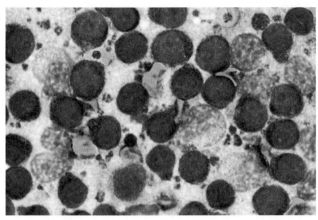

Figure 2-5 Poorly spread-out cells from a different area of the same slide shown in Figure 2-3. The cells are diffusely dark with the nuclei and cytoplasm staining different shades of blue. Compare this with the purple color of the well-spread-out nuclei in Figure 2-3. Also, it is difficult to discern the demarcation between nucleus and cytoplasm.

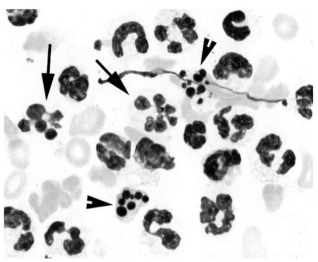

Figure 2-7 Sample from a nonseptic inflammatory lesion. Many of the neutrophils show nuclear hypersegmentation *(arrows)*, an aging artifact. This will ultimately lead to pyknotic change *(arrowheads)* in which the nuclear chromatin condenses and fragments into several discrete, dense spheres.

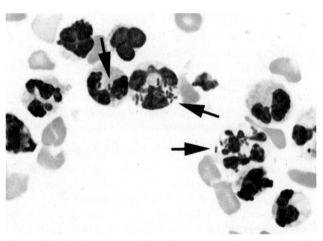

Figure 2-6 Septic neutrophilic inflammation. Many neutrophils are present, some of which contain phagocytized bacterial rods *(arrows)*.

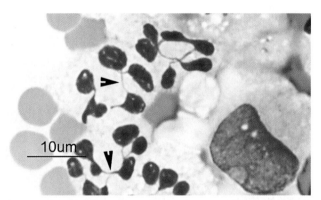

Figure 2-8 Hypersegmentation of neutrophils in which elongated thin filaments connect the nuclear lobes *(arrowheads)*. This is a common manifestation of aged neutrophils in fluid samples.

animals generally do not stain prominently with cytologic stains. Sometimes, however, these granules will be discernable as elongated, faintly eosinophilic structures, and they must not be confused with bacteria or lightly staining eosinophil granules.

In thick preparations or in viscous fluids (e.g., synovial fluid), neutrophils may not spread out well and the segmented nature of their nucleus may be less evident. Sometimes, the nucleus will be essentially round mimicking a lymphocyte, but the cell can still be identified as a neutrophil by the lobulated outline of the nucleus. More normal neutrophil morphology can be observed in the thinner areas (often along the edges) of the smear.

Neutrophils may undergo several morphologic changes in tissues. Aging change is a commonly encountered phenomenon. The initial change seen is hypersegmentation of the nucleus (Figure 2-7). Sometimes, an elongated thin strand of nuclear material (Figure 2-8) connects the nuclear lobes of aged neutrophils. This is especially

common in neutrophils from fluid samples and is more commonly seen on cytocentrifuged preparations than in direct smears. The end result of aging change is pyknosis of the nucleus. Pyknosis is condensation of the nuclear chromatin into one or more small discrete, densely staining spheres lacking any nuclear chromatin pattern (see Figure 2-7). Aging artifact simply represents neutrophils dying of "old age" and must not be confused with degenerative change, described subsequently.

Degenerative change occurs when neutrophils are present in an environment that is damaging to the cell. It is commonly seen in neutrophils from lesions in which endotoxin-producing bacteria are present. The presence of many neutrophils with marked degenerative change should prompt a diligent search for bacteria. Degenerative change is an acquired change and is distinct from the toxic changes noted in peripheral blood neutrophils. Degenerative change occurs when the neutrophil is unable to control water homeostasis and undergoes hydropic

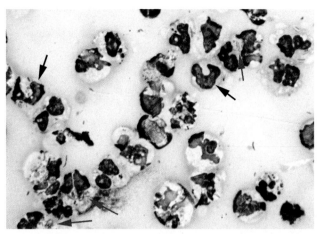

Figure 2-9 Neutrophils showing degenerative change. Degenerative change is evidenced by nuclear swelling *(black arrows)*, which leads to loss of distinct segmentation. As the nucleus swells the neutrophils may appear band shaped, or in more severe change, the nucleus may appear round or overtly lytic. Degenerative change is commonly associated with the presence of endotoxin-producing-bacteria. Many bacterial rods *(red arrows)* were present on this slide.

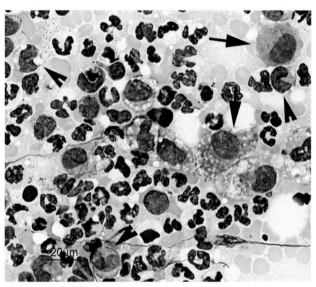

Figure 2-10 Pyogranulomatous inflammatory response demonstrating many macrophages. Some macrophages resemble peripheral blood monocytes *(arrowheads)*. Other macrophages are variably increased in size resulting from increased amounts of cytoplasm that is sometimes vacuolated *(arrows)*.

degeneration. The hallmark of degenerative change is nuclear swelling (Figure 2-9). The nucleus of the cell swells and appears thicker, stains a lighter eosinophilic color, and loses nuclear lobulation. Degenerative neutrophils often resemble large band cells.

Macrophages

Macrophages in inflammatory lesions are derived from peripheral blood monocytes. Many tissues have low numbers of fixed tissue macrophages as normal resident

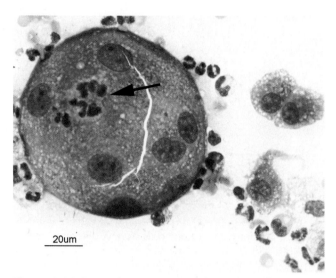

Figure 2-11 Smear from a pyogranulomatous inflammatory reaction (*Actinomyces* infection). An extremely large, multinucleated macrophage is present. The macrophage has phagocytized several neutrophils.

cells (e.g., Kupffer cells in the liver). Macrophages may display extremely variable morphology in tissues, which can be somewhat confusing for the beginning cytologist. Initially, they may resemble peripheral blood monocytes (Figure 2-10). With time, the nucleus becomes round and the cell enlarges as the cytoplasm becomes greatly expanded and, sometimes, extremely vacuolated. Macrophages are also phagocytic cells, typically phagocytizing larger structures like fungal organisms and other cells. Many times, the cytoplasm of macrophages will contain partially phagocytized debris that cannot be identified, but must not be misinterpreted as an infectious agent.

Binucleated or multinucleated macrophages are commonly encountered in long-standing inflammatory lesions (Figure 2-11). Multinucleated macrophages can get very large and are referred to as inflammatory giant cells. In some chronic inflammatory lesions, epithelioid macrophages may be encountered (Figure 2-12). This term is applied to macrophages that are enlarged with expansive cytoplasm that stains uniformly basophilic, giving the cell the look of an epithelial cell. Because these cells often show variation in size and multinucleation (both commonly seen in macrophages) they could potentially be misinterpreted as neoplastic epithelial cells. Extreme caution should be used when diagnosing malignancy in the face of inflammation because of the potential for macrophages to display atypical criteria.

Lymphocytes (Small, Medium, and Large)

Small lymphocytes are smaller than neutrophils with rounded nuclei and scant basophilic cytoplasm (Figure 2-13). The nucleus is generally not perfectly round, but will have a flattened or indented area on one side. The nuclear chromatin has a smudged appearance. Nucleoli are not visible; however, darker areas (heterochromatin) and lighter areas (euchromatin) are often visible. Generally, the cytoplasm does not appear to completely encircle the

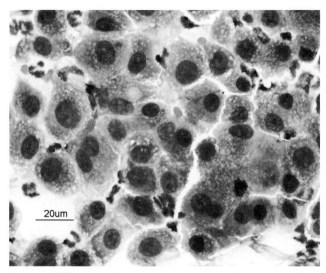

Figure 2-12 Impression smear of a nodule on pleural surface of a dog with pyothorax caused by *Actinomyces* spp. infection. Numerous large epithelioid macrophages are present. These cells have abundant basophilic cytoplasm that may be nonvacuolated to minimally vacuolated. They may also occur in large aggregates resembling epithelial cell clusters.

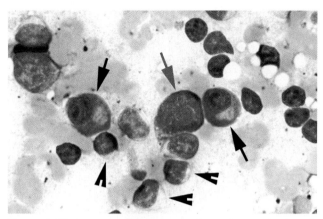

Figure 2-13 Smear made from an aspirate of a reactive lymph node. Many small lymphocytes are present *(arrowheads)*. These cells have scant amounts of cytoplasm that do not appear to encircle the nucleus. Two plasma cells *(arrows)* are also present. One large, immature lymphoid cell (lymphoblast) is present *(red arrow)*. Note that the lymphoblast and plasma cells are similar in size. However, the lymphoblast has a larger nucleus, whereas the nucleus of the plasma cell is similar in size to a small lymphocyte.

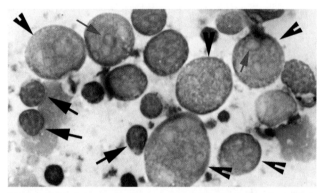

Figure 2-14 Image of a fine-needle aspirate smear of a lymph node from a dog with lymphoma containing numerous lymphoblasts *(arrowheads)* and lymphocytes *(arrows)*. The lymphoblasts are larger, have more abundant cytoplasm, and often show prominent nucleoli *(red arrows)*.

nucleus, because it is visible for only a portion of its way around the nucleus. Medium sized lymphocytes may be present and are similar to small lymphocytes, but they have moderately increased amounts of cytoplasm and may have nucleoli visible. Large, blastic lymphocytes (lymphoblasts) (Figure 2-14), commonly encountered in aspirates of lymphoid tissue and lymphoid neoplasms, may be present in low numbers in inflammatory lesions. Lymphoblasts are large cells with large nuclei and more abundant cytoplasm, which typically stains basophilic. Nuclei can be variably shaped and have stippled nuclear chromatin, which stains somewhat lighter than that of mature lymphocytes. Distinct nucleoli are often visible, and multiple nucleoli may be observed.

Reactive lymphocytes are lymphocytes that have been antigenically stimulated. They have moderately increased amounts of basophilic cytoplasm. Plasma cells are differentiated B-lymphocytes stimulated to produce antibodies. Plasma cells have a round, eccentrically placed nucleus, moderate amounts of deeply basophilic cytoplasm, and usually a distinct clear area located next to the nucleus (see Figure 2-13). This clear area represents the Golgi apparatus and is often located between the nucleus and the greatest volume of cytoplasm. Plasma cells and lymphoblasts are both larger than small lymphocytes, but in the plasma cells most of the increase in size is due to more abundant cytoplasm, whereas in the lymphoblast the nucleus has enlarged (see Figure 2-13).

Some plasma cells (termed *Mott cells*) have numerous large clear vacuoles (termed *Russell bodies*) filling their cytoplasm (Figure 2-15). These vacuoles represent retained immunoglobulin.

Eosinophils

Eosinophils are slightly larger than neutrophils. Their nuclei are segmented, but commonly less lobulated than that of neutrophils and often divided into only two distinct lobes (Figure 2-16). Rarely, eosinophils with perfectly round nuclei will be identified in cytologic specimens. The cytoplasm of eosinophils contains prominent orange to pink granules. In dogs, eosinophil granules are round and vary widely in size and number (Figure 2-17). Eosinophil granules are numerous, small, and rod shaped in cats (Figure 2-18). The delicate, densely packed granules of feline eosinophils are often less obvious than those of the dog, particularly in thick specimens that may not stain well (i.e., transtracheal washes). Also, neutrophils in exudates will occasionally have mild eosinophilic stippling. Care must be taken not to confuse neutrophils and poorly stained eosinophils when trying to differentiate eosinophilic from neutrophilic inflammatory reactions

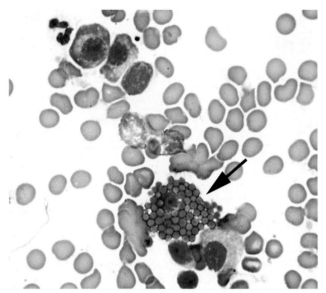

Figure 2-15 Image from a lymph node aspirate demonstrates small lymphocytes, plasma cells, and one Mott cell with numerous Russell bodies *(arrow)*. The Russell bodies may range from appearing as clear vacuoles or may be somewhat basophilic as in this image. *(Courtesy Dr. Robin Allison, Oklahoma State University.)*

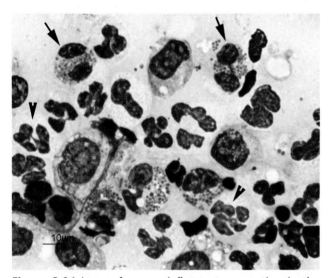

Figure 2-16 Image from an inflammatory reaction in the intestines of a dog containing a mixture of neutrophils, eosinophils, and macrophages. The nuclei of the eosinophils are typically less lobulated *(arrows)* than those of the neutrophils *(arrowheads)*.

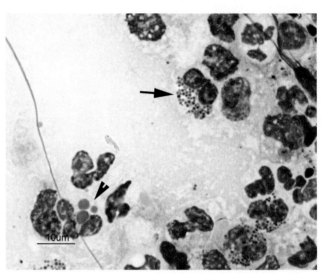

Figure 2-17 Image from the same slide as Figure 2-16. In the dog, eosinophils have numerous small granules *(arrow)* or just a few large granules *(arrowhead)*.

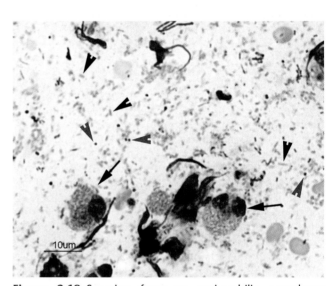

Figure 2-18 Scraping from an eosinophilic granuloma complex lesion in a cat. Cat eosinophils *(arrows)* have densely packed granules, often making it difficult to see the individual granules in intact cells. Numerous free granules *(black arrowheads)* released from ruptured cells are present and demonstrate the slender rod shape typical of feline eosinophil granules. Numerous bacteria *(red arrowheads)* are also present free in the background.

in cats. Eosinophils are slightly larger than neutrophils and their nuclei less lobulated. Often, it is easier to identify feline eosinophils that have been traumatized during slide preparation as their granules spread out and become more obvious. If many eosinophils have been ruptured during sample collection (such as with scraping of feline eosinophilic granuloma complex lesions) high numbers of eosinophil granules will be present throughout the background of the smear and may be identified before intact cells are seen.

Occasionally, eosinophil granules will not stain well with Diff-Quik stain (similar to what sometimes occurs with mast cells) yet stain prominently with Wright's stain or Wright-Giemsa stain.

IF A SMEAR IS COMPOSED OF TISSUE CELLS RATHER THAN INFLAMMATORY CELLS, WHAT TYPE OF CELLS ARE PRESENT?

A wide variety of specific cells may be encountered from the various normal tissues and tumors sampled cytologically. With experience, most of these cells can be easily

TABLE 2-1

General Cytologic Characteristics of Different Tissue Cell Types

	Round Cells	Epithelial Cells	Mesenchymal Cells
Cellularity of slides	High cellularity	High cellularity	Low to high cellularity Normal mesenchymal cells and many tumors are of low cellularity due to adherence of cell in matrix Malignant tumors may yield high numbers of cells
Cell distribution	Evenly distributed across slide	Typically present in clusters Malignant cells may lose adhesion	Discretely oriented or adhered in aggregates by extracellular matrix
Cell size and shape	Small to medium sized Generally round with distinct cell borders	Small to large, depending on tissue samples Cuboidal to columnar to round depending on specific tissue Generally distinct cell borders when cells are individually oriented or at the edges of cell clusters	Often fusiform or "spindle-shaped" Some cells may be plump or round (particularly cells from bone or bone tumors) Often have indistinct cytoplasmic borders
Other features suggestive of this cell type	Distinctive morphology or select individual cell types	Formation of acini or tubules Extremely large cells with abundant cytoplasm Squamous differentiation	Production of eosinophilic extracellular matrix

recognized, particularly with the knowledge of what structure is being sampled. However, even if the cells are not immediately recognizable, they can generally be classified into one of three major categories based on certain common cytologic features (Table 2-1):

1. Discrete cells (or round cells)
2. Epithelial cells
3. Mesenchymal cells

Categorizing cells into which major group they belong helps the evaluator identify the specific cell type present. Even if precise identification cannot be made, relevant information may be gained, such as the presence of a cell type abnormal for the tissue sampled (e.g., epithelial cells in a lymph node aspirate).

Discrete Cells (Round Cells)

Discrete cells are a group of cells that share certain cytologic features owing to the fact that they are present individually in tissues, not adhered to other cells or connective tissue matrix. The majority of these cells are of hematogenous origin. Aspirates of normal lymphoid tissue, such as spleen and lymph nodes, yield cell populations that have a discrete cell pattern. Other than normal lymphoid tissue, a discrete cell pattern usually indicates the presence of one of a group of tumors termed discrete cell tumors (or round cell tumors). Recognition of discrete cell tumors is important because these are some of the more common neoplasms encountered in small animal practice. Also, cells of most discrete cell tumors have cytologic

characteristics that are sufficiently distinct to allow for a specific diagnosis.

General Cytologic Characteristics of Discrete Cell Populations: Because discrete cells are not adhered to other structures within the tissues, they generally exfoliate very readily during fine-needle biopsy (FNB). Hence, the cellularity of the resulting smears is usually very high. In addition, the individual cells are usually evenly spread throughout the smear (Figure 2-19). Cell clusters or aggregates are not present; however, the extremely high cellularity of the smears may result in cells being piled on top of each other in thicker areas of the smears and this may be misinterpreted as cell adhesion (cell clustering). In the thinner areas of the smears, the cells can be seen to be individually oriented.

The individual cells tend to be small to medium sized and round. If the cells have not been traumatized during sample preparation, they typically have distinct cytoplasmic borders (i.e., the boundary of the cell is well defined).

Specific Discrete Cell Tumors: The discrete cell tumors are mast cell tumor, lymphoma (lymphosarcoma), histiocytoma, malignant histiocytosis, plasmacytoma, and transmissible venereal tumor. In addition, melanomas are the great imitator, yielding cell populations that may appear discrete, epithelial, or mesenchymal.

Mast Cell Tumor: Mast cell tumors are the only lesions that will yield highly cellular smears consisting

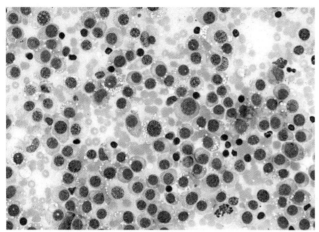

Figure 2-19 This slide, made from an aspirate of a transmissible venereal tumor, shows a typical discrete cell pattern. The slide is highly cellular and the cells are evenly spread out throughout the smear. This pattern can usually be recognized from low-power magnification.

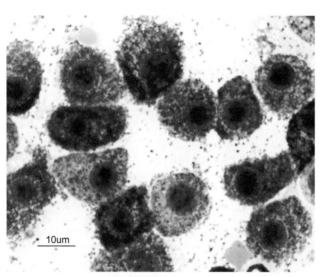

Figure 2-20 Smear made from a mast cell tumor has a pure population of heavily granulated mast cells. The nuclei of these cells are often obscured by the granulation. Numerous free granules are present in the background.

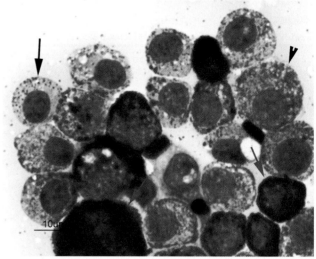

Figure 2-21 Image from a mast cell tumor. Some cells are sparsely granulated and the individual granules are easy to see *(black arrow)*. In some heavily granulated cells, the cytoplasm appears diffusely pink-purple, but some individual granules can be seen and the outline of the nucleus can still be visualized *(black arrowhead)*. Some cells are so densely packed with granules that neither individual granules nor the nucleus can be seen, making the cell appear as a dark purple mass *(red arrows)*.

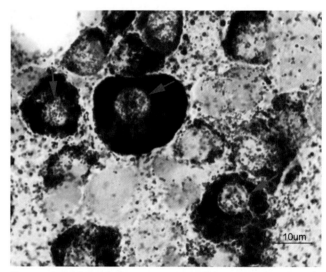

Figure 2-22 Image from a mast cell tumor. The densely packed granules in the cytoplasm have a high affinity for the stain and the nuclei of many cells are understained, giving the cells the look of a photographic negative.

entirely (or predominantly) of mast cells. Mast cells are recognized by their distinctive small, red-purple intracytoplasmic granules (Figure 2-20). The number of granules in mast cells varies tremendously, even within cells from the same tumor (Figure 2-21). Most mast cell tumors yield cells that contain a sufficient number of granules to be easily recognized as mast cells. Sometimes, the cells are so densely packed with granules that the cytoplasm will appear diffusely dark purple and the individual granules difficult or impossible to discern. In this situation, the granules will be evident in cells that have been ruptured. Since mast cell granules have such a high affinity for most cytologic stains, the nucleus of a heavily granulated mast cell may appear pale or even totally unstained, giving the cell a photographic negative look (dark cytoplasm with pale nucleus) (Figure 2-22). Some of the components of

mast cell granules are chemotactic for eosinophils. The number of eosinophils present in smears from a mast cell tumor varies from very few to many. Occasionally, an aspirate from a mast cell tumor will yield predominantly eosinophils with lesser numbers of mast cells (Figure 2-23). In this case, it can be difficult to differentiate a mast cell tumor from a hypersensitivity response. Generally, if there are areas on the slides containing large sheets or aggregates of mast cells, mast cell tumor is most likely.

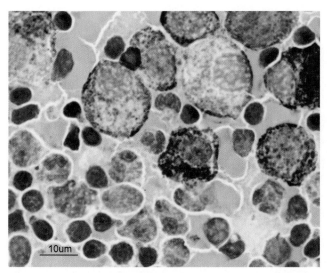

Figure 2-23 Mast cell tumor metastasis to a lymph node. Many mast cells are present, but there are greater numbers of eosinophils, which are attracted by constituents of mast cell granules. In some cases, the number of eosinophils can be greater than the number of mast cells in an aspirate from a mast cell tumor.

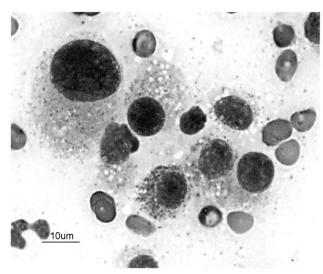

Figure 2-24 Aspirate from a poorly differentiated (Grade III) mast cell tumor. The poorly differentiated cells contain relatively few granules. The individual cells show marked atypia including significant variation of cell size, nuclear size, and N:C ratio.

Cells from some mast cell tumors contain relatively few granules. If a mast cell tumor had degranulated during or prior to aspiration, a percentage of the cells may have relatively few granules. Generally, some granules will still be evident in most cells and some cells will remain heavily granulated. In addition, high numbers of free granules may be present in the background of the slides. Aspirates of degranulated mast cell tumors may be of lower than normal cellularity because of resultant tissue edema. Anaplastic (poorly differntiated) mast cell tumors may yield cells virtually devoid of granules because the cells have not differentiated sufficiently to produce them (Figure 2-24). In this case, the cells generally display marked atypia (see section entitled, "Do the Tissue Cells Present Display Significant Criteria of Malignancy?"). Finally, Diff-Quik sometimes fails to stain the granules of mast cells tumors. Slides from the same tumor stained with Wright's stain may be heavily granulated (Figure 2-25). This is an inconsistent event, occurring only in some mast cell tumors and not others. When it occurs, mast cells may resemble plasma cells or macrophages. A diligent search of the slides will usually reveal low numbers of identifiable, although poorly stained, granules in some cells. A person routinely using Diff-Quik should always consider this possibility when evaluating a discrete cell population.

Cells from mast cell tumors should be evaluated for criteria of malignancy as described later in this chapter. Evaluation of cells for criteria of malignancy is often limited by the fact that the mast cell granules can obscure nuclear detail. In addition, cytology cannot evaluate tissue invasion by neoplastic cells.

The majority of tumors composed of poorly granulated cells (Wright's stained) that display marked cytologic atypia (criteria of malignancy) will have an aggressive biological behavior. A small percentage of tumors composed of heavily granulated, well-differentiated cells will be behaviorally malignant, and thus all mast cell tumors should be removed with wide surgical excision, if possible.

Examination of peripheral blood smears or buffy coat preparations, bone marrow aspirates, and aspirates of any enlarged lymph nodes or abdominal organs (particularly liver and spleen) can be useful in detecting systemic spread of the mast cell tumor.

Lymphoma (Lymphosarcoma): Most cases of lymphoma in dogs and cats are high-grade tumors composed predominantly of large blastic lymphoid cells (Figure 2-26). If large, blastic lymphoid cells compose greater than 50% of the cells in a highly cellular smear from lymphoid tissue containing mostly intact cells, a diagnosis of lymphoma can reliably be made. Lymphoblasts are usually easy to differentiate from the cells of other discrete tumors, based on their higher nuclear-to-cytoplasmic (N:C) ratio and intensely basophilic cytoplasm. Also, in aspirates from lymphoma there are usually numerous small but variably sized basophilic fragments of cytoplasm (lymphoglandular bodies) scattered amongst the cells (see Figure 2-26). Lymphoid cells, particularly lymphoblasts, are fragile cells and easily ruptured during slide preparation. If an overwhelming majority of the cells on the smears are ruptured, it is difficult to be confident that the remaining cells accurately represent the cell population in the lymph node. In this situation, additional samples must be collected for a diagnosis.

Occasionally, low-grade, well-differentiated lymphoma will be encountered. Such tumors may yield predominantly small lymphocytes. Such tumors are difficult to differentiate from normal or reactive lymphoid tissue based solely on cytology and often require histologic biopsy (which can demonstrate architectural effacement and capsular invasion) for a definitive diagnosis.

Canine Cutaneous Histiocytoma: Canine cutaneous histiocytomas are benign tumors of dendritic cell origin that are common in young dogs (Figure 2-27). Tumor cells are medium sized, slightly larger than neutrophils.

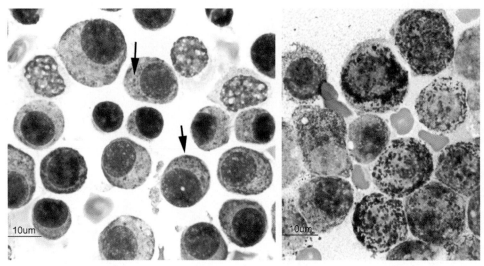

Figure 2-25 Two different slides from the same mast cell tumor were stained with either Diff-Quik *(left)* or Wright-Giemsa *(right)*. Although the sample stained with Wright-Giemsa shows that the cells are heavily granulated, Diff-Quik did not stain the granules of the cells well in this tumor. Some granules can be seen in the Diff-Quik–stained specimen *(arrows)*.

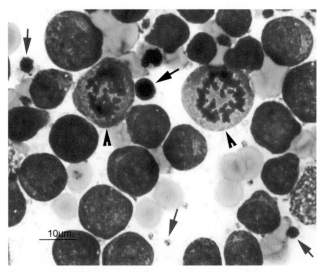

Figure 2-26 Aspirate of the lymph nodes of a dog with lymphoma. The slide consists almost entirely of large blastic lymphoid cells. One poorly spread-out small lymphocyte is present *(black arrow)*. Two mitotic figures are present *(arrowheads)* and numerous cytoplasmic fragments of lymphoid cells (lymphoglandular bodies) are present in the background *(red arrows)*.

Nuclei are generally round to oval but may be indented to irregular in shape. The nucleus has finely stippled chromatin and may have indistinct nucleoli. They have a moderate amount of light blue-gray cytoplasm. If there is a significant amount of protein-rich tissue fluid present between cells, the cytoplasm of the cells may appear lighter than the background, or cell borders may be indistinct.

Histiocytomas usually regress spontaneously within a few weeks to months. Regression is associated with an infiltration of small lymphocytes into the tumor. Therefore, aspirates from these tumors will sometimes contain a mixture of tumor cells and small lymphocytes (Figure 2-28). The presence of small lymphocytes amongst the larger

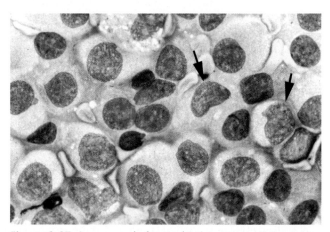

Figure 2-27 Smear made from a histiocytoma. Histiocytoma cells have moderate amounts of light colored cytoplasm. Nuclei are usually round to oval but may be indented, kidney shaped, or irregular *(arrows)*.

tumor cells sometimes leads to misidentification of histiocytoma cells as lymphoblasts. The irregularly shaped nuclei, light color and volume of the cytoplasm, and lack of lymphoglandular bodies help differentiate histiocytoma cells from lymphoid cells.

Malignant Histiocytosis/Histiocytic Sarcoma/ Systemic Histiocytosis: Systemic and malignant proliferations of histiocytes represent a group of disorders whose classification is ongoing. They result from a proliferation of either dendritic cells or bone marrow origin macrophages. Cytology alone may not be able to differentiate these diseases from each other or from inflammatory proliferations of macrophages (granulomatous inflammation).

Cytologic appearance of samples from histiocytic proliferative diseases varies from a population of relatively benign looking cells (Figure 2-29) to populations of histiocytic cells with marked atypia (Figure 2-30, *A*). Common features include large discrete cells with abundant vacuolated

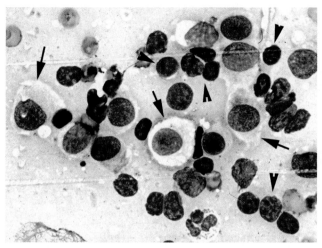

Figure 2-28 Smear made from a histiocytoma. Regression of a histiocytoma is associated with an infiltration of small lymphocytes *(arrowheads)*, which may be more numerous than the histiocytoma cells *(arrows)*.

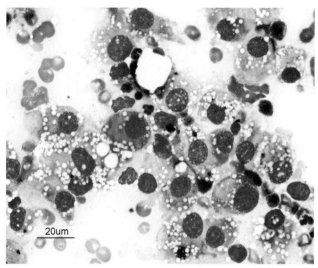

Figure 2-29 Splenic aspirate from a dog with malignant histiocytosis. The spleen was markedly enlarged and consisted almost entirely of a population of discretely oriented, heavily vacuolated histiocytic cells. Most of the cells were fairly uniform, although a small percentage of cells shows significant atypia (see Figure 2-30, *A*). Histopathology confirmed malignant histiocytosis.

cytoplasm, prominent cytophagia, and multinucleation (Figure 2-30, *B*). With tumors of dendritic cell origin, the cytoplasmic vacuoles are often small and of uniform size and may lack the presence of phagocytic debris common in macrophages seen in inflammatory lesions (see Figure 2-29). The cells may demonstrate marked anisocytosis, anisokaryosis, and variation of N:C ratio (Figure 2-31, *A*). Macrocytosis, karyomegaly and the presence of large multinucleated cells are common (Figure 2-31, *B*).

When masses are composed of histiocytic cells showing marked atypia, a diagnosis of malignant histiocytosis/histiocytic sarcoma can be made (Figure 2-32). However, when the cells consist of relatively bland appearing macrophages, definitive diagnosis may not be possible based solely on cytology. It should be noted that many of these lesions with relatively bland cytologic appearance may have an aggressive biological behavior.

Plasmacytoma: Tumors of plasma cell origin include multiple myeloma (plasma cell myeloma), a systemic tumor arising primarily in the bone marrow, and extramedullary plasmacytomas. Extramedullary plasmacytomas are commonly cutaneous tumors but have been described from other sites including the gastrointestinal tract. Cutaneous plasmacytomas are usually benign, although malignant behavior has been reported in some tumors. A higher percentage of plasmacytomas arising from the gastrointestinal tract have been reported as having malignant behavior. Well-differentiated plasmacytomas yield cells that resemble normal plasma cells. Distinguishing features include eccentrically placed small, round nuclei surrounded by a moderate amount of deeply basophilic cytoplasm with or without the characteristic distinct paranuclear clear zone. Poorly differentiated plasmacytomas may yield a less distinct population of discrete cells that demonstrate significant cytologic criteria of malignancy. Binucleate and multinucleated cells are common in both well differentiated and poorly differentiated tumors (Figure 2-33). This and a lack of lymphoglandular bodies help differentiate these tumors from

lymphosarcoma. Some plasma cells have a distinct red color to the periphery of their cytoplasm and are referred to as *flame cells*. Rarely, an eosinophilic extracellular matrix representing amyloid (composed of immunoglobulin light chain) is seen amongst the neoplastic cells.

Transmissible Venereal Tumor: Except in certain geographic areas, transmissible venereal tumors (TVTs) are less commonly encountered than the other discrete cell tumors. These tumors are often present on the external genitalia but may occur in other locations as well.

The cells from a TVT are typically more pleomorphic than from most other discrete cell tumors (Figure 2-34). They have moderate amounts of smoky to light blue cytoplasm with sharply defined cytoplasmic boundaries. A prominent characteristic of TVT cells, which can help distinguish them from other discrete cell tumors, is the presence of numerous distinctly walled, cytoplasmic vacuoles (see Figure 2-34). These vacuoles can also be found extracellularly, appearing as clear areas against a proteinaceous background of tissue fluid. Nuclei show moderate to marked anisokaryosis and have a coarse nuclear chromatin pattern. Nucleoli may be prominent and mitotic figures are common.

Melanoma: Tumors of melanocytic origin are the great imitators; cells may show features of discrete cells, epithelial cells or mesenchymal cells. Melanocytes are usually easily recognized by their pigmentation. Individual melanin granules are rod-shaped granules that typically stain dark green to black. When these granules are densely packed within cells, they appear black. Cells from a melanoma may range from heavily pigmented to sparsely pigmented, depending on the degree of differentiation of the tumor.

With heavily pigmented tumors, the cells often appear simply as dark black circular to spherical objects (Figure

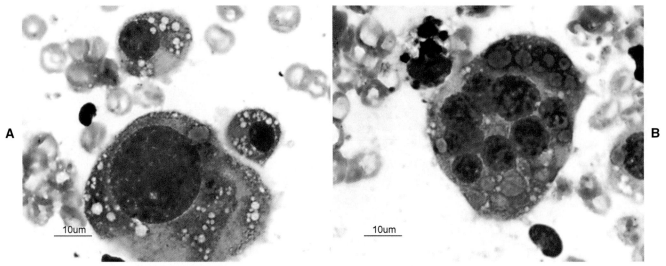

Figure 2-30 Same slide as Figure 2-29. **A,** Some macrocytic, karyomegalic cells were also present. Note the phagocytosis of several red blood cells. **B,** Large multinucleated cell showing erythrophagia.

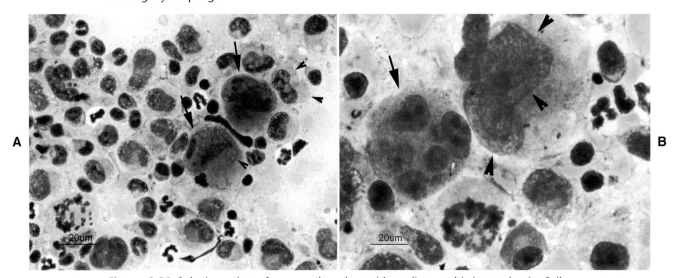

Figure 2-31 Splenic aspirate from another dog with malignant histiocytosis. **A,** Cells from this tumor showed marked atypia including anisocytosis, anisokaryosis, and nuclear pleomorphism. Large, karyomegalic cells with large, prominent, irregularly shaped nucleoli are present *(arrows)*. Many of the cells in this tumor demonstrated erythrophagia *(arrowheads)*. **B,** Both large multinucleated cells and large cells with a single, pleomorphic, karyomegalic nucleus *(arrowheads)* are common in this tumor.

2-35). Visualization of cell detail is often completely obscured by the pigmentation. Nuclei may be seen in cells that are traumatized, and there is often a background containing numerous free melanin granules (see Figure 2-35).

In poorly differentiated tumors, pigmentation may be sparse (Figure 2-36) to absent requiring a lengthy search to find any pigment granules at all. These cells typically show marked criteria of malignancy (see subsequent section in this chapter) (see Figure 2-36).

Most poorly pigmented tumors with marked cytologic atypia have a malignant biological behavior. It is difficult to assess the malignant potential of heavily pigmented tumors because the individual cells cannot be evaluated. Although many heavily pigmented tumors are benign,

some of these may also have an aggressive biological behavior. Anatomic location of the tumor greatly affects the likelihood of malignancy.

Epithelial Cells

Normal epithelial cells are commonly encountered in many cytologic preparations. Surface epithelium will be present in most surface scrapings/swabs (e.g., squamous cells from skin scrapings and nasal/vaginal swabs), in washings (e.g., columnar cells from transtracheal washes), and as the result of normal exfoliation (transitional cells from urine sediments). In addition, epithelial cells will be the major cellular component of smears made from FNB of many parenchymal organs (e.g., hepatocytes and bile

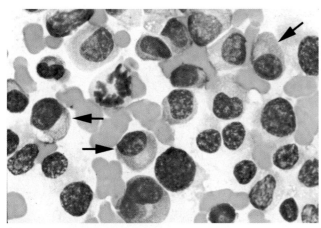

Figure 2-32 Smear made from an extramedullary plasmacytoma. Cells show a typical discrete cell pattern. Many cells resemble mature plasma cells having eccentric nuclei and distinct perinuclear clear areas *(arrows)*.

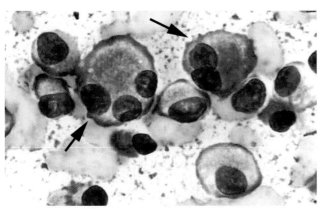

Figure 2-33 Smear made from an extramedullary plasmacytoma. Binucleated and multinucleated cells *(arrows)* are common in tumors of plasma cell origin.

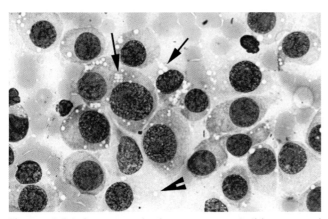

Figure 2-34 Smear made from a transmissible venereal tumor (TVT). Cells from a TVT are characterized by numerous clear vacuoles within the cytoplasm of the cells *(arrows)* and free in the background *(arrowhead)*. Many of the cells have coarse nuclear chromatin and large nucleoli.

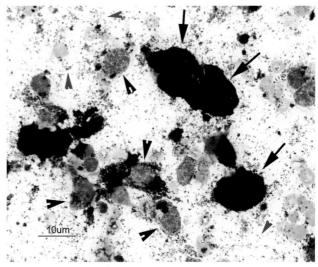

Figure 2-35 Aspirate of a heavily pigmented cutaneous melanoma from a dog. In most of the intact cells *(arrows)*, the cellular detail is completely obscured by the pigmentation, preventing evaluation of these cells. Nuclei can be seen in some cells *(arrowheads)* that appear partially ruptured. Numerous free melanin granules *(red arrowheads)* are present in the background of the smear.

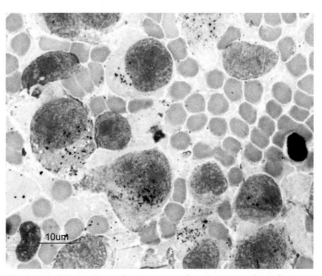

Figure 2-36 Aspirate from a poorly pigmented malignant melanoma from the oral cavity of a dog. The slide consists of large, pleomorphic cells with a high N:C ratio and large prominent nucleoli. Most cells have a few cytoplasmic melanin granules that are easily recognizable.

duct epithelium from liver aspirates, renal tubular cells from kidney aspirates) and glandular aspirates (e.g., mammary, prostate).

Epithelial cells may also originate from a hyperplastic proliferation or neoplasm. Cells from benign epithelial tumors may be difficult to impossible to differentiate from their normal, or hyperplastic, counterparts based solely on cytology. However, combining clinical and cytologic findings can often allow the diagnosis of a benign epithelial proliferation to be made. For example, a discrete wartlike mass on an older dog that yields numerous clusters

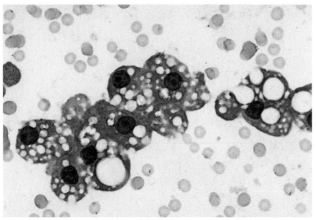

Figure 2-37 Smear made from an aspirate of a feline kidney. Numerous renal tubular epithelial cells are present. Epithelial cells tend to form cell clusters. Feline renal tubular cells may have numerous lipid vacuoles within their cytoplasm.

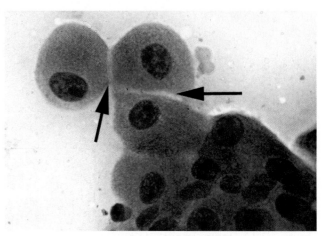

Figure 2-38 Aspirate from a perianal adenoma. The areas of cell adhesion can be seen in some cells *(arrows).*

of normal appearing sebaceous epithelial cells suggest a sebaceous adenoma or sebaceous gland hyperplasia.

Epithelial cells that display sufficient cytologic criteria of malignancy indicate the presence of a carcinoma/adenocarcinoma. A specific diagnosis of cell type may or may not be possible based solely on cytology, depending on how well differentiated and characteristic the cells are. Histopathology may be required for a more specific diagnosis of cell type. However, the ability to confirm the presence of a malignant epithelial tumor by cytology is often sufficient to guide clinical management of a case.

General Cytologic Characteristics of Epithelial Cell Populations: A main feature of epithelial cells is cell-to-cell adhesion (Figure 2-37). Normal epithelial cells are typically present in variably sized sheets or clumps. Sometimes, the area of adhesion between individual cells can be seen (Figure 2-38). True cell clustering from cell-to-cell adhesion must be differentiation from crowding of cells in highly cellular aspirates of any cell type. This can usually be accomplished by looking at thinner areas of the smear. In thin areas, if the cells are still present in clusters but are separated by acellular areas, cell to cell adhesion is documented.

Mesenchymal cells are sometimes held together by an extracellular matrix, resulting in large aggregates of cells, which resembles cell adhesion. Often, this extracellular matrix is apparent as a brightly eosinophilic, homogenous material between the cells and can be used to identify the type of cell present.

Epithelial cells can be very large cells and have abundant cytoplasm. Although normal epithelial cells vary in size from small (basal cells) to large depending on the specific type, the presence of extremely large cells on a cytologic smear suggests an epithelial origin. Epithelial cells are round to columnar to caudate and have distinct, sharply defined cytoplasmic borders. Cytoplasmic borders within cell clusters may be difficult to discern; however, the outer edges of the cells in the clusters typically are

clearly demarcated. Nuclei of epithelial cells are generally round to somewhat oval.

Epithelial Criteria Specific to Certain Cell Types: Mature squamous epithelial cells, often found in samples collected from surface swabs or scrapings, tend to be more individually oriented and may not show prominent cell clustering (Figure 2-39). Fully mature (cornified or keratinized) squamous cells have abundant cytoplasm with angular (squared off) cytoplasmic borders. Their nuclei become small and pyknotic, and eventually the cell becomes anucleate (see Figure 2-39). Less differentiated squamous cells, often present in swabs/scrapings along with mature cells, are more cohesive and have a greater tendency to be in clusters (Figure 2-40). These cells tend to be round and have variable amounts of cytoplasm (increasing as the cell matures). Nuclei of these cells are large and round with functional (nonpyknotic) chromatin (see Figure 2-40).

Normal epithelial cells from the respiratory and gastrointestinal tract are distinctly columnar. Cell clusters may show long rows of cells, with nuclei lined up at the basal end of the cell (Figure 2-41). Often, cilia can be seen at the apical surface of samples from the respiratory tract (Figure 2-42). Normal epithelial cells from the gastrointestinal tract are often present in large pavemented clusters, often with clear cytoplasm suggesting their secretory nature (Figure 2-43). The columnar nature of the cells may be evident only at the sides of the clusters, where the cells have arranged on their sides (rather than a "top down" view seen in the middle of the clusters) (Figure 2-44).

Although most tissue architecture is lost during fine-needle aspiration, some architectural arrangements may endure. Epithelial cells of glandular origin may show evidence of tubular or acinar formation (Figures 2-45 and 2-46). Papillary or trabecular patterns may also be retained in some epithelial tumors.

Tumors of endocrine epithelial cells (e.g., thyroid carcinoma) and neuroendocrine cells (e.g., pheochromocytoma, chemodectoma) often yield cell populations with characteristic features (Figures 2-47 and 2-48). The slides

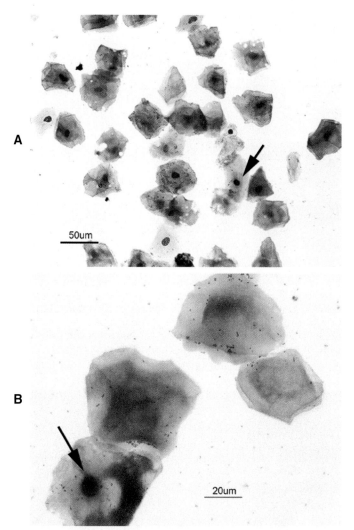

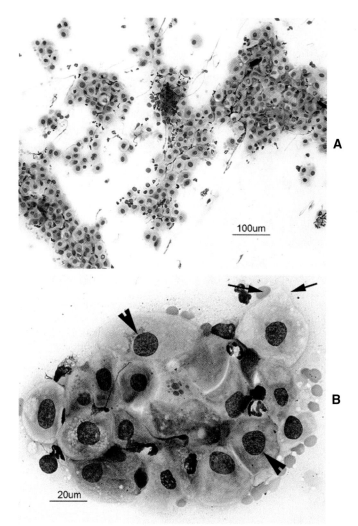

Figure 2-39 Mature, cornified cells from a canine vaginal swab. **A,** Low-magnification image shows that these cells tend to exfoliate individually rather than in cohesive clusters. Individual cells show angular cytoplasmic borders. Nuclei become pyknotic *(arrow)* and eventually disappear, leaving anucleate cells. **B,** High-magnification image showing three anucleate squamous cells and one mature squamous cell with a condensed pyknotic nucleus *(arrow).*

Figure 2-40 Noncornified squamous cells from a canine vaginal swab. These cells are less differentiated than those shown in Figure 2-39. These cells can be seen in surface swabs and scraping and may be intermixed with fully keratinized cells. **A,** Low-magnification image shows that these cells tend to demonstrate cell-to-cell adhesion, being present in cohesive clusters. **B,** High magnification of one cluster of noncornified squamous cells. The cells tend to be round, although some cells are beginning to develop angular borders. Amount of cytoplasm is variable depending on stage of maturation. Cells have functional, nonpyknotic nuclei *(arrowheads).*

are highly cellular and consist of loosely cohesive cells. In addition, these cells tend to be fragile and smears typically contain many bare nuclei admixed with the loosely cohesive intact cells. Bare nuclei of fragile cell populations must be differentiated from bare nuclei occurring from cell rupturing due to poor smearing technique (i.e., excessive pressure during smearing). Bare nuclei from endocrine/neuroendocrine population often have relatively intact nuclear outlines, as opposed to the traumatized, irregular appearance often seen with poor smearing technique.

Mesenchymal Cells

Occurrence of Mesenchymal Cells: Mesenchymal cells are cells that form connective tissue, blood vessels, and lymphatics. Because blood is considered a liquid connective tissue, hematopoietic cells (including many of the

cells described in the section about discrete cells) are typically classified as mesenchymal cells. However, because these hematopoietic cells have a cytologic appearance that is so distinct from the other connective tissues, they are typically considered as a separate classification. Most often, the discussion of mesenchymal cells in cytology texts implies stromal connective tissue cells.

Most normal connective tissues exfoliate no cells when sampled by fine-needle biopsy. Fibroblasts and fibrocytes are normal mesenchymal cells commonly encountered. Clusters of normal stromal cells can be seen in aspirates of internal organs, particularly the spleen. Scattered individual fibroblasts may be seen in aspirates

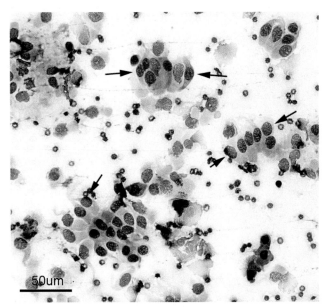

Figure 2-41 Smear of a bronchial brushing from a dog. Low-magnification image shows numerous clusters of columnar epithelial cells. In some of the well-spread-out cells, the columnar nature is evident and the nuclei can be seen lining up on what was the basal surface of the cell.

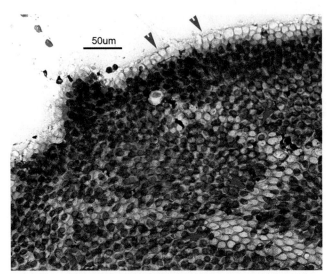

Figure 2-43 Aspirate of intestinal epithelial cells from a cat. Low magnification shows large, tightly cohesive clusters of cells in a pavemented monolayer. The secretory nature of the cells is evident by the clear nature of the cytoplasm of many of the cells *(red arrows)*. The columnar nature of the cells is evident only at the edges of the cluster *(red arrowheads)*.

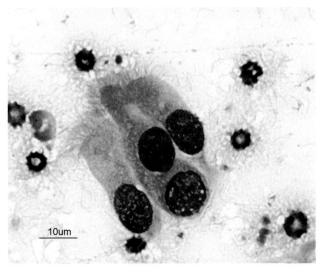

Figure 2-42 Higher magnification of slide from Figure 2-41. Cilia can be seen on the apical surface of the columnar epithelial cells.

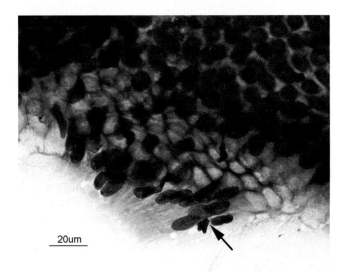

Figure 2-44 Higher magnification of intestinal epithelial cells shown in Figure 2-43. The columnar nature of the cells and palisading nuclear arrangement can be seen on the edge of the cluster *(arrow)*. Again, many of the cells have clear, distended cytoplasm typical of secretory cells.

from virtually any tissue. Reactive fibroblasts may be present in significant numbers in aspirates from areas of inflammation or tissue repair (e.g., surgical scars). Reactive fibroblasts may show many of the cytologic criteria of malignancy, so caution should be taken in evaluating mesenchymal cells when a significant inflammatory response is present. Reactive fibroblasts should be suspected when scattered mesenchymal cells are present along with a population of inflammatory cells (Figure 2-49).

Highly cellular smears that contain predominantly a pure population of mesenchymal cells are likely to indicate a mesenchymal neoplasia. Malignant tumors of mesenchymal origin are by definition sarcomas, although the names of some tumors do not follow the standard nomenclature (e.g., malignant fibrous histiocytoma, hemangiopericytoma).

General Cytologic Characteristics of Mesenchymal Cell Populations: As previously mentioned, aspirates of normal mesenchymal tissue are usually sparsely cellular due to the tightly cohesive nature of connective tissue. Benign mesenchymal tumors tend to exfoliate very few cells, and samples of diagnostic quality may be difficult to obtain. In contrast,

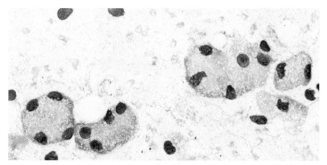

Figure 2-45 Smear from an aspirate of a normal salivary gland (accidentally aspirated instead of the submandibular lymph node). The cells are arranged in an acinar pattern with nuclei at the periphery of the acinus. Individual cells are relatively small with small, round nuclei showing mature chromatin and abundant cytoplasm yielding a low N:C ratio.

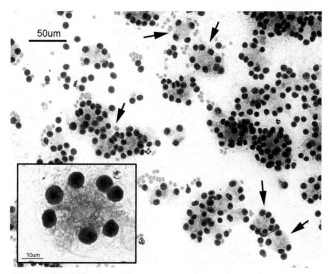

Figure 2-46 Smear of a pancreatic aspirate from a cat. Uniform epithelial cells are in clusters and show acinus formation *(arrows)* indicating a glandular origin. *Inset,* Higher magnification of a single acinus with evidence of secretory material (slightly pink) in the center of the acinus.

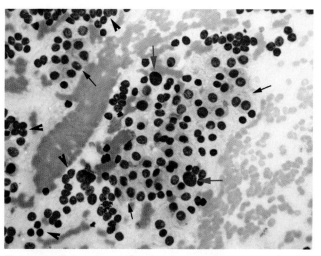

Figure 2-47 Low-magnification image of a neuroendocrine (heartbase) tumor from a dog. The slide is highly cellular and consists of a mixture of loosely cohesive intact cells *(black arrows)* and bare nuclei of ruptured cells *(black arrowheads).* The cells are fairly uniform, although some karyomegalic cells are seen *(red arrows).*

are identified as mesenchymal in nature based on clinical suspicion (i.e., lytic bone lesion), the presence of extracellular matrix, the presence of osteoclasts (Figure 2-54), and the characteristic appearance of the cells (see Figure 2-53).

In contrast to the other cell types (discrete and epithelial), the cytoplasmic borders of mesenchymal cells are often very indistinct (Figure 2-55) and the cytoplasm may blend imperceptibly with the background, making it nearly impossible to distinguish the limits of the cell membrane. Ruptured cells may also have indistinct cytoplasmic borders, but in these traumatized cells the nuclear membrane is usually also disrupted, whereas the nuclear outline of intact mesenchymal cells is well defined. Another characteristic of mesenchymal cells is production of an extracellular matrix (Figure 2-56). This is seen as a variably eosinophilic material present between cells, often holding them in large aggregates.

These descriptions outline general characteristics. The entire cell population present should be carefully evaluated because no single criterion will definitively identify a cell population. Sometimes, particularly with poorly differentiated malignant tumors, the cells will show criteria of more than one category. In these cases, it may be impossible to accurately classify the type of cell present. If cell type cannot be categorized, the cells should be evaluated for criteria of malignancy because identification of a malignant tumor may be sufficient information to direct management of the case. Surgical biopsy and histopathology may be able to provide a more specific diagnosis as to tissue of origin, if needed.

malignant mesenchymal tumors may yield highly cellular aspirates (Figure 2-50). The cells are usually individually oriented, although large aggregates may be present, particularly if held together by an extracellular matrix (see below).

Mesenchymal cells are often elongated cells with cytoplasm that tapers in one or more directions (Figure 2-51). These are commonly referred to as *spindle cells.* Mesenchymal cells may range from extremely elongated, fusiform cells with thin, rod-shaped nuclei (Figure 2-52) to cells that are plump and minimally tapered and have round nuclei. Aspirates from malignant mesenchymal tumors often show a mixture of cells of various shapes, so the entire population must be examined to determine the cell type (see Figure 2-50). Depending on the histologic subtype, cells from primary bone tumors (e.g., osteosarcoma, chondrosarcoma) may show virtually no spindling and may have well-defined cytoplasmic borders mimicking discrete cells or epithelial cells (Figure 2-53). Usually they

DO THE TISSUE CELLS PRESENT DISPLAY SIGNIFICANT CRITERIA OF MALIGNANCY?

Tissue cells should be evaluated for cytologic criteria of malignancy. If sufficient criteria are present, a diagnosis of malignant neoplasia can be made. Cells from normal tissue, hyperplastic tissue, and benign neoplasia generally do not contain significant criteria of malignancy.

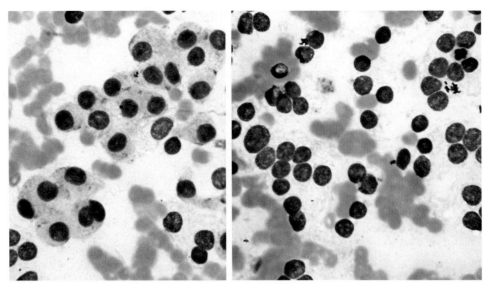

Figure 2-48 Higher magnification of same slide as Figure 2-47. On the left, the intact cells appear fairly uniform and have small nuclei with mature, condensed chromatin and moderate amounts of lightly basophilic cytoplasm. On the right, a different field shows many bare nuclei suggesting the fragile nature of the cells. Note that although the cells are ruptured, the bare nuclei appear intact rather than the nuclear streaming often seen when cells are ruptured from excessive pressure during slide preparation.

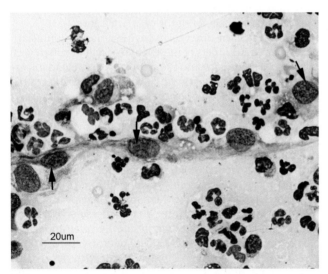

Figure 2-49 Fibroblasts present in an inflammatory reaction. Note that the fibroblasts have prominent nucleoli *(arrows)*. In many cases, reactive fibroblasts will show other atypical features often associated with malignancy such as marked anisocytosis and anisokaryosis. When large numbers of inflammatory cells are present, as with this case, reactive fibroblasts should be suspected and great caution exercised before diagnosis of mesenchymal neoplasia (i.e., biopsy).

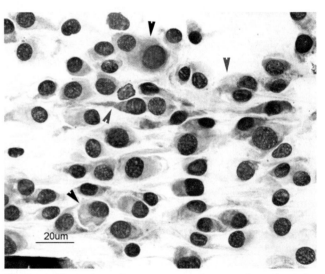

Figure 2-50 Aspirate from a tumor of mesenchymal origin. The slide is highly cellular and the population of mesenchymal cells has a mixture of tapered cells *(red arrowheads)* to cells that are essentially round *(black arrowheads)*, demonstrating the need to evaluate the entire cell population to determine the cell type present. Contrast this with the appearance of the cells in Figure 2-51.

Cytologic Criteria of Malignancy

Although some assessment of the arrangement of cells within cell clusters can be made, cytologic samples often lack the architectural information that is available on histologic sections. Therefore, factors such as disruption of normal architecture and invasion of suspect cells into adjacent normal tissue or lymphatics usually cannot be made. Evaluation of malignant potential in cytology specimens involves evaluating cell populations for lack of differentiation and cellular atypia. In general, benign lesions yield morphologically uniform populations of well-differentiated cells, whereas malignant tumors are characterized by variability of cell features. Cytologic criteria are divided into general criteria of malignancy and nuclear criteria of malignancy (Table 2-2). Nuclear criteria of

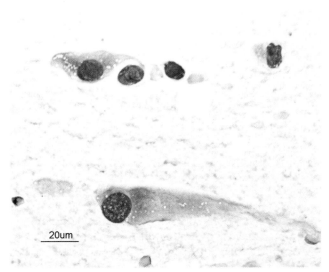

Figure 2-51 Spindle cells from a malignant tumor of mesenchymal origin (myxosarcoma). Note the elongated appearance of the cells with cytoplasm that tapers in one or more directions.

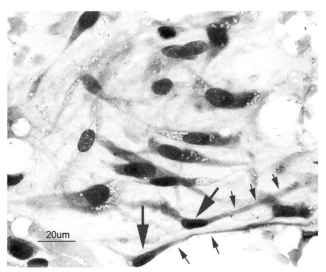

Figure 2-52 Cells from a malignant mesenchymal tumor (fibrosarcoma). Note that most cells are extremely elongated with thin, tapered cytoplasm (red arrows). The majority of the nuclei are also fusiform *(blue arrows).*

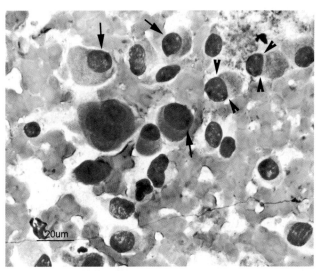

Figure 2-53 Cells from a canine osteosarcoma. The osteoblasts show little to no spindling and have distinct cytoplasmic borders. Note that most of the cells have eccentrically placed nuclei *(arrows).* Often, the nuclei appear to be partially outside the cytoplasmic borders *(arrowheads).* The mesenchymal nature of these cells is suggested by the presence of extracellular matrix.

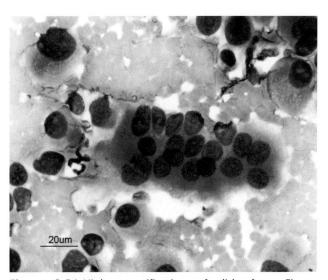

Figure 2-54 High magnification of slide from Figure 2-53. A large osteoclast is present in the center surrounded by osteoblasts. Osteoclasts often have 10 to 20 nuclei or more.

malignancy are more reliable because they are less likely to be induced by nonneoplastic processes such as inflammation induced dysplasia. No single criterion indicates the presence of malignancy and any of the features described below may be seen in certain cells or cell populations.

General Criteria of Malignancy

Anisocytosis and Macrocytosis: *Anisocytosis* (Figure 2-57) refers to variation in cell size, whereas *macrocytosis* (Figure 2-58) refers to exceptionally large cells. Macrocytic cells are most commonly observed in tumors of epithelial origin. Both are atypical findings in most cell populations, although there are exceptions. In samples of

normal or reactive lymphoid tissue, variation in cell size is an expected finding because of the variety of different cell types present (i.e., mature lymphocytes, lymphoblasts, plasma cells). In contrast, lymphoid malignancy (lymphosarcoma) yields a uniform, monotonous population of lymphoblasts. In scrapings from skin surfaces and some vaginal swabs, there can be moderate to marked anisocytosis of the squamous epithelial cells. This relates to the fact that such samples can collect squamous cells of varying degrees of maturation, ranging from small, immature basal/parabasal cells to mature, fully keratinized, superficial squamous cells. Transitional epithelial cells also show moderate anisocytosis as a normal feature of that cell type. Finally, macrophages in inflammatory reactions

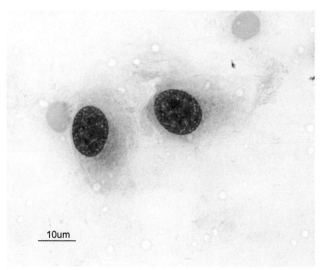

Figure 2-55 Cells from a tumor of mesenchymal origin. The cytoplasmic boundary of these cells is extremely indistinct; the cytoplasm seems to fade gradually into the background. This is another common feature of cells of mesenchymal origin.

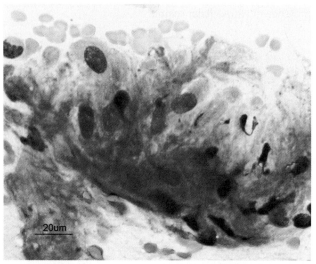

Figure 2-56 Aspirate from a mesenchymal tumor showing extracellular matrix production. Numerous mesenchymal cells are present, which appear to be embedded in a brightly eosinophilic extracellular matrix.

can show marked variation in size (see Figures 2-10 and 2-11) as well as many other atypical features.

Some degree of anisocytosis is normal in any cell population. The tendency of many beginning cytologists is to overinterpret normal variability in cell size rather than to ignore significant variation when it is present; therefore caution is warranted in evaluating subjective parameters. Significant variation in cell size is when one cell is multiple times the size of other cells from the same population. There are no easily defined objective criteria of macrocytosis, although this usually indicates cells that are decidedly larger than what is normal for the cell population. Obviously, this requires having sufficient experience to recognize the limits of normal. If normal cells from the tissue in question are present along with

neoplastic cells, this can give a valuable reference point from which to judge the degree of variability (Figure 2-59).

Hypercellularity: Malignant tumors tend to exfoliate high numbers of cells, even when arising from tissues that would not normally exfoliate any cells. A classic example of this is primary bone tumors, such as osteosarcoma and chondrosarcoma. Normal bone will obviously exfoliate very few, if any, cells. However, aspirates from primary bone tumors are often highly cellular (Figure 2-60). Cells in malignant tumors are often anaplastic and have not differentiated to the point where they develop cell receptors or produce the extracellular matrix that makes them adhesive to other tissues in the body. Therefore, these cells will exfoliate very well by FNB. Similarly, these cells will often demonstrate a loss of cohesion. Highly malignant epithelial tumors may yield cells that distribute in more of a discrete cell pattern, with fewer cell clusters (Figure 2-61).

Obviously, hypercellularity as a criterion of malignancy must be viewed in terms of the tissue sampled. Inflammatory lesions (see Figure 2-1), lymphoid tissue, and some other tissues normally yield high numbers of cells. In these instances, hypercellularity cannot be considered a criterion of malignancy. However, highly cellular slides containing a single population of mesenchymal cells is not a normal finding (see Figure 2-50). Hypercellularity is also important because the sample is more likely to be representative of the lesion than if relatively few cells are present. A definitive diagnosis of malignancy should be made with extreme caution if the sample is of low cellularity.

Pleomorphism: This term refers to variability in the shape of cells. Pleomorphism may be normal if more than one cell type is present on a smear. Also, pleomorphism among cells of a single cell type is seen in some normal tissue, such as transitional cells from the urinary tract and samples containing squamous cells of varying degrees of maturation (skin scrapings and vaginal smears).

Nuclear Criteria of Malignancy

Anisokaryosis and Macrokaryosis (Karyomegaly): These terms refer to variation in nuclear size (see Figure 2-57) and excessively large nuclei (see Figure 2-58), respectively. Nuclei that are multiple times the size of those in other cells within the same population represent significant anisokaryosis. In some malignant tumors, particularly carcinomas, macronuclei, which may be larger than some entire cells of the same population, may be present.

Anisokaryosis is a normal finding in samples containing squamous epithelial cells. As squamous cells mature, the nucleus becomes small and pyknotic, eventually disappearing from the cell.

Multinucleation: Cells with multiple nuclei may be seen in malignant tumors of any cell type. Multinucleation is particularly important when anisokaryosis is present among nuclei within a single cell (Figure 2-62). Multinucleation in neoplastic cells results from nuclear division without cell division. Usually, in multinucleated cells, even numbers of nuclei are present. Odd numbers of nuclei indicate atypical nuclear division and are an important finding (Figure 2-63).

TABLE 2-2

Easily Recognized General and Nuclear Criteria of Malignancy

Criteria	Description	Schematic representation
General criteria		
Anisocytosis and macrocytosis	Variation in cell size, with some cells ≥ 1.5 times larger than normal.	
Hypercellularity	Increased cell exfoliation due to decreased cell adherence.	Not depicted
Pleomorphism (except in lymphoid tissue)	Variable size and shape in cell of the same type.	
Nuclear criteria		
Macrokaryosis	Increased nuclear size. Cell with nuclei larger than 20 μ in diameter suggest malignancy.	RBC
Increased nucleus:cytoplasm ratio (N:C)	Normal nonlymphoid cells usually have a N:C of 1:3 to 1:8, depending on the tissue. Increased ratio (1:2,1:1, etc.) suggests malignancy.	See "macrokaryosis"
Anisokaryosis	Variation in nuclear size. This is especially important if the nuclei of multinucleated cells vary in size.	
Multinucleation	Multiple nucleation in a cell. This is especially important if the nuclei vary in size.	
Increased mitotic figures	Mitosis is rare in normal tissue.	normal abnormal
Abnormal mitosis	Improper alignment of chromosomes.	See "increased mitotic figures"
Coarse chromatin pattern	The chromatin pattern is coarser than normal. It may appear ropy or cord-like.	
Nuclear molding	Deformation of nuclei by other nuclei within the same cell or adjacent cells.	
Macronucleoli	Nucleoli are increased in size. Nucleoli ≥ 5 μ strongly suggest malignancy. For reference, RBCs are 5-6 μ in the cat and 7-8 μ in the dog.	RBC
Angular nucleoli	Nucleoli are fusiform or have other angular shapes instead of their normal round to slightly oval shape.	
Anisonucleoliosis	Variation in nucleolar shape or size (especially important if the variation is within the same nucleus).	See "angular nucleoli"

RBC, Red blood cell.

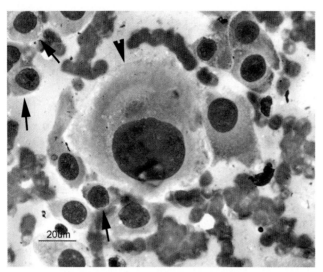

Figure 2-57 Aspirate from a transitional cell carcinoma. The cells show significant anisocytosis and anisokaryosis. Some cells *(arrowhead)* are several times larger than other cells in the population *(arrows)*.

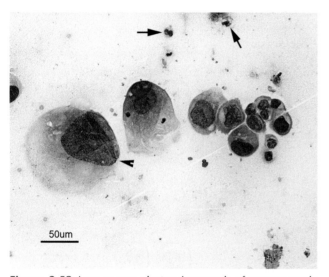

Figure 2-58 Low-power photomicrograph of smears made from thoracic fluid of a cat with a metastatic carcinoma. Atypically macrocytic cells almost 100 μm in diameter with macronuclei (karyomegaly) greater than 50 μm are present. Macrophages *(arrows)* are present for size comparison.

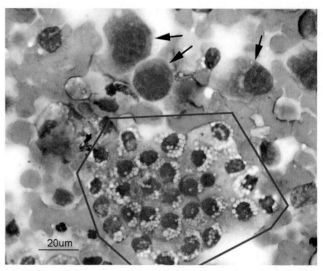

Figure 2-59 Aspirate of a carcinoma from the prostate of a dog. In this case, the presence of relatively normal, uniform prostatic cells in the middle *(surrounded by the red boundary)* allows for easier recognition of the surrounding abnormal larger cells with larger nuclei and prominent nucleoli.

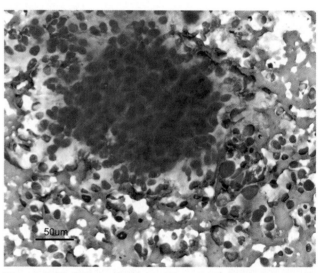

Figure 2-60 Aspirate from a canine osteosarcoma demonstrating the hypercellularity that may be seen with malignant tumors. Normal bone would exfoliate no cells, whereas an osteosarcoma often yields highly cellular slides.

Inflammatory lesions may have macrophages that are multinucleated (multinucleated inflammatory giant cells) (see Figure 2-11). Osteoclasts are also normally multinucleated (see Figure 2-54). Megakaryocytes, which are commonly present in the spleen as a reflection of extramedullary hematopoiesis, may have multiple nuclear lobes (Figure 2-64) that may sometimes appear to be multiple individual nuclei. Binucleate cells are commonly found in aspirates of epithelial tissue undergoing hyperplasia/regeneration (e.g, hepatic nodular hyperplasia). Also, some benign tumors, such as cutaneous plasmacytomas, may have many binucleated and multinucleated cells (see Figure 2-33).

Abnormal Nuclear-to-Cytoplasmic Ratio: The N:C ratio refers to the relative areas occupied by the nucleus and cytoplasm of the cell. A low N:C ratio indicates a cell with a relatively small nucleus and vast amounts of cytoplasm (Figure 2-65). In contrast cells with minimal amounts of cytoplasm have a very high N:C ratio (Figure 2-66). Epithelial and mesenchymal cells having a high N:C ratio are suggestive of malignancy. A high N:C ratio is a particularly important finding in very large cells because some small cells (e.g., mature lymphocytes, basal epithelial cells) normally have a high N:C ratio. A high N:C ratio in a large cell generally indicates a poorly differentiated cell.

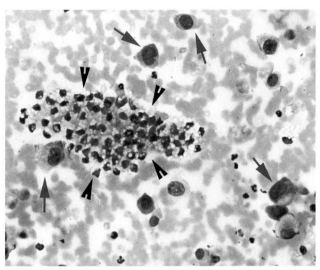

Figure 2-61 Aspirate from a carcinoma in the prostate of a dog. Note that the smaller, uniform cells representing normal prostatic epithelium *(black arrowheads)* are in a tightly cohesive cluster, whereas the larger, neoplastic cells are largely individually oriented due to loss of cellular cohesion *(red arrows)*.

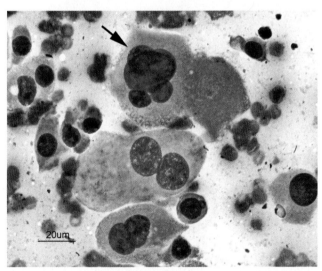

Figure 2-62 Aspirate of a transitional cell carcinoma from a dog. Two binucleate cells are present with equally sized nuclei. However, one multinucleated cell *(arrow)* shows significant variation in nuclear size.

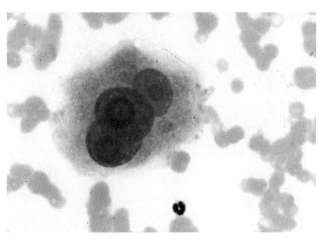

Figure 2-63 A multinucleated cell with an odd number of nuclei. Prominent, large nucleoli of varying size are also present. The erythrocytes and neutrophil can be used for size comparison.

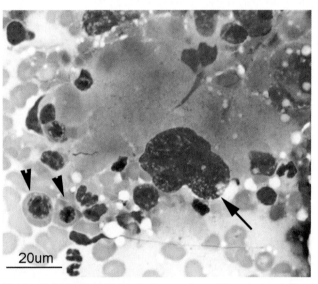

Figure 2-64 Splenic aspirate from a dog with extramedullary hematopoiesis. Two erythroid precursors are present *(arrowheads)*. A single megakaryocyte is present. This large cell has expansive cytoplasm and a single, multilobulated nucleus *(arrow)*.

Marked variation in the N:C ratio of cells within a single population is also abnormal finding (Figure 2-67). Again, there are exceptions. Slides of normal lymphoid tissue and scrapings containing normal squamous cells of varying stages of maturation will demonstrate variation in N:C ratio.

Abnormal Nucleoli: Nucleoli are areas within the nucleus that are responsible for production of RNA. All cells have nucleoli, but they are usually small and often not readily visible. Nucleoli that are large (macronucleoli) that are atypically shaped angular), or that vary in size (anisonucleoliosis) are strong indicators of malignancy. Nucleoli in normal cells are small, approximately 1 to 2 micrometers in diameter. Nucleoli greater than 5

micrometers in diameter are suggestive of malignancy (see Figure 2-66). Erythrocytes can be used as a reference for evaluating the size of nucleoli. Canine erythrocytes are 7 to 8 micrometers, whereas feline erythrocytes are approximately 5 to 6 micrometers in diameter (if well spread out). Normal cells have round nucleoli. Fusiform, pleomorphic, or angular nucleoli are indicative of malignancy (Figure 2-68). Diff-Quik often stains nucleoli more prominently than do other cytologic stains, so this must be considered when evaluating cells for malignant potential. Also, nucleoli may be more prominent than normal in cells that are either ruptured or understained.

Abnormal Mitosis: Mitotic figures are rare in samples from most normal tissue cell populations (except lymphoid tissue and bone marrow). Macrophages can divide

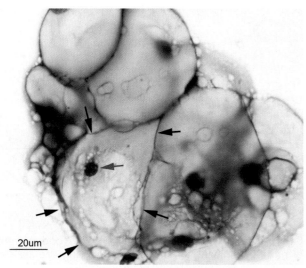

Figure 2-65 Aspirate of mature adipose tissue (lipoma) demonstrates a low nuclear:cytoplasmic ratio. The cells are extremely large *(black arrows outline the cytoplasmic boundaries of a single adipocyte)* yet have very small nuclei *(red arrow).*

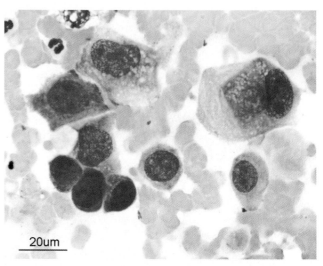

Figure 2-67 Aspirate from a carcinoma. Note the variation in N:C ratio.

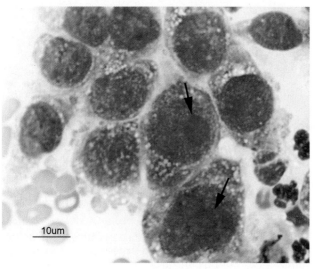

Figure 2-66 Carcinoma from a sample of canine pleural fluid. The neoplastic cells demonstrate a high N:C ratio. Note that the nucleus takes up well over half of the volume of the entire cell. Some cells have only scant amounts of visible cytoplasm. A high N:C ratio is normal in some cells such as lymphocytes and basal epithelial cells, but in large cells such as this, it generally indicates undifferentiated cells. Also note large nucleoli *(arrows).*

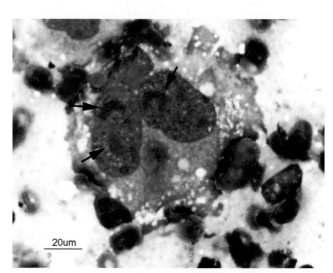

Figure 2-68 Cell from a carcinoma. Note the large, irregularly shaped nucleoli *(arrows).*

in tissues and so mitotic figures are frequently seen in inflammatory responses with numerous macrophages (Figure 2-69). Increased numbers of mitoses or mitotic figures showing abnormal alignment of chromosomes are suggestive of malignancy (Figures 2-70, 2-71, and 2-72).

Coarse or Immature Nuclear Chromatin: Nuclear chromatin patterns are not as distinctive and evident in cells stained with Romanowsky-type stains as they are when cells are wet fixed and stained with Papanicolaou-type stains. Still, an abnormally coarse nuclear chromatin pattern is

often visible in malignant cells. Also, mature cells tend to have nuclear chromatin that is densely or darkly stained.

Abnormal Nuclear Arrangement: Although the majority of tissue architecture is lost when performing a fine-needle aspirate, some cellular structure is still evident in cell clusters. Normal cell clusters tend to have a very uniform arrangement of the nuclei, giving them a honeycomb appearance (Figure 2-73). Because mature cells typically have a lower N:C ratio, the nuclei often appear evenly spaced and not touching each other (see Figure 2-73). In contrast, clusters of neoplastic cells often show irregular arrangement (Figure 2-74). Lack of normal contact inhibition can result in nuclei that are crowded together and piled on top of each other (see Figure 2-74).

Sometimes, the nucleus of one cell can be seen to deform around the nucleus of another cell (or another nucleus within a multinucleated cell). This is referred to as *nuclear molding* and indicates rapid growth and loss of contact inhibition (Figure 2-75).

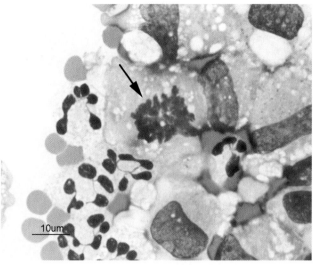

Figure 2-69 Transtracheal wash fluid from a cat. Several neutrophils and macrophages are shown. One macrophage is undergoing mitosis *(arrow)*.

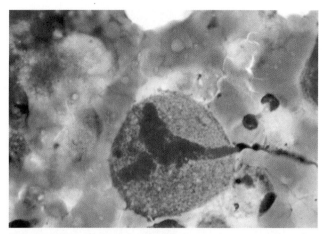

Figure 2-71 Abnormal mitotic figure in a sample of a malignant tumor from a dog. The nuclear material has formed a Y shape rather than forming a straight line.

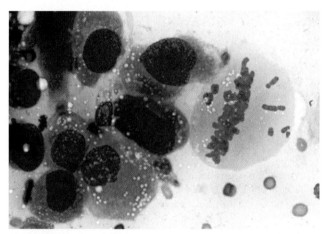

Figure 2-70 Smear from a malignant tumor in the lung of a cat. One abnormal mitotic figure is present, which demonstrates some lagging chromosomes.

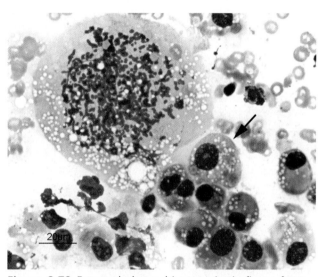

Figure 2-72 Extremely large, bizarre mitotic figure from a spleen aspirate of a dog with malignant histiocytosis. Several other histiocytic cells are present, one of which shows erythrophagocytosis *(arrow)*.

General Cautions Regarding Evaluating Cytologic Criteria of Malignancy

As stated before, there is no single cellular feature that reliably distinguishes malignant from benign cells. A reliable diagnosis of malignancy can usually be made if three or more nuclear criteria of malignancy are present in a majority of the cells present in the smear. If cytologic features of malignancy are not unambiguous, the diagnosis should be confirmed with a biopsy and histologic evaluation. It is imperative that a representative sample (highly cellular) is available and that only intact (nontraumatized), well-spread-out, well-stained cells are evaluated. Nucleoli are often more distinct in understained cells present in thick areas of the smears. When cells are partially ruptured, the nuclear chromatin spreads out and uncoils. This results in the nucleus appearing larger than it really is and also makes nucleoli, normally obscured by the condensed chromatin, more visible.

Also, caution should be used in diagnosing neoplasia in the face of inflammation. Inflammation can induce dysplastic changes in tissue cells that can mimic neoplasia. Inflammatory lesions may also contain large, epithelioid macrophages and proliferating fibroblasts, both of which may have some features that are similar to malignant cells.

Conversely, not every malignant tumor shows marked cellular atypia and variability. Some tumors may yield relatively uniform populations of cells, yet exhibit aggressive biological behavior. This finding is frequently encountered in endocrine tumors. The majority of thyroid tumors in dogs are malignant, yet samples from some thyroid carcinomas contain relatively uniform cells without marked criteria of malignancy. The same situation is described in other tumors of endocrine and neuroendocrine origin. Many other well-differentiated carcinomas (e.g., perianal gland tumors) are difficult to distinguish

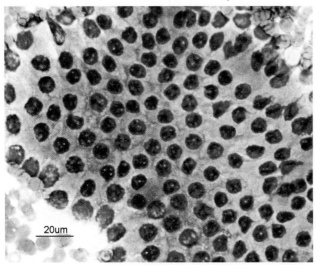

Figure 2-73 Prostatic aspirate from a dog with benign prostatic hyperplasia. The slide consists of mature, well-differentiated prostatic epithelial cells. Note the uniform and even spacing of the nuclei in the center of this cell cluster. The nuclei are round and have densely stained, mature chromatin. Around the edges of the cell cluster, some of the cells have been traumatized, resulting in lighter staining nuclei with irregular outlines.

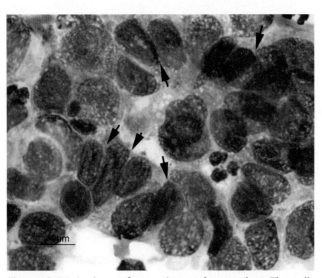

Figure 2-74 Aspirate of a carcinoma from a dog. The cells lack the regular arrangement of benign well-differentiated cells. Nuclei are crowded together and pile on top of each other. The cells have a high N:C ratio and many have prominent nucleoli.

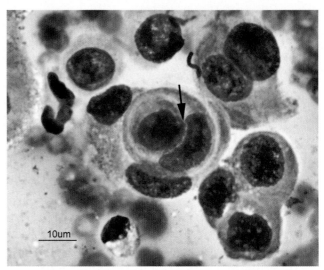

Figure 2-75 Cells from a transitional cell carcinoma from a dog. Nuclear molding is seen in the center where the nucleus of one cell is wrapping around that of another.

from a benign proliferation based solely on cytologic examination. In some cases, this differentiation is also difficult to make on histologic examination. In these cases, experience with the peculiarities of each individual tumor type is helpful in forming a correct interpretation of the sample.

References

1. Raskin RE: General categories of cytologic interpretation. In Raskin RE, Meyer DJ (eds): *Atlas of Canine and Feline Cytology.* Philadelphia, Saunders, 2001, pp 19-33.
2. Lumsden JH, Baker R: Cytopathology techniques and interpretation. In Baker R, Lumsden JH (eds): *Color Atlas of Cytology of the Dog and Cat.* St. Louis, Mosby, 2000, pp 7-20.

Selected Infectious Agents

R.L. Cowell, R.D. Tyler, J.H. Meinkoth, and D. DeNicola

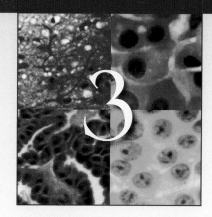

CHAPTER 3

Cytologic evaluation often reveals organisms. Sometimes these organisms are the primary cause of the patient's condition, whereas at other times they are only secondary invaders or normal flora. This chapter is intended to help in recognizing organisms that can be found during cytologic evaluation. Discussions of the conditions that they produce are found in the relevant chapters. Submission of samples for culture is covered in Chapter 1.

IDENTIFICATION OF ORGANISMS

Size, shape, and staining characteristics are important in the cytologic identification of organisms. The remainder of this chapter contains brief descriptions of organisms that can be identified by cytologic analysis and one or more photomicrographs of each organism to aid in their identification. The staining characteristics indicated in this chapter are for Romanowsky-type stains unless otherwise stated.

Bacteria

Staining Characteristics: With the routine Romanowsky-type stains (Wright's, Diff-Quik, Dip-Stat) all bacteria, whether gram-positive or gram-negative, stain blue to purple with a few exceptions such as *Mycobacterium*. The lipid cell wall of *Mycobacterium* spp. prevents uptake of Romanowsky-type stains, causing the organisms to appear as nonstaining small rods.

Gram stains can be used, but it is much more difficult to find bacteria with Gram stains than with Romanowsky-type stains and Gram stains often do not give reproducible, accurate results for bacteria in exudates. Cells, exudative proteins, and bacteria (whether gram-positive or gram-negative) tend to stain red in exudates.

Primary Versus Secondary Infection or Normal Microflora: Intracellular bacteria indicate a bacterial infection (primary or secondary), whereas extracellular bacteria may represent a bacterial infection, normal microflora, or contamination. Bacterial infections often reveal bacteria intracellularly and extracellularly, whereas normal microflora and contamination yields only extracellular bacteria. Also, a monomorphic bacterial population (only one bacterial type present) suggests infection, whereas a pleomorphic population (mixture of rods and cocci or variably sized rods) may be seen with contamination, normal microflora, or a bacterial infection. Pleomorphic bacterial populations may occur with gastrointestinal infections, bite wounds, and foreign bodies.

Bacterial Cocci: Pathogenic bacterial cocci are usually gram positive and of the genera *Staphylococcus, Streptococcus, Peptostreptococcus,* or *Peptococcus* (Figure 3-1). Staphylococci usually occur in clusters of 4 to 12 bacteria, but *Streptococcus, Peptostreptococcus,* and *Peptococcus* spp. tend to occur in short or long chains of organisms. *Staphylococcus* and *Streptococcus* spp. are aerobic, and *Peptostreptococcus* and *Peptococcus* spp. are anaerobic. When cocci are identified in cytologic preparations, aerobic and anaerobic cultures and sensitivity tests should be performed to identify the organism and the optimum antibiotic therapy. Because most cocci are gram-positive, antibiotic therapy effective against gram-positive organisms should be used when it is necessary to start therapy before culture and sensitivity results are received.

Dermatophilus congolensis replicates by transverse and longitudinal division, producing long chains of coccoid bacterial doublets that resemble small, blue railroad tracks (Figure 3-2). It infects the superficial epidermis, causing crusty lesions. Cytologic preparations from the undersurface of scabs from these crusty lesions are most rewarding in demonstrating organisms. The preparations usually contain mature epithelial cells, keratin bars, debris, and organisms. A few neutrophils may also be found.

Small Bacterial Rods: Most small bacterial rods are gram-negative. Some can be recognized as bipolar rods (Figure 3-3). All pathogenic, bipolar bacterial rods are gram-negative. Common small bacterial rods include *Escherichia coli* and *Pasteurella* spp. Infections with bacterial rods are usually associated with a marked neutrophilic inflammatory response. When small bacterial rods are recognized

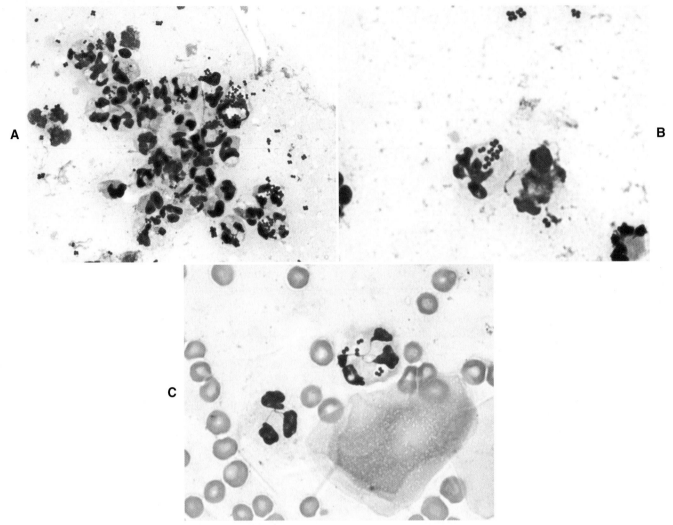

Figure 3-1 A, Neutrophilic inflammation with moderate numbers of bacterial cocci present both intracellularly and extracellularly. (Wright's stain.) **B,** Higher magnification showing a neutrophil containing phagocytized bacterial cocci. (Wright's stain.) **C,** Scattered red blood cells, two neutrophils, and a superficial squamous epithelial cell are shown. One of the neutrophils contains phagocytized bacterial cocci. (Wright's stain.)

in cytologic preparations, the lesion should be cultured to identify the organism, and sensitivity tests should be performed to determine the optimum antibiotic therapy. If it is necessary to institute antibiotic therapy before the culture and sensitivity results are received, the therapy employed should be effective against gram-negative organisms because most pathogenic, small rods are gram-negative.

Filamentous Rods: Pathogenic filamentous rods that cause cutaneous or subcutaneous lesions are usually *Nocardia* or *Actinomyces* spp. Some other anaerobes, such as *Fusobacterium* and *Mycobacterium* spp., may be filamentous, but rarely are. *Nocardia* and *Actinomyces* spp., generally have a distinctive morphology in cytologic preparations stained with Romanowsky-type stains. They are characterized by long, slender (filamentous) strands that stain pale blue and have intermittent small pink or pur-

ple areas (Figure 3-4). This morphology is characteristic of both *Nocardia* and *Actinomyces* spp. and the filamentous form of *Fusobacterium* spp. When these features are recognized cytologically, cultures should be performed specifically for *Nocardia* and *Actinomyces* spp. and for other anaerobes.

On the other hand, *Mycobacterium* spp. often does not stain with Romanowsky-type stains. As a result, negative images (Figure 3-5) may be observed in the cytoplasm of macrophages and/or inflammatory giant cells. When epithelioid macrophages and/or inflammatory giant cells are encountered in cytologic preparations that do not contain any obvious organisms, a careful search for negative images of *Mycobacterium* spp. should be made. *Mycobacterium* spp. stain with acid-fast stains; therefore when negative images are encountered, or when the character of the lesion suggests that *Mycobacterium* spp. be considered, an acid-fast stain can be performed to show the organism

Text continued on p. 52.

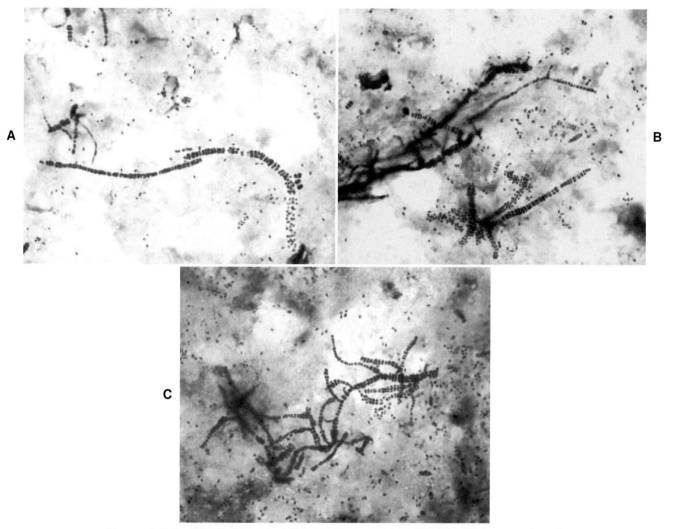

Figure 3-2 A, Skin lesions showing bacterial cocci replicating by transverse and longitudinal division, producing long chains of coccoid bacterial doublets that resemble small, blue railroad tracks. This pattern of bacterial cocci is typical of *Dermatophilus congolensis.* (Wright's stain.) **B,** *D. congolensis* organisms. (Wright's stain.) **C,** Group of *D. congolensis* organisms giving the appearance of railroad tracks. (Wright's stain.)

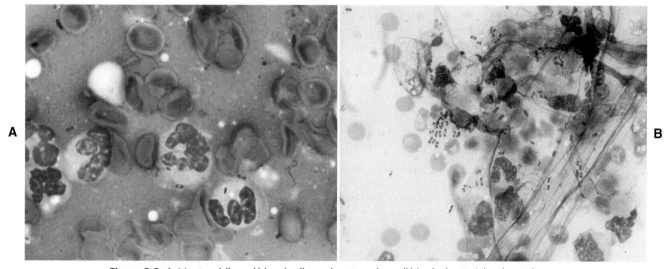

Figure 3-3 A, Neutrophils, red blood cells, and scattered, small bipolar bacterial rods are shown. Whereas all bacteria stain blue-black with Wright's stain, bipolar rods indicate gram-negative bacteria. **B,** Many small bipolar bacterial rods are present extracellularly. (Wright's stain.)

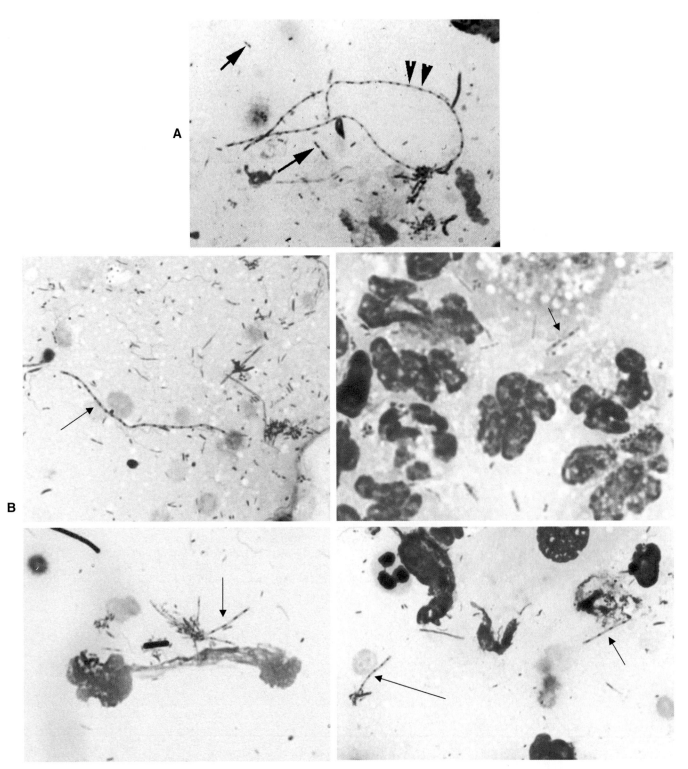

Figure 3-4 A, A long filamentous rod staining pale blue with intermittent small pink or purple dots *(arrowheads)* and smaller filamentous rods *(arrows)* are shown. (Wright's stain). **B,** Composite picture showing filamentous rods *(arrows)* typical of *Actinamyces* or *Nocardia* spp. (Wright's stain.)

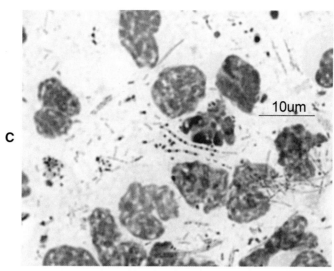

Figure 3-4, cont'd **C,** Multiple filamentous rods and ruptured cells are shown. (Wright's stain.)

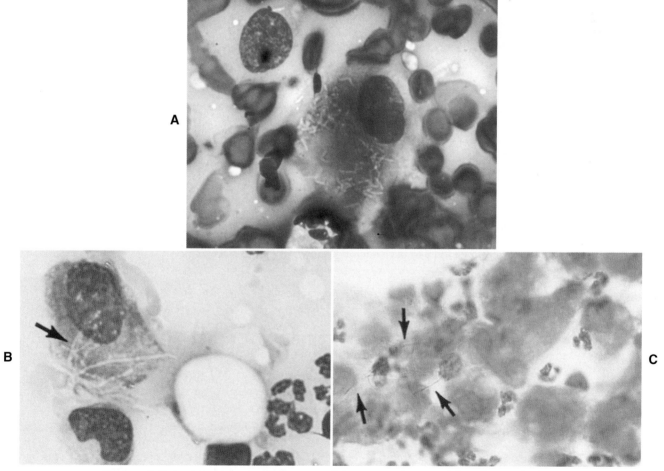

Figure 3-5 A, Large macrophage containing several nonstaining bacterial rods characteristic of *Mycobacterium* spp. (Wright's stain.) **B,** Fine-needle aspirate of a consolidated pulmonary mass. An alveolar macrophage, which contains nonstaining bacterial rods identified as clear streaks through the cell *(arrow),* is indicative of a *Mycobacterium* infection. (Wright's stain.) **C,** Acid-fast stain from the same dog as in **A,** showing reddish filamentous *Mycobacterium* organisms *(arrows).* (Acid-fast stain.)

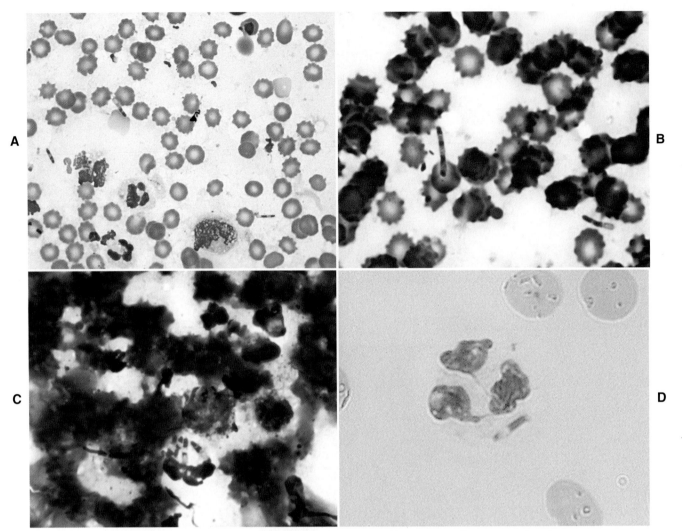

Figure 3-6 A, Scattered inflammatory cells, red blood cells (RBCs), and large spore-forming bacterial rods typical of *Clostridium* spp. are shown. (Wright's stain.) **B,** Higher-power view from same case as in **A.** Scattered RBCs and two large extracellular spore-forming bacterial rods are shown. (Wright's stain.) **C,** Same case as in **A.** Multiple phagocytized spore-forming bacterial rods are shown. (Wright's stain.) **D,** A neutrophil containing a phagocytized spore-forming bacterial rod is shown. (Wright's stain.)

(see Figure 3-5, C), and/or cultures for *Mycobacterium* spp. can be performed for identification.

Because these organisms are often refractory to common antibiotic therapy, and reliable culture has special requirements, cytology is very useful in indicating to the practitioner that special cultures are needed.

Large Bacterial Rods: Large bacterial rods that are pathogenic and sometimes infect the cutaneous and subcutaneous tissues include *Clostridia* spp., and infrequently, *Bacillus* spp. When large bacterial rods are thought to be pathogenic, both aerobic and anaerobic cultures should be performed. Also, the smears should be inspected for large rods containing spores (Figure 3-6). If spore formation is observed, *Clostridium* spp. is most likely present.

Occasionally, the extremely large nonpathogenic bacterial rods of *Simonsiella* spp. are observed in cytologic specimens (e.g., contaminated tracheal washes). *Simonsiella* spp. are bacteria that divide lengthwise, therefore yielding parallel rows of bacteria that give the impression of a single, large bacterium (Figure 3-7).

Yeast, Dermatophytes, Hyphating Fungi, and Algae

General Comments: Mycotic agents produce lesions that tend to have more macrophages present than do bacterial lesions. However, neutrophils may still be the predominant cell type, and eosinophils may be plentiful with certain hyphating fungi. Mycotic lesions often contain low numbers of lymphocytes, plasma cells, and fibroblasts. Mycotic agents tend to be phagocytized by macrophages, but may also be found in granulocytes. The infectious agent, the location of the lesion, the

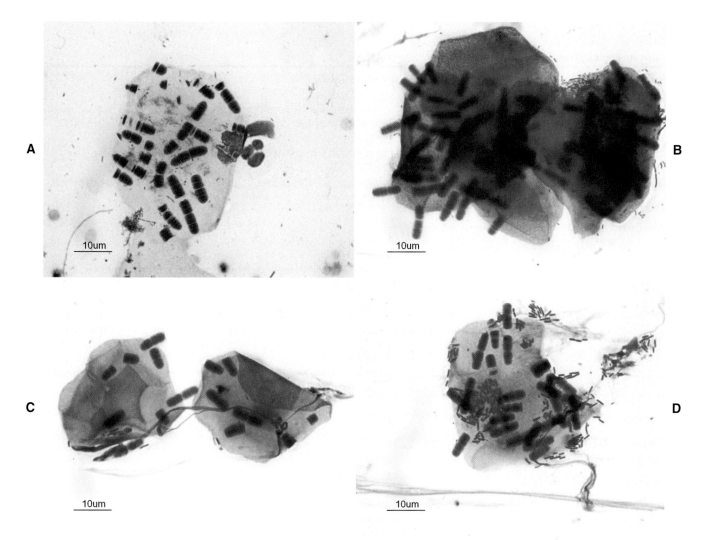

Figure 3-7 A, Superficial squamous epithelial cell with adherent bacteria. *Simonsiella* organisms are large striated rodlike organisms. Other bacteria are present, adhered to the squamous cell and free in the background of the smear. (Wright's stain.) **B,** Two superficial squamous epithelial cells with many *Simonsiella* organisms. (Wright's stain.) **C,** Two superficial squamous epithelial cells with many *Simonsiella* organisms. (Wright's stain.) **D,** One superficial squamous epithelial cell with many *Simonsiella* organisms and bacterial rods. (Wright's stain.)

chronicity of the lesion, and the immune status of the animal all influence the character of the lesion. A comparison of the common fungi that form only yeasts in tissues is presented in Table 3-1.

Sporothrix schenckii: A *Sporothrix schenckii* infection *(sporotrichosis)* can cause raised proliferative lesions that are often ulcerated on the skin of dogs and cats. In cats, many organisms are produced, and cytologic evaluation leads to an easy diagnosis. In dogs, however, organisms are scarce, and cytologic preparations must be carefully screened. If organisms are not found, the lesion should be cultured or a biopsy of the lesion should be submitted for histopathologic evaluation.

In cytologic preparations stained with Romanowsky-type stains, *S. schenckii* (Figure 3-8) are round to oval or

fusiform (cigar-shaped). They are about 3 to 9 microns long and 1 to 3 microns wide and stain pale to medium blue with a slightly eccentric pink or purple nucleus. They may be confused with *Histoplasma capsulatum* if only a few organisms are found and they are not classically fusiform.

Histoplasma capsulatum: Although *H. capsulatum* usually infects the lungs and/or other internal organs, it can infect the skin, with or without concurrent involvement of internal organs. Cutaneous histoplasmosis lesions are typically raised and proliferative and may ulcerate. On rare occasions, they may produce draining tracts. These lesions usually yield many organisms within macrophages and some extracellular organisms. A few organisms may be found in neutrophils. In cytologic preparations stained

TABLE 3-1

Common Fungi That Form Yeasts in Tissue

Yeast	Distinguishing Characteristics
Small Yeasts	
Sporothrix spp.	Round to oval to fusiform (cigar-shaped) organisms that are about 3-9 microns long and 1-3 microns wide, and stain pale to medium blue with a slightly eccentric pink or purple nucleus.
Histoplasma spp.	Round to oval but not fusiform; yeasts are about 2-4 microns in diameter (one fourth to one half the size of an RBC), and stain pale to medium blue with an eccentric pink-to-purple staining nucleus that is often crescent shaped. There is usually a thin, clear halo around the yeast.
Medium-sized Yeasts	
Blastomyces spp.	Organisms are blue, spherical yeasts that are about 8-20 microns in diameter and thick-walled. Occasional organisms showing broad-based budding are found. *Blastomyces* organisms are differentiated from *Cryptococcus neoformans* by their color, lack of a clear-staining capsule, and broad-based budding. They are distinguished from *Coccidioides immitis* by their smaller size and lack of endospores.
Cryptococcus spp.	Extremely pleomorphic yeast that ranges from spherical to fusiform shape, has a smooth (encapsulated) and rough (nonencapsulated) form, and is about 4-15 microns in diameter (not including the capsule). The yeast stains pink to blue-purple and may be slightly granular. *Cryptococcus* spp. demonstrate narrow-based budding. The smooth form usually is easily recognized because of its thick mucoid capsule, which usually is clear and homogenous.
Large Yeasts	
Coccidioides spp.	These organisms are scarce in many cytology specimens; therefore cytologic preparations from suspected coccidioidomycosis lesions should be examined carefully. When present, the organisms are large (10-100 microns in diameter), double-contoured, blue or clear spheres with finely granular protoplasm, and will often appear folded or crumpled. Round endospores from 2-5 microns in diameter may be seen in some of the larger organisms. The tremendous variation in the size and presence of endospores differentiates *Coccidioides immitis* from nonbudding *Blastomyces dermatitidis*.

with Romanowsky-type stains, *Histoplasma* organisms (Figure 3-9) are round or slightly oval, but are not fusiform. They are about 2 to 4 microns in diameter (one fourth to one half the size of a red blood cell), stain pale to medium blue, and contain an eccentric pink-to-purple staining nucleus that is often crescent shaped. There is usually a clear halo around the yeast.

Blastomyces dermatitidis: A *Blastomyces dermatitidis* infection *(blastomycosis)* can involve the skin, eyes, and internal organs. Cutaneous lesions of blastomycosis are usually raised and proliferative, and often ulcerate. Cutaneous lesions should be sought when any form of blastomycosis is suspected. Aspirates from these lesions or impression smears of ulcerated lesions usually have a cell composition characteristic of pyogranulomatous inflammation and organisms ranging in number from a few to many. In cytologic preparations stained with Romanowsky-type stains, the organisms (Figure 3-10) are blue, spherical, 8 to 20 microns in diameter, and thick-walled. Most organisms are single, but occasionally,

organisms showing broad-based budding are found. These organisms are distinctly larger than *S. schenckii* or *H. capsulatum* and are differentiated from *Cryptococcus neoformans* by their color, lack of a clear-staining capsule, and broad-based budding. They are distinguished from *Coccidioides immitis* by their smaller size and lack of endospores.

Cryptococcus neoformans: A *Cryptococcus neoformans* infection (cryptococcosis) can involve the subcutaneous tissues causing subcutaneous swellings, but more commonly involves the upper respiratory and central nervous systems. Cryptococcosis usually elicits a granulomatous response (epithelioid macrophages and/or inflammatory giant cells). In some cytologic preparations, *Cryptococcus* organisms may outnumber inflammatory cells and tissue cells. The organism (Figure 3-11) is extremely pleomorphic, ranging from spherical to fusiform, but usually is easily recognized because of its thick mucoid capsule. Occasionally, nonencapsulated, or rough, forms are found. The organism is about 4 to 15 microns in diameter

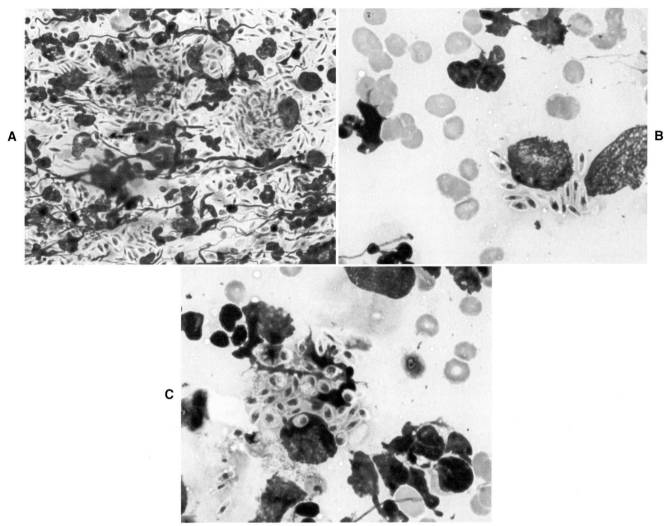

Figure 3-8 A, Scraping from a skin lesion in a cat. Pyogranulomatous inflammation and high numbers of sporotrichosis organisms are present in the smear. (Wright's stain.) **B,** A ruptured macrophage containing many fusiform sporotrichosis organisms. (Wright's stain.) **C,** Macrophage containing round, oval, and fusiform sporotrichosis organisms. (Wright's stain.)

without its capsule and about 8 to 40 microns in diameter with its capsule. In cytologic preparations stained with Romanowsky-type stains, the organism stains pink to blue-purple and may be slightly granular. The capsule is usually clear and homogenous, but on some occasions, it may stain light to medium pink. Unlike *Blastomyces* spp., *Cryptococcus* spp. demonstrates narrow-based budding. Although India ink is often proposed as an aid in identifying *C. neoformans*, air bubbles and fat globules can be mistaken for organisms, particularly by inexperienced microscopists.

Coccidioides immitis: *Coccidioides immitis* infections generally involve the lungs and bones of dogs. In some cases, however, cutaneous lesions (masses) and draining tracts from bony lesions develop. Cytologic preparations usually have a cell composition characteristic of pyogranulomatous or granulomatous inflammation. *Coccidioides* organisms (Figure 3-12) may be scarce in some

lesions; therefore cytologic preparations from suspected coccidioidomycosis lesions should be examined carefully. In cytologic preparations stained with Romanowsky-type stains, the organisms are large (10 to 100 microns in diameter), double-contoured, blue or clear spheres with finely granular protoplasm and will often appear folded or crumpled. Round endospores from 2 to 5 microns in diameter may be seen in some of the larger organisms. The tremendous variation in the size and presence of endospores differentiates *C. immitis* from nonbudding *B. dermatitidis*.

Malassezia spp.: *Malassezia canis*, also called *Malassezia pachydermatis*, *Pityrosporum canis*, and *Pityrosporum pachydermatis*, is a broad-based, budding, gram-positive, nonmycelioid yeast, typically peanut-shaped, but may be globose or ellipsoidal (Figure 3-13). It is a common problem in the ear canal, and occasionally *Malassezia dermatitis* occurs on the skin.

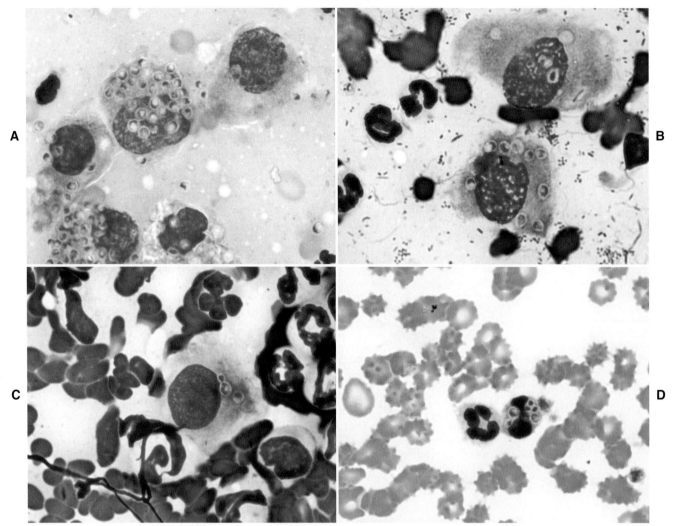

Figure 3-9 A, Lung aspirate showing macrophages containing high numbers of *Histoplasma* organisms. (Wright's stain.) **B,** Scraping from an ulcerated mass in the mouth of a cat. High numbers of mixed bacteria, blood, pyogranulomatous inflammation, and many *Histoplasma* organisms are shown. (Wright's stain.) **C,** Pyogranulomatous inflammation and a macrophage containing a budding *Histoplasma* organism and a round nonbudding *Histoplasma* organism. (Wright's stain.) **D,** Peripheral blood from a dog with disseminated histoplasmosis. A neutrophil containing several *Histoplasma* organisms, including a budding *Histoplasma* organism, is shown. (Wright's stain.)

Dermatophytes: The dermatophytes *Microsporum* and *Trichophyton* spp. commonly cause ringworm in dogs and cats. Scrapings from the edge of lesions are the best cytologic samples for finding dermatophytes. They can be identified in cytologic preparations using the standard 10% potassium hydroxide stain for hair, in wet-mount preparations stained with new methylene blue, or air-dried preparations stained with Romanowsky-type stains. Cytologically, fungal mycelia and spores are found adhered to the surface of epithelial cells and free in the background of the smear, as well as within hair shafts (*Trichophyton* spp.) or on the hair shaft surface (*Microsporum* spp.). With Romanowsky-type stains, the mycelia and spores stain medium to dark blue with a thin, clear halo (Figure 3-14). An inflammatory reaction of an admixture of neutrophils, macrophages,

lymphocytes, and plasma cells may be seen in cytologic preparations from skin scrapings.

Rhinosporidium seeberi: Rhinosporidiosis in dogs is characterized by polypoid nasal growths. The fungal organism, *Rhinosporidium seeberi*, is diagnosed by finding round to oval, approximately 7-μm-diameter spores in nasal exudates or tissue imprints. The spores stain bright pink, have internal eosinophilic globules, and are surrounded by thin bilamellar cell walls (Figure 3-15). Finding large sporangia containing numerous endospores supports the diagnosis; however, these structures are infrequently seen.

Pneumocystis carinii: This opportunistic fungal pulmonary pathogen may be observed in either cyst (5 to 10 μm

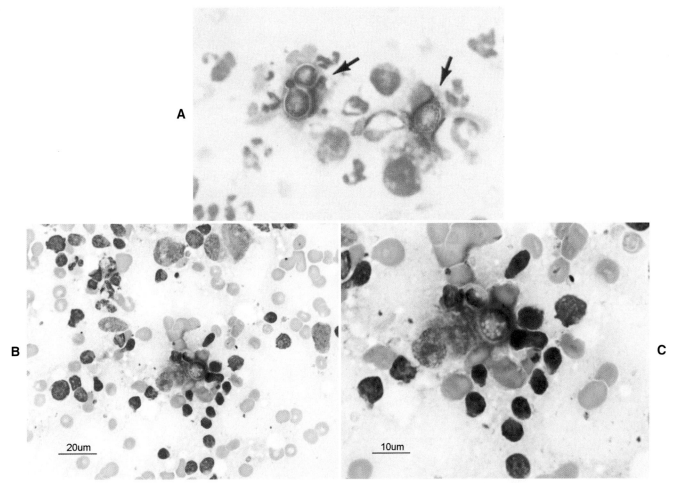

Figure 3-10 A, *Blastomyces dermatitidis* is a bluish, spherical, thick-walled, yeast-like organism in Romanowsky-stained smears *(arrows.)* The organisms are about 8 to 20 μm in diameter. Occasionally, a single broad-based bud may be present. (Wright's stain.) **B,** A budding *Blastomyces* organism in a lymph node aspirate is shown. (Wright's stain.) **C,** Higher-power, magnification of **B**. (Wright's stain.)

diameter that may contain up to eight intracystic bodies) or troph form (1 to 2 μm). With Romanowsky-stains, intact cysts are distinctive in appearance (Figure 3-16), but the free troph form is difficult to differentiate from debris. Cytologically, *Pneumocystis* organisms may appear morphologically similar to a protozoal organism.

Fungi That Form Hyphae in Tissues: Many different fungi can infect the cutaneous and subcutaneous tissues or internal organs and form hyphae (Figure 3-17). With cutaneous lesions, these fungi usually cause small to large raised, proliferative lesions that often ulcerate. They often induce a granulomatous, inflammatory response that is charactcrized by epithelioid macrophages and inflammatory giant cells. The number of neutrophils, lymphocytes, plasma cells, and eosinophils varies. Some hyphating fungi do not stain well with hematologic-type stains and are recognized as negative images (Figure 3-18). The organisms that cause the disease phycomycosis typically do not stain with hematologic stains and induce an eosinophilic, granulomatous response in the infected tissue. A fungal culture or histopathology with special immunohisto-chemical stains may be used to definitively classify the organism involved.

Algae: *Prototheca* spp. (*P. zopfii* and *P. wickerhami*) are colorless algae that are ubiquitous in the southern regions of America, but only rarely cause disease (i.e., protothecosis). In dogs, the disease is often disseminated, but only cutaneous protothecosis has been reported in cats. Cytologic preparations reveal an inflammatory response characteristic of pyogranulomatous or granulomatous inflammation and organisms ranging in number from a few to many. The organisms (Figure 3-19) are round to oval and are from 1 to 14 microns wide and 1 to 16 microns long. When stained with Romanowsky-type stains, they have granular basophilic cytoplasm and a clear cell wall about 0.5 micron thick The organisms, except those that are small and immature, contain a small nucleus that stains pink to deep purple. A single organism may consist of 2 or 4 or more endospores. Most organisms are extracellular, but small forms may be found in macrophages and neutrophils.

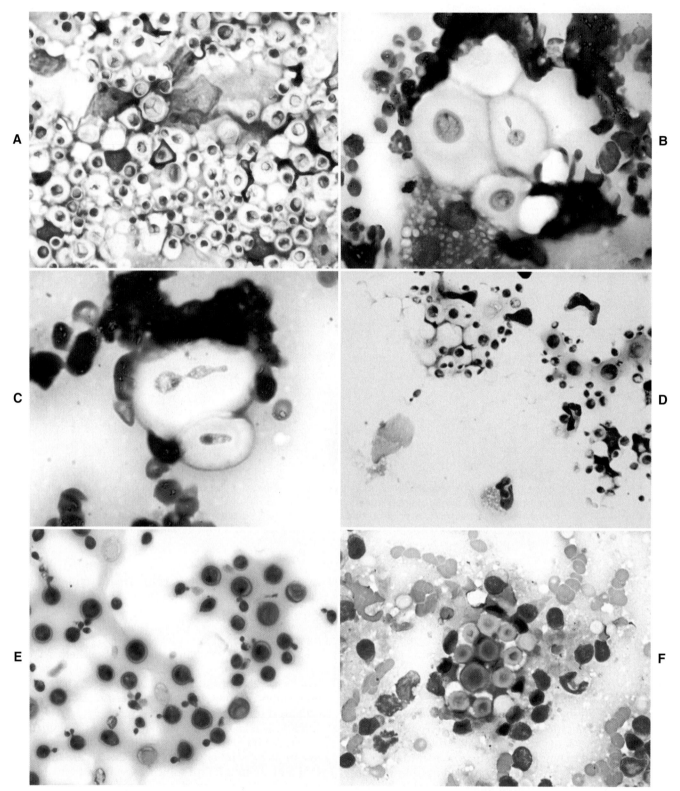

Figure 3-11 A, Low-power view of high numbers of *Cryptococcus* organisms characterized by medium-sized yeasts with clear capsules. Note the lack of an inflammatory response. (Wright's stain.) **B,** *Cryptococcus* organisms with large clear capsules and narrow-based budding. (Wright's stain.) **C,** Two *Cryptococcus* organisms showing narrow-based budding. (Wright's stain.) **D,** *Cryptococcus* organisms found in cerebrospinal fluid. (Wright's stain.) **E,** Higher-power magnification from same case as shown in **D.** (Wright's stain.) **F,** Lymph node aspirate showing a group of *Cryptococcus* organisms, scattered lymphocytes, a single neutrophil, and scattered red blood cells. (Wright's stain.)

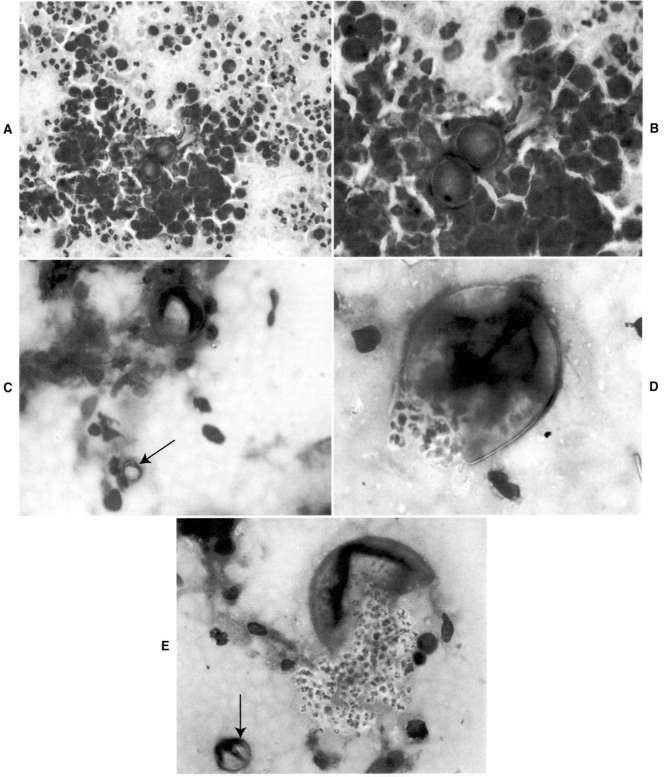

Figure 3-12 A, Low-power view showing pyogranulomatous inflammation and two large *Coccidioides immitis* organisms. These organisms are differentiated from *Blastomyes* organisms by their large size and production of endospores. (Wright's stain.) **B,** Higher-power magnification of same organisms as shown in **A.** (Wright's stain.) **C,** Two *C. immitis* organisms *(arrows)* showing the marked variation in size that can occur with the organisms. (Wright's stain.) **D,** Large *C. immitis* organism with endospores. (Wright's stain.) **E,** Large *C. immitis* organism with endospores that has ruptured, releasing the endospores. Also, a small *C. immitis* organism *(arrow)* is present. (Wright's stain.)

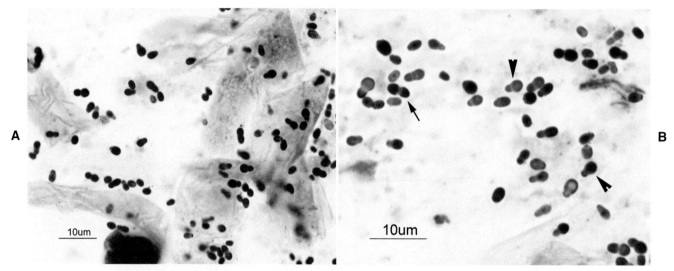

Figure 3-13 A, Canine ear swab showing numerous *Malassezia canis* organisms (*Malassezia* overgrowth) adhered to cornified epithelial cells and free in the background. **B,** Individual *Malassezia* organisms are spherical, but broad-based budding produces figure-8 *(arrow)* and snowman *(arrowheads)* shapes.

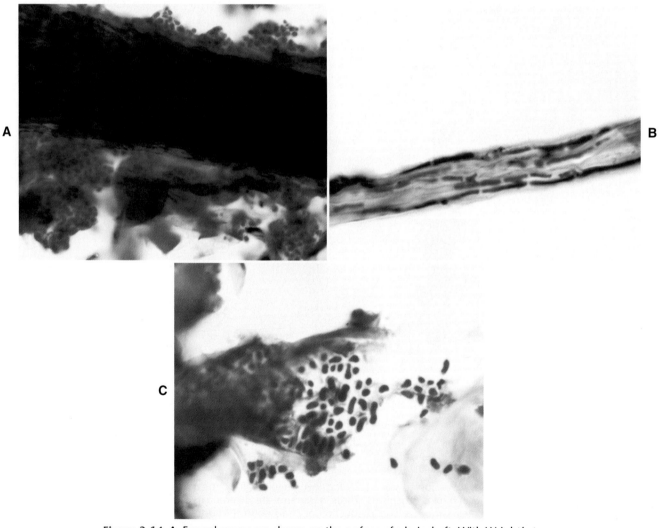

Figure 3-14 A, Fungal spores are shown on the surface of a hair shaft. With Wright's-type stains, the mycelia and spores stain medium to dark blue with a thin, clear halo. (Wright's stain.) **B,** Fungal mycelia and spores are shown on a hair shaft. (Wright's stain.) **C,** Fungal mycelia and spores are found adhered to the surface of epithelial cells and free in the background of the smear. (Wright's stain.)

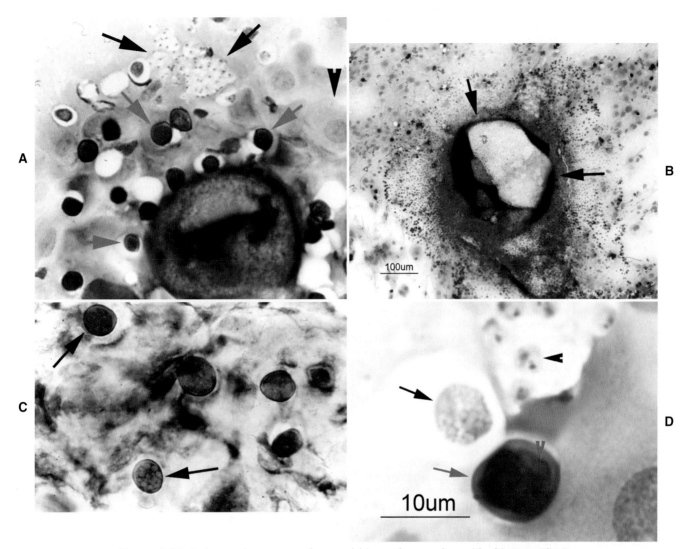

Figure 3-15 A, Impression smear of a nasal biopsy from a dog with rhinosporidiosis. Three distinct forms of the organism can be seen along with nasal epithelial cells *(black arrowhead).* The large circular structure at the bottom is a relatively small sporangium. Surrounding this are numerous spores/endospores *(blue arrows),* which stain dark when not well spread out but pink to pink-purple when well spread out. Also present are small immature spores/endospores *(black arrows).* (Wright's stain.) **B,** Low-magnification image showing a large, ruptured sporangium surrounded by hundreds of developing spores/endospores *(arrows).* (Wright's stain.) **C,** Canine rhinosporidiosis. Numerous well-spread-out spores/endospores are present among cellular debris *(arrows).* (Wright's stain.) **D,** Higher magnification of a mature spore/endospore *(blue arrow)* demonstrating thick cell wall and eosinophilic globular bodies *(blue arrowhead).* Also present are immature spores/endospores *(black arrowhead)* as well as an intermediate form *(black arrow).* (Wright's stain.)

Continued.

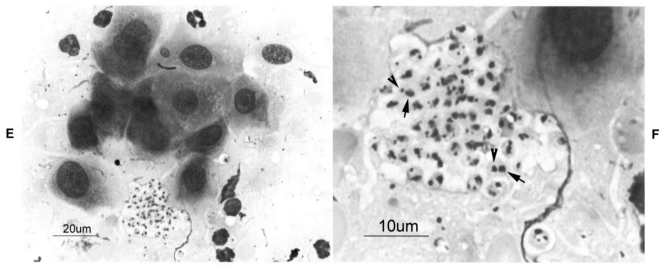

E

F

Figure 3-15, cont'd E, Immature spores/endospores of *Rhinosporidium seeberi*. Low-magnification image showing numerous epithelial cells with a cluster of immature spores/endosperes near the bottom of the image. (Wright's stain.) **F,** Higher magnification from same field as shown in **E** shows details of the immature spores/endospores. They are spherical, lightly basophilic structures that contain purple areas thought to be nuclear material *(arrows)* and one or more darker blue spherical structures *(arrowheads)*. (Wright's stain.)

Protozoa

Leishmania spp.: *Leishmania donovani* can infect the skin and subcutaneous tissues of the dog, producing small to large thickened, ulcerated areas. Imprints, scrapings, and aspirates yield numerous cells, which are an admixture of neutrophils, macrophages, lymphocytes, and plasma cells, with neutrophils or macrophages generally predominating. Usually, numerous organisms are found within macrophages and free in the preparation. *Leishmania* organisms are small (2 to 4 microns) and oval (Figure 3-20). They have an oval, light purple nucleus and a small, dark purple, rod-shaped kinetoplast. The position of the kinetoplast with respect to the nucleus is variable; however, the kinetoplast tends to be located between the nucleus and greatest volume of cytoplasm. The presence of a kinetoplast distinguishes this organism from *Toxoplasma* spp. and small, fungal yeasts, such as *Histoplasma* spp.

Toxoplasma gondii: *Toxoplasma gondii* is a coccidial organism that is found in contaminated water, soil, and other substances. It causes toxoplasmosis, which can affect most mammals, including dogs and humans, but most often affects unborn kittens and cats with compromised immune systems. Although it is uncommon for infection to lead to serious clinical disease, toxoplasmosis can result in damage to the eye. In addition, it can cause gastrointestinal, respiratory, and neurologic disorders that may be fatal. In cats *T. gondii* infection is common, although disease caused by *T. gondii* is uncommon. In general, around 50% of all cats are believed to have been infected with this organism at some point in their lives, although the prevalence of infection varies according to the cat's lifestyle.

T. gondii may be found in tissue or fluid samples from animals with toxoplasmosis. Tachyzoites are spindle- to crescent-shaped, 2 to 4 μ in length, with light blue cytoplasm and red-purple nuclei (Figure 3-21). Tachyzoites of *T. gondii* and *Neosporum caninum* cannot be distinguished cytologically. Polymerase chain reaction is the most reliable method for definitively identifying these organisms.

Neospora spp. (Neosporum caninum): *Neosporum caninum* is a coccidian parasite very similar to *T. gondii*. Infection, in the dog, is usually congenital and often lethal. Ocular lesions, (e.g., chorioretinitis, uveitis, and myositis) may occur. Tachyzoites of *N. caninum*, which may be found in tissue or fluid samples, have the same cytologic appearance as *T. gondii* tachyzoites. PCR is the most reliable method for definitively differentiating these organisms.

Cytauxzoon felis: Cytauxzoonosis is a commonly fatal disease of cats caused by the protozoan parasite *Cytauxzoon felis*. In tissues, developing merozoites may be seen in macrophages. The macrophages are typically large with visible nucleoli and contain either small, dark-staining bodies or larger irregularly defined clusters of developing merozoites of *Cytauxzoon* (Figure 3-22). The macrophages may contain other cellular and phagocytic debris also. It is important not to confuse these macrophages with neoplastic cells. Red blood cells in the background of the smear may contain *Cytauxzoon* organisms appearing as signet-rings.

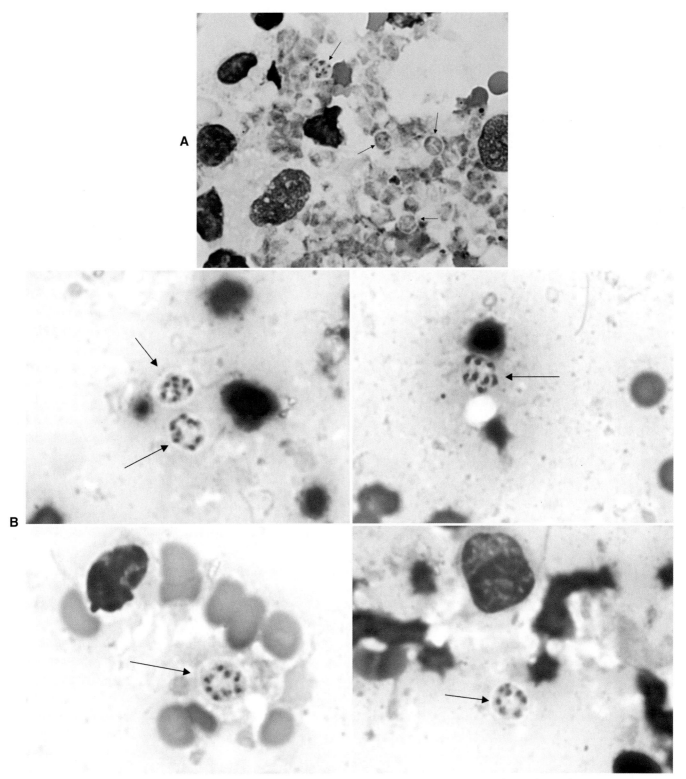

Figure 3-16 A, Transtracheal wash from a dog with pneumocystosis. High numbers of *Pneumocystis carinii* cysts *(arrows)* are present. *Pneumocystis carinii* cysts are 5 to 10 microns in diameter and usually contain four to eight intracystic bodies that are 1 to 2 microns in diameter. (Wright's stain.) **B,** Composite showing *P. carinii* cysts *(arrows).* (Wright's stain.)

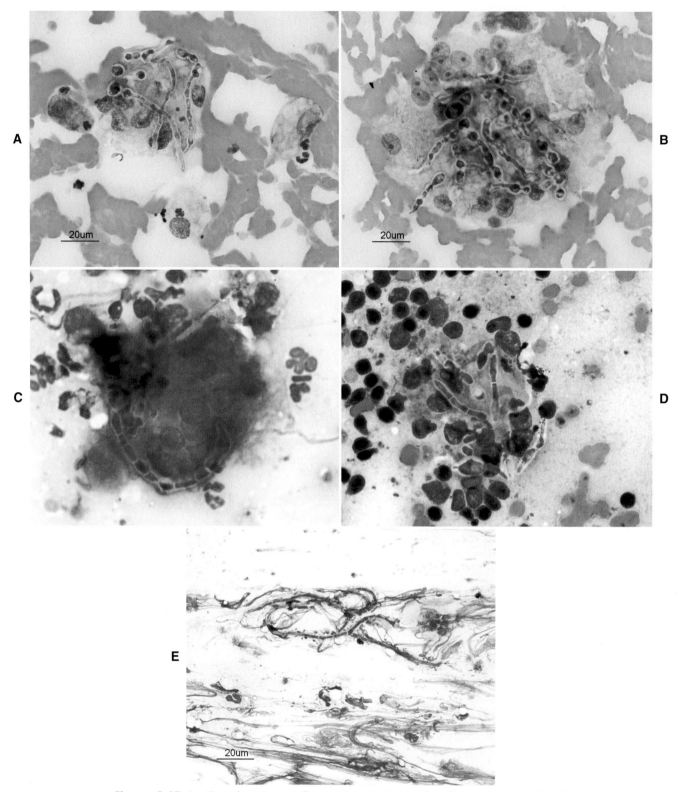

Figure 3-17 A, Granulomatous inflammation, red blood cells, and a giant cell (macrophage) containing several fungal hyphae are shown. (Wright's stain.) **B,** Multinucleated inflammatory giant cell containing several fungal hyphae. (Wright's stain.) **C,** Pyogranulomatous inflammation and a giant cell containing fungal hyphae. (Wright's stain.) **D,** Lymph node aspirate. High numbers of lymphocytes and a group of macrophages containing several fungal hyphae are shown. (Wright's stain.) **E,** Nasal swab showing strands of DNA from ruptured cells and a fungal hyphae. (Wright's stain.)

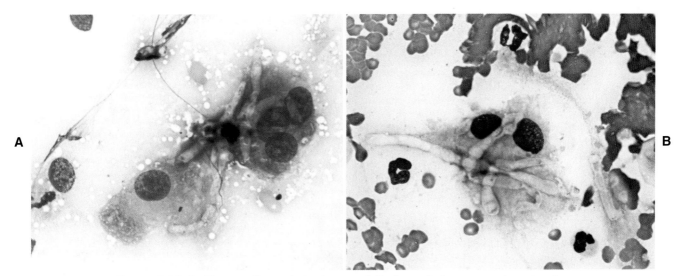

Figure 3-18 A, Fine-needle aspirate from a lytic bone lesion on a dog showing granulomatous inflammation and negative images of fungal hyphae. (Wright's stain.) **B,** Fine-needle aspirate from a mass in the nose of a cat showing negative images of fungal hyphae within macrophages and free in the background of the smear. (Wright's stain.)

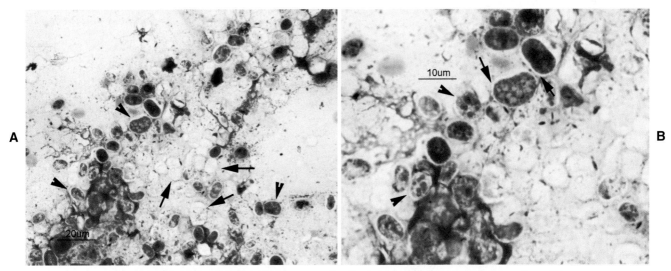

Figure 3-19 A, Ocular (fluid from areas of retinal separation) aspirate from a dog with prototothecosis. Numerous round to oval organisms are present *(arrowheads)* as well as clear, negatively staining areas representing empty casings of ruptured organisms *(arrows).* (Wright's stain.) **B,** Higher magnification of same slide as **A,** shows numerous round to oval organisms, many of which contain endospores *(arrowheads).* A thin, clear cell wall can be seen surrounding most organisms *(arrows).* (Wright's stain.)

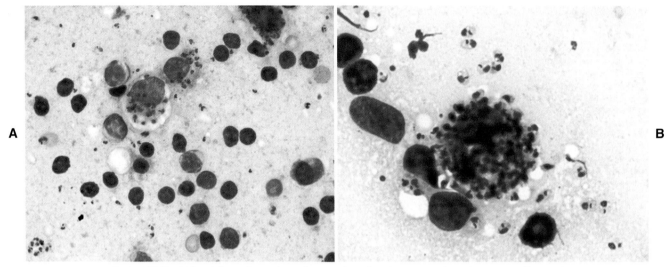

Figure 3-20 A, Lymph node aspirate from a dog showing many lymphocytes, a few red blood cells, and macrophages. *Leishmania* organisms are present within the macrophages and in the background of the smear. (Wright's stain.). **B,** Higher magnification showing *Leishmania* organisms in a macrophage and free in the background of the smear. (Wright's stain.)

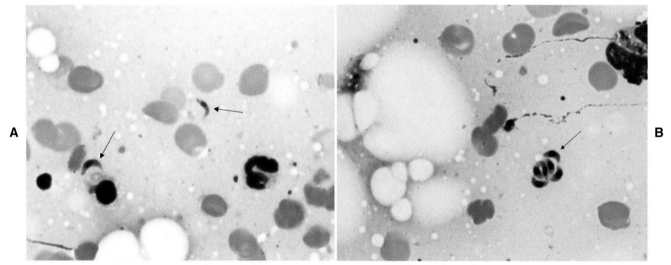

Figure 3-21 A, Bronchoalveolar lavage (BAL) from a cat showing two small crescent-shaped bodies with light blue cytoplasm and dark-staining pericentral nucleus typical of *Toxoplasma* tachyzoites *(arrows).* (Wright's stain.) **B,** A group of Toxoplasma tachyzoites *(arrow)* in a BAL. (Wright's stain.)

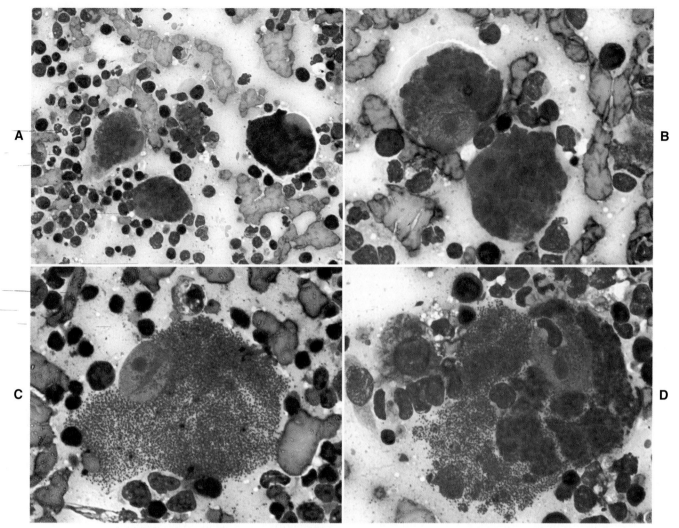

Figure 3-22 A, Lymph node aspirate from a cat with cytauxzoonosis. Many lymphocytes, red blood cells, scattered neutrophils, and three macrophages containing developing merozoites of *Cytauxzoon* are shown. (Wright's stain.) **B,** Same case as **A.** Two macrophages with large prominent nucleoli are shown. Both macrophages contain intracytoplasmic irregularly defined clusters of developing *Cytauxzoon* organisms. (Wright's stain.) **C,** Same case as **A.** A single macrophage containing high numbers of small, dark-staining bodies of *Cytauxzoon* merozoites. (Wright's stain.) **D,** Same case as **A.** A macrophage containing a mixture of irregularly defined clusters and small, more-defined, dark-staining bodies of *Cytauxzoon* merozoites. (Wright's stain.)

Selected References

1. Bottles K, et al: Fine needle aspiration biopsy: Has its time come? *Am J Med* 81:525-531, 1986.
2. Easley JR, et al: Nasal rhinosporidiosis in the dog. *Vet Pathol* 23:50-56, 1986.
3. Dubey JP, Lappin MR: Toxoplasmosis and neosporosis. In Greene CE (ed): *Infectious Diseases of the Dog and Cat*, ed 2. Philadelphia, Saunders, 1998, pp 493-503.
4. Foil CS: Miscellaneous fungal infections. In Greene CE (ed): *Infectious Diseases of the Dog and Cat*. Philadelphia, Saunders, 1990, pp 731-741.
5. Kline TA, Neal HS, Holroyde CP: Needle aspiration biopsy: Diagnosis of subcutaneous nodules and lymph nodes. *JAMA* 235:2626, 2848-2849, 1976.
6. Lappin MR, et al: Primary and secondary *Toxoplasma gondii* infection in normal and feline immunodeficiency virus–infected cats. *J Parasitol* 82:733-742, 1996.
7. Mosier DA, Creed JE: Rhinosporidiosis in a dog. *J Am Vet Med Assoc* 185:1009-1010, 1984.
8. McCully RM, et al: Canine *Pneumocystis pneumonia*. *J South Afr Vet Assoc* 50:207-213, 1979.
9. Rebar AH: Diagnostic cytology in veterinary practice. *Proceedings of the 54th Annual Meeting of the AAHA,* 1987, pp 498-504. In Kirk RW (ed): *Current Veterinary Therapy VII.* Philadelphia, Saunders, 1980, pp 16-27.
10. Rebhar AH:
11. Seybold I, Goldston RT, Wikes RD: Exfoliative cytology. *Vet Med Small Anim Clin* 77:1029-1033, 1982.

Round Cells

D. DeNicola

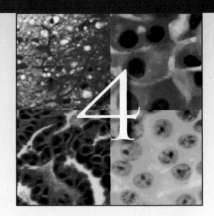

CHAPTER 4

The category of discrete round cell neoplasms is composed primarily of cells of the hemolymphatic system. The title of these types of neoplastic conditions is highly descriptive of the cytomorphologic presentation. Neoplastic cells in this category are typically discrete in nature and round in shape; however, the round shape of these cells is not distinguishing. There are many other neoplastic processes where the neoplastic cells are predominantly round in shape. Most epithelial neoplastic processes and many of the more poorly differentiated mesenchymal neoplastic processes consist of round to oval shaped cells. Even few well-differentiated mesenchymal neoplastic processes, namely, osteoblastic osteosarcoma and chondrosarcoma, may be round to oval in shape.

The distinguishing morphologic feature of the discrete round cell neoplasms is the discrete nature of the neoplastic processes. Because there are no cellular junctions connecting individual neoplastic cells as with epithelial neoplasms, this becomes a highly distinguishing feature. With mesenchymal neoplasms with round to oval cells, there is often an extracellular matrix material produced by the neoplastic cells that sometimes causes loosely packed groupings of cells that resembles cohesion between cells. This apparent grouping is not typically seen with discrete round cell neoplasms.

General comments on the cytomorphologic features, tissue distribution, and biological behavior of discrete round cell neoplasms are outlined next:

Cell Shape – As was noted above, these cells are typically round to oval in shape; however, an amoeboid or irregular shape may be seen particularly with cells of histiocytic lineage.

Nuclear Shape – Cell nuclei of discrete round cell neoplasias are generally round to slightly oval; however, irregularly shaped nuclei are often present within the histiocytic group of discrete round cell neoplasms.

Cytoplasmic Characteristics – The cytoplasmic features of the various discrete round cell neoplasms are among the most important morphologic features used to differentiate one from the other. The presence or absence

of cytoplasmic vacuoles, the presence or absence of cytoplasmic granules, and the color and distribution of cytoplasmic granules prove extremely helpful in making a definitive diagnosis.

Tissue Distribution – Discrete round cell neoplasms can be found essentially in any anatomic location including both cutaneous and visceral tissue distributions. Some have relatively consistent locations of origin, which will be discussed later with each neoplasm type, and other chapters will highlight various visceral locations for discrete round cell neoplasms.

Biological Behavior – Discrete round cell neoplasms have dramatically variable biological behaviors. In many instances, although cytomorphologic atypia may be seen, these morphologic features often do not prove helpful in predicting potential biological behavior.

The list of processes included in the discrete round cell neoplasm varies in the literature because of either including or excluding melanocytic neoplasms from the group. Since many of the cutaneous melanocytic neoplasms have a prominent round cytologic presentation, these are often included. A brief comment on the clinical and cytologic presentation of melanoma is included in this chapter. The entire group of discrete round cell neoplasms follows[3,4,8,9,20,21]:

Mast Cell Tumor
Histiocytic Tumors
Lymphoproliferative Disease
Melanocytic Tumors
Transmissible Venereal Tumor

TRANSMISSIBLE VENEREAL TUMORS

Presentation and Biological Behavior

Transmissible venereal tumors (TVTs) were the first described transplantable neoplastic process. They are more commonly seen in more tropic urban areas where there are large numbers of free-roaming dogs. Young sexually active dogs are most commonly affected because of direct contact and transplantation of neoplastic cells; external genitalia are most commonly affected. The typical social

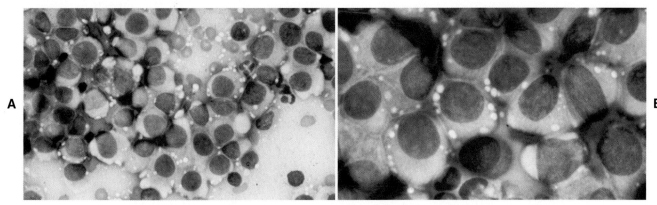

Figure 4-1 Transmissible venereal tumor. Aspirates of a transmissible venereal tumor on the prepuce of a dog. **A,** Highly cellular specimen containing a monotonous population of discrete round mononuclear cells mixed with small amounts of peripheral blood. (Wright's stain.) **B,** Higher magnification of a similar field of view demonstrating the discrete round nature of the cells, the eccentric round to slightly oval nuclei, the uniform chromatin patterns and the moderate amounts of pale blue cytoplasm with multiple, discrete, clear vacuoles at the periphery of the cell. (Wright's stain.)

behavior of dogs licking and sniffing result in transplantation in other locations including the oral and nasal cavities. The TVT is considered mostly to be a benign neoplastic process that, with the aid of a competent immune system, will often spontaneously regress; however, metastatic disease, particularly to the intraocular space, may rarely occur.[10,26]

Cytologic Presentation

Aspirates and touch preparations of a TVT generally yield a large number of neoplastic cells. The typical TVT cell is the epitome of the discrete round cell neoplasm group. The distinctive discrete round cells have eccentric round nuclei with uniform granular chromatin patterns and, oftentimes, a single round prominent nucleolus. Mitotic figures are common and abnormal mitotic figures may be present, but these abnormal figures are not useful in predicting biological behavior. Neoplastic cells range from 12 to 24 µm in diameter and they have moderate amounts of granular and moderately blue staining cytoplasm. Distinguishing cytoplasmic granules are not present; however, low to moderate numbers of TVT cells have distinguishing, clear, distinct, punched-out cytoplasmic vacuoles. These vacuoles are commonly similar in size and arranged in a linear array along the inner surface of the cell membrane (Figure 4-1).[20,22]

In addition to the neoplastic cells, normal-appearing small lymphocytes, few well-differentiated plasma cells, and rarely seen histiocytes/macrophages are commonly present.[20] These cells tend to increase in relative numbers during spontaneous regression of the neoplastic process; a localized immune response is the cause for the regression.

MAST CELL TUMORS

Presentation and Biological Behavior

Mast cell tumors are among the most common cutaneous neoplasms of dogs and cats; however, they may occur at any anatomic location both as primary and secondary neoplastic disease.[26] They are most commonly seen in middle aged dogs and cats, but any age animal is susceptible. In the dog, mast cell tumors are considered malignant with potential of wide-spread dissemination. A histologic grading scheme has been used to help predict biological behavior; however, even well-differentiated Grade I mast cell tumors have the potential for dissemination. Cytologic identification of metastatic or disseminated mast cell tumor, regardless of degree of differentiation, is of great value. Recently, investigators have suggested that detection of agyrophilic nucleolar organizer regions (AgNORs), which are an indirect measurement of cellular proliferation, may prove more subjective in predicting biological behavior. This staining process can be applied to both cytologic specimens and formalin-fixed and paraffin-embedded tissue sections. High AgNOR counts correlate well with poor prognosis.

The general features of the histologic grading system with canine cutaneous mast cell tumors are outlined next:[10,20]

Grade I – well-differentiated, generally well-defined, superficial, low mitotic index

Grade II – moderately differentiated, moderate to poorly circumscribed, mild to moderate infiltration into deeper dermal tissues, moderate mitotic index, potential slight cytomorphologic atypia

Grade III – potentially poorly differentiated, poorly circumscribed, deep infiltration into subcutis, potential high mitotic index, potential moderate cytomorphologic atypia

Feline mast cell tumor has multiple presentations. Isolated cutaneous mast cell tumor is generally considered a benign lesion in the cat and complete excision typically proves curative; however, dissemination may even be seen in cases with suspected isolated cutaneous mast cell tumor.[6,12,25] A guarded prognosis with short median survival times is reported in cats with multiple cutaneous mast cell tumors, recurring mast cell tumors and primary splenic disease. Degree of differentiation is

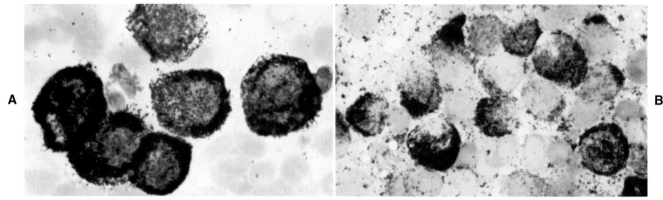

Figure 4-2 Mast cell tumor. Aspirates of two well-differentiated mast cell tumors on the skin of two different dogs. **A,** Moderately cellular specimen with significant peripheral blood contamination, which is common with mast cell tumor aspirates. The neoplastic cells are uniform and well differentiated. Nuclei are almost obscured from view because of the many coarse purple granules. Note the one eosinophil in the center left of the field of view. (Wright's stain.) **B,** Highly cellular preparation with densely packed sheets of mast cells where neoplastic cell nuclei are stained very pale blue because of the heavy degree of granulation and lack of stain penetration to the nucleus. (Wright's stain.)

commonly considered a poor prognostic finding; however, the literature is contradictive related to the more poorly differentiated mast cell tumor in the cat. One study found no correlation between degree of cell differentiation and prognosis.[3,13]

Cytologic Presentation

The diagnosis of mast cell tumor in the dog and cat is relatively straightforward in most cases. Cytologic specimens are commonly very cellular and peripheral blood contamination is common. In addition to the distinctive discrete round cell characteristics, mast cell tumors have distinguishing fine to coarse purple granules when stained with a Romanowsky-type stain (Figure 4-2).[3] These granules allow a definitive diagnosis in most cases; however, it is reported that one of the most commonly used stains in practice, Diff-Quik, often fails in staining these granules making accurate identification of mast cell tumor from other discrete round cell tumors difficult or impossible. Anecdotal reports suggest that approximately 15% of canine mast cell tumors will not stain with Diff-Quik (Figure 4-3). In reality, if one examines the specimen very carefully, although staining may be significantly less with Diff-Quik, there are still identifiable purple granules in neoplastic cells. Additional anecdotal reports suggest that prolonged fixation of mast cell tumors in the first solution of the Diff-Quik stain improves staining of mast cell granules.

Although canine mast cell tumor grading is based upon histologic evaluation where comments on degree of tissue invasion becomes an important criterion, degree of differentiation of mast cell tumor cells is possible cytologically and correlation to histologic grading is good. The less differentiated cells are less granulated and have greater variability of cell size, nuclear size, and nuclear-to-cytoplasmic ratios. Prognosis should be considered guarded for the less differentiated canine neoplasms; however, it

should be noted that well-differentiated mast cell tumors may disseminate also. Identification of metastasis to possible regional lymph nodes or parenchymal organs) proves most beneficial in characterizing the biological behavior of mast cell tumors in the dog and cat (Figure 4-4). With the feline mast cell tumor, the distribution of neoplasms (isolated or multiple or disseminated) and the degree of circumscription of the neoplasm is potentially more predictive on biological behavior than degree of differentiation (Figure 4-5).

Mast cell tumor cell nuclei are generally round to slightly oval and paracentral in location. If discernable, nuclear chromatin patterns are finely stippled and uniform; however, irregularly clumped chromatin patterns may be seen in less differentiated mast cell tumors. Nuclei are often obscured from view with heavily granulated mast cells or they are extremely pale staining due to the high affinity of the cytoplasmic granules to the stain. Eosinophils may be present in the background and these are more commonly seen in canine mast cell tumors than feline mast cell tumors (Figure 4-6). They are not predictive of biological behavior. Low numbers of normal appearing small lymphocytes may be seen in feline cutaneous mast cell tumors.

In addition to the mast cell tumor cells and the potential of eosinophils, many cutaneous mast cell tumor cytologic preparations also have significant numbers of hyperplastic fibroblasts. Collagenolysis and reactive fibroplasia are common histologic findings. Fibroblasts are identified as nongranulated, large, plump spindle to polygonal mononuclear cells with large oval central nuclei, uniform chromatin patterns, potentially prominent nucleoli, and moderate to abundant amounts of deeply blue staining granular cytoplasm (Figure 4-7). These cells are often embedded in densely packed groups of mast cell tumor cells and may be incorrectly identified as a component of the mast cell tumor population or a potential second neoplastic process. If an area of fibroplasia is aspirated and there are high numbers of the hyperplastic fibroblasts

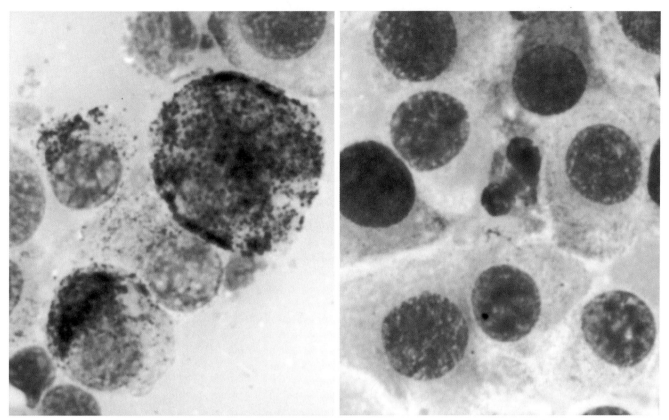

Figure 4-3 Aspirates of a cutaneous mast cell tumor on a dog. The image on the left is from a Wright's-stained preparation, and the image on the right is from a Diff-Quik–stained preparation from the same aspirate. Based upon the Wright's-stained preparation *(left)*, the tumor is characterized as moderately well differentiated with neoplastic cells containing variable numbers of fine to coarse, purple to pink granules. On the Diff-Quik–stained preparation *(right)*, only extremely few cytoplasmic granules are distinguishable. The eosinophil in the center of the field of view gives a possible clue to an underlying poorly differentiated mast cell tumor or one of those mast cell tumors that do not stain well with Diff-Quik stain.

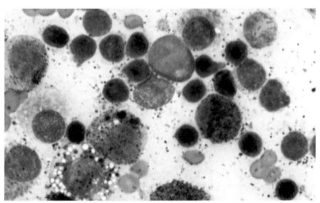

Figure 4-4 Aspirate of a popliteal lymph node from a cat with multiple cutaneous mast cell tumors. Note the mixture of moderately well-differentiated mast cells mixed with many normal appearing small lymphocytes, which represent a population of residual normal lymphoid elements in the lymph node. A single eosinophil is noted in the top right region of the field of view; eosinophils are not as commonly seen in as feline mast cell tumor as in the canine counterpart. (Wright's stain.)

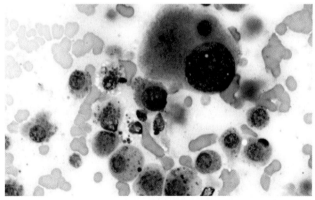

Figure 4-5 Aspirate of an isolated and well-defined cutaneous mast cell tumor in the skin of a cat. Intermixed with moderate amounts of peripheral blood, there are many poorly granulated mast cells. There is marked cytomorphologic atypia; however, upon complete surgical excision, this animal was disease free with no recurrence of neoplastic disease. (Wright's stain.)

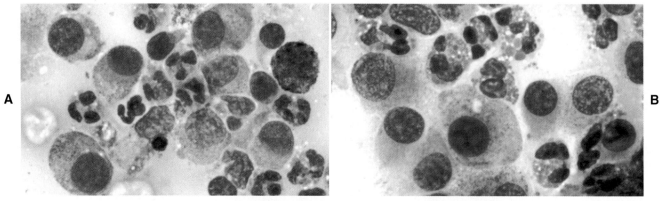

Figure 4-6 Aspirates from cutaneous mast cell tumors on two different dogs. **A,** Wright's-stained specimen. **B,** Diff-Quik–stained specimen. The samples are highly cellular, containing a mixture of poorly granulated mast cells and numerous eosinophils. The high number of eosinophils may help in suggesting that the underlying discrete cell neoplastic process is a poorly differentiated mast cell tumor.

and fewer well-differentiated mast cells, a diagnosis of a primary mesenchymal neoplasm with mast cell infiltration is possible also. Specimen collection ensuring sampling from different areas of the primary mass can help minimize this possibility.

HISTIOCYTIC TUMORS

Presentation and Biological Behavior

Histiocytic neoplastic disease is extremely complex, particularly in the dog. There is a wide range of clinical presentation and biological behavior dependent upon the cell of lineage. In many cases, cytomorphologic features of the neoplastic histiocytes is very predictive of biological potential; however, tissue distribution of two of the benign histiocytic proliferative diseases cannot be predicted based upon cytomorphologic features alone. In recent years, there have been tremendous advances in the understanding of canine histiocytic neoplastic processes, and the reader is directed to the laboratory at the School of Veterinary Medicine, University of California, Davis, California (www.histiocytosis.ucdavis.edu) for a detailed review of canine histiocytic disease.[2,15,16,17] The four basic presentations for histiocytic neoplasia in the dog are presented next.

Canine Cutaneous Histiocytoma: This is typically a benign solitary cutaneous lesion in young dogs; however, it may be seen in dogs of any age. Most commonly it is seen in dogs less younger 1.5 to 3.0 years of age. Complete excision is typically curative; and spontaneous regression is reported. These neoplasms may be found anywhere on the body but extremities and ears are common locations.

Cutaneous Histiocytosis: This is considered a benign process even though multiple lesions are common.[17] Lesions are present in the cutaneous and subcutaneous tissues and distribution of lesions is relatively widespread on the body. The lesions may wax and wane, and spontaneous regression is reported. These lesions most likely represent a reactive histiocytosis of dendritic cells rather than a true

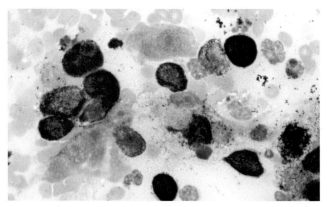

Figure 4-7 Aspirate from a cutaneous well-differentiated mast cell tumor on a dog. There are many well-granulated mast cells mixed with peripheral blood, low numbers of eosinophils, and plump spindle to irregularly shaped hyperplastic fibroblasts. Fibroplasia is commonly seen in mast cell tumors of the skin and should not be interpreted as a second neoplastic process. (Wright's stain.)

neoplastic process.[2] Local and systemic immune modulation prove helpful in lesion management in many cases.

Systemic Histiocytosis: In the past, this has been considered a separate entity from cutaneous histiocytosis because in addition to the possible multiple cutaneous lesions, peripheral lymph nodes and occasionally visceral organs may be affected. Recent studies suggest that systemic histiocytosis and cutaneous histiocytosis are variants of the same reactive histiocytic proliferative process.[2,14] Because of the apparent disseminated nature of this disease process, euthanasia was commonly suggested in the past. Clinical management is more difficult than with cutaneous histiocytosis; immunosuppression therapy directed toward inhibition of T-cell activation is recommended more for patients with systemic histiocytosis than with cutaneous histiocytosis.

Histiocytic Sarcoma Complex: This group of neoplastic processes in the dog encompasses the histiocytic sarcoma, which is typically a solitary lesion, and malignant

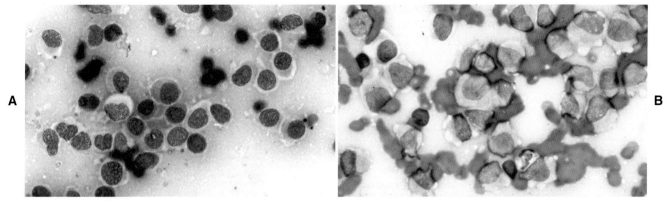

Figure 4-8 Aspirates of two canine histiocytomas from the skin of two different dogs. **A,** Aspirates are from an early developing canine histiocytoma containing many relatively uniform discrete round mononuclear cells with eccentric round to oval to slightly indented nuclei with finely stippled and uniform chromatin patterns. Cytoplasm is moderate in amount, pale blue and granular. Erythrocytes are found in the background. **B,** Aspirates are from a late-stage resolving canine histiocytoma containing slightly larger discrete round mononuclear cells compared with cells from **A.** Nuclei are more irregularly shaped, and the nuclear chromatin pattern resembles chromatin patterns of peripheral blood monocytes.

histiocytosis or disseminated histiocytic sarcoma, which is when the disease process extends beyond regional lymph nodes and involves various visceral tissues.[1] This disease complex is best described in the Bernese Mountain Dog but has been seen in many breeds of dogs.[1,11] This disease complex presents with cytomorphologic distinguishing features of cellular atypia and in many cases, multinucleated giant pleomorphic neoplastic cells.

Feline histiocytic disorders are less common and much less understood than the canine counterparts. A benign cutaneous histiocytoma, as is seen in the dog, does not exist in the cat. Histiocytic disease in the cat appears progressive in nature both with a morphologically benign appearing neoplastic cell population and a population of histiocytes with significant cytomorphologic atypia. Lesions often present as solitary cutaneous nodules with either gradual progression and possible eventual multiple cutaneous lesions or potential progression to involve regional lymph nodes and terminally, visceral organs. A cytomorphologically malignant appearing histiocytic neoplastic process, histiocytic sarcoma, resembles the canine counterpart. These tumors are typically locally invasive, and metastatic disease primarily to regional lymph nodes is possible.

Cytologic Presentation

Although there are significant variations in clinical presentation for histiocytic proliferative disease in the dog and cat, there are relatively few cytomorphologic variations, which makes it difficult sometimes to make a definitive diagnosis on cytologic presentation alone. All of the different variants of histiocytic proliferative disease typically present with moderate to high cellularity with varying amounts of peripheral blood contamination.

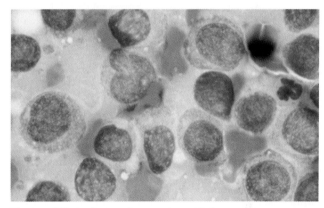

Figure 4-9 Aspirate of one of multiple cutaneous masses on a dog. Morphologic features of the primary neoplastic cell population are similar to those of the typical cutaneous histiocytoma commonly found in young dogs. Erythrocytes are present in the background. This aspirate is from a case of cutaneous histiocytosis. (Wright's stain.)

Canine Cutaneous Histiocytoma, Cutaneous Histiocytosis, and Systemic Histiocytosis: The proliferative histiocytes in these lesions in the dog have similar morphologic features.[1,5,18] These discrete cells are relatively round and range from 12 to 30 µg in diameter. They may present with an irregular or amoeboid cell shape; this is seen more in later stages of resolution, particularly in the canine cutaneous histiocytoma of young dogs. Nuclei are mostly round to oval and eccentric in location, but blunt indentations of the nucleus or irregular shapes may be seen also. Nuclear chromatin patterns are finely stippled and uniform and in many cases resemble the nuclear chromatin patterns of normal appearing peripheral blood monocytes. Cytoplasm is variable in amount but generally moderate to abundant. Cytoplasm is pale blue staining and granular with no distinguishing granules or vacuoles (Figures 4-8 and 4-9).

Low numbers of normal appearing small lymphocytes and rarely seen macrophages and well differentiated plasma cells may be distributed among the histiocytic cells. These nonhistiocytic cells may increase in number during phases of resolution.

Histiocytic Sarcoma Complex: Neoplastic cells within this group of neoplasms are distinctively different from the more benign appearing counterparts noted previously. Anisocytosis, anisokaryosis, variation in nuclear-to-cytoplasmic ratios, and overall pleomorphism are common. In addition, multinucleated giant cell formation is often seen. Nuclear chromatin patterns can be irregularly clumped and prominent; multiple or irregularly shaped nucleoli may be seen. Cytoplasm is typically moderate to abundant in mount, pale blue staining, granular, and someimes vacuolated (Figures 4-10 and 4-11). Phagocytosis of erythrocytes, leukocytes, and other neoplastic cells may be seen and is particularly common in a variant of the histiocytic sarcoma complex called *hemophagocytic histiocytic sarcoma*. A hemophagocytic syndrome with observed anemia and possible other peripheral cytopenias may occur.

LYMPHOPROLIFERATIVE DISEASE

Presentation and Biological Behavior

Detailed discussion of lymphoproliferative disease is found in Chapter 11; however, some general comments related to the discrete round cell nature of this group of neoplastic diseases is warranted because anatomic locations for lymphoproliferative disease overlap locations of origin for other discrete round cell neoplasms. Morphologic distinction between the different types of tumors is important because biological behavior is potentially very dramatically different from one tumor to the next. Malignant lymphoma or lymphosarcoma presenting with classic localized or generalized lymphadenomegaly itself has a variety of potential biological behavior patterns. There are forms of smoldering malignant lymphoma and the opposite extreme, high-grade and rapidly progressive malignant lymphoma. Cutaneous and other nonlymphoid tissue originating lymphoproliferative disease is generally considered malignant, and progressive disease with eventual dissemination.[10]

A variant of lymphoproliferative disease, plasma cell neoplasia, commonly presents differently from malignant lymphoma. Cutaneous and other extramedullary plasmacytomas are most commonly considered benign lymphoproliferative disease, and complete excision typically proves curative.[24] This is in significant contrast to the predominating pattern for multiple myeloma, a plasma

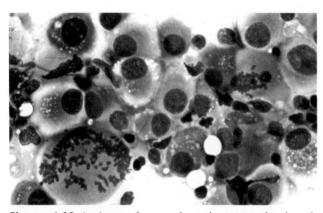

Figure 4-10 Aspirate of an enlarged prescapular lymph node on a dog with multiple skin and internal organ space-occupying lesions. The sample is highly cellular, containing a population of discrete round and mostly mononuclear cells with moderate anisocytosis, anisokaryosis, and variation in nuclear-to-cytoplasmic ratios. Two abnormal mitotic figures are present. This aspirate is from a case of histiocytic sarcoma complex.

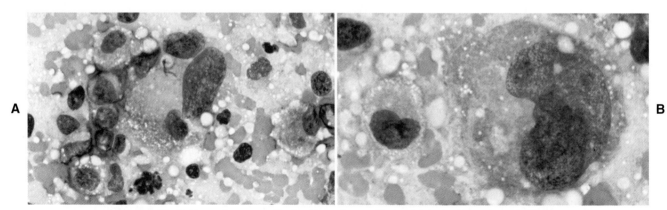

Figure 4-11 Aspirates from a mediastinal mass from a dog with histiocytic sarcoma complex. **A,** The specimen is highly cellular and has much peripheral blood contamination mixed with the neoplastic cell population. There is significant cytomorphologic atypia consistent with this malignant variant of histiocytic disease in the dog. A single mitotic figure is noted in the bottom center region of the field of view. (Wright's stain.) **B,** *Higher-magnification field* of view of a different area of the same lesion as presented in **A.** Cytomorphologic atypia is characterized by the presence of a giant cell with a giant nucleus. Nuclear chromatin patterns are open with irregular clumping of chromatin. (Wright's stain.)

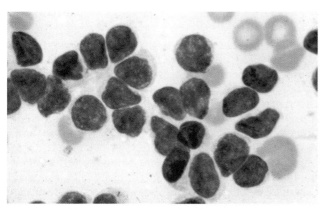

Figure 4-12 Aspirate from a case of cutaneous malignant lymphoma in a dog. Aspirates of multiple cutaneous lesions yielded highly cellular specimens containing primarily a single population of normal appearing small lymphocytes mixed with peripheral blood. The lack of heterogeneity within the lymphoid cell population is strong support for a lymphoproliferative process because most reactive lymphoid reactions result in the finding of many lymphocytes in different stages of reactivity and maturation. (Wright's stain.)

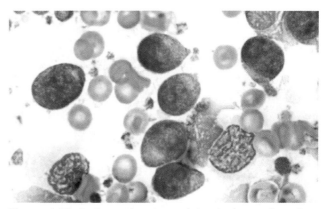

Figure 4-13 Aspirate of an intra-abdominal mass in a dog. This specimen is highly cellular containing a primarily monotonous population of intermediate-sized to large and immature-appearing lymphocytes, often with eccentric round nuclei with single and sometimes multiple prominent nucleoli. Cytoplasm is moderate in amount, deeply blue, and granular with no distinguishing granules or vacuoles. The relative high nuclear-to-cytoplasmic ratios are supportive of lymphoid lineage. Many erythrocytes and lymphoglandular bodies are present in the background. (Wright's stain.)

cell tumor originating in the bone marrow. These latter neoplastic processes may present with isolated lesions, but more commonly present with multiple lesions within the marrow resulting in multiple lytic lesions that can be identified radiographically. Even though most cutaneous or isolated extramedullary plasmacytomas are considered benign, the potential for disseminated disease exists regardless of cytomorphologic presentation (atypia or no atypia) and investigation into possible systemic disease is always warranted. Complete excision of the extramedullary plasmacytomas is typically curative.

Cytologic Presentation

The key cytologic feature of malignant lymphoma other than the discrete round nature of the neoplastic cells is that these tumors are generally composed of a homogeneous population of lymphocytes at one state of differentiation. Cytologic specimens are typically highly cellular, even when presented with aspirates of plaque-like lesions in the skin of a dog. Inflammatory lesions with high numbers of infiltrating lymphocytes are also highly cellular, but these specimens typically contain a highly heterogeneous population of lymphocytes. Normal small lymphocytes typically predominate and there are many prominent reactive lymphocytes, plasmacytoid lymphocytes, well-differentiated plasma cells, and very few large and immature appearing lymphocytes.

The neoplastic lymphocytes are commonly very similar to the primary tissue's normal appearing cellular elements. A small cell malignant lymphoma is composed mostly of relatively normal appearing small lymphocytes with potentially slightly greater than normal amounts of pale blue staining cytoplasm or clefted nuclei. The nuclear-to-cytoplasmic ratios are high and the nuclear chromatin patterns are somewhat smudged and dense in contrast to the cells of a TVT or canine cutaneous histiocytoma (Figure 4-12).

Intermediate sized to large cell type malignant lymphomas are composed of a vastly predominating population of morphologically normal appearing intermediate sized to large lymphocytes commonly seen in reactive lymphoid tissues or in very low numbers in normal lymphoid tissue. Even these lymphocytes have distinctively high nuclear-to-cytoplasmic ratios, which helps distinguish them from other discrete round cell tumors (Figure 4-13). In some cases of malignant lymphoma, there is potential for significant variation in cell size and shape as well as significant cellular atypia; however, many malignant lymphoma cases have no significant cytomorphologic criteria of malignancy beyond the lack of heterogeneity typically found in normal or reactive lymphocytic tissue. The mitotic activity (mitotic index) is better classified with histopathologic evaluation of fixed tissue specimens; however, both normal and abnormal mitotic figures may be easily seen in cases of malignant lymphoma with a histologically identified high mitotic index.

A special morphologic variant of lymphoproliferative disease is the plasma cell tumor. Cutaneous plasmacytoma, noncutaneous extramedullary plasmacytoma, and multiple myeloma present with a similar cytologic picture.[3,19,23] Neoplastic cells have morphologic features of differentiated plasma cells. These cells are round to oval mononuclear cells mixed with potentially low numbers of binucleated cell forms. The cells mostly range from 15 to 30 μg in diameter. Nuclei are commonly round with uniform and sometimes coarse but regular chromatin patterns. Nuclei are peripherally located and unlike other lymphoid tumor cells, plasmacytoma cells typically have moderate amounts of cytoplasm giving the cells a moderate rather than a high nuclear-to-cytoplasmic ratio. Cytoplasm is commonly deeply blue staining because of the density of cytoplasmic RNA. A prominent perinuclear clear zone

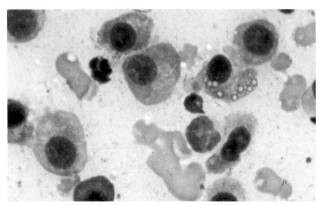

Figure 4-14 Aspirate of a solitary, well-defined, cutaneous, extramedullary plasmacytoma on a dog. The sample is highly cellular containing a primary population of well-differentiated plasma cells with eccentric round dense nuclei and moderate to abundant amounts of deeply blue cytoplasm often with poorly defined perinuclear clear zones. The monotony of the plasma cell population with no other significant inflammatory process is highly supportive of a diagnosis of extramedullary plasmacytoma.

representing the Golgi apparatus of cytoplasmic organelles is commonly seen (Figure 4-14). Extramedullary plasmacytomas and multiple myelomas may present with a monotonous population of very uniform well-differentiated plasma cells or with neoplastic cells with some plasmacytoid differentiation and moderate cellular atypia or a combination of these presentations. Morphologic features are not predictive of biological behavior but, the more atypia present, the greater the concern for disseminated disease and investigation into possible other anatomic locations of disease is strongly warranted.

MELANOCYTIC TUMORS

Presentation and Biological Behavior

Benign and malignant melanoma can originate from any pigmented location; however, the haired skin and oral cavity are among the most common locations of occurrence.[26] Biological behavior is dramatically variable and in many cases, cytomorphologic criteria of malignancy are helpful indicators of the biological behavior; the more cytomorphologic atypia, the greater the potential for metastatic potential. In the dog, anatomic location or origin also plays a significant role in predicting biological behavior. Regardless of the cytomorphologic presentation, melanomas originating from the lips, oral mucocutaneous junctions, and interdigital skin are given a guarded prognosis because most of the melanomas from these locations prove to be malignant. Isolated cutaneous melanomas are commonly small, well-defined, easily removed neoplastic processes with a benign biological behavior.

Cytologic Presentation

As was mentioned in the overview, melanocytic tumors actually belong to a distinct class of neoplastic tissue, neuroendocrine tumors; however, they often have a presentation cytologically that can be confusing to even the expert cytologist. Melanoma cell morphology ranges from round to polygonal to plump spindle or even stellate; however, if there is a predominance of the more round shaped cells, a poorly differentiated melanoma can resemble other round cell tumors. It is important to examine the entire specimen because in most cases, there will be a mixture of cellular morphologic presentations if one looks at many of the neoplastic cells. Typically, these neoplasms exfoliate well, so there are many cells available for evaluation. Cell sizes can be quite variable ranging from as small as 12 to 20 micrometers in greatest dimension and as large as 20 to 30 µg or more in dimension. Nuclei are commonly paracentral in location and round to oval in shape. Nuclear chromatin patterns in the benign neoplasms are uniform and finely stippled; however, in the malignant variants, chromatin patterns are often coarsely and irregularly clumped. Nucleoli can be multiple, prominent, and irregularly shaped. Good nuclear criteria of malignancy are easily documented in many of the malignant melanomas. A moderate to high number of mitotic figures may be seen with the more malignant variants of melanoma, and rarely seen abnormal mitotic figures may be present.

Cytoplasm is typically moderate to abundant in amount, giving the cells a moderate to low nuclear-to-cytoplasmic ratio. It is granular and lightly to moderately blue staining. One of the distinguishing features of this class of neoplasms is the presence of variable numbers of melanin pigment granules. In contrast to normal melanin granules, these are often rounded and variably sized and sometimes clumped to varying degrees. The granules stain black to green-black with commonly used Romanowsky stains in contrast to the purple staining granules of mast cell tumors (Figure 4-15). Histologically there is a class of melanocytic tumors identified as *amelanotic melanomas* because of the apparent absence of melanin pigment granules with standard histologic staining procedures. Cytologically, even in the least pigmented melanomas, few melanin granules can be identified with deliberate microscopic review of the specimen (Figure 4-16). It should be noted that simple identification of melanin granules does not allow the making of a diagnosis of melanoma. The novice cytologist commonly misidentifies a pigmented basal cell tumor as melanoma; normal melanocytes pass melanin to epithelial cells of the epidermis. Additionally, some may confuse the presence of hemosiderin granules in a macrophage as melanin granules in a melanocyte; hemosiderin typically stains more brown to brown-black with commonly used Romanowsky stains.[20]

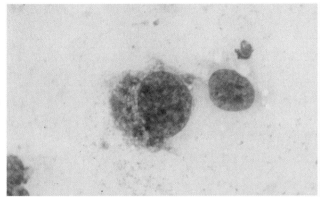
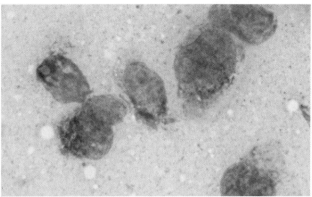

A

B

Figure 4-15 Aspirates of a lip mass on a dog. **A,** There is one intact round to polygonal mononuclear cell adjacent to a broken mononuclear cell. The intact cell has an eccentric round to oval nucleus with slightly irregularly clumped chromatin. Cytoplasm is moderate in amount and filled with fine, black melanin granules. (Wright's stain.) **B,** A different field of view from the same aspirate as **A.** Slightly greater amounts of cellular pleomorphism are noted. (Wright's stain.)

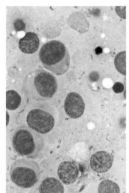
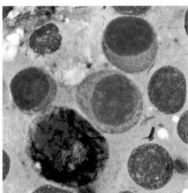

Figure 4-16 Aspirate of an amelanotic melanoma on the lip of a dog. Low-magnification view *(left)* of the specimen reveals a primary population of apparent discrete round mononuclear cells with no obvious melanin pigment (Wright's stain). Upon evaluation of the complete specimen at high-magnification field of view *(right),* isolated neoplastic cells have obvious delicate needle-like melanin granules in the cytoplasm and few other cells have only a minimal dusting of the cytoplasm with melanin granules (Wright's stain).

References

1. Affolter VK, Moore PF: Histiocytosis. In *Proceedings of the 14th Annual Congress ESVD-ECVD,* Pisa, Italy, Sept 5–7, 1997.
2. Affolter VK, Moore PF: Canine cutaneous and systemic histiocytosis: Reactive histiocytosis of dermal dendritic cells. *Am J Dermatopathol* 22:40-48, 2000.
3. Baker R, Lumsden JH: The skin. In Baker R, Lumsden JH (ed): *Color Atlas of Cytology of the Dog and Cat.* Mosby, St. Louis, 2000, pp 39-50.
4. Barton: Cytologic diagnosis of cutaneous neoplasia: An algorithmic approach. *Comp Cont Ed* 9:20-33, 1987.
5. Bender WM, Muller GH: Multiple resolving cutaneous histiocytoma in a dog. *J Am Vet Med Assoc* 194:535-537, 1989.
6. Buerger RG, Scott DW: Cutaneous mast cell neoplasia in cats: 14 cases:1975-1985. *J Am Vet Med Assoc* 190:1440-1444, 1987.
7. Mays MB, Bergeron JA: Cutaneous histiocytosis in dogs. *J Am Vet Med Assoc* 188:377-381, 1986.
8. Duncan JS, Prasse KW: Cytologic examination of the skin and subcutis. *Vet Clin North Am* 6:637-645, 1976.
9. Duncan JS, Prasse KW: Cytology of canine cutaneous round cell tumors. *Vet Pathol* 16:673-679, 1979.
10. Goldschmidt, Hendrick: Tumors of the skin and soft tissues. In Meuten (ed): *Tumors in Domestic Animals,* ed 4. Ames, Iowa, Blackwell Publishing Company, 2002.
11. Hayden DW, et al: Disseminated malignant histiocytosis in a Golden Retriever: Clinicopathologic, ultrastructural, and immunohistochemical findings. *Vet Pathol* 30:256-264, 1993.
12. Miller MA, et al: Cutaneous neoplasia in 340 cats. *Vet Pathol* 28:389-395, 1991.
13. Molander-McCrary H, et al: Cutaneous mast cell tumors in cats: 32 cases—1991-1994. *J Am Anim Hosp Assoc* 34:281-284, 1998.
14. Moore PF: Systemic histiocytosis of Bernese mountain dogs. *Vet Pathol* 21:554-563, 1984.
15. Moore PF, Rosin A: Malignant histiocytosis of Bernese mountain dogs. *Vet Pathol* 23:1-10, 1986.
16. Moore A, et al: Canine cutaneous histiocytoma is an epidermotropic Langerhans cell histiocytosis that expresses CD1 and specific beta 2-integrin molecules. *Am J Pathol* 148:1699-1708, 1996.
17. Moore PF: Canine histiocytic diseases: Proliferation of dendritic cells is key. *Proceedings of the 55th Annual Meeting of the American College of Veterinary Pathologists,* Amelia Island, Fla, December 2000.
18. Paterson S, Boydell P, Pike R: Systemic histiocytosis in the Bernese mountain dog. *J Small Anim Pract* 36:233-236, 1995.
19. Rakich PM, et al: Mucocutaneous plasmacytomas in dogs: 75 cases: 1980-1987. *J Am Vet Med Assoc* 194:803-810, 1989.
20. Raskin RE: Skin and subcutaneous tissues. In Raskin RE, Meyer DJ (eds): *Atlas of Canine and Feline Cytology,* Philadelphia, Saunders, 2001.
21. Rebar: *Handbook of veterinary cytology.* St. Louis, Ralston Purina Co, 1979.
22. Richardson: Canine transmissible venereal tumor. *Compend Cont Ed Pract* 3:951-956, 1981.
23. Rogers: Diagnostic dilemma of extramedullary plasmacytomas. *Vet Cancer Soc Newsletter* 15:12-14, 1991.
24. Rowland PH, et al: Cutaneous plasmacytomas with amyloid in six dogs. *Vet Pathol* 28:125-130, 1991.
25. Wilcock BP, Yager JA, Zink MC: The morphology and behaviour of feline cutaneous mastocytomas. *Vet Pathol* 23:320-324, 1986.
26. Yager and Wilcock: Tumours of the skin and associated tissues. In Yager and Wilcock (eds): *Color Atlas and Text of Surgical Pathology of the Dog and Cat,* St. Louis, Mosby, 1994.

Cutaneous and Subcutaneous Lesions

R.D. Tyler, R.L. Cowell, and J.H. Meinkoth

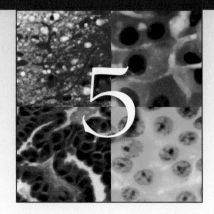

CHAPTER

5

Evaluation of cutaneous and subcutaneous lesions is one of the more common uses of diagnostic cytology and can be an extremely useful clinical tool. Cutaneous and subcutaneous lesions are easily accessible and there are no significant contraindications to collecting samples from them. Tranquilization and/or anesthesia is seldom needed for sample collection. Often the specimen can be collected, prepared, stained, and microscopically evaluated in minutes—providing a diagnosis, prognosis, indication of appropriate therapy, and/or guidance as to the next diagnostic procedure.

COLLECTION TECHNIQUES

Samples may be collected as fine-needle biopsies (FNB) (using either an aspiration or nonaspiration technique), scrapings, imprints, and/or swabs, depending on the characteristics of the lesion and the tractability of the patient. FNBs by an aspiration or a nonaspiration technique (see Chapter 1) are the standard method of collection because they yield the most representative and diagnostic samples in most situations. There are times, however, when alternate techniques or combinations of techniques are warranted, as discussed subsequently.

Fine-Needle Biopsies

Fine-needle biopsy is described in Chapter 1.

Solid Masses: Most cutaneous or subcutaneous solid masses are well suited for both the aspiration and nonaspiration techniques; the primary determinant is the preference of the collector. Sometimes, it is wise to sample the lesion using both techniques, especially if the first method attempted appears to have obtained little material or resulted in marked blood contamination. If large enough, the mass should be sampled several times in different areas to increase the chance of obtaining diagnostic material. FNBs can be collected along with impression smears or swabs, if desired.

Aspirates of Fluid-Filled Masses and Cysts: Aspirates can be collected from fluid-filled masses and cysts with a 22 to 25-gauge needle attached to a 3-ml syringe. When possible, enough fluid should be aspirated to prepare several cytologic smears, perform a nucleated cell count and total protein analysis, and perform or submit a culture. Usually 1 to 3 ml is sufficient.

The lesion is prepared as solid masses are prepared (see Chapter 1). Using the blood smear, line smear, and/or squash prep technique(s) described in Chapter 1, smears can be prepared directly from the aspirated fluids or from the sediment of centrifuged fluids.

When lesions contain both solid and fluid areas, separate aspirates of each should be collected because the cell populations obtained may be markedly different. Neoplasms that are cystic or that contain pockets of inflammation may not exfoliate recognizably neoplastic cells into the fluid portions. Direct fine-needle aspiration of the solid tissue component often yields the most diagnostic samples.

Scrapings

Generally, scrapings are the collection technique of choice when FNBs are inappropriate because they can collect cells that do not exfoliate readily with swabs or imprints. Scrapings of lesions or excised tissues may also help collect cells from lesions that do not easily exfoliate cells (e.g., mesenchymal lesions).

Scrapings of cutaneous lesions are made by rubbing the edge of a blunt instrument, such as a glass slide or the back of a scalpel blade, across the lesion. This results in an accumulation of cells along the edge of the blunt instrument. These cells are then spread onto a clean, dry, glass slide by one of the techniques described in Chapter 1.

Imprints

Although impression smears are easy and are not painful for patients, they have limitations similar to those of swabs. Depending on the types of cells present, in the lesion may not yield enough cells for evaluation. Discrete cells, such as inflammatory cells and cells of round cell tumors, exfoliate well with imprints. Mesenchymal lesions generally do not exfoliate many cells; however, highly malignant mesenchymal tumors may yield very cellular specimens. The cells retrieved from imprints, as with swabs, may not be representative of the lesion. Impression smears of ulcerated neoplasms often yield only surface inflammation. Conversely, in inflammatory lesions, impression smears may yield surface epithelial cells that are dysplastic secondary to the inflammatory process present. Impression smears of exudative or ulcerative lesions are most useful for identifying the presence of infectious agents (e.g., fungal organisms).

Imprints can be made from ulcerated lesions or surgically removed tissue. Imprints of lesions are made by removing any scab that covers the lesion and then touching the dry surface of a clean, glass slide to the surface of the lesion. If a *Dermatophilus congolensis* infection is suspected, the underside of the scab is also imprinted. The lesion is then cleaned with a nonirritating antiseptic, blotted dry with a sterile gauze sponge or other clean absorbent material, and reimprinted. If the tissue is not blotted dry before impressions are made, the slides will usually contain only blood/tissue fluid.

Swabs

Other than for vaginal cytology (see Chapter 25), swabs are generally collected only when imprints, scrapings, and aspirates cannot be made (e.g., fistulous tracts). Swabbing (with a moist, sterile, cotton swab) the ulcerated surface of cutaneous lesions (especially neoplasms) often yields only surface inflammation. Sterile isotonic fluid, such as 0.9% NaCl, should be used to moisten the swab, although very moist lesions do not require that the swab be moistened. Moistening the swab helps minimize cell damage during sample collection and smear preparation. After sample collection, the swab is gently rolled along the flat surface of a clean, glass slide. (The swab should not be rubbed across the slide surface because this causes excessive cell damage.) If a hematologic-type stain is used (e.g., Wright's), the smears are air-dried and stained as described in Chapter 1.

GENERAL APPEARANCE OF THE LESION

The general physical appearance of the lesion is helpful in interpreting the cytologic findings.

Fistulous Tracts

Fistulous tracts are usually caused by infectious agents or foreign bodies. They should be probed for foreign bodies, and culture and swab samples should be collected from deep within the tracts. Cytologic preparations should be carefully perused for filamentous rods that stain light blue with intermittent pink to purple areas. This morphology is characteristic of *Nocardia* and *Actinomyces* spp. which often cause fistulous tracts, but occasionally occurs with some other anaerobic bacteria, such as *Fusobacterium* spp.

Ulcerated Lesions

Ulcerated lesions may be areas of skin that have been injured or infected and become ulcerated and indurated because of the subsequent inflammatory reaction, or may be areas of ulcerated skin overlying a cutaneous or subcutaneous mass. Generally, examination of the lesion indicates whether there is an underlying mass. Ulcerated lesions can result from infectious, foreign body, allergic, parasitic, or neoplastic causes.

Nonulcerated Lesions

Nonulcerated masses may be solid or fluid-filled. Nonulcerated solid masses may be neoplastic or inflammatory in origin. Nonulcerated fluid-filled masses are often nonneoplastic in origin, but occasionally represent cystic neoplasia.

GENERAL EVALUATION OF CYTOLOGIC SMEARS

The first step in the cytologic evaluation of a smear is to determine if an adequate number of intact cells are present and if the sample is spread and stained adequately to allow cell morphology to be evaluated. If collection attempts repeatedly fail to yield sufficient numbers of cells for cytologic evaluation, an alternative procedure, such as biopsy or culture (depending on the character of the lesion), may be necessary.

Once a suitable cytologic preparation is achieved, the number and type of cell populations present are determined. Smears are evaluated for evidence of inflammation and/or neoplasia (Figure 5-1). If all the cells from a solid mass are tissue cells (i.e., no inflammatory cells are present), the lesion is either due to neoplasia or hyperplasia or it was missed. If all the cells are inflammatory cells, an inflammatory process is occurring and is most likely the cause of the lesion, but an inflamed neoplasm cannot be ruled out. An admixture of inflammatory cells and dysplastic tissue cells can be caused by inflammation with secondary tissue cell dysplasia or neoplasia with secondary inflammation; therefore caution must be used in making the diagnosis of malignancy if evidence of inflammation is detected.

EVALUATION OF AN INFLAMMATORY CELL POPULATION

Figure 5-2 provides an algorithm to aid in the evaluation of the inflammatory cell component of cutaneous and subcutaneous lesions, and Table 5-1 gives general considerations for some inflammatory responses. If most of the inflammatory cells are neutrophils (see Figure 5-7 later in the chapter), especially when degenerate neutrophils are present, but no bacteria are found, a covert infection may be present, or the neutrophilic inflammatory response may be due to one of the conditions listed in Table 5-1 under "Marked predominance of neutrophils." The lesion can be cultured to identify a covert infection. If the culture reveals an infectious agent, appropriate therapy can be instituted. If the culture does not reveal an infectious agent or if therapy for the infectious agent identified by culture is not effective, cytology can be repeated or a biopsy can be submitted for histopathologic evaluation.

When >15% of the inflammatory cells present are macrophages (Figure 5-3, *A*), and/or inflammatory giant cells are present (Figure 5-3, *B*), fungal infection, infection with

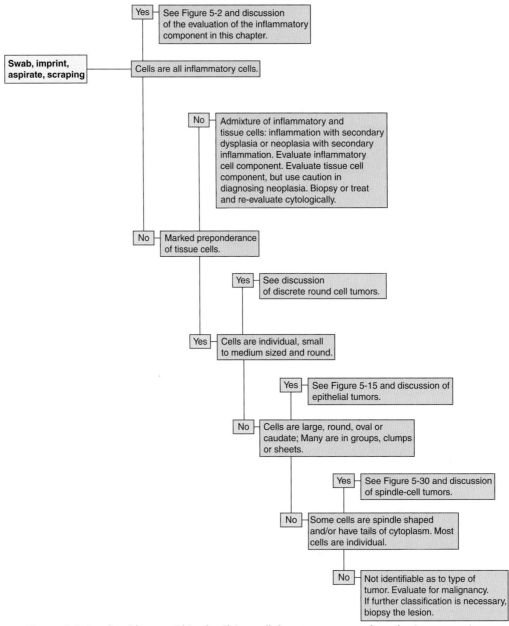

Figure 5-1 An algorithm to aid in classifying cellular components of cytologic preparations from solid lesions.

Actinomyces or *Nocardia* spp., foreign-body granuloma, or other causes of granulomatous inflammation (e.g., lick granuloma) should be considered. The slide should be carefully studied for organisms (Figure 5-3, *C*) or signs of a foreign body, such as refractile debris (Figure 5-4). Also, historical information about the possible introduction of foreign material should be sought. If no organisms are found and no historical information indicates the introduction of a foreign substance into the area, the tissue can be cultured, or a biopsy can be submitted for histopathologic examination.

If the proportion of eosinophils exceeds 10% (Figure 5-5), an allergic, parasitic, or foreign-body reaction or an eosinophilic granuloma complex lesion should be considered. The slide should again be carefully searched for organisms or signs of foreign material. If no organisms

or signs are found, the lesion can be cultured (including fungal cultures), or a biopsy can be submitted for histopathologic evaluation. If the lesion is cultured, but not biopsied, and the culture fails to yield an organism, the lesion may be treated as an eosinophilic granuloma if the historical and clinical evidence is indicative of an eosinophilic granuloma complex lesion. In this situation, the lesion should be watched carefully. If the response to therapy is not appropriate, a biopsy of the lesion should be submitted for histopathologic evaluation.

When tissue cells showing criteria of malignancy are accompanied by inflammatory cells (Figure 5-6), the sample should be interpreted cautiously. Dysplasia occurring in tissue adjacent to inflammatory reactions can alter tissue cell morphology. As a result, tissue cells undergoing

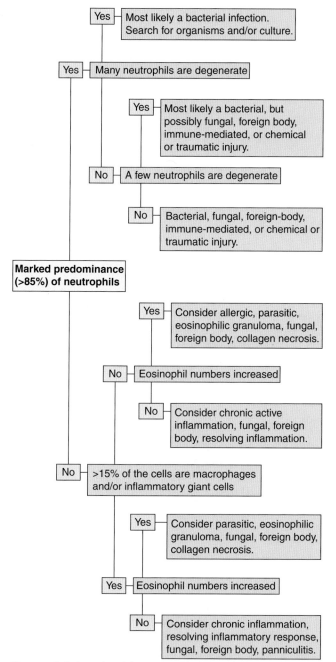

Figure 5-2 An algorithm to aid in evaluating aspirates containing a preponderance of inflammatory cells.

dysplasia in response to a local inflammatory process can be erroneously classified as neoplastic cells. As the intensity of the inflammatory reaction increases, the assurance with which a diagnosis of neoplasia can be made decreases.

INFECTIOUS AGENTS

See Chapter 3 for more photographs of infectious agents. Infectious agents invariably cause lesions characterized by the presence of inflammatory cells. Bacterial agents usually produce lesions characterized by being composed of more than 85% neutrophils (Figure 5-7)—many of which may be degenerate. When bacteria are pathogenic,

some can usually be found phagocytized within neutrophils in addition to those that may be present extracellularly. Mycotic agents produce lesions that tend to have more macrophages present than do bacterial lesions. However, neutrophils may still be the predominant cell type, and eosinophils may be plentiful with certain hyphating fungi. Cytologic evaluation often reveals the type of infectious agent (e.g., bacteria, yeast, protozoa) and in some cases yields a definitive diagnosis (e.g., histoplasmosis, cryptococcosis). Size, shape, staining characteristics, and internal structures are helpful in classifying the type of organism and in some cases, specific identification of the organism.

Bacteria

Staining Characteristics of Bacteria: With the routine Romanowsky-type stains (Wright's, Diff-Quik, Dip-Stat) all bacteria, whether gram positive or gram negative, stain blue to purple with a few exceptions such as *Mycobacterium*.

Bacterial Cocci: Pathogenic bacterial cocci (Figure 5-8) are usually gram positive and of the genera *Staphylococcus* or *Streptococcus*. Staphylococci usually occur in clusters of 4 to 12 bacteria, but *Streptococcus* spp. tend to occur in short or long chains of organisms. When cocci are identified in cytologic preparations, aerobic and anaerobic cultures and sensitivity tests should be performed to identify the organism and the optimum antibiotic therapy. Because most cocci are gram positive, antibiotic therapy effective against gram-positive organisms should be used when it is necessary to start therapy before culture and sensitivity results are received.

D. congolensis replicates by transverse and longitudinal division, producing long chains of coccoid bacterial doublets that resemble small, blue railroad tracks. It infects the superficial epidermis, causing crusty lesions. Cytologic preparations from the undersurface of scabs from these crusty lesions are most rewarding in demonstrating organisms. The preparations usually contain mature epithelial cells, keratin bars, debris, and organisms (Figure 5-9). A few neutrophils may also be found.

Small Bacterial Rods: Most small bacterial rods are gram negative. Some can be recognized as bipolar rods (Figure 5-10). All pathogenic, bipolar bacterial rods are gram negative. Infections with bacterial rods are usually associated with a marked neutrophilic inflammatory response. When small bacterial rods are recognized in cytologic preparations, the lesion should be cultured to identify the organism, and sensitivity tests should be performed to determine the optimum antibiotic therapy. If it is necessary to institute antibiotic therapy before the culture and sensitivity results are received, the therapy employed should be effective against gram-negative organisms because most pathogenic, small rods are gram negative.

Filamentous Rods: Pathogenic filamentous rods that cause cutaneous or subcutaneous lesions are usually *Nocardia* or *Actinomyces* spp. Some other anaerobes, such as *Fusobacterium*

TABLE 5-1

Some Conditions Suggested by Certain Proportions of Inflammatory Cells

Inflammatory Cell Population	First Considerations	Second Considerations
Marked predominance (85%) of neutrophils		
Many neutrophils are degenerate	Gram-negative bacteria Gram-positive bacteria	Abscess secondary to neoplasia, foreign bodies, etc.
A few neutrophils are degenerate	Gram-positive bacteria Gram-negative bacteria Higher bacteria (*nocardia, Actinomyces, etc.*)	Fungi Protozoa Foreign body Immune-mediated chemical or traumatic injury
No neutrophils are degenerate	Gram-positive bacteria Higher bacteria (*nocardia, Actinomyces,* etc.) Chemical or traumatic injury Panniculitis	Abscess secondary to neoplasia Gram-negative bacteria Fungi Foreign body Abscess secondary to neoplasia
Admixture of inflammatory cells		
15% to 40% macrophages	Higher bacteria (*Nocardia, Actinomyces,* etc.) Fungi Protozoa Neoplasia Foreign body Panniculitis Any resolving inflammatory lesion	Nonfilamentous gram-positive bacteria Parasites, chronic allergic inflammation and eosinophilic granuloma if eosinophil numbers are increased
>40% macrophages	Fungi Foreign body Protozoa Neoplasia Panniculitis Any resolving inflammatory lesion	Parasites, chronic allergic inflammation, and eosinophilic granuloma if eosinophil numbers are increased
Inflammatory giant cell present	Fungi Foreign body Protozoa Collagen necrosis Panniculitis Parasites (if eosinophils are present)	—
>10% eosinophils	Allergic inflammation Parasites Eosinophilic granuloma Collagen necrosis Mast cell tumor	Neoplasia Foreign body Hyphating fungi

and *Mycobacterium* spp. may be filamentous, but rarely are. *Nocardia* and *Actinomyces* spp. are characterized by long, slender (filamentous) strands that stain pale blue and have intermittent, small, pink or purple areas (Figure 5-11; see Figure 5-3). This morphology is characteristic of both *Nocardia* and *Actinomyces* spp. and the filamentous form of *Fusobacterium* spp. When these features are recognized cytologically, cultures should be performed specifically for *Nocardia* and *Actinomyces* spp. and for other anaerobes.

On the other hand, *Mycobacterium* spp. often do not stain with Romanowsky-type stains. As a result, negative images (Figure 5-12, *A*) may be observed in the cytoplasm of macrophages and/or inflammatory giant cells. When epithelioid macrophages and/or inflammatory giant cells are encountered in cytologic preparations that do not contain any obvious organisms, a careful search for negative images of *Mycobacterium* spp. should be made. *Mycobacterium* spp. stain with acid-fast stains; therefore when negative images are encountered, or when the character of the lesion suggests that *Mycobacterium* spp. be considered, an acid-fast stain can be performed to show the organism (Figure 5-12, *B*) and/or cultures for *Mycobacterium* spp. can be performed for identification.

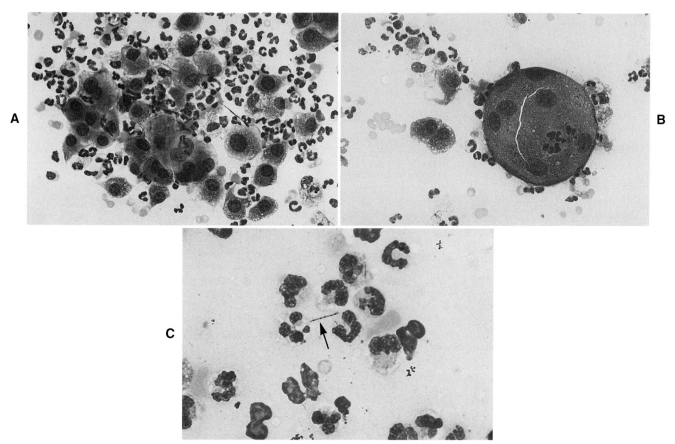

Figure 5-3 Impression smears of a granulomatous nodule from a dog. **A,** Pyogranulomatous inflammatory cell population. Macrophages comprise more than 15% of the cells present. (Diff-Quik, original magnification 160×.) **B,** Large, multinucleate, inflammatory giant cell with scattered neutrophils and macrophages from the same lesion shown in **A.** (Diff-Quik, original magnification 132×.) **C,** Long, slender, filamentous bacterial rod *(arrow)* present among inflammatory cells. Notice the dark granules interspersed along the length of the bacterium. This morphological presentation is suggestive of *Actinomyces* or *Nocardia* spp. (Diff-Quik, original magnification 400×.)

Because these organisms are often refractory to common antibiotic therapy, and reliable culture has special requirements, cytology is very useful in indicating to the practitioner that special cultures are needed.

Large Bacterial Rods: Large bacterial rods that are pathogenic and sometimes infect the cutaneous and subcutaneous tissues include *Clostridia* spp., and infrequently, *Bacillus* spp. When large bacterial rods are thought to be pathogenic, both aerobic and anaerobic cultures should be performed. Also, the smears should be inspected for large rods containing spores (Figure 5-13). If spore formation is observed, *Clostridium* spp. is most likely present. Occasionally, extremely large nonpathogenic bacterial rods *(Simonsiella)* are observed in cytologic specimens (e.g., contaminated tracheal washes; Figure 5-14).

Yeast, Dermatophytes, Hyphating Fungi, and Algae

Sporothrix schenckii: A *Sporothrix schenckii* infection (sporotrichosis) can cause raised, proliferative lesions that are often ulcerated on the skin of dogs and cats. In cats,

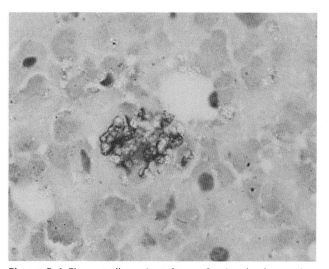

Figure 5-4 Fine-needle aspirate from a foreign-body reaction in a dog. Refractile foreign material is scattered throughout the photomicrograph. A large clump of cell debris and refractile foreign-body material is in the center. (Wright's stain, original magnification 100×.)

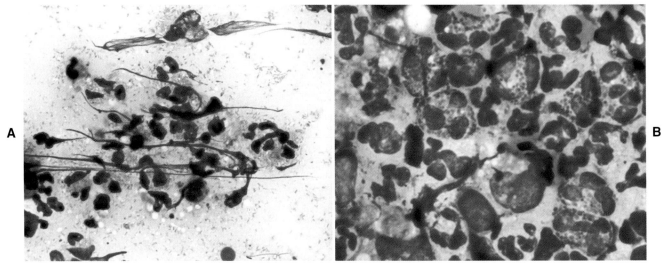

Figure 5-5 A, Skin scraping from a cat with allergic dermatitis. Eosinophilic inflammation, characterized by large numbers of eosinophils, is shown. Free eosinophil granules are observed in the background of the smear. (Wright's stain.) **B,** Aspirate from a mass on a dog. High numbers of eosinophils and neutrophils, scattered macrophages, and low numbers of lymphocytes are observed. These mixed inflammatory reactions are sometimes called *mixed eosinophilic inflammation.* (Wright's stain.)

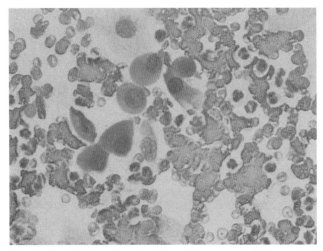

Figure 5-6 Aspirate from a dog with a nasal polyp caused by *Rhinosporidium seeberi.* Note the dysplastic epithelial cells (mild anisocytosis, anisokaryosis, prominent nucleoli, coarse chromatin, cytoplasmic basophilia) and the numerous neutrophils. *Rhinosporidium* organisms were found in other areas of the smear. (Wright's stain, original magnification 100×.)

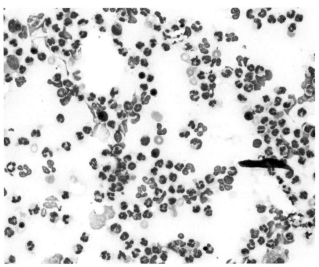

Figure 5-7 Neutrophilic inflammation is characterized by the marked predominance of neutrophils. (Wright's stain.)

many organisms are produced, and cytologic evaluation leads to an easy diagnosis. In dogs, however, organisms are scarce, and cytologic preparations must be carefully screened. If organisms are not found, the lesion should be cultured or a biopsy of the lesion should be submitted for histopathologic evaluation.

In cytologic preparations stained with Romanowsky-type stains, *S. schenckii* (Figure 5-15) are round to oval or fusiform (cigar-shaped). They are about 3 to 9 microns long and 1 to 3 microns wide and stain pale to medium blue with a slightly eccentric pink or purple nucleus. They may be confused with *Histoplasma capsulatum* if only a few organisms are found and they are not classically fusiform.

Histoplasma capsulatum: Although *Histoplasma capsulatum* usually infects the lungs and/or other internal organs, it can infect the skin, with or without concurrent involvement of internal organs. Cutaneous histoplasmosis lesions are typically raised and proliferative, and may ulcerate. On rare occasions, they may produce draining tracts. These lesions usually yield many organisms within macrophages and some extracellular organisms. A few organisms may be found in neutrophils. In cytologic preparations stained with Romanowsky-type stains, *H. capsulatum* organisms (Figure 5-16) are round or slightly oval, but are not fusiform. They are about 2 to 4 microns in diameter (a fourth to half the size of a red blood cell [RBC]), stain pale to medium blue, and contain

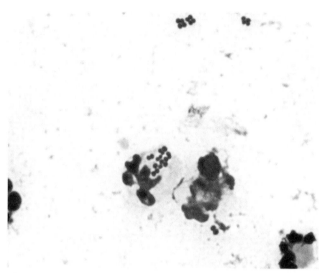

Figure 5-8 A neutrophil containing phagocytized bacterial cocci and scattered extracellular bacterial cocci are shown. (Wright's stain.)

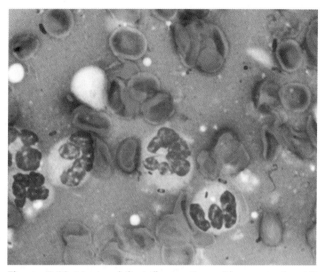

Figure 5-10 Neutrophilic inflammation with one neutrophil containing a phagocytized bacterial rod and scattered extracellular bipolar bacterial rods. (Wright's stain.)

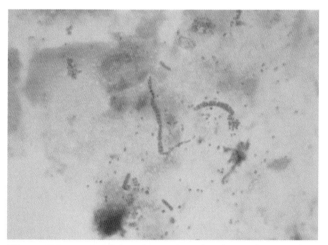

Figure 5-9 Imprint from the underside of a scab caused by *Dermatophilus congolensis*. There is a background of squamous debris and two chains of bacterial doublets. (Wright's stain, original magnification 250×.)

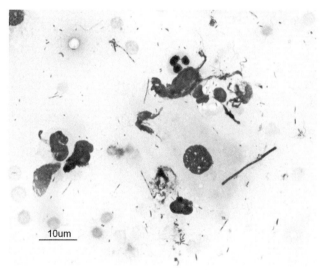

Figure 5-11 The filamentous bacterial rods staining bluish with reddish dots are characteristic of the *Actinomycetes* family. (Wright's stain.)

an eccentric pink to purple staining nucleus that is often crescent shaped. There is usually a clear halo around the yeast.

Blastomyces dermatitidis: A *Blastomyces dermatitidis* infection (blastomycosis) can involve the skin, eyes, and internal organs. Cutaneous lesions of blastomycosis are usually raised and proliferative, and often ulcerate. Cutaneous lesions should be sought when any form of blastomycosis is suspected. Aspirates from these lesions or impression smears of ulcerated lesions usually have a cell composition characteristic of pyogranulomatous inflammation (see Figure 5-3) and organisms ranging in number from a few to many. In cytologic preparations stained with Romanowsky-type stains, the organisms (Figure 5-17) are blue, spherical, 8 to 20 microns in diameter, and thick-walled. Most organisms are single, but

occasionally, organisms showing broad-based budding are found. These organisms are distinctly larger than *S. schenckii* or *H. capsulatum* and are differentiated from *Cryptococcus neoformans* by their color, lack of a clear-staining capsule, and broad-based budding. They are distinguished from *Coccidioides immitis* by their smaller size and lack of endospores.

Cryptococcus neoformans: A *Cryptococcus neoformans* infection (cryptococcosis) can involve the subcutaneous tissues causing subcutaneous swellings, but more commonly involves the upper respiratory and central nervous systems. Cryptococcosis usually elicits a granulomatous response (epithelioid macrophages and/or inflammatory giant cells). In some cytologic preparations, *Cryptococcus* organisms may outnumber inflammatory and tissue cells. The organism (Figure 5-18) is extremely

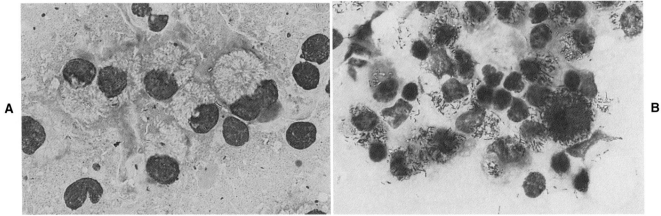

Figure 5-12 A, Impression smear of a lesion induced by *Mycobacterium* spp. Many large macrophages contain nonstaining bacteria that appear as negative images. Numerous negative images are also present extracellularly. (Wright's stain, original magnification 400×.) **B,** Acid-fast stain of a slide from the same lesion. Many red-staining bacterial rods can be seen extracellularly and within macrophages. (Acid-fast stain, original magnification 250×.)

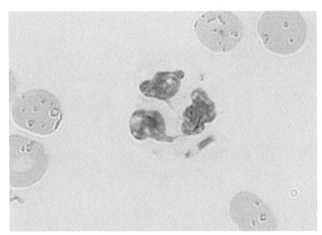

Figure 5-13 A neutrophil containing a phagocytized spore-forming bacillus. The spore is recognized as a clear area in the bacterium. This slide is from a dog with a clostridial infection.

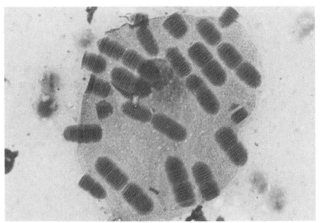

Figure 5-14 A large superficial squamous cell with many adherent *Simonsiella* bacteria on its surface and a few bacterial cocci *(lower center)*. *Simonsiella* organisms appear microscopically as a single large bacterium but are actually several bacterial rods lying side by side, giving the striated appearance. (Wright's stain.)

pleomorphic, ranging from spherical to fusiform, but usually is easily recognized because of its thick mucoid capsule. Occasionally, nonencapsulated, or rough, forms are found. The organism is about 4 to 15 microns in diameter without its capsule and about 8 to 40 microns in diameter with its capsule. In cytologic preparations stained with Romanowsky-type stains, the organism stains deep pink to blue-purple and may be slightly granular. The capsule is usually clear and homogenous, but on some occasions, it may stain light to medium pink. Unlike *Blastomyces* spp., *Cryptococcus* spp. demonstrate narrow-based budding.

Coccidioides immitis: *Coccidioides immitis* infections generally involve the lungs and bones of dogs. In some cases, however, cutaneous lesions (masses) and draining tracts from bony lesions develop. Cytologic preparations usually have a cell composition characteristic of pyogranulomatous or granulomatous inflammation. *Coccidioides* organisms (Figure 5-20) may be scarce in some lesions;

therefore cytologic preparations from suspected coccidioidomycosis lesions should be examined carefully. In cytologic preparations stained with Romanowsky-type stains, the organisms are large (10 to 100 microns in diameter), double-contoured, blue or clear spheres with finely granular protoplasm and will often appear folded or crumpled. Round endospores from 2 to 5 microns in diameter may be seen in some of the larger organisms. The tremendous variation in the size and presence of endospores differentiates *C. immitis* from nonbudding *B. dermatitidis*.

Dermatophytes: The dermatophytes *Microsporum* and *Trichophyton* spp. commonly cause ringworm in dogs and cats (Figure 5-21). Scrapings from the edge of lesions are the best cytologic samples for finding dermatophytes. They can be identified in cytologic preparations using

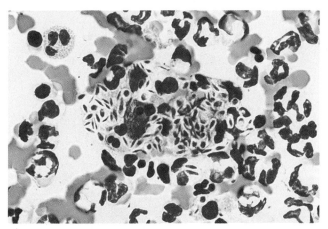

Figure 5-15 Impression smear from an ulcerative lesion on the leg of a cat. Many *Sporothrix* spp. are present in a large macrophage in the center of the field. Both oval and cigar-shaped organisms are present. (Wright's stain, original magnification 250×.)

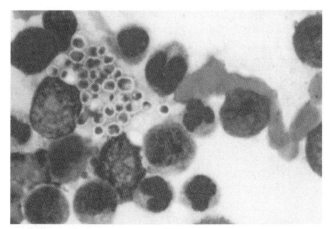

Figure 5-16 A large macrophage containing numerous *Histoplasma capsulatum* organisms is shown. (Wright's stain.)

the standard 10% potassium hydroxide stain for hair, in wet-mount preparations stained with new methylene blue, or air-dried preparations stained with Romanowsky-type stains. Cytologically, fungal mycelia and spores are found within hair shafts (*Trichophyton* spp.) or on the hair shaft surface (*Microsporum* spp.). With Romanowsky-type stains, the mycelia and spores stain medium to dark blue with a thin, clear halo. An inflammatory reaction of an admixture of neutrophils, macrophages, lymphocytes, and plasma cells may be seen in cytologic preparations from skin scrapings.

Fungi That Form Hyphae in Cutaneous and Subcutaneous Tissues: Many fungi can infect the cutaneous and subcutaneous tissue and form hyphae (Figure 5-22). These fungi usually cause small to large raised, proliferative lesions that often ulcerate. They also induce a granulomatous, inflammatory response that is characterized by epithelioid macrophages and inflammatory giant cells (see Figure 5-3). The number of neutrophils, lymphocytes, plasma cells, and eosinophils varies. Some hyphating fungi do not stain well with hematologic-type stains and are recognized as negative images (Figure 5-23). The organisms that cause the disease phycomycosis typically do not stain with hematologic stains and induce an eosinophilic, granulomatous response in the infected tissue (Figure 5-24). A fungal culture or histopathology with special immunohistochemical stains may be used to definitively classify the organism involved.

Prototheca zopfii and P. wickerhamii: *Prototheca* spp. are colorless algae that are ubiquitous in the southern regions of America, but only rarely cause disease (i.e., protothecosis). In dogs, the disease is often disseminated, but only cutaneous protothecosis has been reported in cats.[1-4] Cytologic preparations reveal an inflammatory response characteristic of pyogranulomatous or granulomatous inflammation and organisms ranging

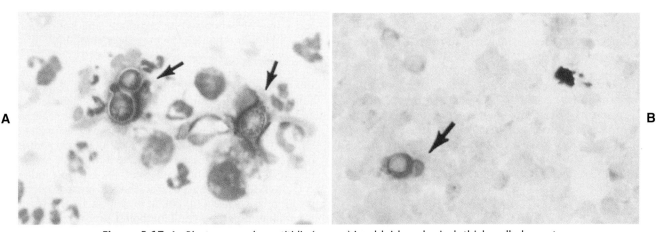

Figure 5-17 A, *Blastomyces dermatitidis (arrows)* is a bluish, spherical, thick-walled, yeast like organism in Romanowsky-stained smears. The organisms are 8 to 20 μm in diameter. Occasionally, a single, broad-based bud may be present (Wright's stain.) **B,** A budding *Blastomyces* organism *(arrow)*. (Wright's stain.)

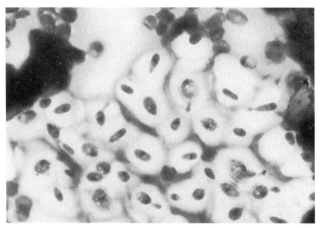

Figure 5-18 *Cryptococcus neoformans* is a spherical, yeast like organism that frequently has a thick, clear-staining mucoid capsule. The organism with its capsule ranges in size from 8 to 40 µm. Occasionally, a single narrow-based bud may be present. Numerous budding and nonbudding *Cryptococcus* organisms with prominent nonstaining capsules are shown. (Wright's stain.)

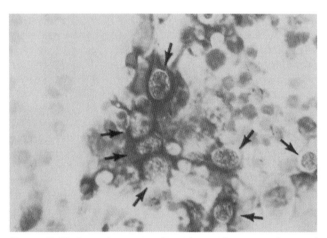

Figure 5-19 *Prototheca* organisms *(arrows)* are round to oval and have a granular basophilic cytoplasm and a clear cell wall. (Wright's stain.)

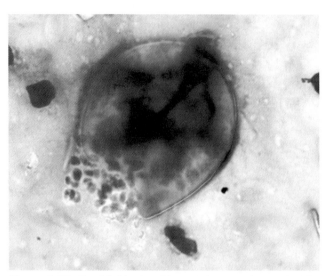

Figure 5-20 *Coccidioides immitis* organisms are large, double-contoured, clear to blue-staining, spherical bodies that range in size from 10 microns to greater than 100 microns. Occasionally endospores varying from 2 to 5 microns in diameter may be seen within some of the larger spherules. (Wright's stain.)

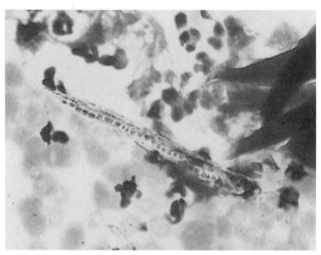

Figure 5-21 Scraping from a dog with ringworm. Several degenerating neutrophils are present with red blood cells and a row of dermatophyte organisms attached to a hair shaft. (Wright's stain, original magnification 330×.)

in number from a few to many. The organisms (Figure 5-19) are round to oval and are from 1 to 14 microns wide and 1 to 16 microns long. When stained with Romanowsky-type stains, they have granular basophilic cytoplasm and a clear cell wall about 0.5 micron thick. The organisms, except those that are small and immature, contain a small nucleus that stains pink to deep purple. A single organism may consist of two or four or more endospores. Most organisms are extracellular, but small forms may be found in macrophages and neutrophils.

Protozoa

***Leishmania* spp.:** *Leishmania donovani* can infect the skin and subcutaneous tissues of the dog, producing small to large thickened, ulcerated areas. Imprints, scrapings, and aspirates yield numerous cells, which are an

admixture of neutrophils, macrophages, lymphocytes, and plasma cells, with neutrophils or macrophages possibly predominating. Usually, numerous organisms are found within macrophages and free in the preparation. *Leishmania* organisms are small (2 to 4 microns) and oval (Figure 5-25). They have an oval, light purple nucleus and a small, dark purple, rod-shaped kinetoplast. The position of the kinetoplast with respect to the nucleus is variable; however, the kinetoplast tends to be located between the nucleus and greatest volume of cytoplasm. The presence of a kinetoplast distinguishes this organism from *Toxoplasma* spp. and small, fungal yeasts, such as *Histoplasma*.

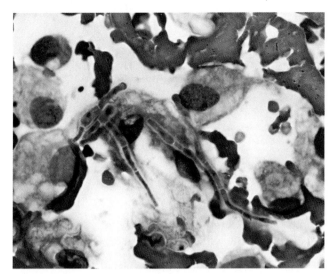

Figure 5-22 Fungal hyphae and a granulomatous inflammatory reaction are shown. (Wright's stain.)

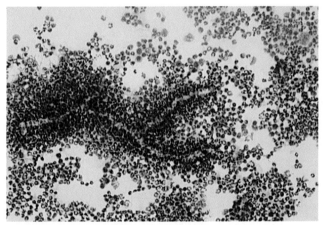

Figure 5-23 The negative image of a nonstaining fungal hyphae can be seen in the background of inflammatory cells. Some fungi do not stain with the routine Romanowsky stains. (Wright's stain.) *(Courtesy of Dr. K. Latimer.)*

NONINFECTIOUS INFLAMMATORY LESIONS

Some inflammatory lesions are not due to infectious agents but to conditions such as immune-mediated diseases, allergic reactions, and sterile foreign-body reactions. Cytologic and clinical evaluation may be helpful to diagnose these lesions. Often, the history and the clinical presentation suggest the nature of the lesion (e.g., injection reaction or insect bite) and a cytologic examination is used to help rule out the presence of neoplasia or infection.

Injection Site Reactions

Inflammatory reactions at the site of previous injections, most typically vaccinations, are common. Sometimes there is a known history of recent vaccination; other times, an injection reaction is suspected based on the anatomic location. In cats, such lesions are frequently aspirated and cytologically evaluated to differentiate them from postvaccinal sarcomas. The cytologic findings in these lesions primarily consist of high numbers of mononuclear inflammatory cells (Figure 5-26). Depending on the lesion and the site of sampling from the lesion, the slides may primarily consist of small, mature lymphocytes (Figure 5-26, *A*), macrophages, or a mixture of both. Neutrophils may be present but usually are not the predominant cell type.

The most characteristic feature of these lesions is the presence of large amounts of amorphous, homogenous, brightly eosinophilic material that is both extracellular and within macrophages. When present within macrophages, this material may be concentrated in phagosomes and appear as round spheres (see Figure 5-26, *C*) that can be differentiated from mast cell granules because they are larger, more variable in size, and different in color (i.e., more brightly eosinophilic).

Clusters of reactive mesenchymal cells (see Figure 5-26, *B*) may be present in the samples. Such cells may have features similar to those of neoplastic mesenchymal cells, raising concerns about the possibility of neoplasia. The mesenchymal cells in an injection-site reaction make up a small percentage of the total cell population. If there is strong concern about the possibility of mesenchymal neoplasia, a tissue biopsy should be taken for histologic examination, or the lesion should be closely monitored clinically and reevaluated if it continues to enlarge or does not regress over time.

Linear Eosinophilic Granulomas and Eosinophilic Plaques: Linear granulomas and eosinophilic plaques (lesions of the eosinophilic granuloma complex) occur most commonly in cats, but may occur in dogs. Cytologically, eosinophilic granulomas are characterized by a predominance of eosinophils with a few neutrophils and macrophages (Figure 5-27). High numbers of eosinophilic granules, the result of cell rupture, are often present in the background. A few lymphocytes, plasma cells, and fibroblasts also may be present. Some of the fibroblasts may have anaplastic characteristics including cytomegaly, basophilic cytoplasm, large nuclei, and large prominent nucleoli (Figure 5-27, *B*). Occasionally, aspirates from eosinophilic granulomas fail to yield eosinophils. Biopsies from these lesions may be submitted for histopathologic evaluation to confirm clinical suspicion of eosinophilic granuloma.

Cytologically, eosinophilic granulomas cannot always be differentiated from allergic and parasite-induced inflammatory reactions. If the clinical evidence in conjunction with cytologic findings is not sufficient to establish the diagnosis, a biopsy of the lesion can be submitted for histopathologic evaluation.

Sterile, Foreign-Body-Induced Inflammation

Cytologic preparations from inflammatory lesions induced by sterile foreign bodies usually contain an admixture of neutrophils and macrophages. Many of the macrophages present in foreign-body reactions may be epithelioid macrophages, but inflammatory giant cells may also be present. Eosinophils are occasionally present, and

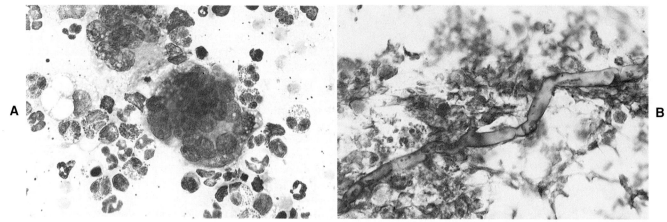

Figure 5-24 Aspirates from a dog with phycomycosis. **A,** The organisms that cause phycomycosis do not stain with hematologic stains and cannot be seen on the slides. Many eosinophils, macrophages, and multinucleate giant cells are present. Sometimes the organisms can be seen as negative images against a proteinaceous background. (Wright's stain, original magnification 250×.) **B,** Slides stained with periodic acid–Schiff reveal thick, branching, nonseptate hyphae. (Original magnification 250×.)

lymphocytes and plasma cells may be present in variable numbers. Sometimes, refractile material (see Figure 5-4) can be found. When a sterile foreign body is suspected, the smear can be polarized. Some foreign material refracts polarized light, but endogenous debris (e.g., hemosiderin), which might be mistaken as particulate foreign-body material, does not refract polarized light.

Panniculitis (Fat Necrosis, or Steatitis): Panniculitis refers to necrosis and inflammation of the subcutaneous adipose tissue and may occur in dogs or cats. Panniculitis can result from many different causes and does not constitute a specific disease. Physical damage (e.g., trauma or foreign body), infectious conditions (e.g., bacterial or fungal), pancreatic disease (e.g., pancreatitis or pancreatic carcinoma), nutritional diseases (e.g., vitamin E deficiency in cats), and immune-mediated conditions have been reported as causes of panniculitis in dogs and cats. Idiopathic, sterile, nodular panniculitis is a term applied to sterile panniculitis of unknown etiology.

Cytologic preparations from areas of panniculitis usually contain variable numbers of macrophages, inflammatory giant cells, and reactive spindle cells (Figure 5-28) interspersed with many clusters of fat cells and free fat droplets. Lymphocytes and neutrophils may be present in variable numbers. The inflammatory cells, giant cells, and reactive spindle cells may contain clear vacuoles indicating ingestion of fat. The spindle cells are often dysplastic and, if caution is not used, can be misclassified as neoplastic.

Allergic Inflammatory Reactions

Cytologically, allergic inflammatory reactions are characterized by numerous eosinophils (see Figure 5-5). The number of neutrophils and mast cells varies. Lymphocytes, plasma cells, and macrophages may also be present if the condition is chronic.

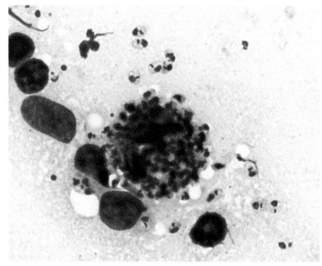

Figure 5-25 Numerous *Leishmania donovani* organisms within a macrophage and extracellularly. (Wright's stain.)

Parasite-Induced Inflammatory Reactions

Parasite-induced inflammatory reactions are characterized by numerous eosinophils, neutrophils ranging in number from few to many, and possibly large numbers of macrophages as well. The number of lymphocytes and plasma cells varies, and, occasionally, the parasitic organism is found.

Immune-Mediated Skin Lesions

Cytologic preparations from immune-mediated skin lesions, such as pemphigus, usually contain neutrophils and necrotic debris. A few lymphocytes and plasma cells may occasionally be present, and the lesion may be secondarily infected. Because there are no specific cytologic findings, histopathologic evaluation of a properly collected and prepared biopsy is necessary for diagnosis of immune-mediated skin lesions.

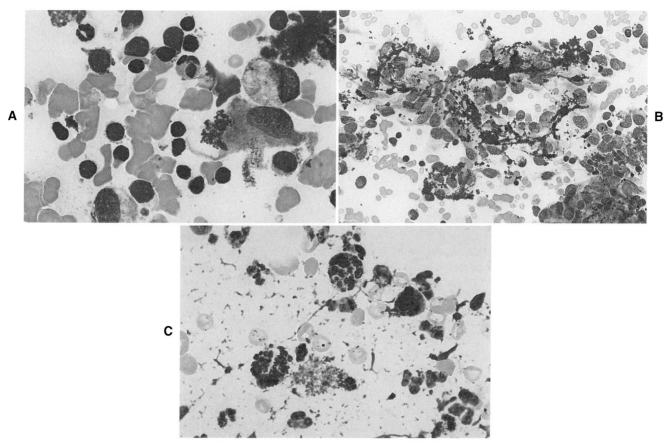

Figure 5-26 Cytologic appearance of injection site reactions. **A,** Vaccine reaction from a cat. The slide consisted primarily of small mature lymphocytes with lesser numbers of macrophages. Extracellular eosinophilic material can be seen. (Wright's stain, original magnification 330×.) **B,** Different field from the same slide as in **A.** A large aggregate of eosinophilic material surrounded by reactive fibroblasts, which compose a small minority of the cells present and do not display prominent nuclear criteria of malignancy. In some cases, it is difficult to distinguish reactive fibroblasts from neoplastic cells. (Wright's stain, original magnification 132×.) **C,** Injection reaction from a dog. Macrophages are more plentiful on these slides, many of which contain phagocytized material, and must not be confused with mast cells. (Wright's stain, original magnification 330×.)

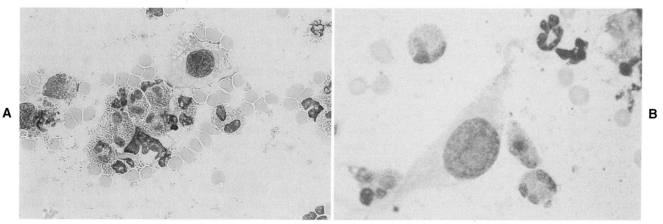

Figure 5-27 Aspirates from an eosinophilic granuloma. **A,** Eosinophils and free eosinophil granules are present along with a single macrophage and scattered red blood cells. (Wright's stain, original magnification 250×.) **B,** A large, reactive fibroblast is present along with several eosinophils and a neutrophil. (Wright's stain, original magnification 250×.)

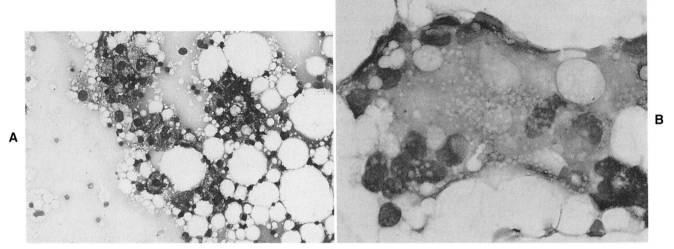

Figure 5-28 Aspirates of a cutaneous nodule from a dog with panniculitis (steatitis). **A,** Many macrophages, which have foamy appearances from phagocytizing lipids, are scattered among lipid droplets. (Wright's stain, original magnification 100×.) **B,** Higher magnification of dysplastic cells with small to large vacuoles in their cytoplasm. Cell borders are indistinct. (Wright's stain, original magnification 250×.) *(Courtesy the University of Georgia, College of Veterinary Medicine.)*

Traumatic Skin Lesions

Traumatic skin lesions may be caused by physical trauma or caustic injury. The cytologic findings in preparations from traumatic skin lesions are nonspecific and usually consist of numerous neutrophils and, possibly, an abundant amount of necrotic material and/or bacteria from secondary infection. History and physical examination usually help establish the suspicion of either physical or caustic injury.

Collagen Necrosis

Collagen necrosis elicits an inflammatory response characterized by a marked infiltration of eosinophils and monocytes and development of epithelioid macrophages and inflammatory giant cells. As a result, cytologic preparations from areas of collagen necrosis contain numerous eosinophils and varying numbers of macrophages, epithelioid macrophages, and inflammatory giant cells. Lymphocytes and plasma cells are scarce. Histopathologic evaluation of a biopsy from the lesion is usually necessary for definitive diagnosis.

Insect Bites

Cytologic preparations from welts caused by acute allergic reactions (i.e., bee stings) usually contain only a few local tissue cells and a few neutrophils and/or eosinophils. Older lesions from insect bites may contain a mixture of neutrophils, eosinophils, macrophages, lymphocytes, and plasma cells, along with a few local tissue cells.

Snake Bites

Cytologic preparations from recent snake bites tend to be of low cellularity; only local tissue cells and a few neutrophils are present. Neutrophilic infiltration of the area bitten is very rapid. Within a few hours of a bite, the number of neutrophils begins to increase markedly, so the number of neutrophils in cytologic preparations from older snake bites increases accordingly. Within a couple days, such preparations contain necrotic debris, numerous neutrophils, and variable numbers of macrophages.

EVALUATION OF NONINFLAMMATORY CELL POPULATIONS

Tissue cells found on cytologic samples may arise from normal, hyperplastic, dysplastic, and/or neoplastic tissue. The skin is the most common site for neoplasms in dogs and cats.[5,6] In one survey, neoplasms of the cutaneous and subcutaneous tissues accounted for 67.5% of all canine tumors.[5] Cutaneous and subcutaneous neoplasms may be of epithelial, mesenchymal (spindle cell tumors), or discrete cell (round cell) origin. Cytologic findings often indicate the cell of origin and the malignant potential of the tumor. Epithelial tumors generally yield medium to large, round to caudate cells with distinct cytoplasmic borders. Cells are often in clumps, groups, or sheets. Mesenchymal tumors yield a few to many cells, some of which are fusiform or stellate in shape. Most of the cells exfoliate individually, but there may be cells present in large aggregates. Individual cells that are well spread out often have indistinct cell borders. Multinucleation and the production of extracellular matrix are also commonly found. Discrete cell (round cell) tumors yield high numbers of small to medium round cells that are individually distributed across the smear. Cell borders are usually distinct.

The cellular morphology should be evaluated for criteria of malignancy (see Table 2-2). When no inflammatory cells are present, criteria of malignancy are more meaningful than when inflammatory cells are present. If many of the cells show three or more nuclear criteria of malignancy

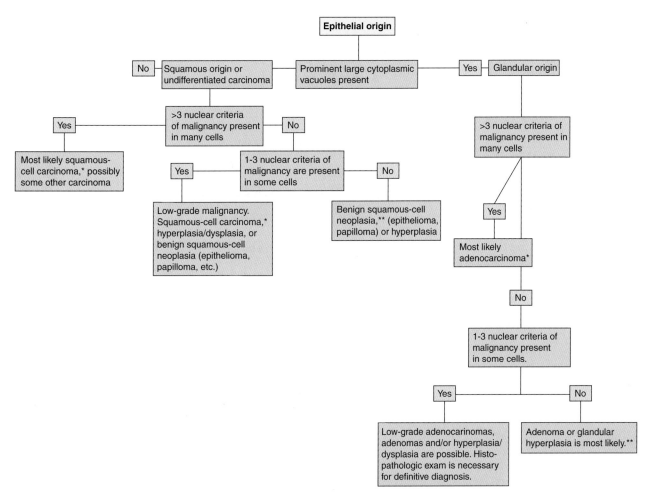

* If evidence of inflammation or other causes of dysplasia are
present, dysplasia cannot be ruled out.
** Well-differentiated malignant neoplasia cannot be totally
ruled out.

Figure 5-29 An algorithm to aid in evaluating cytologic smears containing epithelial cells (large, round to caudate cells with many cell clumps) from cutaneous or subcutaneous tissues.

and no inflammatory cells are present, the lesion is most likely a malignant neoplasm. If fewer significant criteria of malignancy are present or only a few cells are affected, the cytologic preparation should be referred for interpretation, or a biopsy of the lesion should be submitted for histopathologic examination. Sometimes tumors cannot be cytologically classified as to the cell of origin; however, these tumors often demonstrate sufficient criteria of malignancy for them to be recognized as malignant.

Figures 5-29 and 5-30 provide flow charts to aid in evaluating cytologic smears containing epithelial cells and spindle cells, respectively. The typical cytologic characteristics of selected tumors are discussed in subsequent sections.

Discrete Cell (Round Cell) Tumors

Discrete or round cell tumors yield cytologic preparations containing numerous individually oriented, small to medium sized, round cells. Lymphoma, histiocytoma, mast cell tumors, transmissible venereal tumors (TVTs), and extramedullary plasmacytoma are the most common

discrete cell tumors.[7-10] Occasionally, other tumors such as melanomas and basal cell tumors mimic discrete-cell patterns. Selected discrete cell tumors are briefly discussed later. See Chapter 4 for a more complete discussion of round cell tumors and for an algorithm to aid in evaluating aspirates containing primarily discrete (round) cells.

Lymphoma (Lymphosarcoma): Several forms of lymphoid neoplasia can occur in the skin of dogs and cats. They usually produce multiple plaque-like lesions, but occasionally produce solitary nodules[9,11,12] Aspirates of these lesions usually yield highly cellular cytologic preparations (Figure 5-31).

Preparations from histiocytic lymphoma contain lymphoid cells with some histiocytic cell characteristics. The epitheliotropic form of cutaneous lymphoma (i.e., mycosis fungoides) often comprises such cells. Similar to monocytes, they have pleomorphic, indented to lobular nuclei (Figure 5-32). They also tend to have more abundant, somewhat lighter, basophilic cytoplasm. Histiocytic lymphomas typically occur as multiple, rapidly growing, plaque-like lesions in middle-aged or older dogs. In

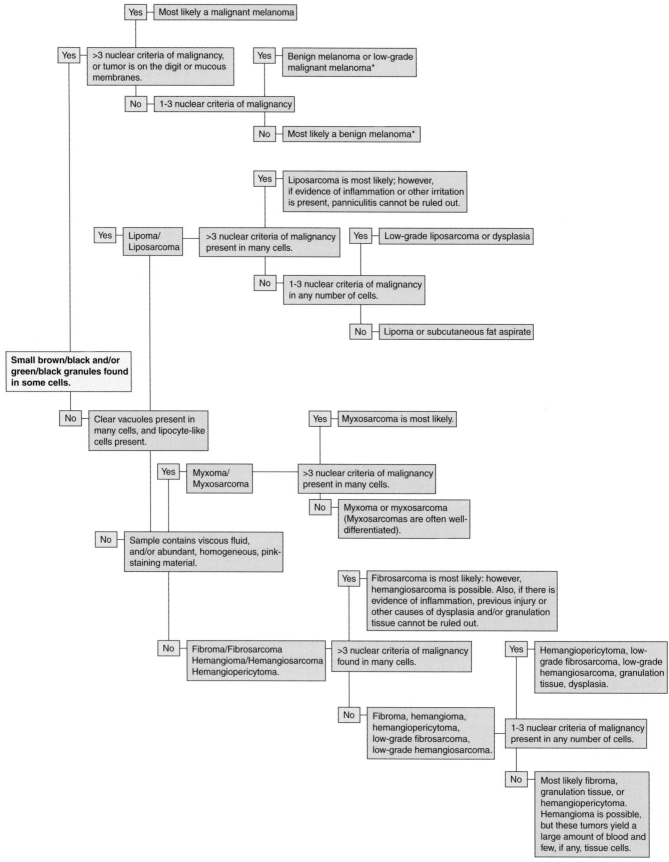

* All melanomas of the digits, oropharynx, and mucous membranes should be considered potentially malignant.

Figure 5-30 An algorithm to aid in evaluating aspirates containing spindle cells.

contrast, histiocytomas typically occur as solitary nodular lesions on the heads and extremities of young dogs. Cells from a benign histiocytoma are cytologically distinct (see section on histiocytomas later in this chapter).

Preparations from lymphoblastic lymphomas contain numerous lymphoblasts. Lymphoblasts are larger than neutrophils and have a moderate amount of cytoplasm that stains light to medium blue and is usually displaced to one side of the nucleus. Lymphoblasts have a higher nuclear-to-cytoplasmic ratio than other discrete cell tumors and have indented to irregular nuclei that have smudged to stippled chromatin patterns and often contain several prominent nucleoli.

Preparations from lymphocytic lymphomas are composed of small lymphocytes that cannot be readily differentiated from normal lymphocytes. These tumors require histopathologic analysis for definitive diagnosis.

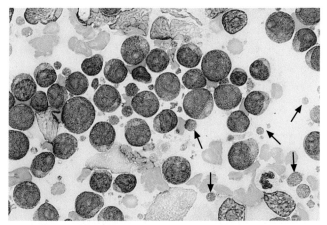

Figure 5-31 Smear consisting primarily of large lymphoblasts from a dog with lymphoma. Scattered lymphoglandular bodies *(arrows)* are present in the background of the smear. (Wright's stain.)

Mast Cell Tumors: Mast cell tumors generally exfoliate high numbers of cells with moderate amounts of cytoplasm containing small, red-purple granules. Most mast cell tumors yield cells that contain many granules (Figure 5-33, *A*). These cells may be so densely packed that individual granules are difficult to discern, except in ruptured cells. The cells usually have round nuclei, which often stain palely because the highly granulated cytoplasm stains so intensely. Variable numbers of eosinophils are usually present among the mast cells and occasionally may be almost as numerous as mast cells.

If a tumor has degranulated, cell numbers may be low because of tissue edema. Also, the cells present may contain few granules, but have many free granules present in the background. Occasionally, anaplastic mast cell tumors contain only rare granules and often display numerous cytologic criteria of malignancy including anisocytosis, anisokaryosis, nuclear pleomorphism, and variable nuclear-to-cytoplasmic ratio. Sometimes, Diff-Quik fails to stain mast cell granules, making the cytologic picture confusing (see Figure 5-33, *B*). Such mast cells may resemble lymphoid cells, plasma cells, or macrophages; although some granules are generally evident if the slides are thoroughly examined. A person using Diff-Quik as a cytologic stain should always consider this possibility when a discrete cell population is encountered.

Mast cell tumors should be evaluated for criteria of malignancy. This may be difficult to do in heavily granulated tumors because the granules often totally obscure nuclear detail. All mast cell tumors should be considered potentially malignant, and surgical removal with wide borders is indicated. A small percentage of tumors with uniform, heavily granulated cells (i.e., well-differentiated tumors) will be behaviorally malignant. The majority of tumors with poorly granulated cells that demonstrate significant cytologic criteria of malignancy will be malignant. Examination of buffy coat preparations, bone marrow aspirates, and any enlarged lymph nodes or abdominal organs (especially the spleen) may be helpful in determining systemic disease. Aspiration of thickened incision lines can help detect local recurrence.

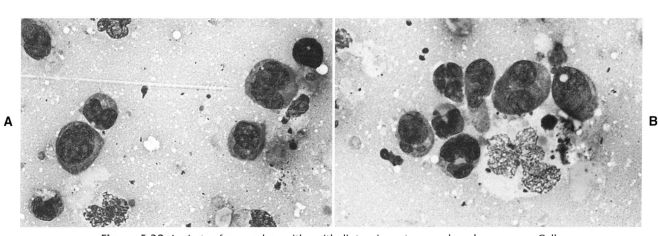

Figure 5-32 Aspirates from a dog with epitheliotropic, cutaneous lymphosarcoma. Cells from this form of lymphosarcoma often have a histiocytic appearance. **A** and **B,** Blasts with irregularly shaped, monocytoid nuclei and more typical lymphoblasts. Lymphoglandular bodies are present in the background. Cells with phagocytic activity are present in adjacent fields. (Wright's stain, original magnification 250×.)

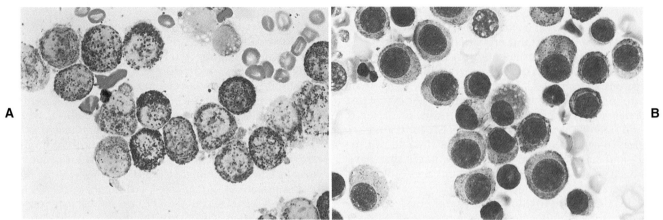

Figure 5-33 Aspirates of a heavily granulated mast cell tumor from the leg of a dog. **A,** Wright's-stained slide reveals many cytoplasmic granules that take the stain so well that the slides may be understained, and the nucleus of the cells may appear as a negative image. (Wright's stain, original magnification 250×.) **B,** Diff-Quik–stained slide from the same lesion as in **A.** The granules of some mast cell tumors do not stain well with Diff-Quik, so these cells can resemble plasma cells or macrophages. If the smears are carefully examined, faint granules can usually be seen in some of the cells. (Diff-Quik, original magnification 250×.)

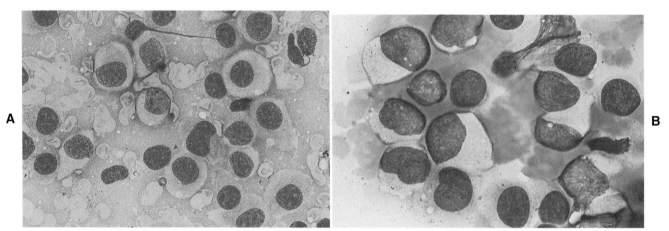

Figure 5-34 Aspirates from a benign cutaneous histiocytoma. **A,** Pale-staining cytoplasm stains lighter than the proteinaceous background in this slide of many histiocytoma cells. (Wright's stain, original magnification 250×.) **B,** Numerous histiocytoma cells show irregularly shaped nuclei and light blue-gray cytoplasm. (Wright's stain, original magnification 400×.)

Histiocytomas: Histiocytomas are common tumors of young dogs (Figure 5-34). Cells from a histiocytoma show a discrete cell pattern, are somewhat larger than neutrophils, and have a moderate amount of pale blue cytoplasm that may stain lighter than the background if a significant amount of protein-rich tissue fluid is present (Figure 5-34, *A*). When a proteinaceous background is present, cell borders may be difficult to discern. Histiocytoma cells have round, oval, or irregularly shaped nuclei with finely etched, lacy, or finely stippled chromatin patterns. These cells may contain multiple small, indistinct nucleoli (Figure 5-34, *A*). Mitotic figures may be seen, but are not as characteristic as in the histologic findings of these tumors. The amount and color of the cytoplasm and the lack of lymphoglandular bodies are useful in distinguishing these cells from lymphoid cells.

Histiocytomas are benign and usually regress spontaneously within a few weeks to months. Regression is associated with an infiltrate of small lymphocytes into the tumor, so cytologic preparations taken from some tumors may yield a mixture of histiocytoma cells and small, mature lymphocytes.

Plasmacytomas (Extramedullary Plasmacytomas): Cutaneous plasmacytomas are tumors of plasma cell origin, but they are not associated with systemic multiple myeloma. They are usually hairless, small, smooth, raised tumors and tend to occur in older dogs, with large breeds possibly being overrepresented. The majority of reported plasmacytomas have been benign; however, we have encountered plasmacytomas with malignant characteristics including recurrence, local invasion, and distant metastasis.

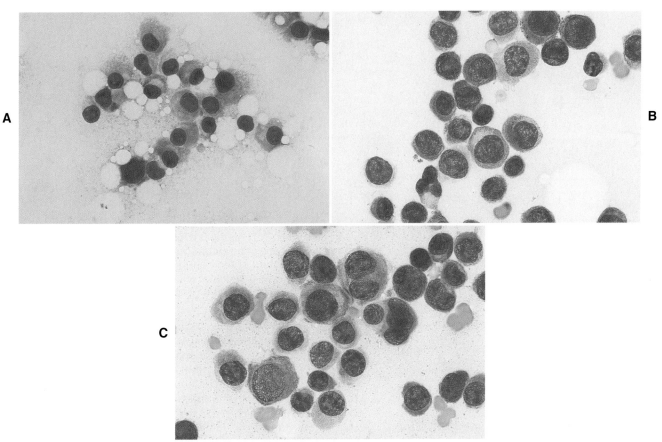

Figure 5-35 Aspirates from extramedullary plasma cell tumors. **A,** A population of uniform, well-differentiated plasma cells from a mass on a dog. The cells have the characteristic eccentric nucleus, and some also have a distinct, perinuclear clear area (i.e., Golgi zone). (Wright's stain, original magnification 250×.) **B,** Aspirate from a malignant extramedullary plasma cell tumor on the neck of a dog. Compared with the cells in **A,** these cells show more variability, a higher nuclear-to-cytoplasmic ratio, and coarse nuclear chromatin. Most of the cells are not as obviously plasmacytoid. When viewed histopathologically, this tumor had areas of amyloid deposition and stained positively for immunoglobulin light chain. Pulmonary metastases were present. (Wright's stain, original magnification 250×.) **C,** Same slide as **B.** Binucleate and multinucleate cells are present. (Wright's stain, original magnification 250×.)

Aspirates from plasmacytomas, like those from other discrete tumors, yield high numbers of cells that are evenly spread throughout the smear. The morphology of the individual cells varies between tumors (Figure 5-35). In some tumors, the cells are obviously plasmacytoid, resembling typical mature plasma cells (Figure 5-35, *A*), but in other cases, they are a less distinct population of discrete cells (Figure 5-35, *B* and *C*). These cells usually have a round nucleus with a moderate amount of deeply basophilic cytoplasm. Perinuclear clear areas (e.g., Golgi areas) often may not be present despite characteristically eccentric nuclei. Binucleate and multinucleate cells are common (Figure 5-35, *C*) and, along with a lack of lymphoglandular bodies, help differentiate these tumors from lymphomas.

Transmissible Venereal Tumors: Transmissible venereal tumors (TVTs) exfoliate many cells on scrapings, aspirates, and imprints. These cells are more pleomorphic than those of most other discrete cell tumors (Figure 5-36). TVT cells have a moderate amount of smoky to medium light blue cytoplasm that has distinct boundaries. A prominent feature of TVT cells is the presence of many clear, distinctly walled vacuoles both within the cytoplasm and extracellularly. The nuclei of TVT cells are round, show moderate to marked variation in size, and have coarse, cord-like chromatin with one or sometimes two very prominent, large nucleoli.

Epithelium

Epithelial cells tend to adhere cell-to-cell, so epithelial cell tumors typically exfoliate clumps of cells, but usually some individual cells are also present. Acinar or ductal arrangements may be seen in samples from adenomas and adenocarcinomas. Cells from epithelial cell tumors tend to be large or very large and have moderate to abundant cytoplasm and round nuclei. The nuclei generally have smooth to slightly coarse chromatin patterns that often become more coarse and ropy as malignant potential increases. The nuclei usually contain one or more prominent nucleoli that

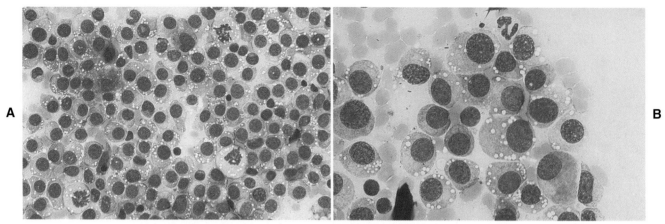

Figure 5-36 Aspirates of a transmissible venereal tumor (TVT) on the prepuce of a dog. **A,** Highly cellular slide of pleomorphic, discrete cells with two visible mitotic figures. (Wright's stain, original magnification 132×.) **B,** Higher magnification of the cells in **A.** Many clear vacuoles with distinct borders are present in these cells, as is characteristic of TVTs. Note the coarse nuclear chromatin. (Wright's stain, original magnification 250×.)

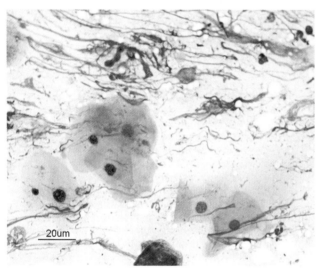

20um

Figure 5-37 Normal superficial squamous epithelial cells are very large, appear flattened, have an abundant amount of cytoplasm that stains light blue or aqua, and have a small, contracted, dark-staining nucleus without a discernible nucleolus or are anucleate.

become larger and more irregular in shape as malignant potential increases. Malignant epithelial cell tumors often show marked variations in cellular, nuclear, and nucleolar size and shape. These variations are most significant when occurring within the same cell or group of cells. Malignant epithelial cell tumors often display nuclear molding and a markedly increased and variable nuclear-to-cytoplasmic ratio. Highly malignant, poorly differentiated carcinomas tend to exfoliate more cells individually than in clusters.

Local inflammation or other irritation can cause epithelial cells to become dysplastic. Epithelial cells undergoing dysplasia may show mild to moderate variations in cellular, nuclear, and nucleolar size and shape; increased nuclear-to-cytoplasmic ratio; and coarse chromatin (in a few cells). Dysplasia usually does not cause bizarre nuclear and nucleolar morphology. When there is concern

that the abnormal tissue cell morphology observed in a cytologic sample is caused by dysplasia instead of neoplasia, a biopsy from the lesion should be submitted for histopathologic evaluation, or the cause of dysplasia should be treated and the lesion reevaluated cytologically.

Neoplasms of epithelial origin are often ulcerated and may have a superficial secondary infection. Imprints of ulcerated areas on epithelial cell tumors often yield only inflammatory cells—with or without bacteria. When impression smears are collected from ulcerated areas, the changes in cellular morphology caused by neoplasia are difficult to distinguish from the dysplastic changes caused by inflammation. Therefore it is more rewarding to collect cytologic samples from ulcerated lesions by deep aspiration because aspirates from deep within a lesion are advantageous because they are collected farther from the site of possible inflammation.

Figure 5-29 provides an algorithm to aid in the identification of epithelial tumors. Some specific epithelial tumors are discussed subsequently.

Tumors Involving Superficial Squamous Epithelial Cells

Normal superficial squamous epithelial cells (Figure 5-37) are very large, appear flattened, have an abundant amount of cytoplasm that stains light blue or aqua, and are anucleate or have a small, contracted, dark-staining nucleus without a discernible nucleolus. Normal squamous epithelial cells from the basal layer tend to be round with a moderate amount of light to medium blue cytoplasm. They have a single nucleus that stains medium to dark purple and has a smooth or slightly coarse chromatin pattern. Their nuclei may contain a small, round, indistinct nucleolus. As squamous epithelial cells mature, their morphology changes from that of basal squamous epithelial cells to that of mature superficial squamous epithelial cells. As a result, cells with varying morphologies may be collected from cutaneous lesions, depending upon the manner of collection and the erosiveness of the lesion.

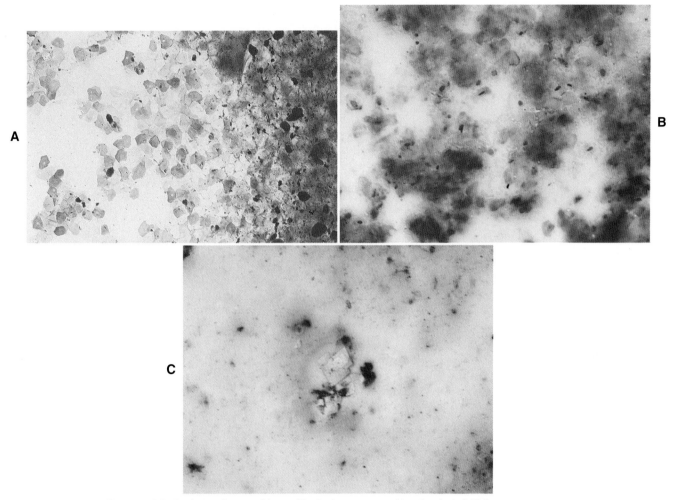

Figure 5-38 Aspirates from epidermal inclusion cysts and benign hair follicle tumors appear similar cytologically. **A,** Abundant, amorphous, cellular debris and mature, anucleate, squamous cells from a soft, fluctuant, cutaneous nodule on a dog. (Wright's stain, original magnification 33×.) **B,** Aspirate from an epidermal cyst in a dog that shows many squamous cells and much blue, amorphous debris. (Wright's stain, original magnification 25×.) **C,** Aspirate from an epidermal cyst in a dog. Several cholesterol crystals are located in the center. (Wright's stain, original magnification 25×.)

Benign Tumors of Squamous Epithelium: Benign tumors of squamous epithelium (e.g., papillomas) that are not undergoing dysplasia subsequent to local inflammation or other irritation usually exfoliate cells that cannot be distinguished from normal cells of the tissue of origin, or they exfoliate cells that may be slightly more active than normal cells from the tissue of origin (i.e., nucleoli may be more prominent, but still round and of reasonable size; cytoplasm may be slightly more basophilic; and the nuclear-to-cytoplasmic ratio may be mildly increased).

Benign tumors of squamous epithelium yield cytologic samples predominantly composed of mature squamous epithelial cells. A few basal and intermediate stages of squamous maturation may also be present. If there is any concern that the lesion might be a well-differentiated squamous-cell carcinoma, a biopsy of the lesion should be submitted for histopathologic evaluation.

Epidermal Cysts and Benign Hair Follicle Tumors: Epidermal cysts and benign hair follicle tumors (e.g., trichoepithelioma and pilomatricoma) yield a similar cytologic pattern characterized by a predominance of mature, cornifying, squamous epithelial cells and amorphous cellular debris (Figure 5-38). Cytologic preparations are usually thick and range from a predominance of mature, anucleate squamous epithelial cells to a predominance of amorphous, basophilic debris, or are a mixture of the two (Figure 5-38, *A* and *B*). Free melanin granules may be present in the background, and a few small, uniform, basal-type epithelial cells can occasionally be seen. Sometimes, cholesterol clefts and/or crystals are present (Figure 5-38, *C*). Such crystals develop from cholesterol that accumulates from degradation of cells exfoliating into the cyst. Cholesterol clefts are the negative images left after cholesterol crystals have been dissolved by the alcohol in Romanowsky-type stains.

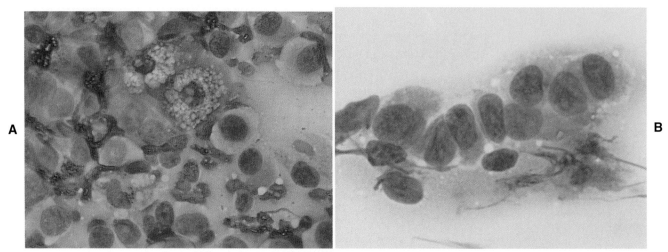

Figure 5-39 Aspirates from a trichoblastoma (basal cell tumor) in a dog. **A,** Many of the basal cells are morphologically similar to histiocytoma cells. The two cells containing numerous cytoplasmic vacuoles are probably sebaceous cells. (Wright's stain, original magnification 250×.) **B,** These basal cells show row formation sometimes seen in cytologic preparations from basal cell tumors. (Wright's stain, original magnification 400×.)

If they rupture, such lesions can release keratinized material into the surrounding tissues and become inflamed. In these cases, a population of neutrophils will be present along with the squamous cells and cellular debris.

Tumors of Basal-Type Epithelial Cells (Trichoblastoma):
Tumors of basal-type epithelial cells, trichoblastoma or basal cell tumors, are usually benign, but can represent a low-grade malignancy. The term basal cell tumor has long been used to refer to a group of tumors presumed to arise from cells of the basal epithelium of the epidermis or adnexal structures. Many subtypes of basal cell tumors have been reclassified as trichoblastoma or basal cell carcinoma (basal cell epithelioma) to reflect their tendency to show follicular differentiation and potentially aggressive behavior, respectively. Basal cell tumor is still used to refer to a specific benign tumor in cats. These various tumors cannot be reliably differentiated cytologically and are still referred to here as basal cell tumors. Basal cell tumors yield some cells in groups and some as individuals. Sometimes a row or ribbon of several cells is found (Figure 5-39) and is caused by the tendency of basal cells to line up along basement membranes within the tumor. This gives the characteristic ribbon-like histologic pattern of some of these tumors.

The individual cells of basal cell tumors have a morphology similar to normal basal cells; they are small, fairly uniform epithelial cells and they may appear cytologically similar to histiocytoma cells. Identification of cell-to-cell adhesion or the presence of rows or ribbons of cells is helpful in differentiating them from histiocytomas. Because aspirates from basal cell tumors do not always contain rows or ribbons of cells, the absence of such rows and ribbons does not totally rule out basal cell tumors. The cells should be evaluated for standard criteria of malignancy.

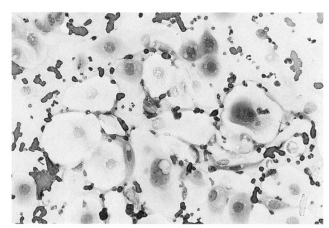

Figure 5-40 Well-differentiated squamous cell carcinoma from a dog. Note the cell showing a large, nonpyknotic nucleus with large nucleoli despite a mature cornified appearance to the cytoplasm. (Wright's stain, original magnification 100×.)

Squamous Cell Carcinomas: Squamous cell carcinomas may occur anywhere in the skin of the dog and cat. They are often ulcerated with a secondary superficial bacterial infection. Imprints of ulcerated areas may yield only bacteria and inflammatory cells, but scrapings of cleaned and débrided ulcerated areas may yield numerous tissue cells, although interpretation is often impaired by the secondary inflammation. Deep aspirates from squamous-cell carcinomas are helpful in diagnosis, because interpretation is usually not impaired by local inflammation.

Squamous cell carcinomas tend to yield a mixture of cell clusters and more mature individual cells. Many of the clusters may be too thick to evaluate, but thinner groups and individual cells can be evaluated to determine the cell of origin and the malignant potential. Individual cellular morphology varies from normal, large, mature, squamous

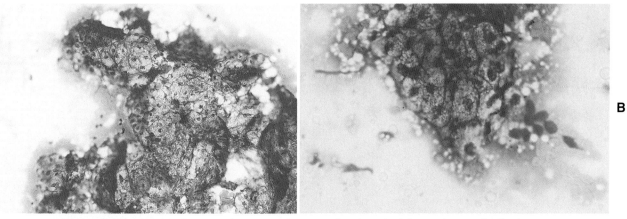

Figure 5-41 Aspirates from a sebaceous adenoma of a dog. **A,** A large cluster of cohesive sebaceous epithelial cells is present. (Wright's stain, original magnification 80×.) **B,** Higher magnification of cells in **A.** The cells resemble normal sebaceous cells. Nuclei are uniform, and the nuclear-to-cytoplasmic ratio is low. Note the fine vacuolation of the cytoplasm. (Wright's stain, original magnification 160×.)

cells to small or medium round cells with a small amount of very basophilic cytoplasm and large, round nuclei that may have a very coarse, ropy chromatin pattern and contain multiple prominent, irregularly shaped and sized nucleoli (Figure 5-40).

The cytologic picture of squamous-cell carcinomas varies greatly depending on the degree of differentiation of the tumor. In well-differentiated carcinomas, the majority of cells may be fairly normal, making a diagnosis of neoplasia difficult. Usually, small clusters of less mature cells with nuclear criteria of malignancy can be found. Biopsies for histologic analysis should be obtained if the cellular features are not diagnostic. Poorly differentiated tumors may contain a population of cells with obviously malignant features, but lacking evidence of keratinization.

Often, there are standard cytologic criteria of malignancy: marked variation in cell, nuclear, and nucleolar size; nucleolar number and shape; variation in nuclear-to-cytoplasmic ratio; and increased cytoplasmic basophilia. Some cells may also contain small, clear vacuoles that may occasionally aggregate around the nucleus (i.e., perinuclear vacuolation) and appear to coalesce, forming a clear ring around the nucleus; these cells are strongly suggestive of carcinoma. The cytoplasm of some keratinizing cells may homogeneously stain blue-green, and occasionally an individual cell has a blunted cytoplasmic tail and its cytoplasm displaced to one side. These cells have been called *tadpole cells* and are suggestive of squamous cell carcinoma. Another feature common in squamous cell carcinomas is large cells with abundant cytoplasm and angular cell borders that have retained a large, functional, nonpyknotic nucleus (i.e., asynchronous maturation of the nucleus and cytoplasm).

Adnexal Tumors

Sebaceous Adenomas: Sebaceous adenomas, which are most common in older dogs, usually appear as wart-like growths. They generally exfoliate cells in groups; however, a few individual cells may be present, and occasionally a group of cells may be arranged in an acinar pattern. The morphology of sebaceous adenoma cells is very similar to that of normal sebaceous cells (Figure 5-41). Sebaceous adenomas cannot be cytologically differentiated from sebaceous gland hyperplasia, but this is of no clinical significance. Cells from a sebaceous adenoma are large with foamy cytoplasm and a small, central or slightly eccentric nucleus that usually stains darkly and has a slightly coarse chromatin pattern. The nucleolus is typically indistinct or indiscernible. In preparations from sebaceous adenomas, some cells may have a slightly larger nucleus that stains with less intensity and has a slightly coarse chromatin pattern and a small or medium round, discernible nucleolus.

Basilar reserve cells, which are immature and contain little or no secretory material, may also be found. They have basophilic cytoplasm and a higher nuclear-to-cytoplasmic ratio, which may result in a misimpression of malignancy.

Sebaceous Epitheliomas: Sebaceous epitheliomas are relatively common in dogs and arise from basal-type reserve cells. Cytologic preparations consist primarily of small, fairly uniform, epithelial cells with low numbers of recognizable sebaceous cells. A lack of prominent criteria of malignancy differentiates these sebaceous epitheliomas from sebaceous carcinomas. The basal-type epithelial cells of these tumors may contain variable numbers of melanin granules. They are of low malignant potential,[13] may be locally aggressive, and may, less commonly, show metastatic behavior.

Sebaceous Carcinomas: Sebaceous carcinomas are rare neoplasms, occurring much less frequently than sebaceous epitheliomas or sebaceous cell adenomas. The cytologic characteristics of malignancy are similar to those of other carcinomas, and cytologic preparations usually consist of groups of extremely basophilic reserve cells that show numerous criteria of malignancy. Cells containing secretory material are scarce; however, signet ring cells (i.e., cells containing large secretory vacuoles that press the nucleus against the cell membrane) may occasionally be found.

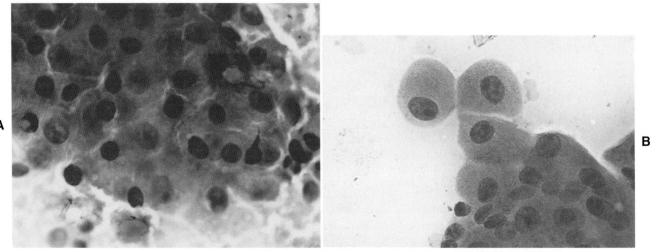

Figure 5-42 Aspirates from a perianal adenoma from an intact male dog. **A,** A cluster of uniform cohesive epithelial cells. (Wright's stain, original magnification 100×.) **B,** Higher magnification of the cells in **A.** Cells that are spread out well have abundant basophilic, granular cytoplasm, giving them a hepatoid appearance. Note that one or two prominent, but small and round, nucleoli are visible, which is typical of perianal adenoma cells. (Wright's stain, original magnification 250×.)

Perianal Gland Adenomas and Adenocarcinomas: The perianal glands are modified sebaceous glands that encircle the anus of dogs. A few perianal gland cells are also located in the skin of the tail, the prepuce, the thigh, and the dorsum of the back. Perianal adenomas and adenocarcinomas can occur at any of these locations and often ulcerate, possibly becoming secondarily infected. Perianal gland hyperplasia is difficult to differentiate from benign neoplasia both cytologically and histopathologically.[9]

Perianal gland adenomas and/or hyperplasia usually yield very cellular cytologic samples (Figure 5-42). Most cells are in clumps, but a few individual cells are typically present. These are medium cells with a moderate to large amount of gray or tan cytoplasm and uniform, round nuclei that may contain one or two small, round nucleoli (Figure 5-42, *B*). At high magnification, the cytoplasm may appear granular. Because these cells resemble hepatocytes, perianal gland neoplasms are sometimes called hepatoid tumors. A few flattened reserve cells may also be present. The reserve cell cytoplasm is more basophilic and the nucleus-to-cytoplasm ratio is between 1:1 and 1:2.

Perianal gland adenocarcinomas may show many criteria of malignancy or may be well differentiated and difficult to differentiate from perianal gland adenomas. Variation in the size of nuclei and nucleoli and the number of nucleoli per cell are the most common malignant features of perianal gland adenocarcinomas.[9]

Apocrine Gland Adenomas, Adenocarcinomas, and Carcinomas: Apocrine gland tumors are uncommon in both dogs and cats. In cats, sweat gland tumors are most often located at the base of the ear, the dorsum of the head and neck, and the base of the tail.[6] They are usually 1 to 2 cm in diameter, attached to the skin, and, in some cases, cystic. In cats, they frequently ulcerate and may resemble a chronic inflammatory process.

Apocrine gland adenomas usually yield poorly cellular cytologic preparations; most cells are in clumps. The cells are medium sized, round or oval, and have a slightly eccentric nucleus. They may contain one or more large droplets of secretory material.

Apocrine gland adenocarcinomas yield groups of small, basophilic, epithelial cells, which have a high nuclear-to-cytoplasmic ratio because of scant amounts of blue-gray cytoplasm and may often be arranged in elongated papillary structures. The majority of the cells are fairly uniform in size and appearance. A small population of large cells with macronuclei and a prominent nucleolus can typically be found along with the smaller cells. Although the malignant nature may be evident, apocrine carcinoma cannot be definitively determined cytologically.

Apocrine gland carcinomas can cause significant hypercalcemia in dogs. They exfoliate high numbers of cohesive cells that may be present in long papillary structures. The tumors may remain relatively small, requiring careful palpation of the anal sac to detect and often metastasize to sublumbar lymph nodes. As a result, dogs with unexplained hypercalcemia should be carefully evaluated for apocrine gland carcinoma.

Undifferentiated Carcinomas

Undifferentiated carcinomas are malignant tumors that morphologically appear to be of epithelial origin, but the specific cell of origin (i.e., squamous epithelial cell or glandular epithelial cell) cannot be determined. Obviously, these tumors may vary greatly in cellular morphology. In order for them to be classified as carcinomas, epithelial cell characteristics must be present without spindle cell characteristics. Because of their undifferentiated (anaplastic) nature, many criteria of malignancy are usually present and easily recognized as malignant.

Subcutaneous and Glandular Tissues

Tumors (e.g., salivary, mammary, thyroid) and lesions of subcutaneous and glandular are discussed in Chapter 6.

Tumors of Mesenchymal Origin (Spindle Cell Tumors)

Tumors of mesenchymal origin are commonly referred to as spindle cell tumors. In most cases, it is difficult or impossible to differentiate the various mesenchymal tumors (i.e., hemangiosarcoma or fibrosarcoma) cytologically; however, some tumors do have distinctive cytologic characteristics (e.g., hemangiopericytomas and giant cell tumors). Usually diagnosis is limited to identifying the mass as a mesenchymal neoplasia and evaluating the malignant potential of the tumor. These tumors may yield individual cells, or the cells may be present in large aggregates as well. The term spindle cell arises from the fusiform, or spindled, appearance that a few to many (depending on the specific cell of origin and the malignant potential of the tumor) of the cells may show. Spindle cells are fusiform with cytoplasmic tails that trail away from the nucleus in one, two, or sometimes several directions. These cells are usually small- or medium-sized. They have a moderate amount of light to medium blue cytoplasm, which has indistinct cytoplasmic borders and contains a round or oval nucleus that stains with medium intensity and has a smooth or fine, lacy chromatin pattern. Nucleoli are usually not visible in nonneoplastic spindle cells. As the malignant potential of spindle cell tumors increases, the nucleoli become prominent and the spindle shape becomes less prominent; cellular, nuclear, and nucleolar size and shape markedly vary; the chromatin pattern becomes coarser; and cytoplasmic basophilia and nuclear-to-cytoplasmic ratio increase.

Reactive fibroplasia (i.e., granulation tissue) in areas of inflammation and/or tissue repair also produces plump, young fibroblasts that may have prominent criteria suggestive of malignancy. As a result, fibroplasia can be very difficult to differentiate from spindle cell neoplasms, and, in some cases, histopathologic findings may be necessary for a definitive diagnosis. Cellular morphologic changes noted in reactive fibroblasts are very similar to the changes caused by neoplasia, but usually are only mildly to moderately severe. Nuclear and nucleolar changes are less sensitive than cytoplasmic changes to dysplasia. If high numbers of inflammatory cells are present, or if there is reason to believe that the aspirate is from an area undergoing active tissue repair (e.g., a prior incision site), extreme caution should be used in diagnosing mesenchymal neoplasia cytologically.

Figure 5-30 provides an algorithm to aid in the identification of spindle cell tumors, some of which are discussed next.

Fibromas: Fibromas can occur in the dermis or subcutaneous tissue and seldom ulcerate. Aspirates and imprints yield very few, if any, cells. Scrapings from excised fibromas yield more cells, but even scrapings do not yield many cells. Cells are usually collected individually, but occasionally a group ranging from two to several cells may be found.

Cells from fibromas are uniform in size and shape. They tend to have a very elongated, spindle shape with a moderate amount of light blue cytoplasm streaming away from the nucleus in opposite directions. Their nuclei are round or oval, stain with medium to marked intensity, have a smooth or lacy chromatin pattern, and may contain one or two small, round, indistinct nucleoli.

Fibrosarcomas: Fibrosarcomas can arise from cutaneous or subcutaneous tissues. They may ulcerate and become secondarily infected. Aspirates, imprints, and scrapings from fibrosarcomas tend to collect more cells than they do from fibromas.

Cells from fibrosarcomas are less spindle shaped than cells from fibromas (Figure 5-43). Many cells may be plump and/or oval shaped. Others may be stellate or have only a single, indistinct tail of cytoplasm. Occasionally, multinucleated fibroblasts may be found. Cytoplasmic basophilia, increased nuclear-to-cytoplasmic ratio, enlarged and/or angular nucleoli, and mild to marked variation in cellular, nuclear, and nucleolar size and shape develop as malignant potential increases.

Granulation Tissue: Granulation tissue is composed of proliferating fibroblasts and small vessels. Because fibroblasts are young plump spindle cells with anaplastic characteristics, granulation tissue cannot always reliably be differentiated cytologically from fibrous tissue neoplasia. If granulation tissue is suspected, a biopsy of the lesion should be submitted for histopathologic evaluation to definitively differentiate granulation tissue from fibrous tissue neoplasia.

Lipomas: Lipomas are very common tumors that most frequently occur in the subcutaneous tissue of the shoulders, thighs, and trunk of the body and seldom ulcerate. Aspirates usually yield a few lipocytes and abundant free fat. As a result, cytologic smears have an oily appearance and do not dry. Fat does not stain with Romanowsky-type stains and is dissolved by alcohol in alcohol-containing stains. Therefore, microscopic evaluations of the smears reveal clear areas and lipocyte numbers that range from none to many. Lipocytes have pyknotic nuclei that are pressed against the side of the cell membrane by huge fat globules (Figure 5-44). Fat stains, such as Sudan IV and oil red O, may be used on fresh smears (before alcohol fixation) to establish the presence of lipids. Although lipomas are benign tumors, they occasionally infiltrate between muscle masses,[14] becoming difficult or impossible to remove and possibly leading to the patient's demise.

Lipomas usually do not become secondarily infected; therefore when inflammatory cells are found with lipid and lipocytes, inflammation of fat tissue (i.e., fat necrosis, steatitis, or panniculitis) should be suspected.

Liposarcomas: Liposarcomas occur most frequently in the subcutaneous tissue of the shoulders, thighs, and trunk of the body. Aspirates, imprints, and scrapings from liposarcomas may contain free fat and some mature lipocytes along with lipoblasts, and thus appear greasy, or they may contain very little free fat and few mature lipocytes along with many lipoblasts, and not appear greasy.

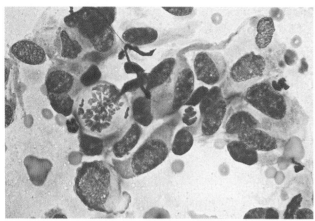

Figure 5-43 Aspirate from a fibrosarcoma from a dog. An aberrant mitotic figure and many pleomorphic mesenchymal cells are present. (Wright's stain, original magnification 250×.)

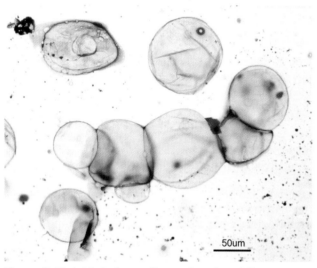

Figure 5-44 Aspirate from a lipoma in a dog. Adipocytes are large and round, with pyknotic nuclei and clear cytoplasm. (Wright's stain.)

Cells from liposarcomas often have very light cytoplasm with indistinct cell borders (Figure 5-45). Within the same tumor, cells may vary from the morphology of lipocytes to that of bizarre blastic cells similar to those found in fibrosarcomas. Small to large lipid globules may be found in any of the cells; in general, however, more immature and anaplastic cells have fewer and smaller fat globules. Smears that have not been exposed to alcohol or other lipid solvents can be stained with fat stains, such as Sudan IV and oil red O, to establish the presence of lipids.

Inflammation can cause fat cells to become dysplastic. The cellular morphology of fat cells undergoing dysplasia can be similar to that of liposarcoma cells. Because liposarcomas do not usually become secondarily infected or inflamed, evidence of inflammation concurrent with cellular changes indicating dysplasia or neoplasia suggests inflammation or necrosis of fat tissue (i.e., fat necrosis, steatitis, or panniculitis) (see Figure 5-28), but secondary

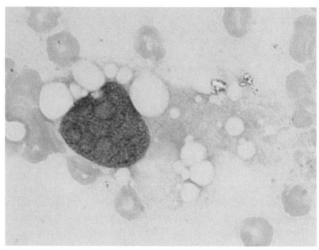

Figure 5-45 Aspirate from a liposarcoma. Note the vacuolated cytoplasm with indistinct borders, large nucleus, ropy chromatin pattern, and multiple prominent nucleoli. (Wright's stain, original magnification 400×.) *(Courtesy the University of Georgia, College of Veterinary Medicine.)*

inflammation of neoplastic fat tissue cannot totally be ruled out. To definitively differentiate neoplasia from dysplasia, a biopsy of the lesion can be submitted for histopathologic evaluation.

Hemangiopericytomas: Hemangiopericytomas most frequently occur in the subcutaneous tissues of the distal portions of dog limbs and seldom ulcerate. Aspirates, imprints, and scrapings usually yield a moderate number of individual cells and a few small groups of cells. Cell morphology varies from very spindled with cytoplasmic tails trailing away in opposite directions from a round or oval nucleus to caudate with a moderate amount of cytoplasm that does not have a distinct tail (Figure 5-46). The cytoplasm of hemangiopericytoma cells stains light to medium blue and is usually devoid of any granules or vacuoles. The nucleus has a lacy to moderately coarse chromatin pattern and contains one or two round nucleoli that can be indistinct or prominent.

Hemangiomas: Hemangiomas may occur in the skin or subcutaneous tissue at any location in dogs and cats and usually do not ulcerate. Hemangiomas are benign neoplasms of blood vessel endothelium and are continuous with the blood vascular system. Aspirates of hemangiomas usually yield a large amount of blood that may contain a few endothelial cells. Because of the tendency for neutrophils to marginate, neutrophil numbers may be higher in blood aspirated from hemangiomas and hemangiosarcomas than in peripheral blood. Even when a few tumor cells are collected, they are difficult to differentiate from nonneoplastic endothelial cells. Hemangioma cells tend to be oval, spindle, or stellate; have a moderate to abundant amount of light to medium blue cytoplasm; and contain a medium round or slightly oval nucleus that usually has a smooth or fine lacy chromatin pattern and may have one or two small round, indistinct nucleoli.

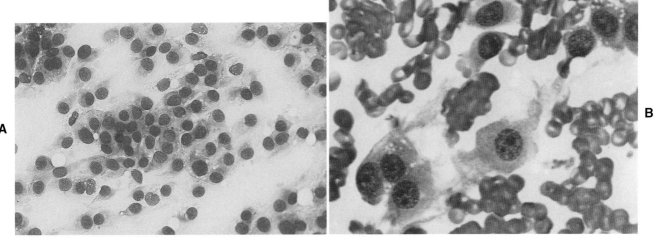

Figure 5-46 Aspirates from a hemangiopericytoma from a dog. **A,** Low-magnification photomicrograph shows a population of plump, spindle-shape cells with round nuclei and indistinct cytoplasmic borders. (Wright's stain, original magnification 132×.) **B,** Higher magnification of cells from a hemangiopericytoma. Notice the extremely wispy, blue-gray cytoplasm. (Wright's stain, original magnification 250×.)

Cytology can be used to differentiate hemangiomas and hemangiosarcomas from hematomas. The blood collected from hemangiomas and hemangiosarcomas contains platelets, whereas aspirates collected from hematomas do not contain platelets unless blood hemorrhaged into the hematoma within a few hours of sample collection or blood contamination occurred during sample collection. Also, aspirates from hematomas usually contain macrophages with phagocytized RBCs and/or RBC breakdown products (Figure 5-47), but blood from hemangiomas and hemangiosarcomas does not.

Hemangiosarcomas: Hemangiosarcomas may occur in the skin and subcutaneous tissue at any location in dogs and cats and seldom ulcerate. They are malignant tumors of the vascular endothelium and are continuous with the vascular system. Aspirates from hemangiosarcomas may yield very few to many mesenchymal cells, depending upon the architecture of the tumor (i.e., solid or cavernous). Usually, an abundant amount of blood is also collected. Because of neutrophils' tendency to marginate, the number of neutrophils in blood collected from hemangiosarcomas may exceed that in the peripheral blood. Neoplastic endothelial cells collected from hemangiosarcomas morphologically range from apparently normal endothelial cells to (more commonly) medium or large cells with marked variation in cellular, nuclear, and nucleolar size and increased nuclear-to-cytoplasmic ratio, nucleolar prominence, nucleolar angularity, and cytoplasmic basophilia (Figure 5-48).

Three or more nuclear criteria of malignancy (see Table 2-2) are prominent in many of the cells collected and there is no evidence of inflammation, the tumor can be classified as malignant. Often, however, sufficient cell numbers are not collected for the tumor to be classified as malignant. Tumors thought to be hemangiosarcomas that do not yield sufficient cells to be recognized as such should be excised and submitted for histopathologic evaluation.

Benign and Malignant Melanomas: Melanomas are very common in dogs, but rare in cats. In dogs, most cutaneous melanomas are benign, but melanomas of the lips, oral cavity, and digits are frequently malignant.

Cytologic preparations from melanomas are usually of moderate cellularity and contain a small to moderate amount of blood, but are occasionally of low cellularity and contain a large amount of blood. Most cells are found as individual cells, but a few small groups of cells may be found. The cells may be round, oval, stellate, or spindle-shaped. Melanomas composed predominantly of round or oval cells may be confused with round cell tumors; however, a few spindle-shaped cells can generally be found. The cells have a moderate to abundant amount of cytoplasm that usually contains granules of brown to green-black pigment (Figure 5-49). In some cells, these granules may be densely packed, obscuring the nucleus, but in other cells, they may be absent. Amelanotic melanomas, which are usually malignant, contain only a small amount of pigment that is often not discernible histopathologically (Figure 5-50); however, a careful search of cytologic preparations invariably identifies a few cells containing a few small pigment granules interspersed throughout the cytoplasm. Some malignant melanomas demonstrate many cytologic criteria of malignancy, but others are well differentiated and do not demonstrate significant criteria of malignancy; therefore caution should be used in classifying melanomas as benign based on cytologic evaluation alone.

Melanocytes must be differentiated from melanophages (i.e., macrophages that have phagocytized melanin), hemosiderophages (i.e., macrophages containing hemosiderin), and mast cells. Melanophages (see Figure 5-49) usually contain a few clear vacuoles along with a few or many large phagocytic

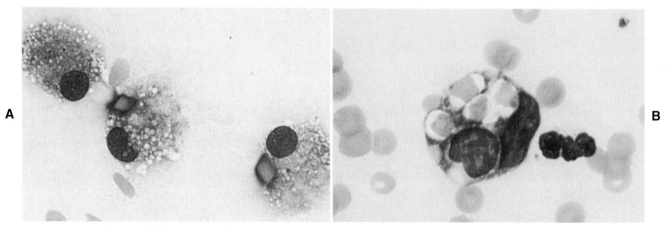

Figure 5-47 A, Large foamy macrophages with intracytoplasmic golden hematoidin crystals. Hematoidin is a product of red blood cell breakdown and is often referred to as *tissue bilirubin.* It indicated intratissue hemorrhage. (Wright's stain.) **B,** A macrophage showing erythrophagocytosis. (Wright's stain.)

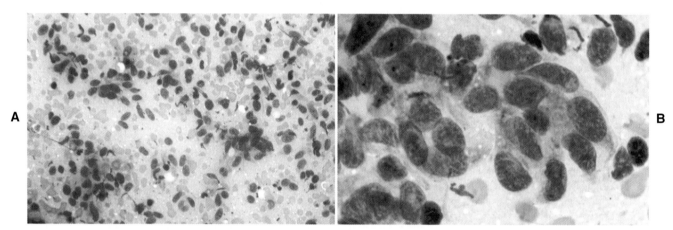

Figure 5-48 A, Scraping from a hemangiosarcoma. Scattered red blood cells, spindle cells, and bare nuclei are shown. **B,** Higher magnification of slide shown in **A.** (Wright's stain.) *(Slide courtesy Dr. D. DeNicola, Idexx Laboratories.)*

vacuoles packed with melanin pigment that are much larger than the small granules in melanocytes and melanoblasts. Hemosiderophages have a few to many phagocytic vacuoles stuffed with hemosiderin, which are blue to brown-black and usually much larger than the small granules of melanocytes and melanoblasts. Mast cells are round or oval and contain a few to many red-purple granules, which are larger than the small green to brown-black granules of melanocytes and melanoblasts but smaller than the melanin laden phagocytic vacuoles of the melanophage and the hemosiderin laden phagocytic vacuoles of hemosiderophages.

Myxomas and Myxosarcomas: Myxomas and myxosarcomas (Figure 5-51) are uncommon tumors of the subcutaneous tissues. On aspiration, a small to large amount of viscid material is usually obtained, and cytologic preparations contain a few to many individual cells in a background of pink homogeneous material. The cells vary in morphology from oval to stellate or spindle-shaped and have a small to abundant amount of cytoplasm that sometimes contains small vacuoles of pink secretory material. The oval cells often have eccentric nuclei and medium to

dark blue cytoplasm, giving them an appearance similar to plasma cells. Myxosarcomas exhibit variable degrees of criteria of malignancy (Figure 5-51, *C*).

Neurofibromas and Neurofibrosarcomas: Neurofibromas and neurofibrosarcomas are rare tumors of the nerve cell sheath that can occur in the subcutaneous tissue. Cytologically, they cannot be reliably differentiated from other spindle-cell tumors, such as fibromas and fibrosarcomas. Histologic demonstration of tumor involvement with a nerve sheath is necessary for a definitive diagnosis.

Malignant Fibrous Histiocytomas: Malignant fibrous histiocytomas, or giant cell tumors of soft parts, occur more commonly in cats than dogs, but are not common in either species. When located in the subcutaneous tissues, they are infiltrative and aggressive, but rarely metastasize.[9]

Preparations from these tumors generally are highly cellular and consist of multinucleated giant cells (Figure 5-52), neoplastic mesenchymal cells (see section on fibrosarcomas earlier in this chapter), and, less

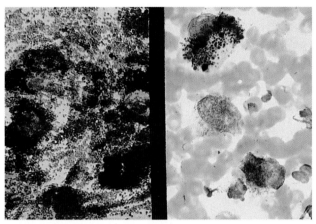

Figure 5-49 Smears from a melanoma that was so heavily pigmented that most cellular and nuclear detail was obscured *(left)*. (Wright's stain.) A melanophage (uppermost cell) and two melanocytes. The melanophage contains granules that are larger than those of the melanocytes *(right)*. (Wright's stain.) *(Left, courtesy Dr. K. Prasse.)*

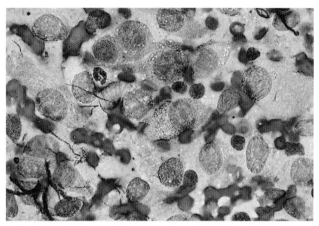

Figure 5-50 Aspirate from a malignant melanoma. Several melanoma cells containing melanin pigment are present. Many criteria of malignancy are present, including anisocytosis; coarse chromatin; increased nuclear-to-cytoplasmic ratio; and prominent, variable sized, and often angular nucleoli. (Wright's stain.)

commonly, low numbers of smaller round cells that resemble histiocytes (see section on histiocytomas earlier in this chapter). The multinucleated giant cells may have a characteristic appearance and contain 20 to 30 nuclei.

Undifferentiated Sarcomas: Undifferentiated sarcomas are malignant tumors that morphologically appear to be of mesenchymal origin, but the specific cell of origin (i.e., fibroblasts, endothelial cells) cannot be determined. Obviously, these tumors may vary greatly in cellular morphology, so there must be some spindling in order for them to be classified as sarcomas. Because of their undifferentiated and anaplastic nature, they usually are easily recognized as malignant. Their cellular characteristics are those discussed in the general description of spindle cell tumors earlier in this chapter.

Carcinosarcomas: Carcinosarcomas are malignant tumors that do not show sufficient cellular differentiation to be classified as either carcinomas or sarcomas. Because of the anaplastic nature of these tumors, they usually are easily classified as malignant. Their cellular characteristics are a variable admixture of the characteristics for carcinomas and sarcomas.

Evaluation of Fluid-Filled Lesions

Fluid-filled lesions may be neoplastic or nonneoplastic in origin. Nonneoplastic fluid-filled lesions of the cutaneous and subcutaneous tissues include hematomas, seromas, hygromas, and abscesses. Cytologic evaluation of fluid from these lesions can be very helpful in their differentiation. Fluid samples should be evaluated for the presence of malignant cells and acute inflammation/infection. Often, cytologic findings from fluid lesions will be nonspecific, containing only mature macrophages, and simply called benign cystic fluid. Figure 5-53 provides an algorithm to aid in the evaluation of fluid-filled lesions, and discussion of some fluid-filled lesions follows.

Hematomas: The fluid from hematomas is red to red-brown. Supernatant from centrifuged samples usually has a total protein content between 2.5 gm/dl and that of peripheral blood. Cytologically, the fluid contains macrophages, nondegenerate neutrophils, and numerous RBCs. A few lymphocytes may also be present. Usually, the macrophages are activated and often contain intact RBCs, hematoidin, and other RBC breakdown products (see Figure 5-47). Platelets are not found in fluid from hematomas unless there has been hemorrhage into the hematoma within a few hours of sample collection or the sample is contaminated with peripheral blood. Differentiation of hematomas from hemangiomas and hemangiosarcomas is discussed in the section on hemangiomas earlier in this chapter.

Seromas/Hygromas: Fluid from seromas/hygromas is typically clear or amber and of low cellularity, and usually has a total protein concentration >2.5 gm/dl. The cell population is predominantly composed of mononuclear cells with macrophage or cyst lining cell characteristics. These cells are medium or large, round, and have moderate or abundant cytoplasm that is often highly vacuolated. Their nuclei may be centrally located, but are often eccentric. Usually, the nucleus is round; has a smooth or fine, lacy chromatin pattern; and may contain one or two indistinct nucleoli. A few nondegenerate neutrophils may also be found. A few cyst lining cells may be spindle-shaped and, occasionally, some cells may be very dysplastic and exhibit criteria of malignancy.

A combination of the cytologic characteristics of hematomas and/or peripheral blood and the cytologic characteristics of seromas/hygromas will be found when there is hemorrhage into the lesion or peripheral blood has contaminated the sample.

Abscesses: Fluid from abscesses is usually creamy, yellow, pink, or brown, and total protein concentration usually cannot be determined because of the opacity of the fluid. Even the supernatant of centrifuged samples is often too

Text continued on p. 111.

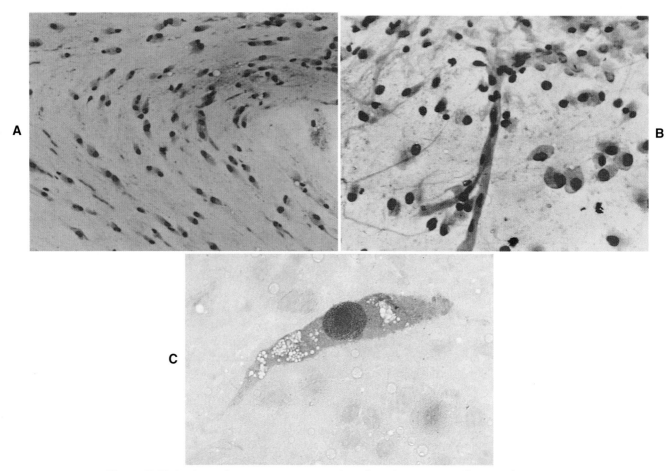

Figure 5-51 Aspirates from a myxosarcoma in a dog. **A,** Low magnification shows many rows of cells embedded in a pink substance. (Wright's stain, original magnification 50×.) **B,** A higher magnification shows many cells with a plasmacytoid appearance and a background of pink material. A few cells are spindle-shaped. (Wright's stain, original magnification 100×.) **C,** Cell from a myxosarcoma showing a large, prominent nucleolus. (Wright's stain, original magnification 250×.)

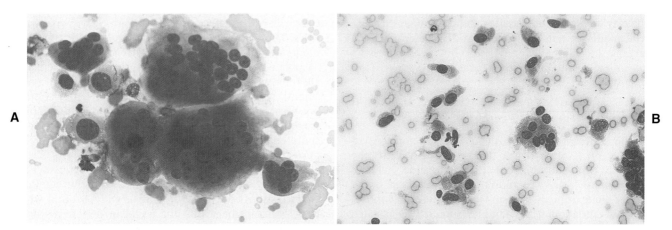

Figure 5-52 Aspirates from a malignant fibrous histiocytoma (giant cell tumor) from a cat. **A,** These tumors contain a mixture of large, multinucleated, giant cells. (Diff-Quik, original magnification 132×.) **B,** Mesenchymal cells. (Wright's stain, original magnification 160×.)

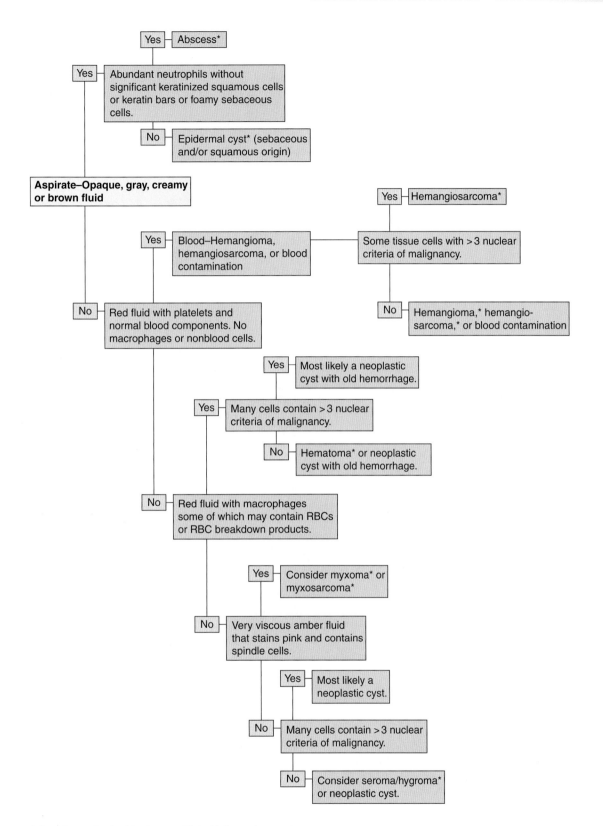

* See discussion in this chapter. Clinical information, such
as the history of the lesion, physical examination and radiographic
findings, may allow further differentiation.

Figure 5-53 An algorithm to aid in evaluating cytologic preparations from fluid-filled lesions.

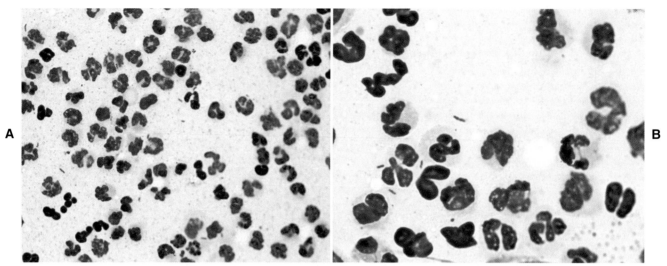

Figure 5-54 A, Neutrophilic inflammation is characterized by the predominance of neutrophils. Many of the neutrophils in this slide are degenerate. Scattered bacterial rods are present. (Wright's stain.) **B,** Higher magnification from same slide as shown in part **A.**

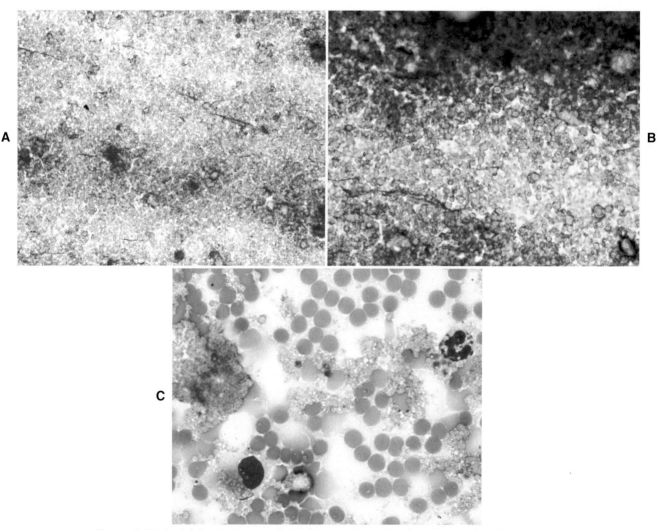

Figure 5-55 A, Calcinosis circumscripta often consists only of small granules of calcareous material. (Wright's stain.) **B,** Higher magnification of area shown in **A.** (Wright's stain.) **C,** Red blood cell macrophage, eosinophil, and moderate amount of calcareous material.

opaque for accurate total protein measurement. When the total protein concentration can be determined, it usually is > 4 gm/dl.

Smears prepared from abscesses are highly cellular, usually composed of more than 90% neutrophils with a few macrophages. Scattered lymphocytes and plasma cells may also be present. Abscesses caused by gram-negative bacteria usually contain many degenerate neutrophils (Figure 5-54), and abscesses caused by gram-positive bacteria often contain a few to many degenerate neutrophils. Other abscesses usually contain no or only a few degenerate neutrophils. Especially with sterile abscesses, macrophages may occasionally compose more than 50% of the nucleated cells. Sterile foreign-body abscesses, such as those caused by oil-based injections, may contain refractile material (see Figure 5-4) in addition to inflammatory cells.

Miscellaneous

Calcinosis Circumscripta (Tumoral Calcinosis): These benign masses may be seen in both dogs and cats. They often occur on the lower extremities of large breed dogs but have been seen in other areas including the neck and tongue in both dogs and cats. The cause of calcinosis circumscripta masses is unknown but is thought to be associated with factors such as trauma, calcium phosphorus disorders, and breed predilection.

Fluid collected from calcinosis circumscripta lesions is often thick and appears chalky white when aspirated. If blood contamination or intralesional bleeding is present, the fluid may appear red. When smears made from the collected material are evaluated microscopically, they may consist only of small granules of calcareous material with no tissue cells present (Figure 5-55), or the smears may consist of calcareous material with macrophages and/or blood (Figure 5-55, *C*).

References

1. Coloe PJ, Allison JF: Protothecosis in a cat. *J Am Vet Med Assoc* 180:78-79, 1982.
2. Kaplan W, et al: Protothecosis in a cat: First recorded case. *Sabouraudia* 14:281-286, 1976.
3. Finnie JW, Coloe PJ: Cutaneous protothecosis in a cat. *Aust Vet J* 57:307-308, 1981.
4. Lorenz. In Ettinger SJ: *Textbook of Veterinary Internal Medicine: Diseases of the Dog and Cat.* Saunders, Philadelphia, 1983, pp 1346-1372.
5. Dorn CR, et al: Survey of animal neoplasms in Alameda and Contra Costa Counties, California. II. Cancer morbidity in dogs and cats from Alameda County. *J Natl Cancer Inst* 40:307-318, 1968.
6. Susaneck: Feline skin tumors. *Comp Cont Ed* 5:251-257, 1983.
7. Duncan JS, Prasse KW: Cytologic examination of the skin and subcutis. *Vet Clin North Am* 6:637-645, 1976.
8. Duncan JS, Prasse KW: Cytology of canine cutaneous round cell tumors. *Vet Pathol* 16:673-679, 1979.
9. Barton: Cytologic diagnosis of cutaneous neoplasia: An algorithmic approach. *Comp Cont Ed* 9:20-33, 1987.
10. Rebar: *Handbook of Veterinary Cytology.* St. Louis, Ralston Purina Co, 1979.
11. Brown, et al: Cutaneous lymphosarcoma in the dog: a disease with variable clinical and histologic manifestations. *J Am Anim Hosp Assoc* 16:565-572, 1980.
12. McKeever PJ, et al: Canine cutaneous lymphoma. *J Am Vet Med Assoc* 180:531-536, 1982.
13. Gross, Ihrke, and Walder: *Veterinary Dermatopathology.* St. Louis, Mosby, 1992.
14. Kramek BA, et al: Infiltrative lipoma in three dogs. *J Am Vet Med Assoc* 186:81-82, 1985.

Subcutaneous Glandular Tissue: Mammary, Salivary, Thyroid, and Parathyroid

R.W. Allison and J.M. Maddux

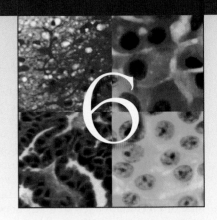

CHAPTER 6

The mammary, salivary, thyroid, and parathyroid glands are located in the subcutaneous fat layer. Knowledge of normal microanatomy of these glands and of other structures in close proximity is important for accurate cytologic interpretation. Except for the thyroid and parathyroid glands, regional locations of these glands differ considerably. Cytologically, normal exocrine glands (mammary and salivary) may appear similar, and differ from normal endocrine glands (thyroid and parathyroid). Lymphoid and adipose tissues may be found near any of these glands; salivary tissue may be inadvertently aspirated when attempting to aspirate submandibular lymph nodes. Thymic tissue may be near the thyroid and parathyroid, especially in young animals or when any of these tissues exist in ectopic locations.

Cytologic evaluation of subcutaneous glandular tissue is a valuable extension of clinical examination. Collection of samples by fine-needle aspiration biopsy is simple and rapid and avoids the trauma and anesthetic risk of surgical biopsy. Most lesions are readily palpable and therefore easily aspirated. Although aspiration is the usual means of obtaining specimens, cytologic evaluation of mammary glands may also be performed on imprints of excised tissue, scrapings of ulcerated surface lesions, and secretions.

A primary goal of aspiration cytology is to distinguish inflammatory from neoplastic lesions and to differentiate, when possible, benign neoplasms from malignant neoplasms. However, endocrine tumors (e.g., thyroid and parathyroid) frequently exhibit few cellular criteria of malignancy, appearing cytologically benign even when malignant. These tumors require histopathologic evaluation of invasion and other features to determine their malignant potential.

Mammary gland lesions present special challenges due to the diversity of cell types that may be involved and the oftentimes overlapping cell populations within hyperplastic, dysplastic, benign, and malignant lesions. Reported diagnostic accuracy for cytologic differentiation of benign from malignant mammary neoplasms in dogs varies from 33% to 79%.[1-3] A cytologic grading system for differentiation of benign from malignant mammary tumors in dogs based on 10 important criteria of malignancy has been proposed.[1] In that study, the predictive value of a positive result was higher (90% to 100%) than that of a negative result (59% to 75%), suggesting that cytologic evaluation tends to underdiagnose mammary gland malignancies. Wet fixation and a Papanicolaou-type stain were used in that study, which are less frequently used by most cytologists, and were thought to allow better appreciation of some criteria of malignancy.

A high rate of false negatives in cases of malignancies may result from several factors. Sampling errors occur if the needle is not directed into a representative area of the tumor. This problem is proportional to tumor size, and sampling of multiple sites in large tumors may increase the likelihood of aspirating neoplastic cells. Multiple mammary tumors in an animal may be of different types, thus requiring examination of all lesions. Tumors containing an abundance of connective tissue may exfoliate poorly, leading to nondiagnostic samples. Many mammary gland malignancies are diagnosed based on histopathologic evidence of tissue invasion regardless of cellular atypia. It is no surprise that cytologic samples from such tumors may be misleading. Conversely, some encapsulated tumors containing areas with significant cell pleomorphism may be considered benign based on absence of tissue invasion. Cytologic samples from these tumors may falsely suggest a malignant process. Accuracy of evaluation will also depend on the experience of the cytologist. Samples yielding equivocal results, such as cyst fluid, nonseptic inflammatory changes, or those cytologically suggestive of benign neoplasia should be evaluated histologically. Presence of marked criteria of malignancy makes malignant neoplasia most likely, but histopathology should still be employed to confirm the diagnosis. Samples yielding definitive nonneoplastic diagnoses may not need to be evaluated histologically.

THE MAMMARY GLANDS

Normal Cytologic Appearance

Mammary tissue of dogs and cats consists of five pairs of modified sweat glands that extend along the ventral body wall from the cranial thorax to the inguinal region. Glands consist of secretory acini and a series of excretory ducts. Myoepithelial cells lie between glandular epithelial cells and the basement membrane. During lactation the glands undergo marked hypertrophy to produce colostrum and then milk. Normal mammary secretions contain large amounts of protein and lipid droplets, and are of low cellularity. The predominant cell type in milk is the foam cell, a large, vacuolated epithelial cell that resembles an active macrophage (Figure 6-1). These cells usually occur singly. Small numbers of lymphocytes and neutrophils may also be present.

Aspirates of normal mammary tissue are frequently acellular or contain only blood. When mammary tissue is present, secretory cells are arranged in an acinar pattern. Individual cells have moderate amounts of basophilic cytoplasm and round, dark nuclei of uniform size. Duct epithelial cells have basal, ovoid nuclei and scanty cytoplasm and are arranged in small sheets or fragments of ductules. Myoepithelial cells appear as dark-staining, naked, oval nuclei or as spindle-shaped cells. Adipocytes and lipid droplets may be present.

Benign Lesions

Mastitis: Mastitis, or inflammation of the mammary glands, may occur either as a diffuse form involving two or more mammae or as a focal lesion. Mastitis is usually associated with postpartum lactation or pseudopregnancy, and may result from ascending or hematogenous infections.[4] Mammary secretions are usually adequate for diagnosis in cases of diffuse inflammation, whereas aspirates may be required for diagnosis of focal lesions. Smears are very cellular and contain large amounts of debris. Inflammatory cells may include neutrophils, lymphocytes, and macrophages in variable numbers, depending on the causative agent (Figure 6-2). Bacteria may be seen within phagocytes. Offending agents are usually coliforms, *Streptococcus* or *Staphylococcus* spp,

although other bacteria and fungi may occasionally be isolated.[5] Nonseptic mastitis, usually affecting the most caudal pair of glands, may occur secondary to milk stasis. Inflammatory cells will be present in variable numbers without accompanying bacteria.[5] Focal, nonseptic inflammatory nodules may occur secondary to lobular hyperplasia. These are characterized by epithelial metaplasia, pigment-laden macrophages, nondegenerate neutrophils, lymphocytes, and plasma cells.[6]

Cysts: Mammary cysts result from a dysplastic process in which dilated ducts expand to form large cavitations.[6] Cyst linings may consist of single layers of flattened epithelium or may have papillary overgrowth. Cysts may be present as single nodules or multinodular masses that grow slowly and have a bluish surface. Cysts are common in middle-aged and older bitches, but may occasionally appear in young dogs. Fluid aspirated is usually yellow, brown, green, or blood-tinged and of low cellularity unless there is concurrent inflammation. Cells are primarily vacuolated or pigment-laden macrophages. Epithelial cells aspirated from cysts lined by papillary projections may occur in dense clusters and exhibit a minor degree of nuclear pleomorphism.[6] Because mammary cysts may be present along with benign or malignant neoplasia, sampling of solid tissue in addition to cystic fluid is recommended.

Solid Masses: Dysplastic lesions and benign epithelial neoplasms of mammary tissue include lobular hyperplasia, adenosis, adenomas, and papillomas, all of which contain similar cell populations.[6,7] Smears made from aspirates contain many epithelial cells occurring singly or arranged in sheets and clusters. These cells generally exhibit little pleomorphism, having evenly dispersed chromatin and small, round nucleoli. However, dilated ducts can contain exfoliated epithelial cells that may have more criteria of malignancy than the rest of the mass.[8] Sampling those cells for cytologic

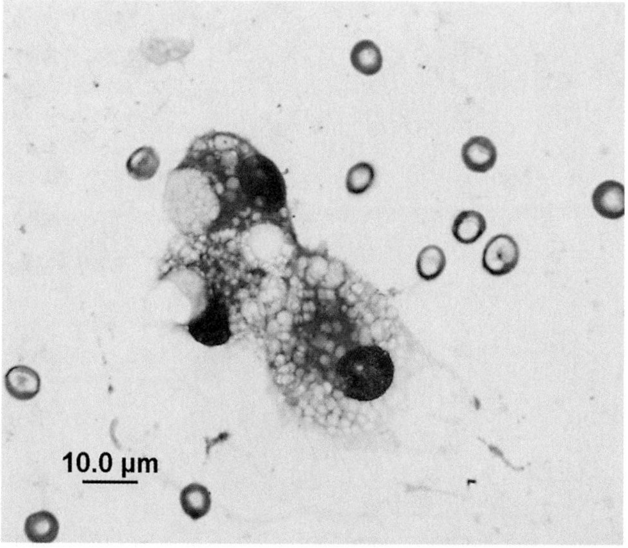

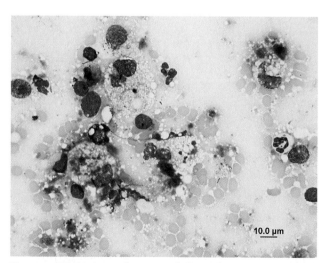

Figure 6-1 Several vacuolated foam cells from a mammary gland aspirate contain eccentric oval nuclei and abundant vacuolated cytoplasm with a variable amount of basophilic secretory product. (Wright's stain, 1000×.)

Figure 6-2 Aspirate from an inflamed mammary gland contains macrophages, foam cells, and neutrophils with amorphous basophilic secretory material in the background. (Wright's stain, 1000×.)

evaluation may result in a false impression of malignancy. Pigment-laden macrophages may be present (Figure 6-3). Some of these processes can also involve myoepithelial cells and connective tissue, further complicating the cytologic picture.[7] Benign tumors involving stromal and epithelial elements, such as complex adenomas, fibroadenomas and benign mixed tumors, are common in dogs and sometimes seen in cats.[6,7] Smears of aspirates from these lesions contain spindle shaped cells of myoepithelial or connective tissue origin in addition to clusters of epithelial cells similar to those described previously (Figure 6-4). These lesions can be difficult to differentiate even with histopathology due to the spectrum of cell types involved. Benign mixed tumors may produce cartilage, bone, or fat, in addition to fibrous tissue and epithelial tissue.[7] Aspirates from these lesions may contain all these elements, but if a single population predominates the cytology can be misleading.[9] Additionally, individual cell pleomorphism is occasionally marked in tumors considered benign due to lack of tissue invasion (Figures 6-5 and 6-6). Spindled mesenchymal cells are not a definitive cytologic characteristic of complex or mixed tumors, because they may also be found in some simple tumors.[1]

A specific form of mammary hyperplasia termed *fibroepithelial hyperplasia/hypertrophy* or *fibroadenomatous change* has been recognized in cats. This condition can affect young female cats that are pregnant or actively cycling or cats of either gender that have received progesterone-containing compounds.[10,11] Typically there is rapid enlargement of multiple glands. Aspirates from affected mammary glands contain both uniform epithelial cells and spindled mesenchymal cells, usually associated with abundant pink extracellular matrix material.[12] The epithelial cells are of ductal origin and have a relatively high nuclear-to-cytoplasmic ratio with dense round nuclei and a small amount of basophilic cytoplasm. The mesenchymal cells may exhibit moderate anisocytosis and anisokary-

osis.[12] Ovariohysterectomy or removal of the progesterone-containing compound is generally curative. Drug therapy with a progesterone antagonist has also been an effective treatment.[13]

Malignant Neoplasms

Mammary gland tumors are common in both dogs and cats; however, the biological behavior of the tumors varies greatly between these species. Mammary tumors comprise

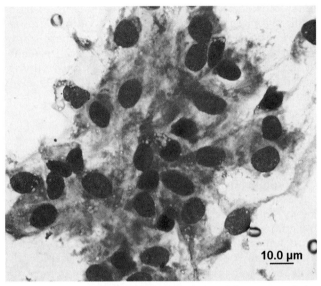

Figure 6-4 Spindled cells and eosinophilic extracellular matrix in an aspirate of a benign mammary complex adenoma from a dog. (Wright's stain, 1000×.)

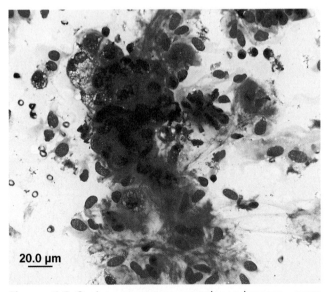

Figure 6-5 Canine mammary complex adenoma, same aspirate as Figure 6-4. Abundant eosinophilic matrix material and spindled mesenchymal cells near a cluster of vacuolated mammary epithelial cells. Epithelial cells exhibit moderate criteria of malignancy. (Wright's stain, 500×.)

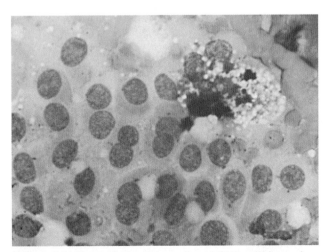

Figure 6-3 Sheet of glandular cells exhibiting little nuclear or cytoplasmic pleomorphism and a fine granular chromatin pattern characteristic of a mammary adenoma. A large, pigment-laden macrophage is present. (Wright's stain, 1250×.)

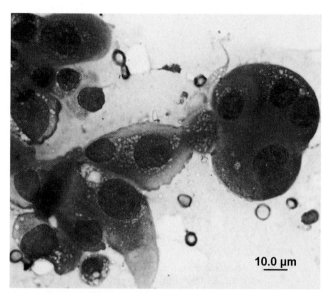

Figure 6-6 Canine mammary complex adenoma, same aspirate as Figure 6-4. These epithelial cells exhibit moderate to marked criteria of malignancy, including anisocytosis, anisokaryosis, and multiple prominent nucleoli. Histopathologic examination revealed this tumor to be well encapsulated and benign, despite individual cell pleomorphism. (Wright's stain, 1000×.)

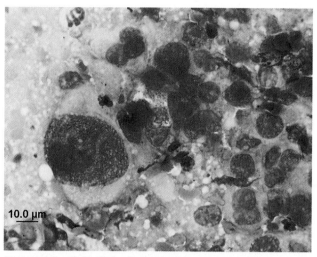

Figure 6-7 Epithelial cells from a feline mammary carcinoma have marked variation in cell and nuclear morphology. One large nucleus contains an abnormally shaped macronucleolus. (Wright's stain, 1000×.)

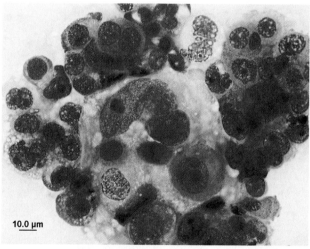

Figure 6-8 Pleural fluid from the same cat as Figure 6-7 contains tightly cohesive clusters of epithelial cells with marked criteria of malignancy, confirming the presence of intra-thoracic metastatic disease. (Wright's stain, 1000×.)

up to 50% of neoplasms in the bitch, and 40% to 50% of those tumors are malignant, with adenocarcinomas the most common histologic type.[6,14] Mammary tumors are the third most common neoplasm in cats and account for about 17% of all neoplasms in queens.[7] By contrast to dogs, up to 80% of feline mammary gland tumors are malignant. Similar to dogs, adenocarcinomas are diagnosed most frequently.[15,16] Mammary tumors are rare in males of both species.[6,17]

Multiple morphologic types of carcinoma are recognized histologically based on the pattern of cell arrangement and degree of cell differentiation.[7] Carcinomas are also graded based on histologic features such as tubule formation, mitotic rate, and cell pleomorphism. Many different types of carcinomas can contain collagenous stroma, sometimes in large amounts. Both histologic type and grade, as well as degree of invasion, have been shown to have prognostic significance in dogs.[18] Dogs frequently have multiple tumors, which are often of different histologic types.[14] In cats with mammary carcinomas, tumor size has been shown to be the single most important prognostic factor.[16,19]

Cytologic criteria that best correlate with malignancy include variable nuclear size, nuclear giant forms, high nuclear-to-cytoplasmic ratio, variable numbers of nucleoli, abnormal nucleolar shape, and the presence of macronucleoli (Figures 6-7 and 6-8).[1] However, as previously discussed, mammary malignancies may be well differentiated and show little cellular pleomorphism, and moderate criteria of malignancy may be present in tumors considered benign due to lack of tissue invasion. Smears of aspirates from adenocarcinomas generally contain epithelial cells occurring singly and in clusters of variable size. Adenocarcinoma cells are

usually round, with round to oval, eccentrically placed nuclei and variable quantities of basophilic cytoplasm that occasionally contains vacuoles that may be filled with secretory product (Figure 6-9). Cell borders are usually distinct, and cells may be arranged in acinar or tubular patterns. Binucleated or multinucleated cells may be seen. Mesenchymal cells may be present in variable numbers.

Anaplastic carcinomas are diffusely infiltrative tumors composed of large, pleomorphic epithelial cells with bizarre nuclear and nucleolar forms.[7] These cells occur singly and in variably sized clusters and have a high nuclear-to-cytoplasmic ratio (Figure 6-10). Multinucleated cells and mitotic figures are common (Figures 6-11 and 6-12). These tumors may contain

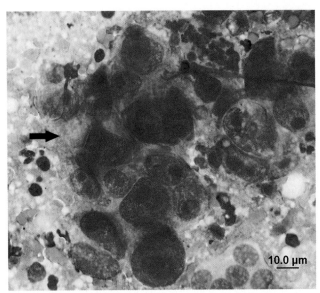

Figure 6-9 Aspirate from a feline mammary carcinoma. Eosinophilic secretory product is visible within the cytoplasm of one cell *(arrow)*. (Wright's stain, 1000×.)

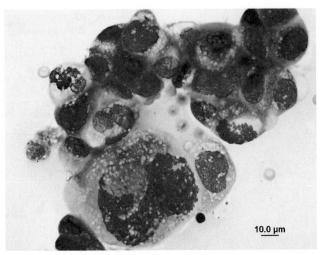

Figure 6-11 Anaplastic mammary carcinoma, same aspirate as Figure 6-10. Malignant epithelial cells have cytoplasmic vacuoles in this cluster, and two mitotic figures are present. (Wright's stain, 1000×.)

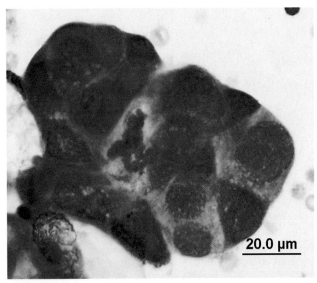

Figure 6-10 Aspirate of an anaplastic mammary carcinoma from a dog. Cohesive cluster of malignant mammary epithelial cells with a high nuclear-to-cytoplasmic ratio and multiple prominent nucleoli. A mitotic figure is visible in the center of the cluster. (Wright's stain, 1000×.)

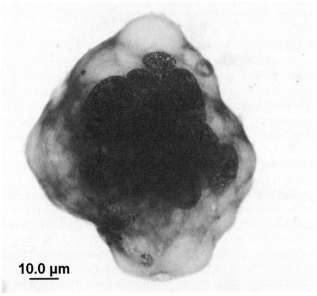

Figure 6-12 A large multinucleated epithelial cell from the same anaplastic mammary carcinoma as Figure 6-10. Notice the nuclear fragments visible in the cytoplasm. (Wright's stain, 1000×.)

abundant collagenous stroma infiltrated by inflammatory cells.[7] Anaplastic carcinomas frequently metastasize and have a poor prognosis.

Inflammatory carcinomas have distinctive clinical and histologic features and are aggressive tumors associated with a poor prognosis. These tumors may be misdiagnosed as mastitis due to the marked inflammation and clinical signs of systemic disease. Inflammatory carcinomas have been reported in dogs and cats, with a variety of histologic types represented.[20-22] In one report, cytology of mammary gland aspirates revealed malignant epithelial cells in 15 of 33 dogs and contributed to

the diagnosis; the other 18 cytologic samples had low cellularity.[21] The hallmark of inflammatory carcinoma was the histologic finding of dermal lymphatic involvement.[21]

Nonglandular carcinomas may be simple, with only epithelial proliferation, or complex, with cells of epithelial and myoepithelial origin. Accordingly, cytology samples may contain predominantly epithelial cells or a mixture of cell types. In contrast to adenocarcinomas, epithelial cells from nonglandular carcinomas may not contain intracytoplasmic vacuoles (Figure 6-13). Squamous cell carcinomas in mammary glands appear cytologically

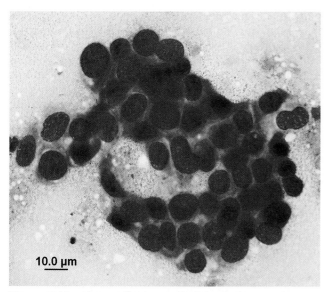

Figure 6-13 These cohesive epithelial cells from an aspirate of a canine papillary mammary carcinoma have no cytoplasmic vacuoles and minimal cellular atypia, emphasizing the need for histopathologic confirmation when neoplasia is suspected. (Wright's stain, 1000×.)

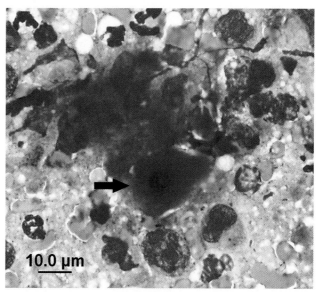

Figure 6-14 Aspirate from a feline mammary carcinoma. A single cell contains glassy dark blue cytoplasm and angular cytoplasm *(arrow)*, consistent with squamous differentiation. (Wright's stain, 1000×.)

similar to those in other body regions. Tumor cells occur singly or in small sheets and may be keratinized or non keratinized. Nuclei are variable in size, from small and pyknotic to large with immature chromatin and prominent nucleoli. Cytoplasm is variably abundant and basophilic, appearing glassy and blue-green with keratinization (see Chapter 5 for further discussion of the features of squamous cell carcinoma). These tumors frequently adhere to the overlying dermis and may be ulcerated, leading to the presence of many inflammatory cells and bacteria in samples taken from ulcerated areas. It is important to realize that squamous metaplasia may occur in other tumor types; thus finding squamous cells on a cytologic sample is not specific for squamous cell carcinoma (Figure 6-14).[7,8]

Mammary sarcomas are less common than carcinomas. They are usually large, firm tumors that have an unfavorable prognosis due to local recurrence and metastasis.[7] Fibrosarcomas and osteosarcomas are the most frequent types in the dog. Cells from sarcomas are often irregular or spindle shaped, occur singly or in small aggregates, and have indistinct cell borders. Pink matrix material may be associated with cell aggregates. The degree of pleomorphism and mitotic activity is variable and indicative of tumor malignancy. In general, cytologic criteria of malignancy described for carcinomas apply to sarcomas. Because mesenchymal cells, collagenous stroma, cartilage, and even bone formation can also be found in benign tumors and malignant mixed mammary tumors, cytologic interpretation of these cell populations can be confusing (Figures 6-15 and 6-16).[9] Histologically (and presumably cytologically), fibrosarcoma may be confused with spindle cell carcinoma, a rare tumor likely of myoepithelial origin.[7] Special stains can be used to differentiate the two. Carcinosarcomas are uncommon tumors of mixed origin, containing both malignant epithelial and malignant mesenchymal populations.[7]

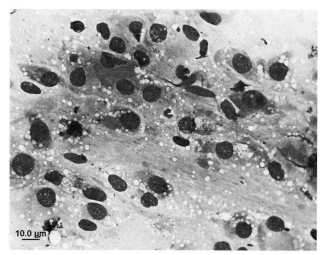

Figure 6-15 Spindled cells and extracellular matrix in an aspirate of a malignant mixed mammary gland tumor in a dog. (Wright's stain, 1000×.) *(Glass slide courtesy Boone et al, Texas A & M University, presented at the 2000 ASVCP case review session.)*

Table 6-1 presents a summary of the most common cytologic findings in aspirates from mammary lesions.

THE SALIVARY GLANDS

Normal Cytologic Appearance

Major salivary glands in dogs and cats are the parotid, mandibular, sublingual, and zygomatic glands. Minor, or buccal, salivary glands are spread over the oral mucosa. Salivary glands are composed of secretory cells arranged

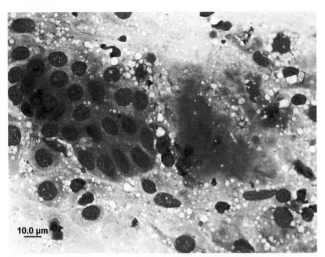

10.0 µm

Figure 6-16 Malignant mixed mammary gland tumor, same aspirate as Figure 6-15. A few clusters of well-differentiated epithelial cells and an abundance of spindled cells and extracellular matrix. Despite the lack of cellular pleomorphism, the presence of neoplastic epithelial cells within lymphatics and evidence of metastases to the lung and lymph node confirmed malignancy in this case. (Wright's stain, 1000×.)

in acini and an extensive ductular network. A layer of myoepithelial cells lies between the glandular cells and basement membrane. Aspirated samples from normal salivary glands reveal secretory epithelial cells with small, round nuclei and abundant cytoplasm distended with clear vacuoles. Acinar cells usually occur in clusters (Figure 6-17). When seen individually, these cells are difficult to differentiate from foamy macrophages. Ductal epithelial cells are seen less frequently and have a higher nuclear-to-cytoplasmic ratio (Figure 6-18). Basophilic mucin may be present in the background. Samples may also include occasional spindle-shaped myoepithelial cells, adipocytes, and lipid droplets. Hemorrhage is frequent upon aspiration of salivary glands. Erythrocytes in smears assume a characteristic linear pattern (windrowing) caused by the mucin content of the sample.

Nonneoplastic Lesions

Sialoceles: The most common salivary gland disorder in dogs is the sialocele.[23] These are nonepithelial-lined cavities filled with salivary secretions. Leakage of salivary secretions into fascial tissues usually follows blunt trauma but may occasionally be secondary to calculi or duct obstruction by bite wounds, abscesses, and ear canal surgery. Swellings occur most commonly on the floor of the mouth (ranulae) or the cranial cervical area, and less frequently in pharyngeal or retrobulbar areas. Aspirated fluid is viscous, clear or blood tinged, and contains low to moderate numbers of nucleated cells.

Cytologic evaluation of sialocele aspirates usually reveals diffuse or irregular clumps of homogeneous eosinophilic to basophilic mucin. Large phagocytic cells

with small round nuclei and abundant foamy cytoplasm may be found individually or in small clusters (Figure 6-19). Salivary gland epithelial cells may be intermixed but are not easily distinguished cytologically from macrophages. Erythrocytes often occur in linear patterns (windrows) because of the mucin content. Nondegenerate neutrophils are present in variable numbers depending upon the extent of the inflammatory response. Neutrophil nuclear segmentation may be difficult to appreciate because the cells often do not spread out well in the viscous fluid. Lymphocytes may increase in number with extended duration of the lesion. Macrophages containing phagocytized erythrocytes or debris may also be present. Golden, rhomboidal hematoidin crystals seen extracellularly or within the cytoplasm of macrophages result from erythrocyte degradation secondary to intracyst hemorrhage and suggest chronicity (Figure 6-20).

Sialadenosis: Idiopathic bilateral enlargement of the mandibular salivary glands (sialadenosis) has been reported in both dogs and cats as a cause of excessive salivation.[24-27] Fine-needle aspirates from affected glands have shown normal salivary epithelium, and histopathologic evaluation has revealed either normal or hypertrophied salivary tissue. Some of these animals have responded to oral phenobarbital therapy, suggesting a neurogenic cause.

Sialadenitis: Inflammatory lesions of the salivary gland are uncommon.[28] Inflammation may be primary or secondary, extending into the gland from surrounding tissues. Primary inflammation is often associated with sialocele, as described previously. or rarely with infarction. In both situations mixed inflammatory cells (neutrophils, lymphocytes, and macrophages) may be present.[28] Sialadenitis may occur with systemic viral infections (canine distemper virus, rabies virus, paramyxovirus).[29] Viral lesions may contain significant numbers of lymphoid cells. Secondary inflammation may occur due to trauma or bacterial infections in surrounding tissues. The inflammatory cell infiltrate will vary dependent upon the primary process. In bacterial infections, degenerate neutrophils with phagocytized bacteria may be observed. Depending upon the extent of the infection, salivary epithelial cells may not be evident in cytologic samples.

Neoplastic Lesions

Salivary gland neoplasia is uncommon in dogs and cats. It occurs most frequently in animals older than 10 years, and there is some evidence that poodles, spaniel breeds, and Siamese cats may be predisposed.[30] Both the parotid and mandibular salivary glands are frequent sites for salivary neoplasia.[28,30] Carcinomas occur most often, and a wide variety of tumor types can be recognized histologically, including acinar cell carcinomas, adenocarcinomas, squamous cell carcinomas, mucoepidermoid tumors, basal cell carcinomas, sebaceous carcinomas, and undifferentiated carcinomas.[31-33] Acinar cell carcinomas and adenocarcinomas represent the most common malignant neoplasms of the salivary glands in dogs and cats.[30,31,34]

TABLE 6-1

Common Cytologic Findings in Mammary Gland Aspirates

Cell Types	Key Features	Differential Diagnoses	Comments

Foam cells
Inflammatory cells:
  neutrophils, lymphocytes,
  plasma cells, macrophages
Epithelial cell clusters
	Predominance of
	  inflammatory cells.
	Proteinaceous debris.
	± Bacteria
	Epithelial cells may
	  be reactive.
		Mastitis
		
		Inflammatory
		  carcinoma
			Mild atypia in epithelial cells
			  expected with inflammation.
			Marked epithelial pleomor-
			  phism with nonseptic
			  inflammation typical for
			  inflammatory carcinoma
			  (requires histopathologic
			  confirmation).

Vacuolated macrophages
± Epithelial cell clusters
	Low-cellularity fluid
	  aspirated.
	Minimal atypia in
	  epithelial cells.
		Cyst	Cysts may occur along or
			  with benign or malignant
			  neoplasia.
			Sample solid tissue as well as
			  cystic fluid.

Epithelial cell clusters
Spindled mesenchymal
  cells
Extracellular matrix
	Uniform epithelial
	  cells, high
	  nuclear-to-cytoplasmic
	  ratio.
	Mildly pleomorphic
	  mesenchymal cells
	  with abundant matrix.
		Fibroepithelial
		  hyperplasia
			Typically affects young
			  intact female cats, or cats
			  previously treated with
			  progesterone drugs.
			Affects multiple glands.
			Rapid growth.
			Cytologic appearance similar
			  to many benign tumors.

Variable numbers of
  epithelial cells and
  mesenchymal cells
± Extracellular matrix,
  cartilage, or bone
  (osteoblasts)
± Inflammatory cells
	Variable depending
	  on specific process.
	Usually mild pleomorphism,
	  but may be moderate
	  to marked.
		Benign neoplasia
		  (adenoma/complex
		  adenoma, benign
		  mixed tumors, etc.)
		Lobular hyperplasia
			Multiple possible cell types
			  result in confusing cytology.
			Inflammatory nodules may
			  occur with lobular hyper-
			  plasia. Tumors exfoliating
			  numerous atypical cells may
			  suggest malignancy despite
			  lack of tissue invasion.
			Histopathologic confirmation
			  required.

Variable numbers of
  epithelial cells and
  mesenchymal cells
± Extracellular matrix,
  cartilage, or bone
  (osteoblasts)
± Inflammatory cells
	Variable depending on
	  specific process.
	Cellular pleomorphism
	  can be minimal or
	  marked.
		Malignant neoplasia
		  (adenocarcinoma,
		  various carcinomas,
		  inflammatory
		  carcinoma,
		  fibrosarcoma,
		  osteosarcoma, etc.)
			Canine: ~50% are malignant.
			Feline: ~80% are malignant.
			Multiple possible cell types
			  result in confusing cytology.
			Marked pleomorphism
			  increases likelihood of
			  malignancy.
			Tumors with minimal atypia
			  may be malignant based on
			  tissue invasion.
			Histopathologic confirmation
			  required.

Cytology samples from salivary carcinomas contain cohesive epithelial cells with round to oval nuclei and basophilic cytoplasm with a relatively high nuclear-to-cytoplasmic ratio. These cells may show little differentiation toward normal vacuolated salivary epithelium (Figures 6-21 and 6-22).[35] Criteria of malignancy may be mild, consisting only of mild anisocytosis and anisokaryosis, or may be more pronounced with the presence of prominent nucleoli and mitotic figures in addition to marked pleomorphism.[36,37] Eosinophilic secretory product may be seen extracellularly or within the cytoplasm of the neoplastic cells in varying amounts (Figures 6-21 to 6-25).

Squamous epithelial cells can be a component not only of salivary squamous cell carcinomas but also of mucoepidermoid carcinomas and necrotizing sialometaplasia.

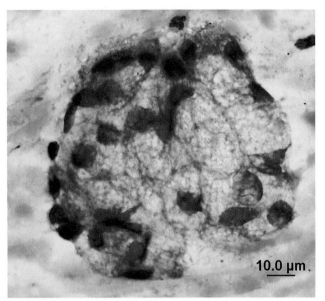

Figure 6-17 Cohesive cluster of vacuolated secretory cells from a normal salivary gland. (Wright's stain, 1000×.)

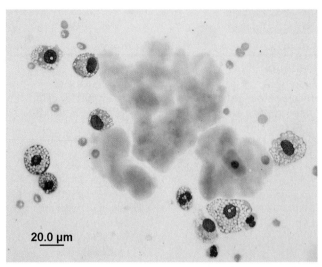

Figure 6-19 Foamy macrophages and/or vacuolated epithelial cells and a few erythrocytes from a salivary sialocele. Notice the extracellular clumps of amorphous basophilic material, consistent with mucin. (Wright's stain, 500×.)

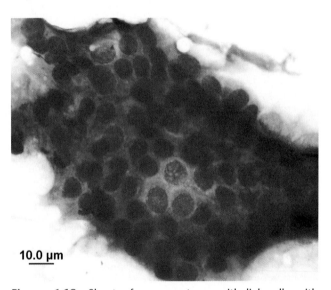

Figure 6-18 Sheet of nonsecretory epithelial cells with a high nuclear-to-cytoplasmic ratio from a normal salivary gland most likely represents ductal epithelium. (Wright's stain, 1000×.)

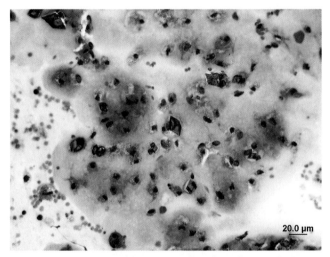

Figure 6-20 Numerous vacuolated cells and large, golden, rhomboidal hematoidin crystals indicating previous hemorrhage in an aspirate from a sialocele. Erythrocytes and basophilic mucin are present in the background. (Wright's stain, 500×.)

Salivary squamous cell carcinomas have a similar cytologic appearance to squamous cell carcinomas in other locations (see Chapter 5 for further discussion of the features of squamous cell carcinoma). Mucoepidermoid carcinomas contain both squamous and mucus-producing cell types. The cytologic appearance of necrotizing sialometaplasia has been described, consisting of mixed salivary glandular cells, pleomorphic spindled cells, and rafts of mononuclear epithelioid cells with increased numbers of neutrophils.[38] In that case, the cytologic diagnosis was

sialadenitis and possible mesenchymal neoplasia, but histopathology revealed necrosis and ductal squamous metaplasia leading to the final diagnosis. Thus, accurate cytologic interpretation may be limited when multiple cell types are present.

Malignant mixed tumors of salivary glands are rare, but have been described in both dogs and cats.[31,39,40] These tumors may be the result of carcinoma arising in a previously benign pleomorphic adenoma. Rarely, true carcinosarcomas have been reported, containing both sarcoma and carcinoma elements. Cytology would be expected to reveal a mixture of epithelial and mesenchymal cell types with criteria of malignancy.

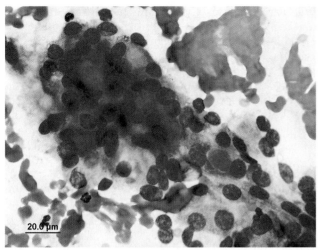

Figure 6-21 Aspirate of a salivary adenocarcinoma from a cat. A cluster of nonvacuolated epithelial cells have a disorganized appearance and indistinct cell borders. A small amount of eosinophilic secretory product is visible. (Wright's stain, 1000×.)

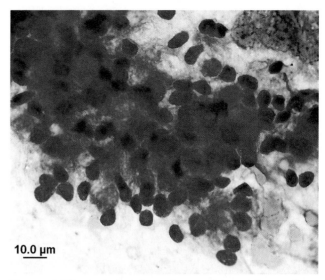

Figure 6-23 Aspirate of a salivary adenocarcinoma from a dog containing abundant extracellular secretory material and monomorphic epithelial cells. (Wright's stain, 1000×.)

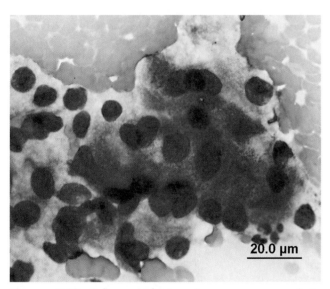

Figure 6-22 Salivary adenocarcinoma, same aspirate as Figure 6-21. Granular, eosinophilic, intracytoplasmic secretory material is present within epithelial cells. (Wright's stain, 1000×.)

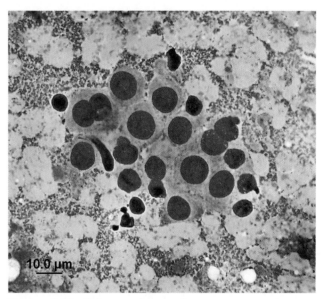

Figure 6-24 Salivary adenocarcinoma, same aspirate as Figure 6-23. Individual epithelial cells with round nuclei and lightly basophilic cytoplasm are present in a thick eosinophilic background of secretory material. Cellular pleomorphism is minimal. (Wright's stain, 1000×.)

Benign salivary tumors are rare in dogs and cats. Pleomorphic adenomas contain epithelial, myoepithelial, and stromal elements and may include areas of cartilage or bone. Sebaceous adenomas and cystadenomas have also been reported.[31]

Table 6-2 presents a summary of the most common cytologic findings in aspirates from salivary gland lesions.

THE THYROID GLANDS

Normal Cytologic Appearance

The thyroid glands of dogs and cats are paired endocrine glands in the ventral cervical region. Their exact location may vary from the laryngeal region to the thoracic inlet. Ectopic thyroid tissue may also occur in the cranial mediastinum near the heart base. The normal thyroid gland is not readily palpated and is, therefore, not usually aspirated for cytologic examination. Palpable abnormalities may occur unilaterally or bilaterally as diffuse swelling, multinodular swelling, or solitary nodular masses. Aspiration cytology may help differentiate benign from malignant lesions and help rule out other causes of cervical masses, including abscesses, lymphadenopathy, sialoceles, and nonthyroid neoplasms.

Thyroid tissue consists of numerous follicles lined by cuboidal to polygonal epithelial cells and filled with colloid. Each gland is enclosed in a connective tissue capsule and has a rich vascular supply. Scrapings or imprints of normal thyroid tissue contain clusters of typical follicular epithelial cells (Figure 6-26). Nuclei are of uniform size with finely stippled chromatin and are located centrally in a moderate amount of lightly basophilic,

granular cytoplasm. Cytoplasmic borders are indistinct, and many naked nuclei from broken cells are often present. Blue-black granular pigment thought to represent tyrosine accumulation and/or thyroglobulin may be seen within the cytoplasm.[35,41] Large macrophages containing variable amounts of pigment believed to be digested colloid are occasionally seen. Amorphous colloid may be present extracellularly, usually appearing pink but occasionally grayish-blue.

Benign Lesions

Inflammation: Chronic lymphocytic thyroiditis is an immune-mediated lesion that is a rare cause of thyroid gland enlargement in dogs.[42,43] Dogs with this syndrome usually have no signs of disease in early stages when the thyroid gland is most likely to be enlarged. When clinical signs of hypothyroidism appear, the thyroid gland has usually atrophied, is not palpable, and therefore is not aspirated. Affected thyroid glands contain numerous lymphocytes, plasma cells, and macrophages in addition to normal and degenerating follicular cells.

Hyperplasia and Adenoma: Functional multinodular (adenomatous) hyperplasia and functional thyroid adenoma are the most common causes of clinical hyperthyroidism in older cats.[44,45] Distinguishing between the two processes requires histopathologic examination to evaluate compression of adjacent thyroid tissue and presence of a capsule, and it is likely that there has

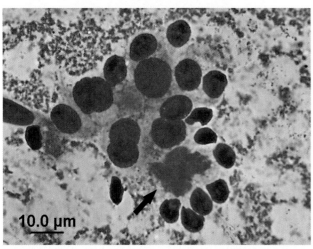

Figure 6-25 Salivary adenocarcinoma, same aspirate as Figure 6-23. The arrow indicates a rare acinar structure containing eosinophilic secretory material. (Wright's stain, 1000×.)

TABLE 6-2

Common Cytologic Findings in Salivary Gland Aspirates

Cell Types	Key Features	Differential Diagnoses	Comments
Secretory epithelium Background RBCs	Clusters and individual cells. Low nuclear-to-cytoplasmic ratio. Abundant cytoplasmic vacuoles.	Normal salivary tissue Sialadenosis	± Clusters of ductal epithelium (high nuclear-to-cytoplasmic ratio, no vacuoles). RBCs often line up (windrowing).
Secretory epithelium and vacuolated macrophages Background RBCs ± Neutrophils, lymphocytes	Viscous sample. Abundant amorphous basophilic mucin background.	Sialocele	Sialocele may have associated inflammation. Hematoidin crystals due to previous hemorrhage indicate chronicity.
Mostly inflammatory cells (neutrophils, lymphocytes) ± Secretory epithelium ± Bacteria	Cell types vary with cause. Degenerate neutrophils suggest bacterial infection.	Sialadenitis	May see bacteria phagocytized by neutrophils. Epithelial cells may be lacking.
Epithelial cell clusters Background RBCs ± Eosinophilic secretory material (intracellular or extracellular)	Clusters of cells with high nuclear-to-cytoplasmic ratio. Cells may not be vacuolated. Pleomorphism variable.	Salivary carcinoma	Carcinomas more common than benign tumors. Malignant cells may have few criteria of malignancy, but often do not resemble normal salivary epithelium. Histopathologic confirmation desirable.

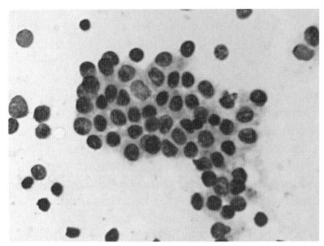

Figure 6-26 Sheet of normal thyroid gland epithelial cells. Cells have centrally located nuclei, with clumped chromatin and a small rim of basophilic cytoplasm. (Wright's stain, 1250×.)

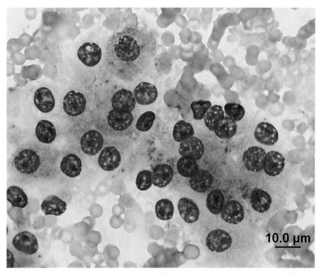

Figure 6-28 Feline thyroid adenoma. Blue intracytoplasmic pigment is present within some of these follicular cells. (Wright's stain, 1000×.)

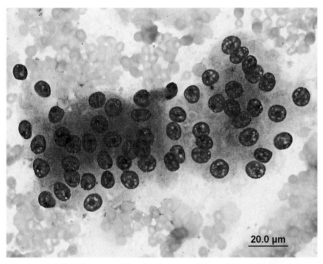

Figure 6-27 Cluster of cells from a feline thyroid adenoma. Cells have monomorphic nuclei and abundant granular cytoplasm. Cells at the edge of the cluster have lysed. (Wright's stain, 1000×.)

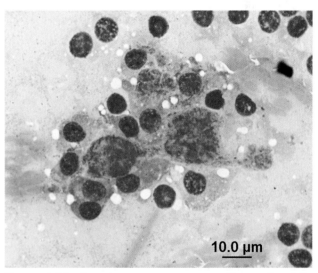

Figure 6-29 An acinar structure surrounding eosinophilic colloid in an aspirate of a thyroid adenoma. Notice the naked nuclei and lightly basophilic background from ruptured cells. (Wright's stain, 1000×.)

been considerable overlap in these histologic diagnoses. In contrast to these typically functional masses in cats, thyroid adenomas in dogs are less common and generally nonfunctional.[44,46] In dogs, the majority of thyroid adenomas are incidental findings at necropsy. Cytologic specimens have variable cellularity with clusters of follicular cells and scattered naked nuclei as the predominant finding. Aspirates are often bloody because of extensive vascularity. Follicular cells are uniform in appearance, with small round nuclei placed centrally in a moderate amount of basophilic cytoplasm (Figure 6-27). The presence of blue-black intracytoplasmic granules is variable (Figure 6-28). Follicular cells may form acinar arrangements, sometimes surrounding central colloid (Figure 6-29).

Uncommon causes of thyroid hyperplasia in animals include iodine deficiency, iodine excess, and errors of thyroid hormone synthesis (dyshormonogenesis).[44,47,48] Thyroid follicular cells may appear hyperplastic, and the amount of colloid present is variable.[44]

Malignant Neoplasms

The vast majority of clinically evident thyroid tumors in dogs are carcinomas (80% to 90%), in contrast to only 5% in cats.[46] Thyroid carcinomas usually occur in older dogs, with no sex predilection. A breed predisposition has been shown for Boxers, Beagles, and Golden Retrievers.[44]

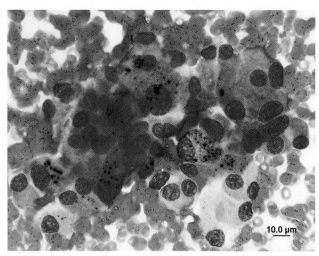

Figure 6-30 Aspirate of a functional follicular thyroid carcinoma from a dog. Neoplastic thyroid epithelial cells are present in a cohesive cluster along with abundant erythrocytes. Some of these cells contain blue-black cytoplasmic pigment. These cells exhibit more criteria of malignancy than is typical for most thyroid carcinomas. (Wright's stain, 1000×.)

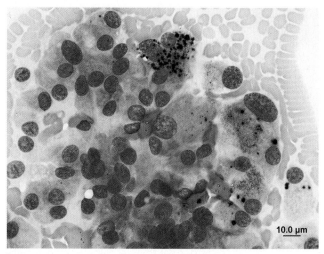

Figure 6-32 Thyroid carcinoma, same aspirate as Figure 6-30. Some cells contain blue-black cytoplasmic pigment, although others do not. (Wright's stain, 1000×.)

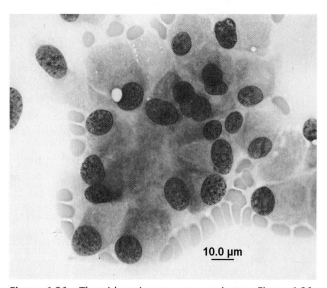

Figure 6-31 Thyroid carcinoma, same aspirate as Figure 6-30. An acinar structure without colloid is present. (Wright's stain, 1000×.)

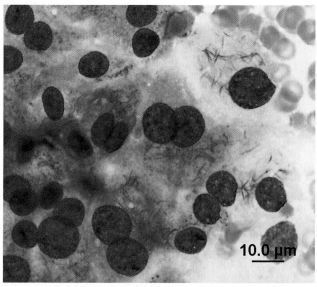

Figure 6-33 Aspirate of a nonfunctional follicular thyroid carcinoma from a dog demonstrating needle-shaped intracytoplasmic inclusions in many cells. The significance of these inclusions is not known. (Wright's stain, 1000×.)

Malignant tumors are poorly encapsulated and usually tightly adherent to underlying tissues because of extensive local invasion. Pulmonary metastases are frequent due to early invasion into thyroid veins.[44] Larger tumors may have a greater potential for metastasis.[49] Areas of mineralization and bone formation may be present within the tumor. Most thyroid carcinomas are nonfunctional in both dogs and cats.

A good correlation between results of aspiration cytology and histopathologic examination has been found with thyroid carcinomas.[50] The problem of excessive

blood contamination in many specimens may require repeated aspirations. In the absence of excessive blood contamination, smears tend to be highly cellular and may or may not contain colloid. Follicular thyroid carcinomas yield cells that occur both singly and in dense clusters, sometimes forming acinar structures (Figures 6-30 and 6-31). Typical blue-black cytoplasmic granules may be seen, and fine needle-shaped cytoplasmic inclusions have also been observed (Figures 6-32 and 6-33). Anisocytosis and anisokaryosis are variable. Cytologic criteria of malignancy are subtle or completely lacking in many carcinomas. Nuclei may be mildly enlarged and have indistinct nucleoli; mitotic

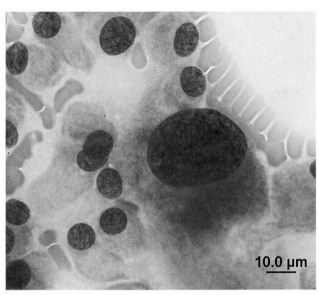

10.0 μm

Figure 6-34 Marked anisocytosis and anisokaryosis are present in this aspirate of a follicular thyroid carcinoma from a dog. (Wright's stain, 1000×.)

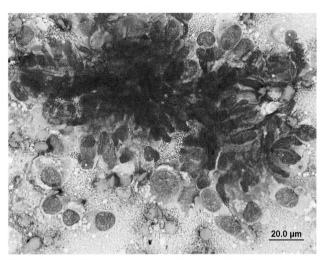

20.0 μm

Figure 6-36 This aspirate of a malignant mixed thyroid tumor from a dog contains only pleomorphic mesenchymal cells and an abundant extracellular eosinophilic matrix, suggesting a diagnosis of sarcoma. Histopathologic examination revealed neoplastic epithelial cells as well. (Wright's stain, 1000×.)

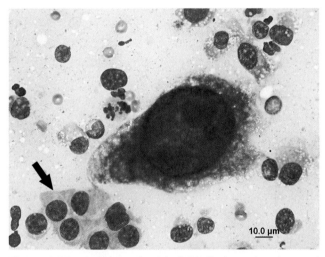

10.0 μm

Figure 6-35 A cluster of epithelial cells *(arrow)* and several pleomorphic mesenchymal cells in a malignant mixed thyroid tumor from a dog. The central mesenchymal cell contains a macronucleus with two macronucleoli. (Wright's stain, 1000×.) *(Glass slide courtesy Juopperi et al, North Carolina State University, presented at the 2002 ASVCP case review session.)*

figures are uncommon. When marked anisocytosis and anisokaryosis are present, a diagnosis of carcinoma can be made with confidence (Figure 6-34). Otherwise, histopathologic evaluation of tumor encapsulation and invasion is required to distinguish adenoma from carcinoma.

Although most carcinomas arise from follicular thyroid epithelium, medullary parafollicular C-cell tumors have also been described in dogs. Previously thought to

be uncommon, there is some evidence that medullary carcinomas may be recognized more frequently with increasing use of immunohistochemical stains (chromogranin A and calcitonin).[49,51,52] Because these tumors tend to be well encapsulated and less likely to metastasize, differentiating them from follicular carcinomas may have prognostic implications.[51] The cytologic features of a medullary carcinoma, recently described by Bertazzolo et al,[53] are virtually identical to follicular carcinomas, with epithelial cells occurring in clusters and acinar patterns. Pink amorphous material consistent with colloid was observed, but blue-black intracytoplasmic pigment was not.[53]

Undifferentiated carcinomas of the thyroid are rare in dogs and cats.[54] These tumors may contain spindle-shaped cells, suggestive of a sarcoma. Malignant mixed thyroid tumors are also rare, being composed of epithelial and mesenchymal elements (Figures 6-35 and 6-36).[44]

Cystic Lesions

Cystic lesions have been reported in association with both thyroid adenomas and carcinomas in dogs and cats.[44,55-57] Aspirated fluid may appear serous but is more commonly brown and turbid because of previous hemorrhage and necrosis. Foamy, pigment-laden macrophages, lymphocytes, erythrocytes, and occasionally cholesterol crystals are seen along with clusters of follicular cells (Figures 6-37 and 6-38). Thyroid hormone levels in the cystic fluid can be measured to confirm thyroid origin.[57]

THE PARATHYROID GLANDS

The parathyroid glands are located adjacent to the thyroid glands. Tumors involving the parathyroid chief cells are uncommon but have been reported in both dogs and cats.[58-60] Parathyroid tumors in dogs are not usually palpable due to their small size and location, but are

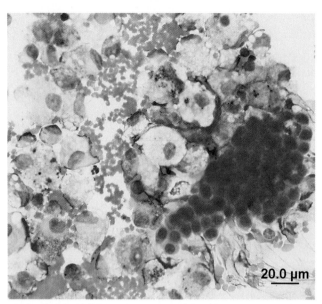

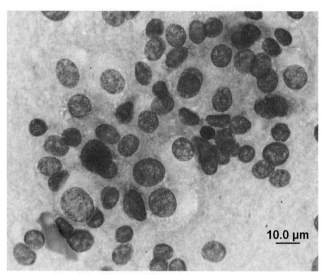

Figure 6-37   Aspirate of a cystic thyroid mass from a cat with hyperthyroidism. A cohesive cluster of thyroid epithelial cells is present along with numerous vacuolated macrophages and erythrocytes. (Wright's stain, 1000×.) (*Glass slide courtesy Theresa Rizzi, Oklahoma State University.*)

Figure 6-39   Aspirate from a functional parathyroid carcinoma (dog). Sheets and small clusters of cells with round nuclei, stippled chromatin, and lightly basophilic cytoplasm. Many cells are ruptured, and basophilic cytoplasm fills the background. (Wright's stain, 1000×.)

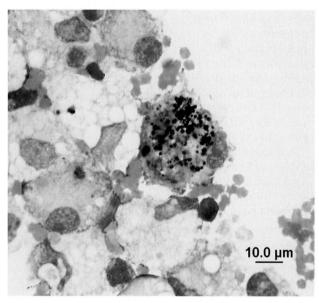

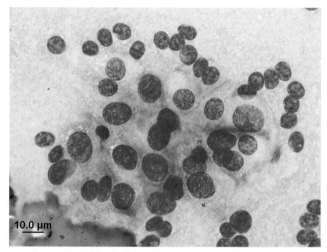

Figure 6-38   Cystic thyroid mass, same aspirate as Figure 6-37. Many macrophages contain blue-black phagocytized pigment, likely representing thyroglobulin. (Wright's stain, 1000×.)

Figure 6-40   Parathyroid carcinoma, same aspirate as Figure 6-39. Moderate anisocytosis and anisokaryosis are seen in the intact cells. (Wright's stain, 1000×.)

more often identified using ultrasound during a search for causes of hypercalcemia in animals showing clinical signs of primary hyperparathyroidism.[61] Cats may be more likely to have a palpable parathyroid nodule.[60,62] Adenomas are diagnosed more frequently than carcinomas in both dogs and cats, and either may be functional, producing excess parathormone. Adenomas are usually encapsulated and compress adjacent normal parathyroid and thyroid tissues. Carcinomas are generally larger than adenomas and are fixed to underlying tissues due to local

infiltration.[63] Because both tumors are composed of well-differentiated chief cells, differentiating adenoma from carcinoma relies on a combination of gross appearance and microscopic evidence of invasion, although cells from carcinomas may exhibit greater pleomorphism.[63]

Cells from both adenomas and carcinomas have a similar cytologic appearance. Many naked nuclei are seen in a background of lightly basophilic cytoplasmic material (Figure 6-39). Nuclei are round to oval and generally uniform in size; mild anisokaryosis may be noted in carcinomas (Figure 6-40). When present in clusters these cells have indistinct cytoplasmic borders, and may

TABLE 6-3

Common Cytologic Findings in Thyroid or Parathyroid Aspirates

Cell Types	Key Features	Differential Diagnoses	Comments
*Follicular epithelium Abundant RBCs ± Colloid	Naked nuclei in background. Intact cells in clusters or singly. ± Acinar structures. ± Blue-black cytoplasmic granules. ± Needle-shaped cytoplasmic inclusions. Colloid eosinophilic or basophilic.	Thyroid follicular hyperplasia Thyroid follicular tumor	Hyperplasia, adenoma, and many carcinomas appear identical with cytology. Carcinomas often exhibit little or no atypia, but can show marked pleomorphism. Feline: most are functional and benign. Canine: most are nonfunctional and malignant. Histopathologic confirmation desirable.
*Parafollicular epithelium (C cells) Abundant RBCs	Naked nuclei in background. Intact cells in clusters or singly. ± Acinar structures.	Thyroid medullary tumor	Less common than follicular tumors. Animal may be hypocalcemic. Colloid may be present. Histopathologic confirmation desirable. Special stains assist identification.
*Epithelial cells (Chief cells)	Naked nuclei in background. Intact cells in clusters or singly. ± Acinar structures. ± Needle-shaped cytoplasmic inclusions. May have fewer RBCs than thyroid tumors.	Parathyroid tumor	Less common than thyroid tumors. Adenomas or carcinomas may be functional. Animal may be hypercalcemic. Carcinomas may exhibit little or no atypia. Histopathologic confirmation desirable.

*Cytologically identical.

form acinar structures. Eosinophilic needle-like structures were noted within the cytoplasm in one report of a canine parathyroid carcinoma.[64] The significance of these inclusions is not known, but they have also been seen in aspirates of follicular thyroid neoplasia (see Figure 6-33).

Table 6-3 presents a summary of the most common cytologic findings in aspirates from thyroid and parathyroid gland lesions.

References

1. Allen SW, Prasse KW, Mahaffey EA: Cytologic differentiation of benign from malignant canine mammary tumors. *Vet Pathol* 23:6649-655, 1986.
2. Griffiths GL, Lumsden JH, Valli VE: Fine needle aspiration cytology and histologic correlation in canine tumors. *Vet Clin Pathol* 13:113-17, 1984.
3. Hellmen E, Lindgren A: The accuracy of cytology in diagnosis and DNA analysis of canine mammary tumours. *J Comp Pathol* 101:4443-450, 1989.
4. Linde-Forsberg C: Abnormalities in pregnancy, parturition, and the periparturient period. In Ettinger SJ, Feldman EC, (eds): *Textbook of Veterinary Internal Medicine.* ed 6, vol 2. St. Louis, Saunders, 2005, pp 1666-1667.
5. Feldman EC, Nelson RW: Preparturient diseases. In Feldman EC, Nelson RW (eds): *Canine and Feline Endocrinology and Reproduction.* ed 3, St. Louis, Saunders, 2004, pp 831-832.
6. Brodey RS, Goldschmidt MH, Roszel JR: Canine mammary gland neoplasms. *J Am Anim Hosp Assoc* 19:61-81, 1983.
7. Misdorp W: Tumors of the mammary glands. In Meuten DJ (ed): *Tumors of Domestic Animals.* ed 4, Ames, Iowa, Iowa State Press, 2002, pp 575-606.
8. Klaassen JK: Cytology of subcutaneous glandular tissues. *Anim Pract* 32:61237-1266, v-vi, 2002.
9. Fernandes PJ, Guyer C, Modiano JF: Mammary mass aspirate from a Yorkshire terrier. *Vet Clin Pathol* 27:379, 1998.
10. Hayden DW, Barnes DM, Johnson KH: Morphologic changes in the mammary gland of megestrol acetate-treated and untreated cats: A retrospective study. *Vet Pathol* 26: 2104-113, 1989.
11. MacDougall LD: Mammary fibroadenomatous hyperplasia in a young cat attributed to treatment with megestrol acetate. *Can Vet J* 44:3227-229, 2003.
12. Mesher CI: What is your diagnosis? Subcutaneous nodule from a 14-month-old cat. *Vet Clin Pathol* 26:14, 1997.
13. Wehrend A, Hospes R, Gruber AD: Treatment of feline mammary fibroadenomatous hyperplasia with a progesterone-antagonist. *Vet Rec* 148:11346-347, 2001.

14. Sorenmo K: Canine mammary gland tumors. *Vet Clin North Am Small Anim Pract* 33:3573-596, 2003.

15. Hayes HM Jr, Milne KL, Mandell CP: Epidemiological features of feline mammary carcinoma. *Vet Rec* 108:22476-479, 1981.

16. MacEwen EG, et al: Prognostic factors for feline mammary tumors. *J Am Vet Med Assoc* 185:2201-204, 1984.

17. Skorupski KA, et al: Clinical characteristics of mammary carcinoma in male cats. *J Vet Intern Med* 19:152-155, 2005.

18. Karayannopoulou M, et al: Histological grading and prognosis in dogs with mammary carcinomas: Application of a human grading method. *J Comp Pathol* 133:4246-4252, 2005.

19. Viste JR, et al: Feline mammary adenocarcinoma: Tumor size as a prognostic indicator. *Can Vet J* 43:133-137, 2002.

20. Pena et al: Canine inflammatory mammary carcinoma: Histopathology, immunohistochemistry and clinical implications of 21 cases. *Breast Cancer Res Treat* 78:2141-2148, 2003.

21. Perez Alenza MD, Tabanera E, Pena L: Inflammatory mammary carcinoma in dogs: 33 cases—1995-1999 *J Am Vet Med Assoc* 219:81110-81114, 2001.

22. Perez-Alenza MD, et al: First description of feline inflammatory mammary carcinoma: Clinicopathological and immunohistochemical characteristics of three cases. *Breast Cancer Res* 6:4R300-4R307, 2004.

23. Smith MM: Oral and salivary gland disorders. In Ettinger SJ, Feldman EC (eds): *Textbook of Veterinary Internal Medicine.* ed 6, vol 2, St. Louis, Elsevier, 2005, pp 1290-1297.

24. Boydell P, Pike R, Crossley D: Presumptive sialadenosis in a cat. *J Small Anim Pract* 41:12573-12574, 2000.

25. Boydell P, et al: Sialadenosis in dogs. *J Am Vet Med Assoc* 216:6872-6874, 2000.

26. Sozmen M, Brown PJ, Whitbread TJ: Idiopathic salivary gland enlargement (sialadenosis) in dogs: A microscopic study. *J Small Anim Pract* 41:6243-6247, 2000.

27. Stonehewer J, et al: Idiopathic phenobarbital-responsive hypersialosis in the dog: An unusual form of limbic epilepsy? *J Small Anim Pract* 41:9416-9421, 2000.

28. Spangler WL, Culbertson MR: Salivary gland disease in dogs and cats: 245 cases—1985-1988 *J Am Vet Med Assoc* 198:3465-3469, 1991.

29. Brown NO: Salivary gland diseases: Diagnosis, treatment, and associated problems. *Probl Vet Med* 1:2281-2294, 1989.

30. Hammer A, et al: Salivary gland neoplasia in the dog and cat: Survival times and prognostic factors. *J Am Anim Hosp Assoc* 37:5478-5482, 2001.

31. Head KW, Else RW: Tumors of the salivary glands. In Meuten DJ (ed): *Tumors of Domestic Animals.* ed 4, Ames, Iowa, Iowa State Press; 2002, pp 410-416.

32. Sozmen M, Brown PJ, Eveson JW: Sebaceous carcinoma of the salivary gland in a cat. *J Vet Med A Physiol Pathol Clin Med* 49:8425-8427, 2002.

33. Sozmen M, Brown PJ, Eveson JW: Salivary gland basal cell adenocarcinoma: A report of cases in a cat and two dogs. *J Vet Med A Physiol Pathol Clin Med* 50:8399-8401, 2003.

34. Carberry CA, et al: Salivary gland tumors in dogs and cats: A literature and case review. *J Am Anim Hosp Assoc* 24:561-567, 1988.

35. Baker R, Lumsden JH: The head and neck. In Baker R, Lumsden JH (eds): *Color Atlas of Cytology of the Dog and Cat.* St. Louis, Mosby, 2000, pp 119-127.

36. Mazzullo G, et al: Carcinoma of the submandibular salivary glands with multiple metastases in a cat. *Vet Clin Pathol* 34:161-164, 2005.

37. Militerno G, Bazzo R, Marcato PS: Cytological diagnosis of mandibular salivary gland adenocarcinoma in a dog. *J Vet Med A Physiol Pathol Clin Med* 52:10514-10516, 2005.

38. Duncan RB, et al: Mandibular salivary gland aspirate from a dog. *Vet Clin Pathol* 28:397-399, 1999.

39. Perez-Martinez C, et al: Malignant fibrous histiocytoma (giant cell type) associated with a malignant mixed tumor in the salivary gland of a dog. *Vet Pathol* 37:4350-4353, 2000.

40. Smrkovski OA, et al: Carcinoma ex pleomorphic adenoma with sebaceous differentiation in the mandibular salivary gland of a dog. *Vet Pathol* 43:3374-3377, 2006.

41. Perman V, Alsaker RD, Riis RC: *Cytology of the Dog and Cat.* South Bend, Ind, American Animal Hospital Association, 1979.

42. Gosselin SJ, et al: Autoimmune lymphocytic thyroiditis in dogs. *Vet Immunol Immunopathol* 3:1-2185-2201, 1982.

43. Graham PA, et al: Lymphocytic thyroiditis. *Vet Clin North Am Small Anim Pract* 31:5915-5933, vi-vii, 2001.

44. Capen CC: Tumors, hyperplasia, and cysts of thyroid follicular cells. In Meuten DJ (ed): *Tumors in Domestic Animals,* ed 4. Ames, Iowa: Iowa State Press, 2002, pp 634-654.

45. Feldman EC, Nelson RW: Feline hyperthyroidism (thyrotoxicosis). In Feldman EC, Nelson RW (eds): *Canine and Feline Edocrinology and Reproduction,* ed 3. St. Louis, Saunders, 2004, pp 152-215.

46. Feldman EC, Nelson RW: Canine thyroid tumors and hyperthyroidism. In Feldman EC, Nelson RW (eds): *Canine and Feline Endocrinology and Reproduction,* ed 3. St. Louis, Saunders, 2004, pp 219-248.

47. Chastain CB, et al: Congenital hypothyroidism in a dog due to an iodide organification defect. *Am J Vet Res* 44:71257-71265, 1983.

48. Fyfe JC, et al: Congenital hypothyroidism with goiter in toy fox terriers. *J Vet Intern Med* 17:150-157, 2003.

49. Leav I, et al: Adenomas and carcinomas of the canine and feline thyroid. *Am J Pathol* 83:161-122, 1976.

50. Thompson EJ, et al: Fine needle aspiration cytology in the diagnosis of canine thyroid carcinoma. *Can Vet J* 21:6186-6188, 1980.

51. Carver JR, Kapatkin A, Patnaik AK: A comparison of medullary thyroid carcinoma and thyroid adenocarcinoma in dogs: A retrospective study of 38 cases. *Vet Surg* 24:4315-4319, 1995.

52. Patnaik AK, Lieberman PH: Gross, histologic, cytochemical, and immunocytochemical study of medullary thyroid carcinoma in sixteen dogs. *Vet Pathol* 28:3223-3233, 1991.

53. Bertazzolo W, et al: Paratracheal cervical mass in a dog. *Vet Clin Pathol* 32:4209-4212, 2003.

54. Anderson PG, Capen CC: Undifferentiated spindle cell carcinoma of the thyroid in a dog. *Vet Pathol* 23:2203-2204, 1986.

55. Wisner ER, Nyland TG: Ultrasonography of the thyroid and parathyroid glands. *Vet Clin North Am Small Anim Pract* 28:4973-4991, 1998.

56. Hofmeister E, et al: Functional cystic thyroid adenoma in a cat. *J Am Vet Med Assoc* 219:2190-2193, 2001.

57. Phillips DE, et al: Cystic thyroid and parathyroid lesions in cats. *J Am Anim Hosp Assoc* 39:4349-4354, 2003.

58. Berger B, Feldman EC: Primary hyperparathyroidism in dogs: 21 cases. 1976-1986 *J Am Vet Med Assoc* 191:3350-3356, 1987.

59. den Hertog E, et al: Primary hyperparathyroidism in two cats. *Vet Q* 19:281-281, 1997.

60. Kallet AJ, et al: Primary hyperparathyroidism in cats: Seven cases. 1984-1989 *J Am Vet Med Assoc* 199:121767-121771, 1991.

61. Feldman EC, et al: Pretreatment clinical and laboratory findings in dogs with primary hyperparathyroidism: 210 cases. 1987-2004 *J Am Vet Med Assoc* 227:5756-5761, 2005.

62. Feldman EC, Nelson RW: Primary hyperparathyroidism in cats. In Feldman EC, Nelson RW (eds): *Canine and Feline Endocrinology and Reproduction*. St. Louis, Saunders, 2004, 711-713.

63. Capen CC: Tumors and nonneoplastic cysts of the parathyroid gland. In Meuten DJ (ed): *Tumors in Domestic Animals*, ed 4. Ames, Iowa, Iowa State Press, 2002, pp 665-669.

64. Ramaiah SK, et al: A mass in the ventral neck of a hypercalcemic dog. *Vet Clin Pathol* 30:4177-4179, pp 2001.

Nasal Exudates and Masses

C.B. Andreasen, P.M. Rakich, and K.S. Latimer

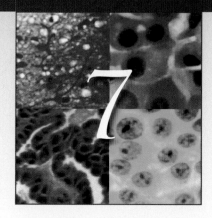

CHAPTER 7

INDICATIONS

Pathologic conditions in the nasal cavity are often characterized by sneezing, nasal discharge, epistaxis, ocular discharge, pawing at the nose, or facial deformity. Epistaxis may also result from primary coagulopathies, secondary coagulopathies (e.g., canine ehrlichiosis), and hyperviscosity syndromes. Cytologic findings are interpreted in light of historical, physical, rhinoscopic, radiographic, and clinical laboratory findings to arrive at a diagnosis. Rhinoscopy and cytologic evaluation are simple noninvasive procedures that may yield a definitive diagnosis. Cytologic evaluation is a method of screening the nasal cavity for the underlying etiology; however, negative or nonspecific findings do not exclude a fungal infection, neoplasm, or foreign body if only superficial inflammatory cells are obtained. The limiting factor for nasal cytology is obtaining a representative sample. In some cases, surgical exploration of the nasal cavity and biopsy/cytologic evaluation may be necessary for definitive diagnosis.

Detailed examination of the nasal cavity and most sample collections are optimally performed while the animal is under general anesthesia, with an endotracheal tube in place and the cuff inflated. Radiographs and rhinoscopy should be performed before biopsy or flushing techniques so that radiographic detail and visualization are not altered by resulting hemorrhage and manipulation of the nasal tissues.[1] The major landmarks and communication of the airways and food passages are schematically indicated (Figure 7-1).

The nasal cavity may be examined with equipment that varies from simple to sophisticated. In some animals, an otoscope may be used to examine the rostral nares; however, a flexible 4-mm fiberoptic endoscope should be used to view the ventral nasal meatus or nasopharynx.[2] The oronasal cavity can be examined by retracting the soft palate with forceps and using a dental mirror or flexible endoscope. These procedures can aid visualization of abnormal tissues but copious exudates or hemorrhage may preclude adequate examination.

SAMPLING TECHNIQUES

Cytologic specimens from the nasal cavity may be obtained by flushing or aspiration techniques. These methods are safe if care is taken not to penetrate the cribriform plate with the instruments used for obtaining samples and if precautions are taken to prevent inhalation of blood and fluids during sampling. Some hemorrhage may occur during manipulation of the nasal cavity, but this should not be a complicating factor unless a coagulopathy is present.

For the nasal flushing technique, the depth of the nasal cavity is estimated and a soft rubber catheter is passed caudad through the external nares or retrograde from caudal to the nasopharynx. A syringe containing about 10 ml of nonbacteriostatic sterile saline is attached to the catheter and multiple flushes are performed using intermittent positive and negative pressure.[1,2] Dislodged particulate matter can be caught in a gauze sponge placed caudal to the soft palate or rostral to the nares, depending on the direction of the flushing procedure. Aqueous cytologic material can be collected within the syringe barrel by aspiration.

Aspiration, the second means of obtaining samples from the nasal cavity, is useful when a mass is localized radiographically or visually. This technique involves use of a large-gauge polypropylene urinary catheter, a Sovereign plastic needle guard (Monoject, Sherwood Medical, St. Louis), or a tomcat catheter cut at a 45-degree angle to form a sharp cutting edge.[3] Proper catheter length is determined by measuring the distance from the external nares to the medial canthus of the eye. Catheter length is important to prevent penetration of the cribriform plate during the procedure. The catheter is attached to a syringe and advanced into the nasal cavity until moderate resistance is felt. Suction is applied while several advances are made into the mass. Gentle negative pressure is maintained as the catheter is removed from the mass and nasal cavity to retain solid tissue fragments.

Alternatively, a biopsy needle (Tru-Cut, Baxter Healthcare Corp., Deerfield, Ill.) may be passed through the nares to the mass and a biopsy obtained. Samples may also be obtained with a biopsy forceps attachment during endoscopic examination. Needle and endoscopic biopsies are large enough for cytologic touch imprint preparations and, if necessary, histopathologic examination.

Nasal swabs often do not yield satisfactory diagnostic material because they cannot be inserted far enough into the nasal cavity and are not abrasive enough to obtain representative samples of deep mucosal lesions. A diagnosis may be obtained using nasal swabs if a causative agent, such as *Cryptococcus neoformans*, is present in the nasal exudate or rostral nares.

Cytologic preparations are made from touch imprints or squash preparations of tissue fragments, smears of flush samples and swabs, and smears of centrifuged nasal flush sediments. These preparations are air-dried, stained, and examined by routine methods. (See Chapter 1 for further discussion concerning specimen preparation and staining.) A portion of the samples can be reserved for

microbiologic culture and sensitivity testing if an infectious agent is suspected or found on stained cytologic preparations. If samples are used for microbiologic testing, a sterile swab or sterile tube should be submitted that does not contain an anticoagulant such as ethylenediaminetetraacetic acid (EDTA), because EDTA can be bacteriostatic. If the fluid is submitted for cytologic examination, EDTA is useful for preservation of cell morphology. After imprinting for cytologic evaluation, tissue fragments can be preserved in 10% neutral buffered formalin for histopathologic evaluation.

Flow charts are provided to aid in the evaluation of nasal cytologic smears containing primarily inflammatory cells (Figure 7-2) and those containing primarily epithelial and/or mesenchymal cells (Figure 7-3).

NORMAL CYTOLOGIC FINDINGS

It is important to distinguish normal from pathologic cells and bacterial populations in cytologic preparations. In nasal flush specimens, oropharyngeal organisms of variable morphology and epithelial cells may be obtained from healthy animals. *Simonsiella* spp. are large, stacked, rod-shaped bacteria that are inhabitants of the oral cavity of dogs and cats and are seen commonly in smears contaminated by oral secretions (Figure 7-4).[4] Epithelial cell morphology varies with the site and depth of the specimen. Nonkeratinized squamous epithelial cells, often with adherent bacteria, are obtained from the external nares and oropharynx. Ciliated pseudostratified columnar epithelial cells and associated mucus originate from the nasal turbinates (Figure 7-5). Basal epithelial cells are smaller and rounded and have darker blue cytoplasm (Figure 7-6). Hemorrhage during sampling results in the presence of red blood cells (RBCs) and white blood cells (WBCs) in similar proportions to peripheral blood (about 1 WBC for every 500 to 1000 RBC).

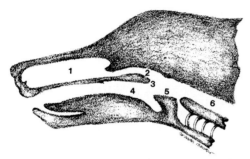

Figure 7-1 Schematic diagram indicating major landmarks and communication of the airways and food passages. **1,** Nasal cavity. **2,** Nasopharynx. **3,** Palate. **4,** Oropharynx. **5,** Epiglottis. **6,** Esophagus. The nasal cavity **(1)** may be sampled rostrad through the nares or caudad through the nasopharynx **(2)** as the soft palate **(3)** is retracted.

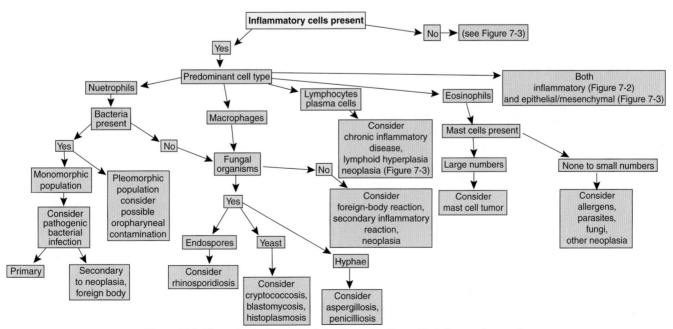

Figure 7-2 Flow chart of nasal cytologic evaluation with inflammatory cells.

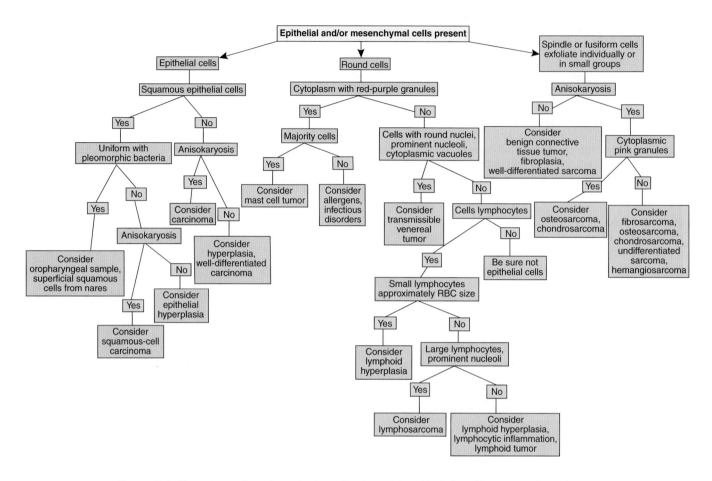

Figure 7-3 Flow chart of nasal cytologic evaluation with epithelial and/or mesenchymal cells.

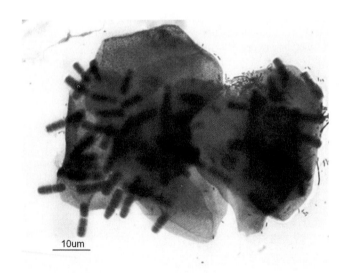

Figure 7-4 Two superficial squamous epithelial cells with many *Simonsiella* organisms and scattered bacterial rods. *Simonsiella* organisms appear as a single large bacterium but are actually several bacterial rods lying side by side, giving the striated appearance. *Simonsiella* organisms are inhabitants of the oral cavity of dogs and cats and are seen commonly in smears contaminated by oral secretions. (Wright's stain.) *(Courtesy Dr. R. L. Cowell.)*

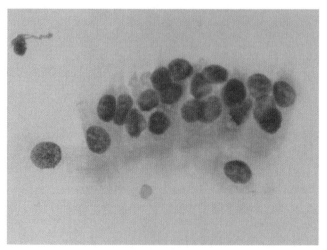

Figure 7-5 A row of normal ciliated columnar respiratory epithelial cells. (Wright's stain, 630×.)

INFECTIOUS AGENTS

Neutrophils usually predominate in exudates associated with bacterial, viral, and some fungal infections (Figure 7-7). In addition to neutrophils, variable numbers of macro-phages, lymphocytes and plasma cells may be present with any inflammatory condition. Pathogenic bacterial infection should be suspected when bacterial organisms are seen within neutrophils as compared with normal bacterial flora that colonize squamous epithelial cells in the absence of neutrophils. Because bacteria from the oral cavity are usually a pleomorphic population, a monomorphic bacterial population suggests infection.[5]

Identification of bacteria only on the basis of a gram-stained exudate is often unreliable. With routine hematologic stains, homogeneous populations of cocci usually represent gram-positive organisms, such as *Staphylococcus* or *Streptococcus* spp., whereas homogeneous populations of rods often indicate gram-negative organisms. Prior treatment with antibiotics may preclude identification of bacteria on cytologic preparations. Samples should be submitted for microbiologic culture, identification, and sensitivity testing.

Bacterial infections are usually secondary to mucosal injury from trauma or foreign bodies, but also may be associated with viral infection, fungal infection, and

neoplasia. Oronasal fistulas can result in chronic bacterial rhinitis. These fistulas most commonly involve canine, premolar, and molar teeth.[6]

Viral inclusions are infrequently seen in nasal cytology specimens. Herpesvirus infection in cats may produce intranuclear inclusions within epithelial cells.[7] Because inclusions are rarely found in Wright's-stained cytologic preparations, definitive diagnosis of viral inclusions is best accomplished by fluorescent antibody examination or viral isolation.

Fungal infections, foreign bodies, and neoplasia of the nasal cavity should be suspected when sinusitis is unresponsive to antibacterial therapy. In the case of mycotic rhinitis, fungal hyphae frequently are present within dense accumulations of cells and debris (Figure 7-8). Hyphae may be difficult to discern because they may not stain well with Romanowsky and new methylene blue stains and appear as clear filamentous structures. If a fungal infection is suspected but no fungal elements are identified on cytologic preparations, slides can be submitted to a laboratory for examination with special stains, such as periodic acid–Schiff (PAS) or Gomori's methenamine silver (GMS), to enhance visualization of fungal organisms. Additionally, fungal cultures are more reliable in identifying a fungal species than are morphologic characteristics.

Aspergillus spp. and/or *Penicillium* spp. produce nasal cavity and sinus infections in dogs and cats. These agents are associated with serosanguineous to mucopurulent nasal exudates, nasal mucosal necrosis, and turbinate destruction.[8-10] Both *Aspergillus* spp. and *Penicillium* spp. appear as 2- to 4.5-μm-wide septate, branching hyphae on cytologic preparations; therefore, specific identification requires fungal culture.[10]

C. neoformans is a saprophytic yeast that causes rhinitis and sinusitis and occurs most commonly in cats.[11,12] The organism may sometimes be found in touch imprints or aspirates of nasal lesions without nasal flushing or biopsy techniques. This basophilic yeast is round to oval, 3.5 to

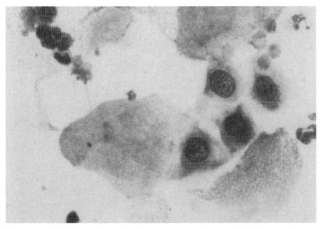

Figure 7-6 Four basal squamous cells and three mature, superficial squamous cells. (Wright's stain, 100×.)

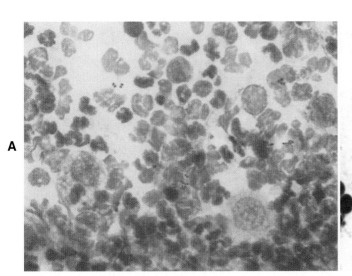

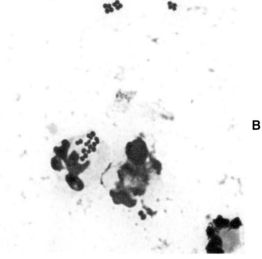

A

B

Figure 7-7 A, Septic purulent exudate with a monomorphic population of intracellular and extracellular paired cocci. (Wright's stain, 400×.) **B,** Degenerate neutrophil containing phagocytized bacterial cocci. (Wright's stain.) (*B courtesy Dr. R. L. Cowell.*)

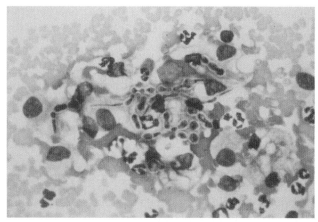

Figure 7-8 Numerous fungal hyphae and pyogranulomatous inflammation. (Wright's stain, 250×.)

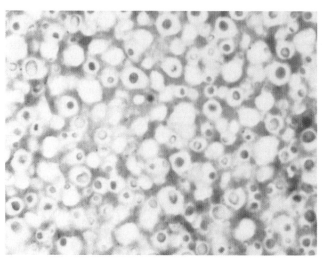

Figure 7-9 Numerous variably sized, spherical yeasts with thick unstained capsules are typical of *Cryptococcus neoformans*. (Wright's stain, 400×.)

7.0 μm in diameter, surrounded by a thick polysaccharide capsule (1-30 μm) that stains poorly with Wright's or Diff-Quik (Baxter Healthcare Corp., Dade Division, Miami) stains (Figure 7-9). Although India ink is often proposed as an aid in identifying *C. neoformans*, air bubbles and fat globules can be mistaken for organisms, particularly by inexperienced microscopists.

Rhinosporidiosis in dogs is characterized by polypoid nasal growths and caused by *Rhinosporidium seeberi*, a fungal organism of uncertain taxonomy and incompletely defined life cycle.[13,14] Diagnosis is based upon finding round to oval, 7-μm-diameter spores in nasal exudates or tissue imprints. The spores stain bright pink, have internal eosinophilic globules, and are surrounded by thin bilamellar cell walls (Figure 7-10). Finding large sporangia containing numerous endospores supports the diagnosis; however, these structures may be infrequently seen.[1]

Although parasitic diseases of the nasal cavity and sinuses are infrequent causes of clinical signs in small animals, infections with the arthropods *Pneumonyssus caninum* and *Linguatula serrata* have been reported in dogs.[6,16] Adult or larval forms of the nasal mite *P. caninum* may be found on the nasal mucosa. The mites may be an incidental finding or may be associated with mucosal irritation and sneezing. *L. serrata* is a penta-stome that attaches to the nasal mucosa and may induce sneezing, coughing, and epistaxis. Adult parasites may be visualized endoscopically or larvated eggs may be found in nasal exudates. Exudates associated with these parasites often contain increased numbers of eosinophils.

The helminth parasite *Capillaria aerophila* usually is found in the distal respiratory tract but may be found within the nasal sinuses.[6,17] Inflammatory exudates may contain characteristic barrel-shaped eggs with bipolar end plugs, neutrophils, and eosinophils (Fig 7-11). Sedimentation of nasal flush samples may be helpful in obtaining ova.

NONINFECTIOUS CONDITIONS

Nasal foreign bodies most frequently consist of inhaled plant material, such as grass awns or foxtails. Cytologic preparations should be examined closely for foreign mate-

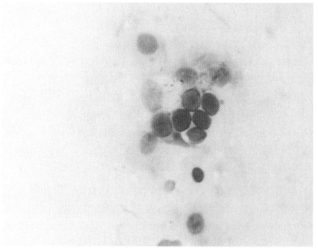

Figure 7-10 Round, eosinophilic, bilamellar-walled spores of *Rhinosporidium seeberi*. (Wright's stain, 400×.)

rial consisting of variably sized and shaped particles with distinct cell walls, fibers, and various degrees of pigmentation. A common sequel to this problem is chronic rhinitis due to persistence of foreign material, with damage to the nasal mucosa.

Exudates with a predominance of eosinophils may result from environmental inhalant allergens (Figure 7-12). Because eosinophils may be present in response to parasites, fungi, bacteria, and neoplasms, these conditions should be ruled out cytologically and/or radiographically before allergic inhalant rhinitis is diagnosed.

NEOPLASTIC DISORDERS

Neoplasia involving nasal passages and sinuses generally occurs in older animals, with a mean age of 8 to 10 years.[6,18,19] Nasal tumors are malignant in 80% to 90% of

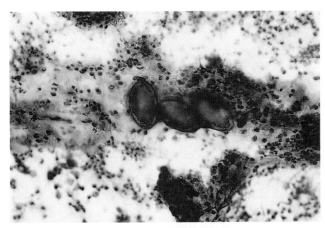

Figure 7-11 Barrel-shaped egg with bipolar end plugs characteristic of *Capillaria* spp. (Wright's stain, 1000×.)

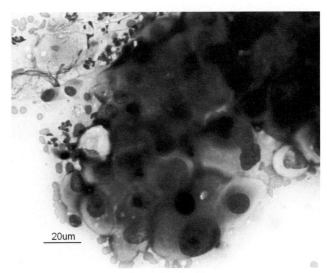

Figure 7-13 Cluster of epithelial cells showing marked criteria of malignancy indicating a nasal carcinoma. (Wright's stain.) *(Courtesy Dr. R. L. Cowell.)*

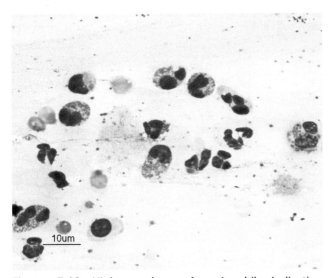

Figure 7-12 High numbers of eosinophils indicating eosinophilic inflammation. (Wright's stain.) *(Courtesy Dr. R. L. Cowell.)*

reported cases, but metastasis is uncommon.[18] Tumors can arise from epithelial or mesenchymal tissues of the nasal cavity, extend from the oral cavity into the nasal passages, or be transplanted into the nasal cavity, (e.g., transmissible venereal tumors).

Clinical presentation, history, and radiographic lesions may lead to presumptive diagnosis of neoplasia; however, cytologic or histologic examination is needed to confirm the diagnosis. Cytologic specimens of any tumor type may contain RBCs, inflammatory cells, bacteria, and necrotic debris. Neoplastic cells may or may not be present. Fine-needle aspiration or catheter biopsy of a tumor is more likely to yield identifiable neoplastic cells than a nasal flush. Usually, only normal superficial nasal epithelial cells or inflammatory cells are obtained from a nasal flush.

Most nasal tumors are of epithelial cell origin. Adenocarcinomas are most common, followed by squamous cell carcinomas and undifferentiated carcinomas.[18,20] Carcinomas usually consist of clusters of round

to oval cells, with variable nuclear:cytoplasmic ratios (Figure 7-13). These characteristics of malignancy are less pronounced in well-differentiated carcinomas, which may be difficult to distinguish from hyperplastic epithelial cells. Adenocarcinomas may be associated with production of mucus, apparent as amorphous to fibrillar deeply pink-staining material. Squamous-cell carcinomas generally consist of various developmental stages ranging from small hyperchromatic cells to large round or angular cells with pale basophilic cytoplasm and large nuclei (Figure 7-14). Perinuclear clearing, if present, strongly suggests squamous-cell origin.

Mesenchymal tumors of the nasal cavity primarily include fibrosarcomas, chondrosarcomas, osteosarcomas, hemangiosarcomas, and undifferentiated sarcomas.[20] As with sarcomas in any location, these tumors do not exfoliate readily. Aspirates or catheter biopsy imprints tend to produce a more cellular sample for evaluation than do nasal flushes. Sarcoma cells range from plump oval to fusiform or spindle shaped, with cytoplasm streaming away from the nucleus. These cells also tend to exfoliate individually or in small clumps, as compared with carcinomas, which often exfoliate in large sheets (see Figure 7-13). In osteosarcomas and chondrosarcomas, cells may have abundant basophilic cytoplasm and pink granules. Reactive fibroplasia and fibrosarcoma may be difficult or impossible to differentiate cytologically. Definitive identification of the type of sarcoma usually requires histologic examination.

Round cell tumors of the nasal cavity include transmissible venereal tumors, lymphosarcomas, and mast cell tumors. Generally these tumors exfoliate as a homogeneous population of individual round cells with distinct cell margins. Lymphosarcoma usually is characterized by a monomorphic population of large immature lymphocytes (Figure 7-15). In contrast, small mature lymphocytes predominate in nonneoplastic conditions with submucosal lymphoid hyperplasia. (See Chapter 11 on lymph node

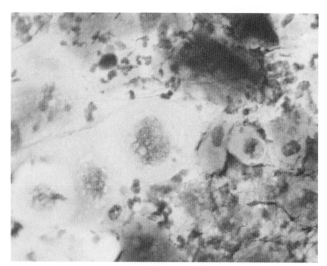

Figure 7-14 Cells from a squamous cell carcinoma with characteristic pale basophilic cytoplasm, large nuclei, and perinuclear clearing. (Wright's stain, 400×.)

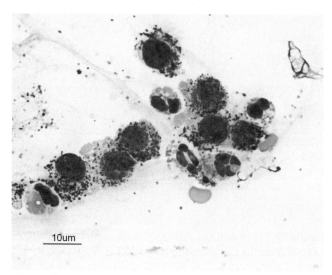

Figure 7-16 Scattered eosinophils and high numbers of moderately to heavily-granulated mast cells indicating a nasal mast cell tumor. (Wright's stain.) *(Courtesy Dr. R. L. Cowell.)*

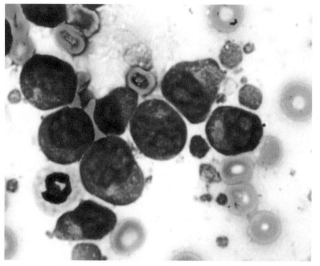

Figure 7-15 High numbers of large lymphoblasts indicating nasal lymphoma. (Wright's stain.) *(Courtesy Dr. R. L. Cowell.)*

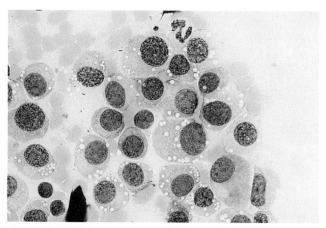

Figure 7-17 Numerous cells from a transmissible venereal tumor with coarse chromatin and smoky gray vacuolated cytoplasm are shown. (Wright's stain.)

cytology for further discussion on differentiating lymphoid hyperplasia from lymphosarcoma.)

Mast cell neoplasia is characterized by bloody aspirates containing numerous mast cells with fewer eosinophils (Figure 7-16). In contrast, allergic rhinitis is characterized by few mast cells and many eosinophils. Other cell types present may include plasma cells and lymphocytes.

Transmissible venereal tumors are more commonly associated with genital neoplasms but may be transplanted to the nasal mucosa because of the social habits of dogs, especially males.[21] The tumor cells have round nuclei, variable chromatin pattern, and a single prominent nucleolus. Cytoplasm is lightly basophilic and moderate in amount and usually contains clear vacuoles (Figure 7-17).

Mitoses may be numerous, and inflammatory cells of mixed type may be present.

References

1. Meyer: The management of cytology specimens. *Comp Cont Ed Pract Vet* 9:10-16, 1987.
2. Rudd and Richardson: A diagnostic and therapeutic approach to nasal disease in dogs. *Comp Cont Ed Pract Vet* 7:103-112, 1985.
3. Withrow et al: Aspiration and punch biopsy techniques for nasal tumors. *J Am Anim Hosp Assoc* 21:551-554, 1985.
4. Nyby MD, et al: Incidence of *Simonsiella* in the oral cavity of dogs. *J Clin Microbiol* 6:87-88, 1977.
5. French: The use of cytology in the diagnosis of chronic nasal disorders. *Comp Cont Ed Pract Vet* 9:115-120, 1987.
6. Smith. In Ettinger SJ: *Textbook of Veterinary Internal Medicine,* ed 4. Philadelphia, Saunders, 1995, p 1090.

7. Perman et al: *Cytology of the Dog and Cat.* Denver, American Animal Hospital Association, 1979.
8. Harvey CE, et al: Nasal penicilliosis in six dogs. *J Am Vet Med Assoc* 178:1084-1087, 1981.
9. Goring et al: A contrast rhinographic diagnosis of nasal and sinusoidal aspergillosis in the dog: A case report. *J Am Anim Hosp Assoc* 19:920-924, 1983.
10. Sharp. In Greene CE: *Infectious Diseases of the Dog and Cat.* ed 2. Philadelphia, Saunders, 1990, pp 714-719.
11. Medleau and Barsanti. In Greene CE: *Infectious Diseases of the Dog and Cat,* ed 2. Philadelphia, Saunders, 1990, pp 687-695.
12. Wolf and Troy. In Ettinger SJ: *Textbook of Veterinary Internal Medicine,* ed 4. Philadelphia, Saunders, 1995, pp 450-453.
13. Foil. In Greene CE: *Infectious Diseases of the Dog and Cat,* ed 2. Philadelphia, Saunders, 1990, pp 731-741.
14. Mosier DA, Creed JE: Rhinosporidiosis in a dog. *J Am Vet Med Assoc* 185:1009-1010, 1984.
15. Easley JR, et al: Nasal rhinosporidiosis in the dog. *Vet Pathol* 23:50-56, 1986.
16. Barsanti and Prestwood. In Kirk RW: *Current Veterinary Therapy VIII.* Philadelphia, Saunders, 1983, pp 241-246.
17. Evinger JV: et al: Ivermectin for treatment of nasal capillariasis in a dog. *J Am Vet Med Assoc* 186:174-175, 1985.
18. Legendre et al: Canine nasal and paranasal sinus tumors. *J Am Anim Hosp Assoc* 19:115-123, 1983.
19. Madewell BR: et al: Neoplasms of the nasal passages and paranasal sinuses in domesticated animals as reported by 13 veterinary colleges. *Am J Vet Res* 37:851-856, 1976.
20. Norris: Intranasal neoplasms in the dog. *J Am Anim Hosp Assoc* 15:231-236, 1979.
21. Nielsen and Kennedy. In Moulton JE: *Tumors in Domestic Animals,* ed 3. University of Berkeley, California Press, 1990, pp 498-502.

The Oropharynx and Tonsils

D.C. Bernreuter

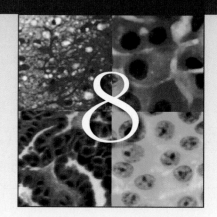

CHAPTER

Cytology is a useful, rapid screening test for lesions in the oropharynx, including masses, ulcers, draining tracts, plaques, and enlarged tonsils. It can be performed alone or in conjunction with biopsy and/or sampling for bacterial and fungal testing. Sedation or anesthesia can be necessary for complete examination of the oropharynx and to obtain adequate, representative samples. For mass lesions and plaques, aspiration of the deeper layers of the lesion to avoid any superficial secondary inflammation is usually most rewarding. If a mass lesion is nonexfoliative, scraping the lesion may yield adequate numbers of cells; however, excisional biopsy is usually necessary for a definitive diagnosis and prognosis. For flat lesions including ulcers, biopsy of the entire lesion or at least of the edge of a lesion, so that the early, primary abnormalities can be evaluated, is usually necessary to obtain an adequate number of representative cells for evaluation. However, impression smears or scrapings of ulcerative lesions can often yield cells or organisms that are distinctive and can be identified as the primary cause of the lesion rather than as secondary opportunists, and eliminate the need for biopsy. Because the oropharynx and tonsils are highly vascular, care must be taken to avoid hemodilution of the sample at the time of collection.

TECHNIQUES

For mass lesions and plaques, fine-needle aspiration should be attempted after the surface has been cleaned with a disinfectant that is nontoxic to the digestive system of the patient. If the lesion is fibrous and nonexfoliative, scraping the lesion with a scalpel blade and transferring the cells to a slide can be rewarding if the cells are immediately thinned into a monolayer by smearing them with another slide, or by using a moistened sterile swab to roll (not rub) the cells along a slide. Draining tracts can also be swabbed and the cells rolled onto a slide for cytologic examination. If a biopsy is performed, impression smears of the cut surface can be made after the surface has been blotted on a paper towel to remove excessive blood and tissue fluids. For flat lesions such as ulcers, any superficial pus and fibrin should be removed before impression smears or scrapings of the surface are made. As for all cytology samples, the smears should be thin enough to dry within 30 to 60 seconds, and they should be completely dry before encasing them in a slide holder for transport to a diagnostic laboratory. Areas of the sample that are more than one cell thick cannot be adequately evaluated, and slow drying causes distortion and disintegration that can ruin otherwise excellent smears.

NORMAL FINDINGS

In order to correctly identify abnormal criteria, recognition of normal findings is essential. The oropharynx and tonsils are covered by mature squamous epithelial cells (Figure 8-1). These are large, flat, and round to slightly angular. They have abundant pale cytoplasm and small round nuclei that exhibit condensed chromatin. Nucleoli are not visible and some cells are anuclear. The presence of occasional intermediate squamous cells with slightly larger, less condensed nuclei is normal (Figure 8-2).

The normal squamous cells frequently exhibit a mixed bacterial population adhered to their surfaces (Figure 8-3). These bacteria are also usually present in the background between cells. The normal flora includes aerobic and anaerobic bacterial rods and cocci. Observation of spirochetes is considered normal. Yeast are never considered to be normal. One bacterium, *Simonsiella* spp., has a characteristic palisading appearance and is a normal inhabitant of the oropharynx (Figure 8-4). It should never be mistaken for a pathogen. If the bacterial population is dominated by only one type of bacteria, that would be considered abnormal.

The normal appearance of smears made from the tonsils is typical of other lymphoid organs. Usually, greater than 80% of the lymphoid cells are small and appear mature. The remaining lymphoid cells are intermediate-sized lymphocytes and occasional lymphoblasts. Plasma cells, neutrophils, macrophages, eosinophils, and squamous cells from the epithelial surface can be rarely observed. Occasional granules of iron pigment can be normal.

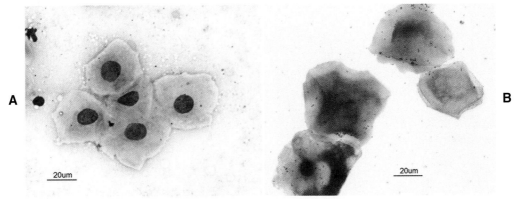

Figure 8-1 Mature squamous cells have cornified cytoplasm that has sharp angular borders. Mature squamous cells may be nucleated or anucleate. **A,** Mature nucleated squamous cells have abundant light blue-gray cytoplasm that has an angular appearance. **B,** Mature squamous cell with a pyknotic nucleus (lower left) and anucleate, mature squamous cells from a scraping of oral tissue.

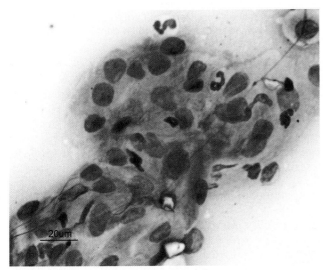

Figure 8-2 Intermediate (less differentiated) squamous cells. These are also a normal finding from the oropharynx, particularly with samples collected by scraping. Cells are more cohesive and have large, noncondensed nuclei and a more deeply basophilic cytoplasm that does not have angular borders.

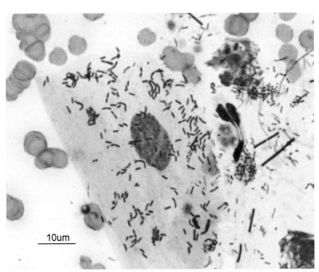

Figure 8-3 Mature squamous cell with adherent bacteria. Extracellular bacteria are also present. Bacteria adherent to squamous cells and bacteria free in the background of the smear that are not associated with an inflammatory response are usually normal flora.

THE OROPHARYNX

Nonneoplastic Lesions

Inflammation: Acute (neutrophilic) inflammation is characterized by a predominance of neutrophils. They can be degenerate or nondegenerate. Neutrophils are most frequently degenerate if bacterial endotoxins are present. Macrophages, occasional lymphocytes, plasma cells, fibrocytes and eosinophils can also be present in low numbers.

Infectious agents can be observed; however, their absence from a sample does not rule out the possibility of an infectious etiology. If the inflammatory lesion is caused by a primary bacterial infection or complicated by secondary bacterial infection, a homogenous population of bacteria is often seen and many will be phagocytized within neutrophils (Figure 8-5).

If the inflammation is superficial, secondary overgrowth of oropharyngeal bacterial flora is common. Secondary opportunistic bacterial inflammation can also be observed in association with primary, noninflammatory lesions. The presence of a heterogeneous population of bacteria that are extracellular or adhered to epithelial cells suggests overgrowth of flora.

If the lesion is granulomatous, such as from a foreign body or yeast/fungal infection, a more evenly mixed population of neutrophils, macrophages, lymphocytes, and plasma cells is observed, with variable numbers of fibrocytes and fibroblasts that are indicative of physiologic fibroplasia (Figure 8-6). In some areas of the country, histoplasmosis in cats can present with oral lesions as the predominant physical examination finding. In these cases, a diagnosis can be made based on identification of organisms from proliferative oral lesions.

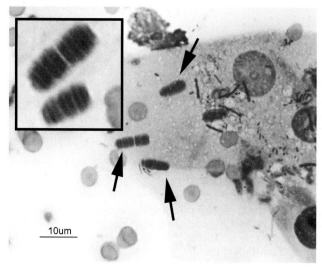

Figure 8-4 Mature squamous cells with *Simonsiella* spp. bacteria *(arrows)*. *Simonsiella* spp. is a normal inhabitant of the oropharynx and must not be mistaken for a pathogen. What appears to be one very large organism is actually numerous slender bacterial rods lined up side to side. *Inset,* Higher magnification of *Simonsiella* organisms in which the individual organisms can be seen.

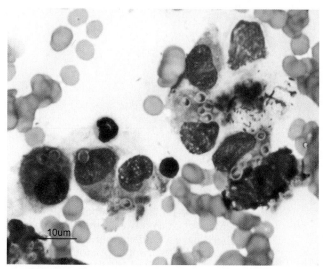

Figure 8-6 Scraping of an oral lesion of a cat with histoplasmosis. The lesion was pyogranulomatous, yielding a mixture of neutrophils and macrophages. In this image, many macrophages are present which contain phagocytized *Histoplasma* organisms.

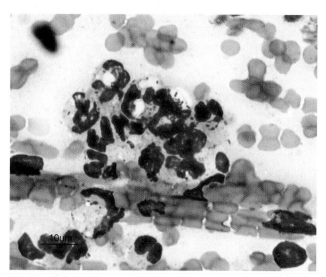

Figure 8-5 Septic, purulent inflammation. Scraping of a lesion in the oral cavity of a cat shows many neutrophils with phagocytized bacteria. Bacteria that are associated with an inflammatory reaction and are phagocytized by neutrophils likely represent pathogens (primary or secondary).

An inflammatory infiltrate characterized by a predominance of mature lymphocytes and plasma cells with scattered other inflammatory cells is seen in samples from cats with chronic gingivitis/stomatitis (i.e., lymphocytic-plasmacytic gingivitis/stomatitis). The characteristic inflammatory cells are typically admixed with normal or dysplastic epithelial cells (Figure 8-7).

Reactive hyperplasia of the tonsils is characterized by a population of lymphoid cells that are predominantly small mature lymphocytes, with variably increased

numbers of plasma cells (Figure 8-8). Lymphoblast numbers remain low. Variable numbers of neutrophils and macrophages may be present, depending on the degree of concurrent inflammation. Bacterial or fungal organisms can be present. Because tonsils have no afferent lymphatics, malignancies and inflammation in the oropharynx drain into the submandibular and pharyngeal lymph nodes rather than the tonsils.

Eosinophilic Granuloma Complex: Eosinophilic ulcers, granulomas, and plaques are common within the oropharynx. Cytologically, they are identified by a predominance of eosinophils (Figure 8-9). Macrophages, fibroblasts, lymphocytes, and plasma cells can also be observed in variable numbers because they are all normal components of eosinophilic granuloma lesions. As with other oropharyngeal lesions, secondary opportunistic bacterial inflammation can be observed if the sample is superficial. Eosinophils can also be the dominant cell type in some mycotic lesions and foreign-body reactions, so these possibilities must be differentiated from eosinophilic granuloma complex by gross appearance of the lesion, fungal culture on serology, or excisional biopsy.

Neoplastic Lesions

Tumors in this region can be classified cytologically as being of epithelial origin, of mesenchymal origin, or as discrete round cell tumors. They can be evaluated for malignant criteria and for any secondary inflammation caused by tissue necrosis from an expanding tumor or by opportunistic bacterial infection. Malignant tumors in the oropharynx usually have a poor prognosis unless they are detected early and can be completely excised, before any microscopic metastasis has occurred.

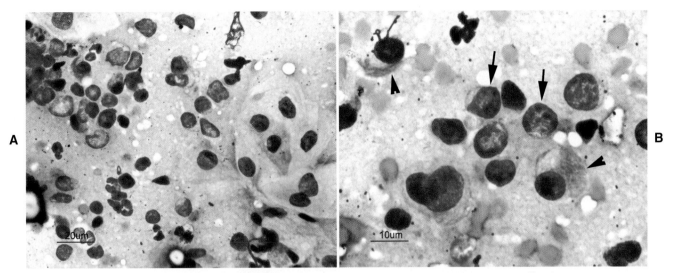

Figure 8-7 Scrapings of a cat with lymphocytic-plasmacytic gingivitis. **A,** Low-magnification image shows normal squamous cells *(right)* and a dense infiltrate of inflammatory cells. **B,** Higher-magnification image of inflammatory cells shows a predominance of small lymphocytes *(arrows)* as well as increased numbers of mature plasma cells *(arrowheads).*

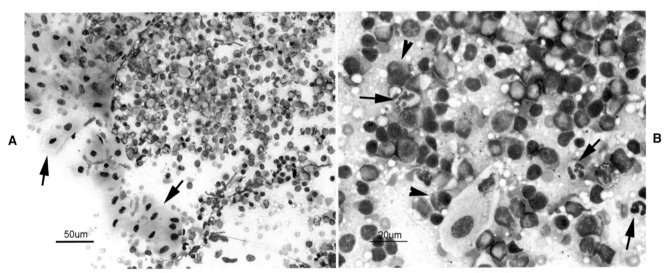

Figure 8-8 Impression smears of a biopsy of an enlarged tonsil from a dog with a hyperplastic, inflamed tonsil. **A,** Low-magnification image shows normal surrounding squamous epithelium *(arrows)* and a lymphoid population from the tonsil itself. **B,** Higher-magnification image shows the lymphoid population to be a predominance of small lymphocytes. Increased numbers of neutrophils *(arrows)* and plasma cells *(arrowheads)* are present.

Tumors of Epithelial Origin: Epithelial tumors of the oropharynx include papillomas, the epulides, squamous cell carcinomas, epithelial odontogenic tumors, and adenocarcinomas. Cytologically, an epithelial origin of a tumor is suggested by cells that display adhesion (i.e., cell clustering, although this may be variable depending on the specific tumor and degree of differentiation), round nuclei with stippled chromatin, and sparse to abundant amounts of cytoplasm with generally distinct cell margins.

Canine oral papillomas are caused by a transmissible papovavirus and usually occur in animals younger than 1 year. They are usually identified by gross appearance. When aspirated, they yield variable numbers of squamous

cells that appear intermediate to mature, with keratinization of the superficial cells.

The epulides are a group of common benign tumors or tumor-like masses that are located on the gingiva. There are several types that are differentiated from each other only by histopathologic examination of the tissue architecture; not by cytology. Because epulides are composed of squamous epithelium and fibrous tissue, aspirates of these tumors are composed of variable numbers of mature squamous cells and occasional small spindle cells. The fibrous portion of the epulis is nonexfoliative or minimally exfoliative, which causes many aspirates to be almost acellular and nondiagnostic. The more cellular

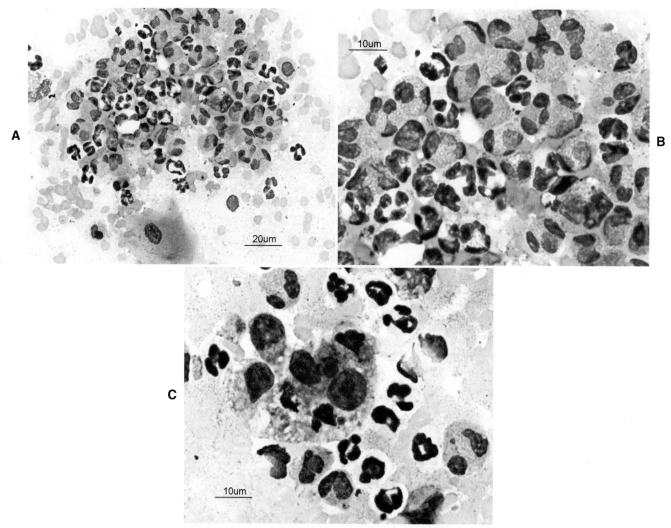

Figure 8-9 Scrapings of an oral lesion from a cat with an eosinophilic granuloma complex lesion ("rodent ulcer"). **A,** Low-magnification image shows one mature squamous cell and many inflammatory cells. **B,** Higher-magnification image of the inflammatory cells shows a predominance of eosinophils and some neutrophils. The eosinophils can be easily differentiated from the neutrophils by the orange appearance of their cytoplasm imparted by the granules. In contrast, the cytoplasm of the neutrophils is clear. The eosinophil granules are so densely packed in the cell that individual granules are often difficult to see. **C,** Another field from the same slide. Although eosinophils predominate in these lesions, variable numbers of macrophages are also present.

samples are usually composed almost entirely of intermediate and mature squamous cells. Ossifying epulides can exhibit some eosinophilic, amorphous, extracellular material representing osteoid. Excisional biopsy is the treatment of choice for epulides so that they can be classified correctly based on the tissue architecture of an adequate number of representative cells. This can lead to complete resolution, although some can recur at the same site and some can invade alveolar bone. Biopsy will also differentiate an epulis from a well-differentiated squamous cell carcinoma and from epithelial odontogenic neoplasms.

Epithelial odontogenic neoplasms are a group of neoplasms that can occur in young or old animals. They usually occur near the teeth. All are characterized by epithelial cells that can exhibit many criteria of malignancy, or can appear rather well differentiated. Examination of the tissue architecture is necessary for accurate classification of these neoplasms and for accurate prognosis. Thus, surgical biopsy and histopathology is needed for these lesions.

Squamous cell carcinomas are common oropharyngeal malignant neoplasms. They can occur in any squamous epithelial tissue, including in the squamous covering of the tonsils. The individual appearance of malignant squamous cells varies widely depending on the degree of differentiation of the tumor. Some squamous carcinoma cells (e.g., from poorly differentiated tumors) are round and exhibit sparse to moderate amounts of moderately to deeply basophilic, finely granular cytoplasm with

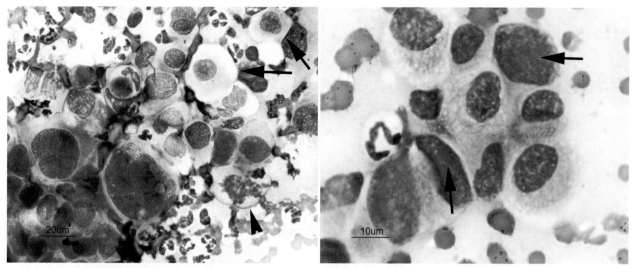

Figure 8-10 Aspirates from a poorly differentiated squamous cell carcinoma in the oral cavity of a cat. A pleomorphic population of epithelial cells is present. Two large, karyomegalic cells are present. Only rare cells show evidence of squamous differentiation having more abundant, lightly colored cytoplasm that is beginning to show angular borders *(arrows)*. A mitotic figure is present *(arrowhead)*.

elevated nuclear:cytoplasmic ratio and prominent large nucleoli (Figure 8-10). In addition, perinuclear, punctate hyaline vacuoles are frequently observed in squamous cell carcinomas (Figure 8-11). Mitotic figures and abnormal nuclear and cellular division can be observed. Other more well-differentiated but malignant carcinomas yield cells that have a more mature squamous appearance with fewer malignant criteria (Figure 8-11). These can exhibit lighter basophilia and more abundant cytoplasm; however, moderate anisocytosis, anisokaryosis, and variability of the nuclear:cytoplasmic ratio remain. With well-differentiated tumors, diligent searching can reveal low numbers of cells with marked criteria of malignancy admixed amongst more well-differentiated cells (Figure 8-11, *B*). Because such cells can be rare to nonexistent, biopsy should be performed on any oropharyngeal squamous cell neoplasm before it is classified as benign. When inflammation is present, epithelial cells can exhibit some criteria that are common to epithelial hyperplasia, dysplasia, and malignancy. Then biopsy can be necessary to differentiate primary malignancy with secondary inflammation from a site of primary inflammation with secondary epithelial dysplasia.

Adenocarcinomas are rarely observed in the oral cavity, although tumors of salivary epithelium are possible. Refer to Chapter 7 for characteristics of benign and malignant salivary epithelial cells.

Tumors of Mesenchymal Origin: Fibrosarcomas are common mesenchymal tumors in cats and dogs, even in young dogs (Figure 8-12). Since they are fibrous, they can be poorly exfoliative. If inadequate numbers of cells are obtained by fine-needle aspiration, a scraping can yield more numerous cells. However, care must be taken to spread the scraped cells into a monolayer for evaluation. Malignant fibroblasts are large spindle cells that exhibit oval nuclei and reticular chromatin and

one or more prominent, large nucleoli. Sometimes, the nucleoli can be larger than erythrocytes. Mitotic figures and abnormal nuclear and cytoplasmic division can be observed. Anisocytosis and anisokaryosis can be moderate to marked. Occasional multinucleated cells can be observed. More primitive fibrosarcoma cells can appear almost round; however, cytoplasmic tails can eventually be found on careful examination. More well-differentiated fibrosarcomas yield cells with fewer malignant criteria. If inflammation is present concurrently, biopsy could be necessary to differentiate a primary, well-differentiated fibrosarcoma with secondary inflammation from primary inflammation with secondary reactive fibroplasia.

Other soft tissue sarcomas can rarely occur in the oral cavity, including liposarcomas and hemangiosarcomas. Most soft tissue sarcomas have a similar cytologic appearance, consisting of poorly exfoliative spindle cells. Histopathologic examination of the tissue architecture is necessary for correct classification and prognosis. Hemangiosarcomas are typically nonexfoliative, and aspirates usually consist entirely of peripheral blood.

The bones and joints around the oropharynx can be the source of osteosarcomas and chondrosarcomas. Their appearance is identical to those described in Chapter 13. Oral squamous cell carcinomas can also metastasize to bone.

Benign fibromas can occur in the oropharynx. They are composed of poorly exfoliative, elongated spindle cells that do not exhibit criteria of malignancy. Because they are very fibrous, they usually require biopsy so that an adequate number of representative cells can be evaluated.

Melanomas are traditionally discussed with tumors of mesenchymal origin, although they are actually of neural crest origin, and many exhibit cytologic morphology that is more epithelioid than spindle-shaped. Greater than 90% of oral melanomas are malignant. If detected early, they

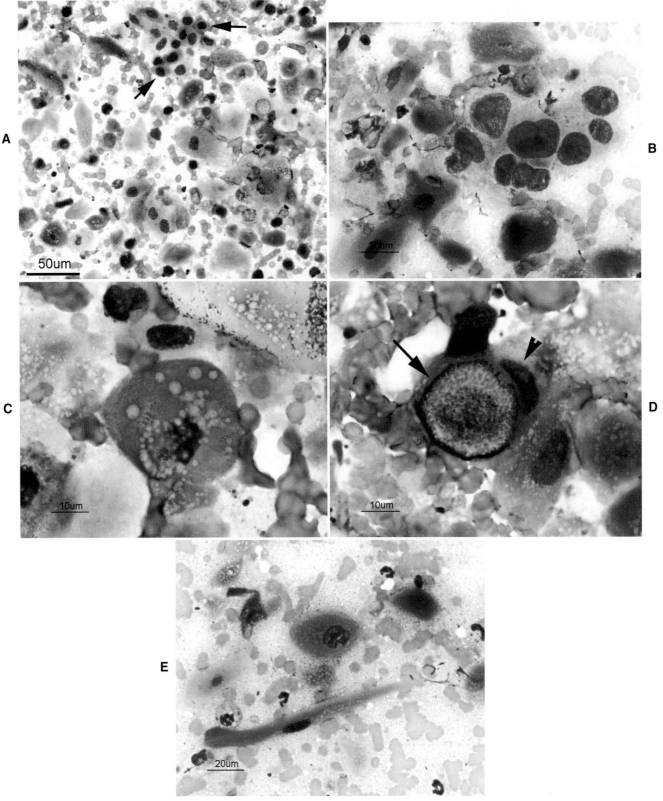

Figure 8-11 Images from an aspirate of a well-differentiated squamous cell carcinoma. **A,** Low-magnification image shows a dense population of squamous cells. The majority of the cells are fully cornified superficial cells, either with pyknotic nuclei or anucleate. A cluster of relatively uniform noncornified cells is present *(arrows).* Overall, the majority of the cells do not show marked criteria of malignancy. **B,** Another image of the same tumor shows some cells with significant atypia including marked anisocytosis, nuclear pleomorphism, and large prominent nucleoli. Although these cells were present, they were in low numbers and required diligent searching to find. **C,** Squamous cell showing perinuclear vacuolation. Note the pink-purple color of the cytoplasm which that is seen in some cells undergoing keratinization. **D,** Large eosinophilic cytoplasmic inclusion. This is a common finding in aspirates from a squamous cell carcinoma. **E,** An elongated cornified epithelial cell. This morphologic presentation is seen in some squamous cell carcinomas.

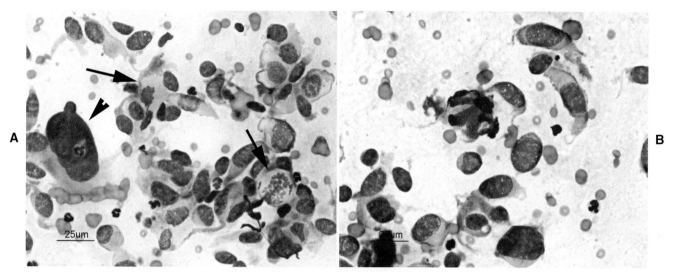

Figure 8-12 Fibrosarcoma from the oral cavity of a cat. **A,** Dense population of mesenchymal cells. A large, karyomegalic cell *(arrowhead)* and two mitotic figures *(arrows)* are present. **B,** Another image from same aspirate shows cellular pleomorphism, moderate anisokaryosis, and variation of N:C ratio.

can be completely excised. However, when detected they have frequently metastasized to the submandibular lymph nodes and then to the thorax. In fact, the ultimate cause of death from malignant melanoma is due to the effect of thoracic metastasis. For this reason, if a melanoma is identified in the oropharynx, evaluation of the submandibular lymph nodes and thoracic radiographs should be included in the workup. If the submandibular lymph nodes are enlarged, cytology or biopsy can be performed to check for metastasis. Individual cellular morphology of malignant melanomas can vary from round to spindle-shaped large cells. They exhibit reticular chromatin, frequently with prominent large nucleoli (Figure 8-13). The nuclear:cytoplasmic ratio is high. The cytoplasm is usually light blue and finely granular, with variable numbers of punctate, round black melanin granules. The nuclear shape varies from round to oval. Some malignant melanomas are very poorly melanotic or completely amelanotic, which can make definitive identification almost totally dependent on histopathologic examination. However, such tumors are readily identified as malignant on cytology, and the possibility of an amelanotic melanoma should be considered if cytology demonstrates malignant tumor cells that have variable characteristics, including some cells that are epithelioid and some slightly more spindle-shaped. Wide excisional biopsy would be warranted. The highly variable cytologic and histologic appearance of melanomas can make their identification and prognosis problematic by both methods. Ancillary diagnostic techniques such as immunohistochemical stains and monoclonal antibodies to melanocytes can be helpful to identify some melanomas. Currently, there is no single diagnostic technique that is always capable of differentiating benign from malignant melanocytic neoplasms or predicting survival time.

Malignant Lymphoma: Malignant lymphoma can be found in any lymphoid tissue, and it is the most common

tumor of the tonsils. In high-grade lymphoma, greater than 50%, and usually greater than 90%, of the lymphoid cells are large lymphoblasts that exhibit one or more, large, prominent nucleoli. The cytoplasm is sparse and deeply basophilic. In some lymphomas, punctate lipid vacuoles are observed in the cytoplasm. The remaining cells are small and intermediate-sized lymphocytes that appear mature. Small cell and intermediate cell lymphomas are less than 10% of canine lymphomas but more frequent in cats. These are characterized by a predominance of small lymphocytes or intermediate lymphocytes (approximately the size of a neutrophil), and for this reason they cannot be identified by cytology alone. By definition, they are identified by abnormalities in the tissue architecture while individual cell morphology remains relatively normal. If small cell or intermediate cell lymphoma is suspected in the oropharynx, biopsy will be necessary for accurate diagnosis and for differentiation from lymphoid hyperplasia due to nonspecific immune stimulation.

Discrete Round Cell Tumors: Histiocytomas can occur in the mouth and in dogs of any age although most are in young dogs. Mastocytomas occur in the mouth; many are poorly granulated. Some are almost agranular, although careful examination will usually lead to the identification of a few granules that are necessary to differentiate mastocytomas from other discrete round cell tumors. When an oral mastocytoma is identified, the submandibular lymph nodes should be checked for any evidence of metastasis. Consultation with an oncologist for possible treatment options would also be warranted, due to the difficulty of obtaining adequate margins when excising a mastocytoma from the oropharynx. Transmissible venereal tumors are occasionally observed in the oropharynx. All discrete round cell tumors in the mouth are cytologically identical to those in the subcutaneous tissues. Refer to the cytologic description of these tumors in Chapter 4.

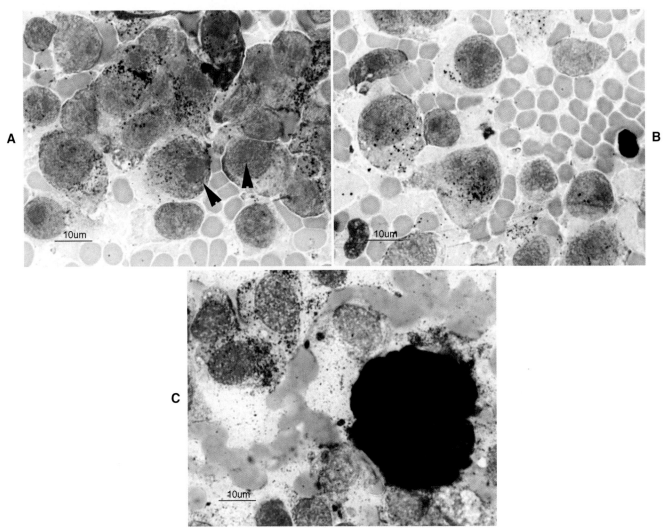

Figure 8-13 Aspirates from a melanoma in the oral cavity of a dog. **A,** A population of melanocytes showing the marked atypia common with oral melanoma. The cells appear poorly differentiated, being large cells with a high N:C ratio, noncondensed chromatin and large prominent nucleoli *(arrowheads)*. Although the tumor is poorly pigmented, melanin granules are present in most cells. **B,** Another image from the same slide as in **A.** In this image, the cells appear to have a discrete cell appearance and are individually oriented. Cells from a melanoma may have features of mesenchymal cells, epithelial cells, or discrete cells. Sometimes, cells with each of these morphologies will be present in the same tumor. **C,** Image from another oral melanoma. In addition to the poorly pigmented cells, rare cells are so densely pigmented that the cellular detail is completely obscured and the cell appears simply as a large black sphere.

ALGORITHMIC INTERPRETATION OF SAMPLES

A logical approach to evaluation of cytology samples is necessary to minimize evaluation time, and especially to ensure that the evaluation is thorough and the interpretation is logical. One example of a logical algorithm is presented in this chapter (Figure 8-14). Ultimately, if cytology determines that a tumor is possible or likely, biopsy (excisional if possible) will be warranted, in addition to evaluation of regional lymph nodes and thoracic radiographs. If inflammation is present, bacterial and/or fungal cultures could be warranted. If appropriate treatment does not lead to complete resolution, biopsy should be performed for further evaluation.

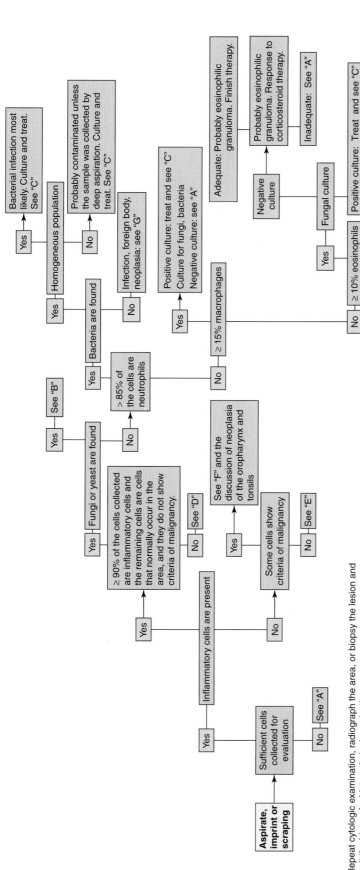

Figure 8-14 An algorithm for cytologic evaluation of oropharyngeal lesions.

A. Repeat cytologic examination, radiograph the area, or biopsy the lesion and submit the biopsy for histopathologic evaluation.

B. Identify as:

Blastomyces dermatitidis (See Figure 3-10, page 57)
Histoplasma capsulatum (See Figure 3-9, page 56)
Cryptococcus neoformans (See Figure 3-11, page 58)
Sporothrix schenckii (See Figure 3-8, page 55)
Coccidioides immitis (See Figure 3-12, page 59)

Culture, or refer the side if unsure of the organism or if specific identification of a hyphating fungus is needed.

C. If there is no response to therapy, the patient should be re-evaluated. Occasionally, tumors become infected and yield cytologic samples containing inflammatory cells and bacteria, but not cells from the tumor. In these cases, antibiotic therapy often eliminates the infection, and subsequent cytologic samples contain sufficient tumor cells to diagnose neoplasia.

D. When there is an admixture of inflammatory cells and noninflammatory cells, the lesion should be evaluated for causes of inflammation and for indications of neoplasia. The more the shift of the admixture is an one direction, the more likely that process is occuring, *ie*, if 85% of the cells are inflammatory cells, then inflammation is very likely and neoplasia is less likely. On the other hand, if 15% of the cells are inflammatory and 85% are noninflammatory cells, neoplasia with secondary inflammation is more likely.

Also, the greater the proportion of inflammatory cells, the stronger the criteria of malignancy must be in cells suspected to be neoplastic for neoplasia to be diagnosed.

Re-evaluation by cytologic, radiographic and/or histopathologic examination after treatment of the inflammatory condition may be necessary.

E. If no inflammatory cells are present and no cells show criteria of malignancy, the lesion is probably due to hyperplasia, benign neoplasia, cyst formation (such as salivary cysts) or collection from normal tissue surrounding the lesion, but malignant neoplasia cannot be ruled out. Re-evaluation by cytologic, radiographic and/or histopathologic examination may be necessary.

F. If no inflammatory cells are present and some of the cells show criteria of malignancy, neoplasia is likely. The morphology of the cells collected should be evaluated to determine, if possible, the tumor cell type and the level of criteria of malignancy. Depending on the tumor cell type and level of criteria of malignancy present, a prediction of the malignant potential of the tumor may be possible. However, histopathologic examination may be necessary for definitive diagnosis.

G. Infection (mycotic or bacterial), neoplasia or foreign body are all possible. At this time, the cytologic preparation may be referred for interpretation, another sample may be collected, the lesion may be cultured and treated accordingly, or radiographic examination or biopsy with histopathologic examination may be performed. If the patient is treated, a cytologic sample collected 1-2 weeks after therapy is begun may reveal the true nature of the lesion.

References

1. Raskin RE Meyer DJ: *Atlas of Canine and Feline Cytology.* St. Louis, Saunders, 2001.
2. Baker R, Lumsden JH: *Color Atlas of Cytology of the Dog and Cat.* St Louis, Mosby, 2000.
3. Bernreuter DC: Cytology of the skin and subcutaneous tissues. In Ettinger SJ, Feldman EC (eds): *Textbook of Veterinary Internal Medicine*, ed 6, 2005, pp 305-307.
4. Smith SH, Goldschmidt MH, McManus PM: A comparative review of melanocytic neoplasms. *Vet Pathol* 39:6651-78, 2002.

The Eyes and Associated Structures

K.M. Young and K.W. Prasse

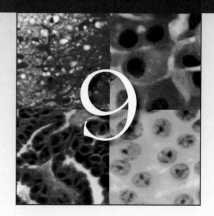

CHAPTER

9

Cytologic evaluation of specimens collected from diseased ocular structures can be a valuable aid in both the diagnosis and management of ocular disease. Although cytologic analysis alone may provide a diagnosis, it is often used in conjunction with other tests, such as culture, immunofluorescent staining, Polymerase chain reaction (PCR) assays, and biopsy. Proper collection (including appropriate cautions when sampling damaged tissue), sample processing (including concentration techniques), slide preparation, and staining are prerequisite to obtaining accurate and useful information from the microscopic evaluation, as is familiarity with the normal cytologic appearance of the sampled site. If possible, several slides containing adequate sample volume should be prepared to permit use of special stains, if indicated. When slides are sent to a cytopathologist, it is essential to identify the source of the specimen (e.g., cornea or conjunctiva). The first slide prepared often contains the best material for evaluation and should be included even if it has been stained. In this chapter, cytologic findings are reviewed by anatomic location following some general considerations. Certain lesions, particularly of the eyelids and orbit, are common to other body systems, and illustrations may appear elsewhere in the text.

GENERAL CONSIDERATIONS

Stains

Romanowsky stains are standard and, in general, are excellent for observing morphologic characteristics of cells, organisms, and other structures. The major artifact is stain precipitate, which can mimic clusters of bacterial cocci. The quick stains (such as Diff-Quik) are often adequate, but do not stain cytoplasmic features as well as the parent stains. In some instances, for example, mast cell granules do not stain with quick stains, and the presence of these cells may go undetected if other stains are not used. Also, quick stains must be maintained well or the stains themselves may contain organisms, such as *Malassezia*, from previously stained specimens or from contamination. Other stains that may be used as adjuncts include stains for fungal organisms, including periodic acid–Schiff (PAS) and Gomori's methenamine silver stain, and Gram's stain

to determine if bacteria are gram positive or negative. Gram-stained slides can be tricky to read and require experience to avoid misinterpretation. Indirect fluorescent antibody (IFA) staining requires special reagents and a fluorescence microscope.

Microscopic Evaluation

Ocular specimens are often small in volume, and, therefore, examination of the entire sample is easy. The observer should be familiar with the normal cytologic characteristics of the tissue sampled and recognize cellular patterns, other structures, and background material. Identification of specific types of inflammatory cells permits classification of inflammation as neutrophilic (synonyms include suppurative and purulent); eosinophilic (often accompanied by mast cells); lymphocytic/plasmacytic; mixed, including pyogranulomatous; and granulomatous. If neoplasia is suspected based on the presence of a mass lesion and a homogenous population of noninflammatory cells, the observer should be able to identify the cell type (epithelial, mesenchymal or connective tissue, and discrete round cells) and the cytologic features of benign and malignant tumors. It is important to recognize that neoplasms can induce an inflammatory response. Finally, the observer should be familiar with the cytologic characteristics of cysts, acute and chronic hemorrhage, and degenerative diseases.

When identifying cell types, it is important to look in an area where individual cells can be evaluated. However, thick collections of material, often consisting of clustered epithelial cells or necrotic material, tend to be understained, and cells with granules that stain more readily than other components (mast cells and eosinophils), naturally pigmented elements (melanin), bacteria, and fungal hyphae may be visualized within or on top of the thick tissue (Figure 9-1). Inclusions found in epithelial or inflammatory cells may be normal elements, artifacts of treatment, or evidence of the pathologic process or etiology (Table 9-1). Normal tissue also may be present.

Once a category is identified, a more specific diagnosis may be possible. For example, a search for an etiologic agent is indicated if inflammation is present. At the very

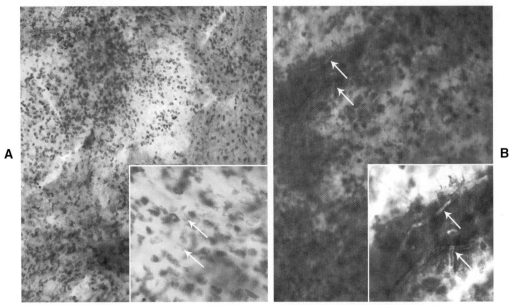

Figure 9-1 Thick understained tissue from two corneal scrapes, in which significant structures/cells can be visualized. **A**, Eosinophils and eosinophil granules *(arrows)*. **B**, Fungal hyphae *(arrows)*. (Wright's stain, original magnification 200×; insets 600×.)

least, the category can guide additional testing or therapy. Special cytologic features of neutrophils, epithelial cells, and extracellular material are listed in Table 9-2 and often provide additional information about the pathologic process; misinterpretation of these features (e.g., mistaking free mast cell granules for bacterial cocci) can lead to erroneous conclusions.

THE EYELIDS

The eyelid comprises layers of skin and mucous membrane (palpebral conjunctiva) separated by muscle and specialized glands, particularly of the sebaceous type. Lesions of the eyelids for which cytologic evaluation is useful include ulcerative and exudative lesions of the epidermal surface (blepharitis) and discrete masses on either the epidermal or conjunctival surface. Conjunctivitis and conjunctival cytology are described later.

Fine-needle aspiration of ulcerated lesions and discrete masses usually provides diagnostic specimens. Frequently, specimens from eyelid lesions contain abundant blood. Scraping may be a reasonable means of sample collection for diffuse exudative epidermal lesions of the eyelid, such as parasitic blepharitis. Touch imprints of exudative skin lesions may reflect the cause of the lesion or may contain only surface debris. Therefore, both touch imprints of the exudate and samples collected after cleaning the surface of the lesion should be examined.

Blepharitis

Blepharitis may be focal or diffuse and acute or chronic. Causes may be bacterial, mycotic, parasitic, allergic, or immune mediated. The objectives in cytologic examination of blepharitis are to characterize the type of exudate (neutrophilic, lymphocytic-plasmacytic, eosinophilic, or granulomatous) and search for the causative agent. Agents that may be encountered in scrapings are *Sarcoptes* spp. *Demodex* spp. dermatophytic yeast, and bacteria. *Demodex folliculorum* causes minimal exudation. Bacterial blepharitis, particularly staphylococcal, has a neutrophilic exudate. Certain fungi, such as *Blastomyces dermatitidis*, cause either a primarily neutrophilic or a pyogranulomatous exudate, whereas others cause a granulomatous exudate (macrophages, including epithelioid forms, and giant cells). Foreign bodies can elicit a pyogranulomatous or granulomatous response (Figure 9-2).

Immune-mediated disease usually is characterized by a neutrophilic exudate, but eosinophilic types also occur. The presence of either bacteria or a primarily neutrophilic exudate does not exclude allergic and immune-mediated causes, especially if the lesion is ulcerated. In cats, eosinophilic plaques may be manifested as periocular blepharitis.[1] A fine-needle aspirate reveals primarily eosinophils, some mast cells, and a mixture of other white blood cell (WBC) types.

Discrete Masses

Discrete masses on the eyelids may be neoplastic (benign or malignant) or nonneoplastic. Among neoplasms, benign sebaceous gland tumors (sebaceous adenoma, sebaceous epithelioma) are the most common type on canine eyelids.[2] The glands of Zeis and Moll at the eyelid margin and the meibomian glands, which lie beneath the palpebral conjunctiva and open at the lid margin, are all of the sebaceous type; tumors arising from them are similar to cutaneous sebaceous gland tumors. The cells are readily recognized by their voluminous vacuolated cytoplasm that nearly obscures small rounded nuclei (Figure 9-3). The malignant counterpart of these tumors is rare on the eyelids.

TABLE 9-1

Inclusions In or On Cells from Ocular Tissue

Inclusions	Significance
Inclusions in or on epithelial cells	
Melanin granules	Normal in pigmented tissue
	Small granules may be confused with *Mycoplasma* organisms.
Mucin or mucin granules	Normal goblet cells
Surface mixed bacteria	Contaminants
Drug inclusions	Artifact of treatment with topical ophthalmic ointments
Mycoplasma spp.	Pathogen
Chlamydophila spp.	Pathogen
Neutrophils	Intact neutrophils within squamous cells: no known significance
Inclusions in neutrophils	
Bacteria	Pathogen
Small fungal organisms (e.g., *Histoplasma* spp.)	Pathogen
Pyknotic nuclei	Aging change or accelerated apoptosis
Inclusions in macrophages	
RBCs (erythrophagia)	Hemorrhage
WBCs (leukophagia): whole or degraded	Long-standing inflammation
Iron pigment (macrophages are termed hemosiderophages)	Chronic or previous hemorrhage
Melanin (macrophages are termed melanophages)	Pigmented tissue with release of melanin from ruptured or degraded epithelial cells
Certain bacteria (e.g. *Mycobacterium* spp.)	Pathogen
Some fungal organisms (e.g. *Histoplasma* spp.)	Pathogen
Protozoal organisms (e.g. *Leishmania* spp.)	Pathogen

Other tumors frequently encountered on the eyelids and readily diagnosed by cytologic examination include melanoma (benign and malignant), histiocytoma (Figure 9-4), lymphoma, mast cell tumor (low and high grade) (Figure 9-5), papilloma, and squamous cell carcinoma. Squamous cell carcinomas are frequently ulcerated. In mast cell tumors, mast cell granules sometimes are not visible if quick stains are used (Figure 9-5, *B*). Other carcinomas and connective tissue tumors (fibrosarcoma, hemangiosarcoma, histiocytic sarcoma) occur less frequently and are discussed in Chapter 2.[2,3]

Nonneoplastic discrete masses unique to the eyelid include the hordeolum, a localized purulent lesion of sebaceous glands, and the chalazion, a lipogranuloma of the meibomian gland. Fine-needle aspiration of these lesions yields numerous foamy macrophages and a few giant cells and lymphocytes. The macrophages are apparently phagocytosing glandular secretory product; cytophagia is not prominent. Variable numbers of sebaceous epithelial cells also are found (Figure 9-6). Differentiating a hordeolum or chalazion from sebaceous gland adenoma by cytologic examination may be difficult if the latter has internally ruptured and caused secondary inflammation. Hordeolum or chalazion may contain inspissated secretory product or mineralized debris that appears as amorphous granular material on cytologic preparations.

Idiopathic ocular adnexal granulomas may simulate neoplasms, be bilateral, and be a component of systemic granulomatous disease.[4] Systemic histiocytosis of Bernese mountain dogs causes periocular granulomatous masses.[5,6] True cysts can occur on the eyelids and typically contain foamy macrophages and cholesterol crystals from epithelial degeneration (Figure 9-7).

THE CONJUNCTIVA

The primary indications for conjunctival cytologic evaluation are to characterize an exudate and to attempt to identify the cause of conjunctivitis.[7] Certain anatomic structures affect the types of cells found on all preparations from normal and diseased eyes. The conjunctiva is composed of two continuous layers of epithelium that lie in apposition. The inner epithelial layer of the eyelid, called the palpebral conjunctiva, is composed of pseudostratified columnar epithelium and interspersed goblet cells (Figure 9-8). Cilia may be found on the columnar cells. At the fornix, deep within the conjunctival sac, the epithelium reflects back over the globe. This bulbar conjunctiva is composed of stratified squamous epithelium (Figure 9-9). Bulbar conjunctiva is continuous with the corneal epithelium at the limbus. The squamous cells are noncornified and often contain melanin granules (Figure 9-10). In most

TABLE 9-2

Special Cytologic Features and Their Significance

Cytologic Feature	Significance
Neutrophils	
Nondegenerate: well-lobulated condensed nuclei, intact nuclear and plasma membranes	Neutrophilic or purulent inflammation: septic or nonseptic
Degenerate: swollen hypolobulated nuclei, fragmented nuclear or cytoplasmic membrane	Septic inflammation likely
Pyknotic: shrunken, condensed, rounded, and disconnected nuclear lobes	Aging change or accelerated apoptosis
Intracytoplasmic bacteria	Usually pathogen(s)
Epithelial Cells	
Dysplastic change: nuclear:cytoplasmic asynchrony	Secondary to inflammation; differentiate from epithelial neoplasia with secondary inflammation
Cornification/keratinization: keratin does not stain with Romanowsky stains; its presence is inferred when squamous cells are angular or folded	Abnormal for corneal epithelial cells; occurs in keratitis
Extracellular material	
Bacteria	Possible contaminants, but may be significant especially if found in corneal samples or if many bacteria of a single morphology are noted
Fungal organisms: yeast forms of *Blastomyces, Cryptococcus, Coccidioidomyces, Histoplasma;* hyphae of *Aspergillus* and other fungi	Pathogens
Parasites: larvae rarely seen cytologically	Pathogens
Free eosinophil, mast cell, or melanin granules	Indicate presence of ruptured eosinophils, mast cells, or epithelial cells; granules may be mistaken for bacteria
Cell fragments, especially stringy nuclear chromatin	Artifact of slide preparation; can resemble hyphae when surrounded by mucus
Cholesterol crystals	Epithelial degeneration
Stain	Artifact; may be mistaken for bacterial cocci
Mucus	Normal in areas where goblet cells are located; may be increased with some pathologic processes

conjunctival scrapings, squamous cells are more numerous than columnar cells.

In animals treated with topical ophthalmic ointments (particularly neomycin), epithelial cells may contain dense basophilic homogeneous cytoplasmic inclusions (Figure 9-11).[8] Such inclusions must be differentiated from infectious agents. At the fornix, conjunctival lamina propria contains lymphoid tissue; various types of lymphoid cells may be found in any conjunctival scraping. Without clinical signs of conjunctivitis, little emphasis should be placed on the observation of lymphocytes or plasma cells among epithelial cells.

Cytologic preparations from the conjunctiva should include freshly derived cells. If external debris within the conjunctival sac is present, imprints of the debris should be made because this material may contain the etiologic agent, such because *Blastomyces* spp. More often, the debris obscures the primary lesion; therefore, after imprints are made the debris should be removed

and conjunctival scraping performed with a flat, round-tipped spatula. Preparation of bulbar conjunctival imprints using filter strips following topical anesthesia has been reported in dogs.[9]

Neutrophilic Conjunctivitis

Canine and feline conjunctivitis frequently is neutrophilic and occurs with bacterial, viral, allergic, or other causes. Pseudomembranous (ligneous) conjunctivitis is neutrophilic.[10] Cytologic evaluation may not reveal the cause. Neutrophils may be nondegenerate or degenerate (Figure 9-12). In cats, the latter are rarely encountered. In both species, intact neutrophils may be found within squamous cells (Figure 9-13), and the significance of this finding is unknown. Mucus is a common component of neutrophilic exudates and may cause cells to appear in rows on the smear.

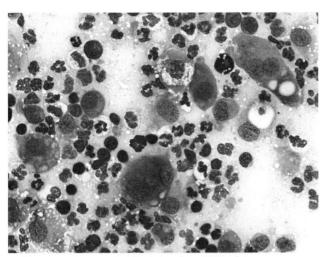

Figure 9-2 Pyogranulomatous inflammation in the eyelid of a dog. Note neutrophils and epithelioid macrophages, including binucleate forms. Lymphocytes and small numbers of red blood cells also are present. (Wright's stain, original magnification 600×.)

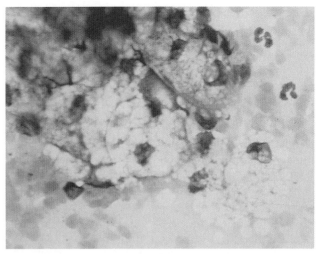

Figure 9-3 Sebaceous gland epithelial cells from a well-differentiated sebaceous gland tumor on a canine eyelid. (Romanowsky-type stain, original magnification 1000×.)

The exudate of canine neutrophilic conjunctivitis often contains bacteria, regardless of primary cause. The bacteria are often large and/or small cocci and less frequently rods (Figure 9-14). The dilemma is whether the bacteria are of primary importance or are merely opportunistic. Normal bacterial flora of the canine conjunctival sac have been described.[11] Keratoconjunctivitis sicca is a common canine disorder causing neutrophilic exudate in which bacteria frequently are encountered. The disease is diagnosed readily by the Schirmer tear test. In contrast to that of dogs, the exudate of feline neutrophilic conjunctivitis rarely contains bacteria. When observed, bacteria should be considered clinically significant in feline conjunctivitis.

Distemper is the most important viral cause of canine neutrophilic conjunctivitis. Canine distemper is diagnosed by its classic clinical signs and fluorescent antibody staining of conjunctival smears. Canine distemper inclusion bodies in epithelial cells are found rarely (Figure 9-15), and a search for them has limited diagnostic value.

A common cause of feline neutrophilic conjunctivitis is herpesvirus infection (Figure 9-16). Diagnosis is confirmed by a PCR assay,[12,13] fluorescent antibody staining of conjunctival smears, or viral isolation. Multinucleated epithelial cells may be found, but intranuclear inclusion bodies rarely are seen.[7,14]

Neutrophils predominate also in the conjunctival exudate of feline chlamydial infection. In experimental *Chlamydophila felis* infections, organisms were found by postinoculation on day 6 when clinical signs first appeared.[15] Solitary, large (3 to 5 μm), basophilic particulate forms initially are found in the cytoplasm of squamous epithelial cells (Figure 9-17). The particulate nature of the initial body is an important observation to distinguish *C. felis* from incidental foci of homogeneous cytoplasmic basophilia found in squamous epithelial cells (see Figure 9-11).[8] Organisms also may appear as aggregates of coccoid basophilic bodies (elementary bodies), 0.5 to 1 μm in diameter (Figure 9-18). In the experimental infections,

organisms rarely were found by day 14 postinoculation,[15] and intracytoplasmic organisms are present only infrequently in chronic conjunctivitis.[7] Chlamydial conjunctivitis may be confirmed by PCR or fluorescent antibody staining. Chlamydiae other than *C. felis* also may play a role in ocular disease in cats.[16]

Feline mycoplasmosis, another cause of neutrophilic conjunctivitis, may be diagnosed by finding the organisms on epithelial cells on routinely stained smears. In one study, mycoplasmosis was diagnosed in nine naturally infected cats by isolation and identification of *Mycoplasma* spp. Of samples from 16 eyes, the organisms were found on Romanowsky-stained smears from 15 eyes. This suggests a high degree of diagnostic sensitivity for routine cytologic evaluation in *Mycoplasma* infection.[17] The basophilic organisms, 0.2 to 0.8 μm long, may be found in clusters adherent to the outer limits of the plasma membrane or over the flattened surface of squamous epithelial cells (Figure 9-19). They also may be seen in clusters between cells. *Mycoplasma* organisms should not be confused with melanin granules (see Figure 9-10).

Lymphocytic-Plasmacytic Conjunctivitis

Conjunctivitis in which lymphoid cells predominate is less common than purulent conjunctivitis. Lymphocytic-plasmacytic conjunctivitis occurs in allergic and chronic infectious conjunctivitis (Figure 9-20). Follicular conjunctivitis yields cells typical of reactive lymphoid hyperplasia (see section on nictitating membrane).

Eosinophilic and Mast Cell Conjunctivitis

Eosinophilic conjunctivitis is encountered in dogs and cats (Figure 9-21). It has been observed in cats as a sole entity and concomitant with eosinophilic keratitis.[18] In conjunctival smears from both dogs and cats, mast cells also may be present. Some cases test positive for feline herpesvirus by PCR.[12] In preparations stained with quick stains, sometimes neither eosinophil granules nor mast cell granules stain well, and eosinophils can be mistaken for neutrophils. In addition, free eosinophil granules, which are rod shaped in cats, and mast cell granules from ruptured cells should not be mistaken for bacterial rods and cocci, respectively (see section on eosinophilic keratitis).

Noninflammatory Lesions of Conjunctiva

Neoplasms that may involve conjunctiva include papilloma, squamous cell carcinoma, melanoma, lipoma, lymphoma (Figure 9-22), and others. A unique form of

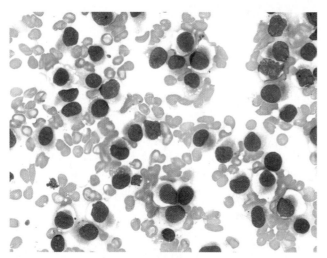

Figure 9-4 Discrete round cell tumor with cytologic characteristics of a histiocytoma on the eyelid of a dog. (Wright's stain, original magnification 600×.)

mast cell neoplasia may involve the canine conjunctiva.[19] It is manifested as severe diffuse swelling of the conjunctiva. Cytologic examination of mast cell tumors is discussed in Chapter 2. Conjunctival hemangioma and hemangiosarcoma occur most frequently within the nonpigmented epithelium of the temporal bulbar conjunctiva in dogs or the nictitating membrane in dogs and cats.[20,21]

Cyst-like swellings of the conjunctiva are uncommon and include dacryops (see discussion of nasolacrimal apparatus later in this chapter), zygomatic mucocele,[22] deposteroid granuloma, tumors, staphyloma, and inclusion cysts. The cytologic findings for a mucocele are identical to salivary cysts described in Chapter 7.

THE NICTITATING MEMBRANE

The nictitating membrane, or third eyelid, is composed of a T-shaped cartilage covered by conjunctiva that is continuous with the bulbar and palpebral conjunctiva on its inner and outer surfaces. The gland of the third eyelid, a seromucous gland, envelops the base of the cartilage. Lymphoid tissue is located on the bulbar surface superior to the gland. Consequently, cells found on nictitans scrapings are determined by which surface is sampled. Scrapings of the bulbar surface of the membrane in normal or diseased eyes may resemble cytologic preparations from lymph nodes, with all expected types of lymphoid cells.

As a conjunctival surface, the nictitating membrane may be affected by most of the diseases of the conjunctiva described in the previous section. Only a few specific

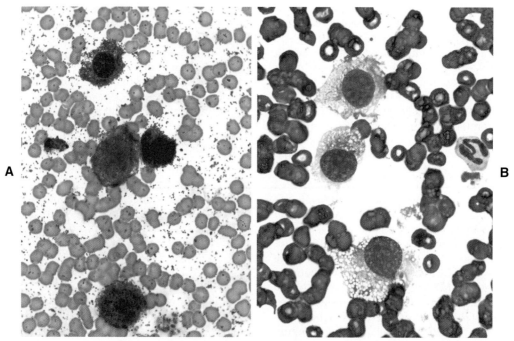

Figure 9-5 **A,** Well-granulated mast cell tumor on the eyelid of a dog. (Wright's stain, original magnification 600×.) **B,** The same specimen stained with a quick stain. Note that mast cell granules did not stain. (Diff-Quik stain, original magnification 600×.)

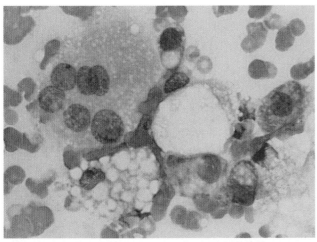

Figure 9-6 A giant cell, macrophages, lymphocytes, and a sebaceous gland epithelial cell *(lower left)* from a chalazion on a canine eyelid. (Romanowsky-type stain, original magnification 1000×.)

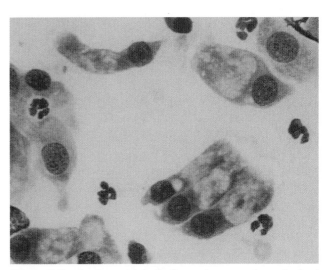

Figure 9-8 Canine conjunctival scraping contains palpebral columnar ciliated cells and goblet cells *(upper right)*. (Romanowsky-type stain, original magnification 1000×.)

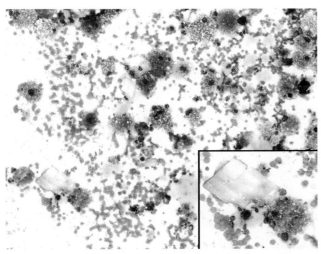

Figure 9-7 Cytocentrifuged material from a cyst on the eyelid of a dog. Note the foamy macrophages and cholesterol crystals. (Wright's stain, original magnification 200×, inset 600×.)

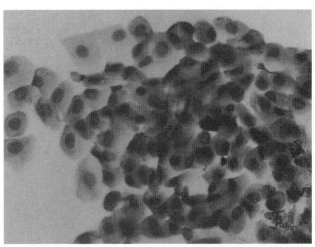

Figure 9-9 Basal, intermediate, and mature noncornified squamous cells typical of bulbar conjunctival epithelium from a canine conjunctival scraping. (Romanowsky-type stain, original magnification 400×.)

lesions of the membrane require cytologic evaluation for differential diagnosis. Cytologic evaluation of follicular hyperplasia reveals lymphoid hyperplasia (Figure 9-23). A specific lesion in German Shepherds is plasmacytic conjunctivitis, in which scrapings of the third eyelid reveal many plasma cells and some lymphocytes (Figure 9-24).[23]

The nictitating membrane may be the site of primary or metastatic tumors, such as squamous cell carcinoma, adenoma/adenocarcinoma of the gland of the third eyelid, melanoma, carcinoma, and apocrine adnexoma.[24] Cytologic examination is helpful to distinguish these lesions. Nodular granulomatous episcleritis (nodular fasciitis) may involve the third eyelid, particularly in collies (see section on the sclera and episclera later in this chapter).[25,26]

THE NASOLACRIMAL APPARATUS

Dacryocystitis

Dacryocystitis is inflammation of the lacrimal sac. Inflammatory exudates composed primarily of neutrophils and macrophages and usually accompanied by bacteria may obstruct the puncta, canaliculi, or nasolacrimal sac. Exudates may be retrieved by flushing the upper or lower punctum with saline through a blunt 22- to 23-gauge cannula. Either the initial plug of material or particularly flocculent material should be examined.

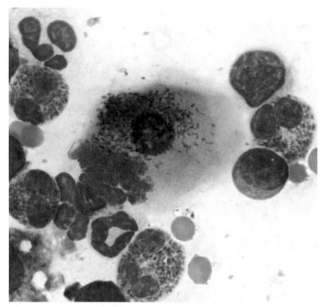

Figure 9-10   Conjunctival scraping from a cat. An epithelial cell contains numerous melanin granules. (Wright's stain, original magnification 1000×.) *(From Young KM, Taylor J: Laboratory Medicine: Yesterday Today Tomorrow: Eye on the cytoplasm. Vet Clin Pathol 35:141, 2006. Reprinted with permission of the American Society for Veterinary Clinical Pathology.)*

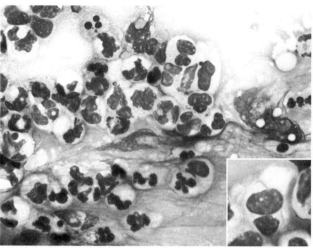

Figure 9-12   Conjunctival scrape from a dog with neutrophilic bacterial conjunctivitis. Both well-segmented nondegenerate neutrophils and degenerate neutrophils with swollen nuclei are present. (Wright's stain, original magnification 600×.) *Inset,* A degenerate neutrophil with two thin bacterial rods. (Wright's stain, original magnification 1000×.)

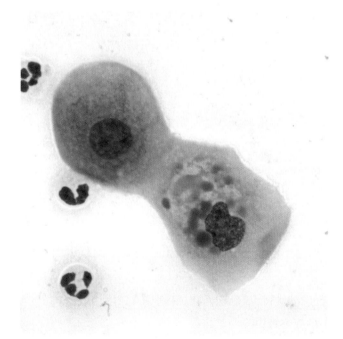

Figure 9-11   A corneal scrape contains squamous cells with dense, homogeneous, blue cytoplasmic inclusions believed to be a consequence of treatment with ophthalmic ointments. (Wright's stain, original magnification 600×.) *(From Young KM, Taylor J: Laboratory Medicine: Yesterday Today Tomorrow: Eye on the cytoplasm. Vet Clin Pathol 35:141, 2006. Reprinted with permission of the American Society for Veterinary Clinical Pathology.)*

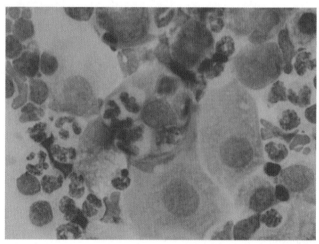

Figure 9-13   Conjunctival smear from a dog with neutrophilic conjunctivitis. Intact neutrophils are found in the cytoplasm of a squamous cell *(center)*, and numerous neutrophils, lymphocytes, and a goblet epithelial cell *(lower left center)* are present. (Romanowsky-type stain, original magnification 1000×.)

Lacrimal Gland Cysts (Dacryops)

A dacryops contains serosanguineous fluid of low cellularity.[22] On smears, red blood cells (RBCs) and small numbers of neutrophils, monocytes, and other WBCs without bacteria are found. Mucus is usually present and may cause the cells to appear in rows (Figure 9-25). There may be a breed predisposition in young Basset Hounds.[22]

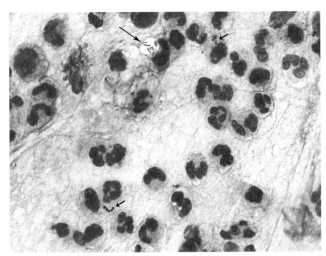

Figure 9-14 Conjunctival scrape from a dog. Note many neutrophils and bacterial rods *(long arrow)* and cocci *(short arrows)*. (Wright's stain, original magnification 1000×.)

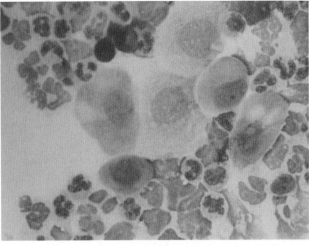

Figure 9-16 Nondegenerate neutrophils, squamous cells, plasma cells (top left center), and a lymphocyte (lower right) from a cat with neutrophilic conjunctivitis. Other smears were fluorescent antibody-positive for feline herpesvirus. (Romanowsky-type stain, original magnification 1000×.)

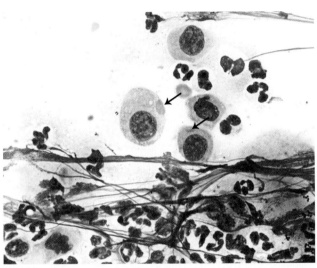

Figure 9-15 Conjunctival scrape from a dog. Variably sized distemper viral inclusions *(arrows)* are found within epithelial cells. Note neutrophils and small bacterial rods and cocci. (Wright's stain, original magnification 1000×.) *(Photomicrograph by Judith Taylor; from Young KM, Taylor J: Laboratory Medicine: Yesterday Today Tomorrow: Eye on the cytoplasm. Vet Clin Pathol 35:141, 2006. Reprinted with permission of the American Society for Veterinary Clinical Pathology.)*

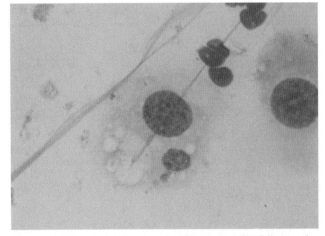

Figure 9-17 Initial body of *Chlamydophila felis* in the cytoplasm of a squamous cell in a conjunctival scrape from a cat. (Romanowsky-type stain, original magnification 1000×.)

Lacrimal Gland Tumors

Neoplasms of the lacrimal gland are rare.[27] Lacrimal adenoma may have a benign cytologic appearance (Figure 9-27) or may be composed of pleomorphic cells. Histopathologic examination provides a definitive diagnosis.

THE SCLERA AND EPISCLERA

The sclera is the noncorneal fibrous tunic of the eye. The scleral stroma is continuous with the corneal stroma. The fibrovascular episclera overlies the scleral stroma and is covered in part by bulbar conjunctiva. These tissues are rich in collagen and nearly free of cells. Fibrocytes and

Parotid Transposition Cysts

A unique noninflammatory cystic lesion may occur in the lateral canthus as a complication of parotid duct transposition. The cyst may occur if the orifice of the transplanted duct becomes occluded. Cyst contents are similar to those of a naturally occurring salivary mucocele and include large foamy macrophages and exfoliated salivary epithelial cells (Figure 9-26). Variable numbers of neutrophils also may be found; bacteria are absent.

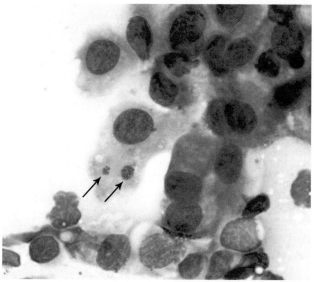

Figure 9-18 Conjunctival scraping from a cat with chlamydial conjunctivitis. Elementary bodies of *Chlamydophila felis* are found in an epithelial cell *(arrows)*. (Wright's stain, original magnification 1000×.) *(From Young KM, Taylor J: Laboratory Medicine: Yesterday Today Tomorrow: Eye on the cytoplasm. Vet Clin Pathol 35:141, 2006. Reprinted with permission of the American Society for Veterinary Clinical Pathology.)*

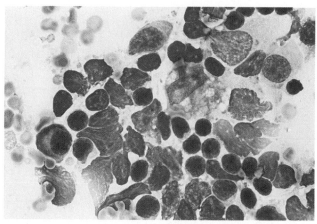

Figure 9-20 Conjunctival scraping from a cat with lymphocytic-plasmacytic conjunctivitis. Note numerous lymphocytes, a plasma cell (left margin), and a macrophage (top right center). (Romanowsky-type stain, original magnification 1000×.)

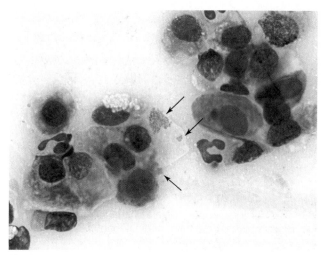

Figure 9-19 Conjunctival scraping from a cat with mycoplasmal conjunctivitis. *Mycoplasma felis* organisms *(arrows)* are visible on the surface of and adjacent to an epithelial cell. Note neutrophilic inflammation. (Wright's stain, original magnification 1000×.) *(From Young KM, Taylor J: Laboratory Medicine: Yesterday Today Tomorrow: Eye on the cytoplasm. Vet Clin Pathol 35:141, 2006. Reprinted with permission of the American Society for Veterinary Clinical Pathology.)*

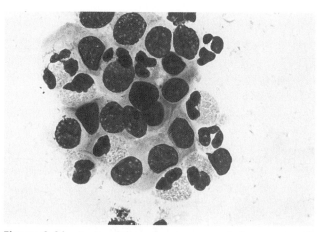

Figure 9-21 Eosinophils and squamous cells in a conjunctival scraping from a cat with eosinophilic conjunctivitis. (Romanowsky-type stain, original magnification 1000×.)

melanocytes increase in number in the inner scleral layers, which merge with the choroid.

A nodular or dome-shaped chronic inflammatory lesion affects the episclera and sclera of dogs.[26,28] It has been called nodular fasciitis, nodular episcleritis, nodular granulomatous episclerokeratitis, fibrous histiocytoma, and proliferative keratoconjunctivitis, among other terms. It primarily involves the episclera and sclera, most often near the limbus deep to the bulbar conjunctiva. Fine-needle aspiration yields lymphocytes, plasma cells, macrophages, multinucleated inflammatory giant cells, and a few neutrophils. Other scleral masses are caused by *Onchocerca* spp. in which the granulomas contain eosinophils,[29,30] and systemic histiocytosis.[5] Neoplasms that involve the sclera or episclera include lymphoma, mast cell tumor, squamous cell carcinoma, and melanoma.

THE CORNEA

The cornea is composed of a thick collagenous stroma covered by noncornified stratified squamous epithelium on the outer surface and a thick basal lamina (Descemet's membrane) deep to a single layer of flattened epithelial cells (endothelium) on the inner surface. The cornea is

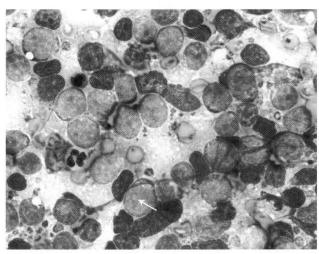

Figure 9-22 Conjunctival lymphoma from a dog. Note the predominance of large lymphoid cells with visible nucleoli *(arrow)*. Free nuclei and cytoplasmic fragments from ruptured cells are present in the background. (Wright's stain, original magnification 1000×.)

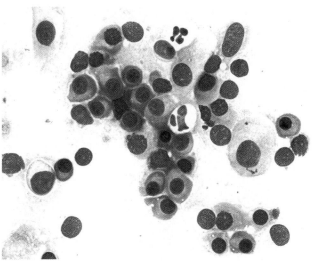

Figure 9-24 Numerous plasma cells in a scraping of the third eyelid from a German Shepherd with plasmacytic conjunctivitis. (Wright's stain, original magnification 600×.)

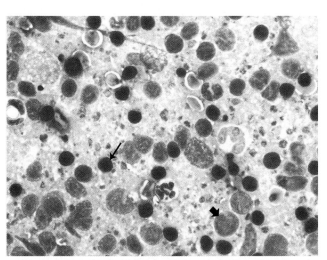

Figure 9-23 Corneal scrape from a dog with follicular conjunctivitis. Small lymphocytes *(thin arrow)* are numerous, and large lymphoid cells *(thick arrow)* also are present. Again, free nuclei and cytoplasmic fragments from ruptured cells are present in the background. (Wright's stain, original magnification 1000×.)

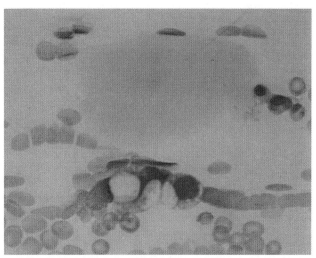

Figure 9-25 A large globule of mucus (top center), macrophages, and red blood cells arranged in rows (caused by mucoid content) in an aspirate of a lacrimal duct cyst in a young Basset Hound. (Romanowsky-type stain, original magnification 1000×.)

subject to a wide variety of lesions, including congenital malformation, opacification, proliferative changes, ulcerations, and exudative keratitis.[31] Many corneal lesions have a classic appearance, and diagnosis is made from the history and by gross examination.

Cytologic examination is most useful to characterize exudative lesions and may aid in differentiation of certain proliferative lesions. After applying a topical anesthetic, samples most often are acquired by scraping or may be obtained with a hypodermic needle if the lesion is very small or focal. Considerable caution must be taken in collecting samples from areas of the cornea that are

very thin secondary to the disease process. Several diseases may affect the cornea and conjunctiva concurrently; some of these are described in the earlier section on conjunctiva.

Infectious Ulcerative Keratitis

The exudate associated with ulcerative corneal lesions is typically neutrophilic and should be examined carefully for organisms. Sometimes, organisms are found only extracellularly, rather than within neutrophils, owing to bacterial defensive mechanisms. If the sample is collected

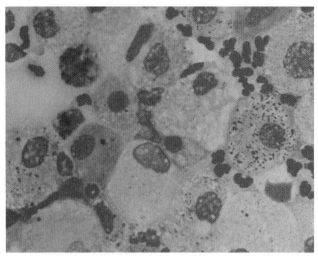

Figure 9-26 Exfoliated foamy salivary epithelial cells, a single melanophage *(top left)*, and neutrophils in a smear of an aspirate from a parotid duct cyst that occluded the opening into the conjunctival sac of a dog. (Romanowsky-type stain, original magnification 1000×.)

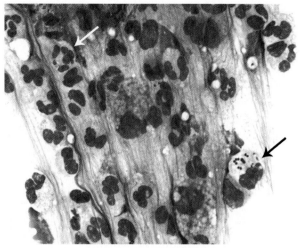

Figure 9-28 Degenerate *(black arrow)* and nondegenerate *(white arrow)* neutrophils in a corneal scrape from a dog with infectious ulcerative keratitis. The degenerate neutrophil contains bacterial cocci. (Wright's stain, original magnification 1000×.)

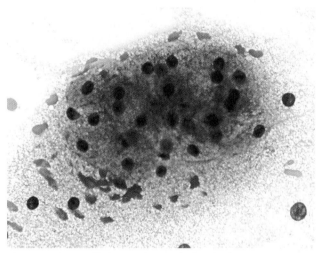

Figure 9-27 Cells from a lacrimal gland adenoma in a dog. Note the cluster of secretory tumor cells with a uniform appearance. (Wright's stain, original magnification 600×.)

dogs.[33] Corneal epithelial cells in areas of intense neutrophilic inflammation may exhibit dysplastic changes that can resemble features of malignancy.

Exudates in keratomycosis may vary in character from being nearly devoid of WBCs to having a neutrophilic or granulomatous composition. Scrapings may reveal such organisms as *Aspergillus* (Figure 9-31) or *Candida* (Figure 9-32), which are the most common species involved in keratomycosis. Pigmented fungi are rare (Figure 9-33), but dematiaceous fungi have been reported in infections involving multiple ocular structures in both the dog and cat.[34] In corneal scrapings with few WBCs, large clumps of corneal epithelium or necrotic cellular debris should be closely studied because hyphae may be embedded in this material (Figures 9-1, *B* and 9-34). Fragmented nuclei, often an artifact of slide preparation, may result in stringy chromatin that, when surrounded by mucus, may resemble hyphae. Hyphae have a definitive internal structure that should be recognized (see Figure 9-31). Special stains for fungi (PAS and Gomori's methenamine silver) may be useful.

Eosinophilic Keratitis

Eosinophilic keratitis is a corneal disease of cats, and cytologic examination is usually diagnostic.[35,36] The raised granular vascular lesion is usually not ulcerated and has small foci of gray-white deposits on the surface. Scrapings reveal an impressive number of mast cells among corneal epithelial cells and eosinophils or free eosinophilic granules (Figure 9-35). When the gray-white surface deposits are examined, cell debris composed primarily of fragmented stringy nuclear material and numerous free eosinophilic granules (and sometimes mast cell granules) are found (Figure 9-36). Free eosinophil and mast cell granules should not be mistaken for bacteria (see Figure 9-36, *inset*). In scrapings from ulcerated lesions or more

appropriately, any bacterial organisms, including ones found extracellularly, are considered significant. The combination of cytologic examination and culture is most effective for diagnosing and managing bacterial diseases.[32] Certain gram-negative rods, such as *Pseudomonas* spp., produce collagenase, which causes keratomalacia, the so-called melting ulcer. Neutrophils may be degenerate if exposure to bacterial toxins is prominent (Figure 9-28), and high numbers of pyknotic neutrophils may be present as an aging change in neutrophils or if apoptosis is accelerated (Figure 9-29). Examination of all samples collected is essential because features may vary from slide to slide (Figure 9-30). Recently, corneal ulceration has been associated with canine herpesvirus-1 infections in

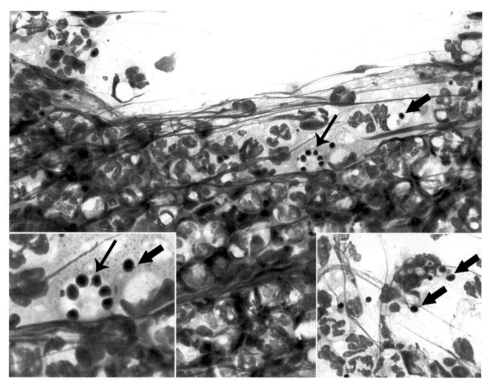

Figure 9-29 Pyknotic neutrophils *(thin arrows)* and free condensed nuclear lobes *(thick arrows)* in a corneal scrape from a dog with infectious keratitis. Pyknosis represents an aging change or accelerated apoptosis. (Wright's stain, original magnification 600×, insets 1000×.)

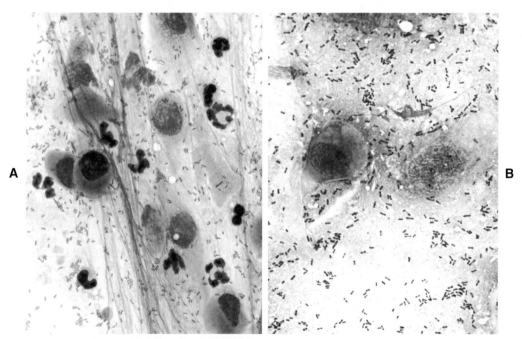

Figure 9-30 Infectious ulcerative keratitis caused by *Pseudomonas* infection in a dog. **A**, The first slide prepared contained numerous neutrophils and many extracellular bacteria of a single morphology. (Diff-Quik stain, original magnification 1000×.) **B**, The second slide prepared had many organisms (similar to those in **A**), but only rare neutrophils. (Wright's stain, original magnification 1000×.)

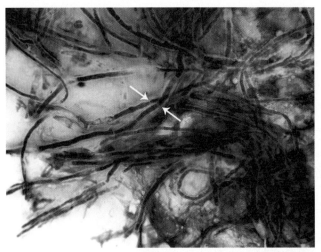

Figure 9-31 Mycotic keratitis caused by *Aspergillus* spp. infection in a dog. Note that the fungal hyphae have internal structure and septa *(arrows)*. (Wright's stain, original magnification 600×.)

deeply scraped nonulcerated lesions, eosinophils predominate, and lymphocytes and plasma cells also may be numerous (Figure 9-37). Eosinophilic keratitis (or keratoconjunctivitis) has been linked to infection with feline herpesvirus type 1.[37]

Chronic Superficial Keratitis

Chronic superficial keratitis, or pannus, is a common proliferative canine corneal lesion seen predominantly in German Shepherds. Scrapings, although not necessary for diagnosis, reveal a mixture of WBC types, including lymphocytes, plasma cells, macrophages, and neutrophils. Lipid corneal degeneration and mineralizing corneal degeneration are two common opacifying corneal lesions of dogs. Each lesion may cause plaque-like or granular thickening of the cornea. Scraping of lipid keratopathy is nondiagnostic and not indicated because the lipid does not readily exfoliate. Scraping of mineralizing corneal degeneration may reveal crystalline unstained granules (Figure 9-38). The granules show a positive reaction with von Kossa stain, a method of demonstrating calcium.

Corneal Tumors

Tumors of the cornea are rare in dogs and cats. Fine-needle aspiration, rather than scraping, is recommended. Corneal neoplasms include squamous cell carcinoma (Figure 9-39),[38] papilloma, melanoma, and various sarcomas.[31] The cytologic characteristics of these tumors are described in Chapter 2. In squamous cell carcinomas, keratin released from ruptured cells can incite neutrophilic inflammation. Distinguishing primary neutrophilic inflammation with secondary epithelial dysplasia from squamous cell carcinoma with secondary inflammation can be challenging, and histopathologic evaluation may be required.

Epithelial Inclusion Cysts

A raised stromal epithelial inclusion cyst occurs in the canine cornea.[39] The cyst is thought to be secondary to trauma. A clear acellular fluid may be aspirated from such cysts.

THE UVEA

The uvea is the layer of the eye that lies between the corneosclera and the retina and collectively consists of the iris and ciliary body, termed the anterior uvea, and the choroid, termed the posterior uvea. The diagnosis of anterior uveitis is made clinically, and aspiration of aqueous humor from the anterior chamber is performed in some cases with the goal of achieving a specific diagnosis. Posterior uveal disease is indicated by changes in the vitreous, which also can be aspirated for diagnostic purposes.

Aqueous Humor

Aspiration of aqueous humor for cytodiagnostic purposes may be indicated when the fluid is cloudy or opaque. However, clinical examination without cytologic examination is sufficient to discern hyphema, hypopyon, flare, and the presence of lipid. In feline anterior uveitis, there are no distinguishing cytologic features among various causes, such as toxoplasmosis and feline infectious peritonitis. Lymphoma may be diagnosed by examination of aqueous or iris aspirates; however, most other intraocular tumors, either primary or secondary, do not exfoliate into aqueous humor (see the following section on the iris and ciliary body). In most cases of infectious endophthalmitis, identification of organisms from aspirates of vitreous is more productive than examining aqueous humor (see later discussion).

Under general anesthesia, aspiration of the anterior chamber is done with a 25-ga or smaller needle attached to a 3-mL syringe. With the exception of hyphema, the protein content of aqueous humor is very low; consequently, in vitro disintegration of cells may be rapid. Sediment smears or cytocentrifuged preparations should be made soon after aspiration. Total cell counts and protein concentration may be determined if enough volume is obtained.[40]

Neutrophilic infiltration of aqueous humor is characteristic of most causes of anterior uveitis, including lens-induced uveitis and viral infections. A few lymphocytes and monocytes may be found. In cases of hypopyon, bacteria may or may not be found among the neutrophils. Infection with *Bartonella* spp. was suspected as a cause of anterior uveitis in cats[41] and of anterior uveitis and choroiditis in a dog based on positive serologic titers.[42] *Blastomyces dermatitidis*, *Prototheca* spp., and *Leishmania donovani* may be found in aqueous humor in certain cases.[43] Ocular toxoplasmosis in cats with anterior uveitis is diagnosed based on serologic testing, and its definitive diagnosis remains challenging.[44] Phagocytosis of melanin by neutrophils is an infrequent finding of unknown significance. Hyphema is characterized by either cells typical

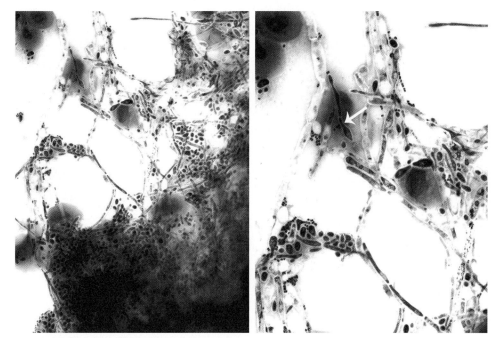

Figure 9-32   Mycotic keratitis caused by *Candida* spp. infection in a dog. Note pseudohyphae with constrictions between segments *(arrow)*. (Wright's stain, original magnification 600× **[A]**, 1000× **[B]**.)

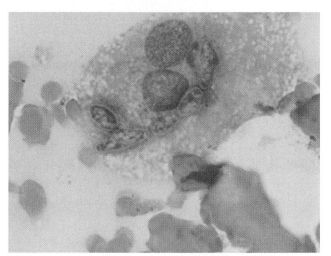

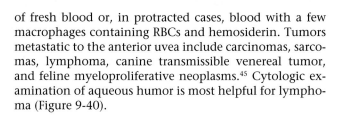

Figure 9-33   A giant cell containing a chain of spherules of *Cladosporium* spp. (a pigmented fungus) in a corneal scraping from a cat with mycotic keratitis. (Romanowsky-type stain, original magnification 1000×.)

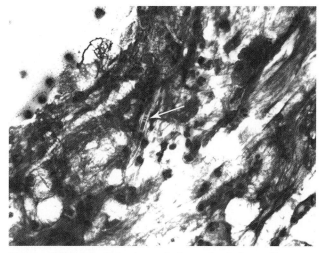

Figure 9-34   Hyphal element *(arrow)* of *Aspergillus* spp. embedded in thick necrotic debris. (Wright's stain, original magnification 600×.)

of fresh blood or, in protracted cases, blood with a few macrophages containing RBCs and hemosiderin. Tumors metastatic to the anterior uvea include carcinomas, sarcomas, lymphoma, canine transmissible venereal tumor, and feline myeloproliferative neoplasms.[45] Cytologic examination of aqueous humor is most helpful for lymphoma (Figure 9-40).

The Iris and Ciliary Body

Space-occupying masses on the anterior uvea may be an indication for cytologic examination of fine-needle aspirates. Direct aspiration of the iris nodule is

accomplished under general anesthesia as described in the previous section on aqueous humor.

Melanoma: Melanoma is the most common primary intraocular tumor. The preparation should contain melanocytes that exhibit cytomorphologic features of malignancy to be diagnostic, because free melanin and some melanocytes are a component of all uveal aspirates. In cats, progressive iris hyperpigmentation may represent diffuse iris melanoma.[46] Melanosis (Figure 9-41), with accumulation of melanocytes forming a freckle, may undergo a transition to iris melanoma,[47] a diagnosis that can be challenging to make. Fine-needle (25-gauge needle or

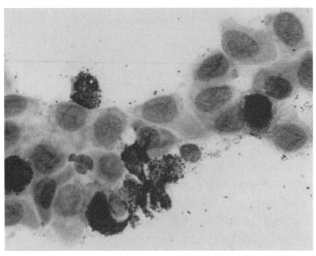

Figure 9-35 Squamous cells, mast cells, and free eosinophilic granules in a corneal scraping from a cat with eosinophilic keratitis. (Romanowsky-type stain, original magnification 1000×.)

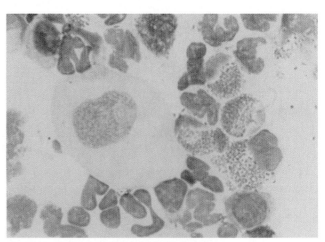

Figure 9-37 Eosinophils, neutrophils, lymphocytes, and squamous cells in a corneal scraping from a cat with eosinophilic keratitis. (Romanowsky-type stain, original magnification 1000×.)

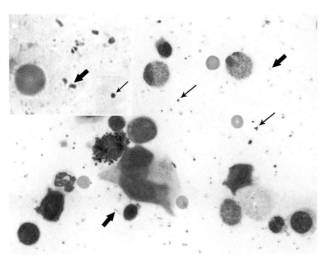

Figure 9-36 Numerous free rod-shaped eosinophil *(thick arrows)* and round mast cell *(thin arrows)* granules are found in a corneal scrape from a cat with eosinophilic keratitis. (Wright's stain, original magnification 1000×.)

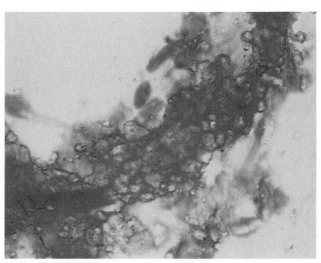

Figure 9-38 Amorphous nonstaining crystalline material and cell debris in a corneal scraping from a dog with mineralizing corneal degeneration. (Romanowsky-type stain, original magnification 1000×.)

smaller) aspiration of the anterior surface of the iris lesion, without needle penetration of the iris, may yield diagnostic cells.[48] Avoid dilution of the sample with aqueous. In iris melanoma the most consistent cytologic findings are variability in the size and shape of nuclei and nucleoli (Figure 9-42). Binucleated cells may be found. Both normal and tumor cells are pigmented. Normal cells have uniform nuclei and small uniform nucleoli (Figure 9-43).

Lymphoproliferative Diseases: Lymphoma also occurs as a diffuse or nodular iris lesion. Whereas lymphoblasts, mitotic cells, and lymphoid cells with broad pseudopodia are present, normal small lymphocytes and plasma cells

also may be seen (see Chapter 8 for discussion and additional photomicrographs of lymphoma). Ocular lymphoma is usually part of multicentric disease. When it is suspected, the disease should be staged by evaluating the animal for systemic lesions that may be more easily sampled for diagnostic purposes. Extramedullary plasmacytoma in the iris of a cat with mandibular lymph node involvement but no other evidence of disease has been reported.[49]

Epithelial Tumors: Adenomas and adenocarcinomas may originate from iris or ciliary body epithelium (Figure 9-44). Among primary intraocular tumors, these are second to melanomas in frequency.[50] The anterior uvea also

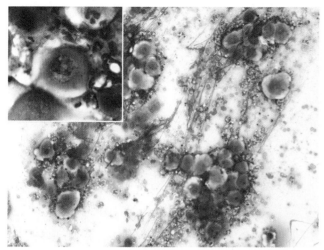

Figure 9-39 Squamous cell carcinoma on the cornea of a dog. Note the monolayer sheets of neoplastic squamous cells and numerous neutrophils. (Wright's stain, original magnification 600×.) *Inset,* Perinuclear vacuolation in a neoplastic squamous cell. (Wright's stain, original magnification 1000×.)

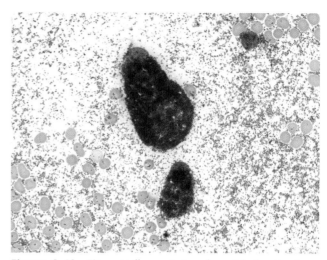

Figure 9-41 Fine-needle aspirate of an iris freckle from a cat. Abundant melanin is found within melanocytes and extracellularly. (Wright's stain, original magnification 600×.)

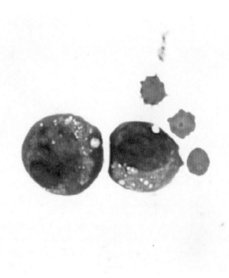

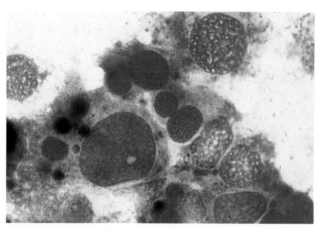

Figure 9-42 Fine-needle aspirate of the surface of a pigmented lesion on a feline iris. Cells have marked anisocytosis and anisokaryosis and contain melanin pigment. The diagnosis is feline iris melanoma. (Romanowsky-type stain, original magnification 1000×.)

Figure 9-40 Aqueous humor aspirate from a dog with lymphoma. Note the large lymphoid cells with bizarre nucleoli and basophilic cytoplasm. (Wright-Giemsa stain, original magnification 1000×.)

is a site for metastasis of systemic carcinomas.[51] Cytologic features of benign and malignant epithelial tumors are described in Chapter 1.

THE VITREOUS BODY

Opacity in the vitreous body is an indication for aspiration and cytologic examination. The diagnostic yield is quite good in our experience. Aspiration of the vitreous body is not an innocuous procedure. If a potentially visual eye is aspirated, care must be taken not to cause

hemorrhage or other sequelae that could jeopardize vision. Under general anesthesia, a 23-gauge or smaller needle is used to penetrate the eye 6 to 8 mm caudal to the limbus: the needle is directed into the middle of the vitreous toward the optic nerve. The lens must be avoided to prevent disruption of the lens capsule and induction of lens-induced uveitis. Aspiration of 0.5 to 1.0 mL of fluid is recommended. Sediment smears or cytocentrifuged preparations should be made immediately after aspiration. After air-drying and before staining, heat the underside of the glass slide by passing it through the tip of a small flame two or three times. Heat fixation helps vitreous body material adhere to the slide.

Vitreous body material is normally acellular, although most samples contain a few RBCs and scattered melanin granules, which, in this location in dogs, are oblong with

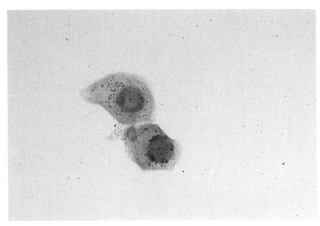

Figure 9-43 Normal melanocytes aspirated from the iris surface of a normal feline eye. Note the uniform size and shape of nuclei and cytoplasmic melanin. (Romanowsky-type stain, original magnification 1000×.)

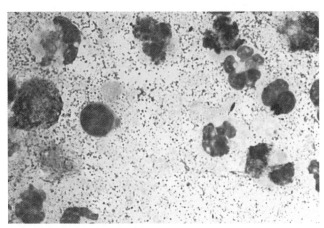

Figure 9-45 Vitreous smear from a dog. Background granular precipitate is characteristic of all vitreous smears. Note the oblong melanin granule (right center) and neutrophils. (Romanowsky-type stain, original magnification 1000×.)

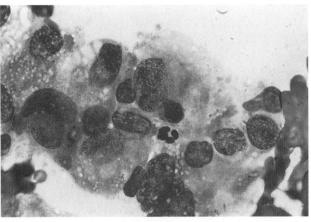

Figure 9-44 Fine-needle aspirate of an iridociliary carcinoma in a cat. Cells exhibit anisokaryosis, irregularly shaped nuclei, nuclear molding, and distinct cytoplasmic vacuoles of variable size. (Romanowsky-type stain, original magnification 1000×.)

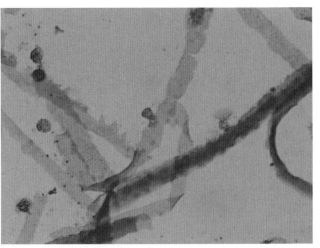

Figure 9-46 Lens fibers in the sediment of a vitreous body aspirate from a dog. Several red blood cells provide a size reference. (Romanowsky-type stain, original magnification 400×.)

pointed ends (Figure 9-45). The background on stained smears is an eosinophilic granular precipitate. Lens fibers may be found in sediment smears in cases of pars planitis (snowbanking) (Figure 9-46). Microfilariae may be found in samples that contain blood from microfilaremic dogs, but they are not associated with ocular disease. Melanin-laden cells may be found in samples from normal or diseased eyes. Asteroid hyalosis is a degenerative disease of the vitreous consisting of calcium and lipid complexes. It is not an indication for cytologic examination.

Endophthalmitis

Bacterial endophthalmitis is purulent, and organisms are usually demonstrable in the exudate on vitreous smears. Neutrophilic exudate without organisms can be seen in lens-induced endophthalmitis and trauma.

Mycotic endophthalmitis with opacification of the vitreous body is relatively common in dogs. Ocular lesions were found in 41% of dogs with blastomycosis.[52] Affected dogs had a neutrophilic exudate and *B. dermatitidis* yeast in vitreous body smears (Figure 9-47). Empty capsules of dead yeast may be the only indication of the infection in some animals (Figure 9-48). Sometimes the organisms are found in the absence of inflammatory cells. Other fungi that may be found in the vitreous body include *Cryptococcus neoformans* (Figure 9-49), *Coccidioides immitis* (Figure 9-50), and *Histoplasma capsulatum*.[53] In cryptococcal infection, in particular, there may be little to no inflammation owing to the protective mechanisms associated with the capsule, and care must be taken not to overlook the yeast forms. The use of India ink to highlight the yeast of *Cryptococcus* is sometimes suggested, but is

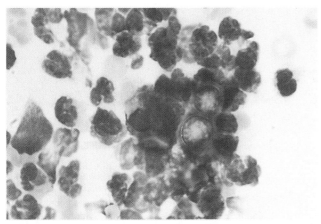

Figure 9-47 Vitreous aspirate from a dog. Note the broad-based budding yeast of *Blastomyces dermatitidis* surrounded by neutrophils. (Romanowsky-type stain, original magnification 1000×.)

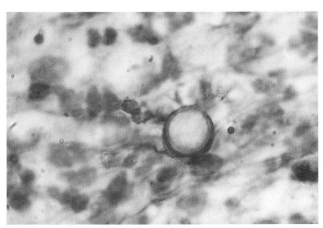

Figure 9-48 Vitreous aspirate from a dog. Note the neutrophils and the empty yeast shell of *Blastomyces dermatitidis*. (Romanowsky-type stain, original magnification 1000×.)

unnecessary and may even result in misinterpretation of a sample. The clear capsule around the yeast can be seen even in the presence of a pale background (see Figure 9-49, *A*), and lipid droplets coated by India ink may be mistaken for organisms. Protothecosis also may affect the vitreous body.[54] The organisms are usually systemic, although ocular manifestations because of chorioretinitis may be the initial clinical problem. A neutrophilic exudate and *Prototheca* organisms may be found on vitreous smears.

Hemorrhage

Cytologic findings in vitreous smears are similar to those in hematomas or other sites of hemorrhage. In addition to RBCs, monocytes and macrophages exhibiting erythrophagia and containing hemosiderin predominate. Causes of hemorrhage can be systemic or local ocular diseases,

such as bleeding disorders, retinal detachment, intraocular tumor, hypertension, or rickettsial disease.

Intraocular Tumors

Posterior segment intraocular tumors can be diagnosed on cytologic examination of vitreous smears. Cats may develop intraocular sarcomas following trauma.[55,56] This may be a consequence of metaplasia of the lens epithelium and subsequent proliferation and migration.[57] Recently, primary intraocular osteosarcoma was reported in a dog.[58] Absence of neoplastic cells does not exclude intraocular tumor from consideration.

THE RETINA

Rarely, cells from the retina are obtained accidentally, if there is retinal detachment, or if the subretinal space is aspirated when cloudy material is visualized in that location. Nuclei of photoreceptor cells from the outer nuclear layer and retinal pigmented epithelial cells were identified in an aspirate of subretinal fluid (Figure 9-51). Hypothetically, inflammatory cells could be identified if retinitis was present, but cytologic examination of the retina is rare.

THE ORBIT
Exophthalmos

Exophthalmos results from a space-occupying lesion in the orbit. Causes include tumors, abscesses, hematomas, foreign bodies, osteomyelitis,[59] mucoceles, or extensions of inflammatory or neoplastic diseases from the sinus or oral cavity. Retrobulbar fine-needle aspiration and cytologic examination are indicated. Orbital cellulitis due to retrobulbar *Toxocara canis* infection with larval migration has been reported in a dog.[60] Traumatic proptosis is not an indication for retrobulbar aspiration.

Imaging by survey radiography or ultrasonographic examination and orbital palpation can help localize the lesion. Aspiration is from the orbit or the mouth, caudal to the last molar. The critical structures to avoid are the optic nerve and globe. The various principles of diagnostic cytology described throughout the text and in detail in Chapter 1 are applicable in differentiation of the various lesions.

Orbital Tumors

Dogs or cats with orbital tumors are presented with either exophthalmos or enophthalmos. The quantity of material obtained from retrobulbar tumors is sparse compared with an abscess or mucocele. Orbital neoplasms include lymphoma, plasmacytoma, squamous cell carcinoma, salivary adenocarcinoma, osteoma and osteosarcoma, chondroma and chondorsarcoma, hemangioma, melanoma, fibrosarcoma, meningioma (Figure 9-52), peripheral nerve sheath tumors (Figure 9-53), and carcinomas and sarcomas of unknown type. The most common orbital tumor in cats is squamous cell carcinoma.[61]

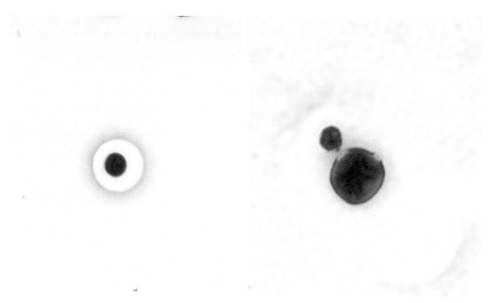

Figure 9-49 Vitreous aspirates from a cat with cryptococcosis. *Cryptococcus* organisms have a capsule and exhibit narrow-based budding *(right)*. The clear capsule is evident even if the background material is pale *(left)*, and staining with India ink is unnecessary. Inflammatory cells often are absent. (Wright's strain, original magnification 1000×.)

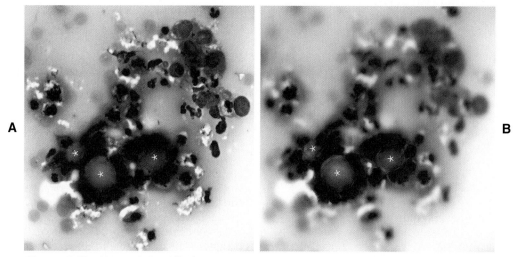

Figure 9-50 Yeast of *Coccidioides* spp. (∗) in a vitreous aspirate from a dog. These large yeast forms appear out of focus when the inflammatory cells are in focus (**A**); conversely, the inflammatory cells are blurred when the yeast wall is in focus (**B**). (Wright-Giemsa stain, original magnification 600×.)

Postenucleation Orbital Lesions

Cysts are an infrequent complication of enucleation.[62,63] A possible mechanism of cyst formation is implantation or incarceration of conjunctival epithelium or the gland of the third eyelid at the time of enucleation. Cytologic examination reveals basal, intermediate, and mature noncornified squamous cells, large foamy macrophages, and abundant mucus (Figure 9-54).

Frontal sinus osteomyelitis may extend into the orbit postenucleation. Osteoclasts, osteoblasts, and leukocytes are found. Mucocele and emphysema may affect the orbit following enucleation.

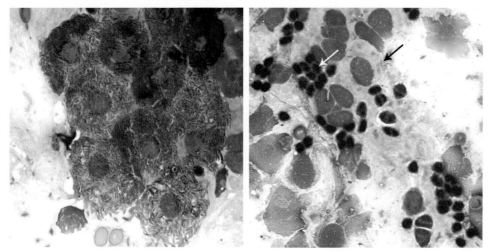

Figure 9-51 Retinal tissue in an aspirate of subretinal fluid from a dog. Note the retinal pigmented epithelial (RPE) cells *(left)*, nuclei of photoreceptor cells *(right, white arrow)*, and free spiculate melanin granules *(right, black arrow)* from RPE cells. (Wright-Giemsa stain, original magnification 1000×.)

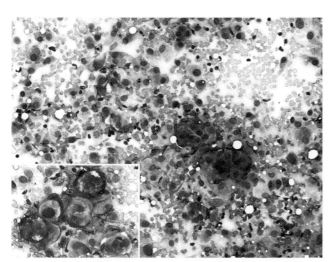

Figure 9-52 Fine-needle aspirate of an orbital mass from a dog with orbital meningioma. Note the large cells with abundant cytoplasm that sometimes form whorls *(inset)*. (Wright's stain, original magnification 200×, inset 600×.)

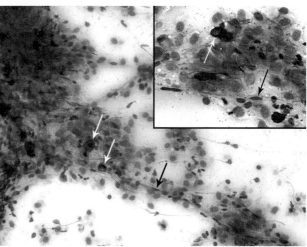

Figure 9-53 Fine-needle aspirate of an orbital mass from a dog with an orbital peripheral nerve sheath tumor. An endothelial-lined vessel *(black arrows)* courses through the polyhedral tumor cells that aggregate around vessels. Mast cells *(white arrows)* are sometimes found in these tumors. (Wright's stain, original magnification 200×, inset 600×.)

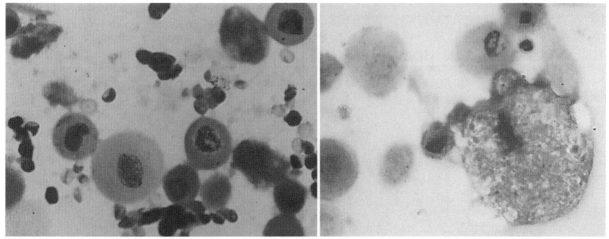

Figure 9-54 Postenucleation orbital cyst in a dog. Note the variably sized noncornified squamous cells, red blood cells, and cellular debris *(left)* as well as the degenerating squamous cells and a large foamy macrophage *(right)*. (Romanowsky-type stain, original magnification 1000×.)

References

1. Latimer and Dumstan: Eosinophilic plaque involving eyelids of the cat. *J Am Anim Hosp Assoc* 23:649-652, 1987.
2. Krehbiel JD, Langham RF: Eyelid neoplasms of dogs. *Am J Vet Res* 36:115-119, 1975.
3. Carlton. In Peiffer RL Jr: *Comparative Ophthalmic Pathology.* Springfield, Ill, Charles C Thomas, 1983, pp 64-86.
4. Collins BK, et al: Idiopathic granulomatous disease with ocular adnexal and cutaneous involvement in a dog. *J Am Vet Med Assoc* 201:313-316, 1992.
5. Scherlie PH Jr, et al: Ocular manifestation of systemic histiocytosis in a dog. *J Am Vet Med Assoc* 201:1229-1232, 1992.
6. Rosin A, et al: Malignant histiocytosis in Bernese mountain dogs. *J Am Vet Med Assoc* 188:1041-1045, 1986.
7. Nasisse MP, et al: Clinical and laboratory findings in chronic conjunctivitis in cats: 91 cases (1983-1991). *J Am Vet Med Assoc* 203:834-837, 1993.
8. Streeten BW, Streeten EA: "Blue body" epithelial cell inclusions in conjunctivitis. *Ophthalmology* 92:575-579, 1985.
9. Bolzan AA, et al: Conjunctival impression cytology in dogs. *Vet Ophthalmol* 8:401-405, 2005.
10. Ramsey DT, et al: Ligneous conjunctivitis in four Doberman pinschers. *J Am Anim Hosp Assoc* 32:439-447, 1996.
11. Gelatt. In Gelatt KN: *Textbook of Veterinary Ophthalmology.* Philadelphia, Lea & Febiger, 1981, pp 206-261.
12. Nasisse MP, et al: The diagnosis of ocular feline herpesvirus-1 (FHV-1) infections by polymerase chain reaction. *Proc ACVO,* 1997, p 83.
13. Stiles et al: Use of nested polymerase chain reaction to identify feline herpesvirus in ocular tissue from clinically normal cats and cats with corneal sequestra or conjunctivitis. *Proc ACVO,* 1997, p 82.
14. Peiffer. In Gelatt KN: *Textbook of Veterinary Ophthalmology.* Philadelphia, Lea & Febiger, 1981, pp 699-723.
15. Hoover EA, et al: Experimentally induced feline chlamydial infection (feline pneumonitis). *Am J Vet Res* 39:541-547, 1978.
16. von Bomhard W, et al: Detection of novel chlamydiae in cats with ocular disease. *Am J Vet Res* 64:1421-1428, 2003.
17. Campbell LH, et al: *Mycoplasma felis* associated conjunctivitis in cats. *J Am Vet Med Assoc* 163:991-995, 1973.
18. Pentlarge: Eosinophilic conjunctivitis in five cats. *J Am Anim Hosp Assoc* 27:21-28, 1991.
19. Johnson et al: Conjunctival mast cell tumor in two dogs. *J Am Anim Hosp Assoc* 24:439-442, 1988.
20. Pirie CG, et al: Canine conjunctival hemangioma and hemangiosarcoma: A retrospective evaluation of 108 cases (1989-2004). *Vet Ophthalmol* 9:215-226, 2006.
21. Pirie CG, et al: Feline conjunctival hemangioma and hemangiosarcoma: A retrospective evaluation of 8 cases (1993-2004). *Vet Ophthalmol* 9:227-231, 2005.
22. Martin et al: Cystic lesions of the periorbital region. *Comp Cont Ed Pract Vet* 9:1022-1029, 1987.
23. Read RA: Treatment of canine nictitans plasmacytic conjunctivitis with 0.2 percent cyclosporin ointment. *J Small Amin Pract* 36:50-56, 1995.
24. Carr AP, et al: Ein ungewohnlicher tumor der nickhautdruse eines hundes—ein fallbericht. *Dtsch Tierarztl Wochenschr* 99:465-466, 1992.
25. Dugan et al: Variant nodular granulomatous episclerokeratitis in four dogs. *J Am Anim Hosp Assoc* 29:403-409, 1993.
26. Paulsen ME, et al: Nodular granulomatous episclerokeratitis in dogs: 19 cases (1973-1985). *J Am Vet Med Assoc* 190: 1581-1587, 1987.
27. Hirayama K, et al: A pleomorphic adenoma of the lacrimal gland in a dog. *Vet Pathol* 37:353-356, 2000.
28. Fischer. In Peiffer RL Jr: *Comparative Ophthalmic Pathology.* Springfield, Ill Charles C Thomas, 1983, pp 272-288.
29. Gardiner CH, et al: Onchocerciasis in two dogs. *J Am Vet Med Assoc* 203:828-830, 1993.
30. Zarfoss MK, et al: Canine ocular onchocerciasis in the United States: Two new cases and a review of the literature. *Vet Ophthalmol* 8:51-57, 2005.
31. Dice. In Gelatt KN: *Textbook of Veterinary Ophthalmology.* Philadelphia, Lea & Febiger, 1981, pp 343-374.
32. Massa KL, et al: Usefulness of aerobic microbial culture and cytologic evaluation of corneal specimens in the diagnosis of infectious ulcerative keratitis in animals. *J Am Vet Med Assoc* 215:1671-1674, 1999.
33. Ledbetter EC, et al: Corneal ulceration associated with naturally occurring canine herpesvirus-1 infection in two adult dogs. *J Am Vet Med Assoc* 229:376-384, 2006.
34. Bernays ME, Peiffer RL Jr: Ocular infections with dematiaceous fungi in two cats and a dog. *J Am Vet Med Assoc* 213:507-509, 1998.
35. Paulsen et al: Feline eosinophilic keratitis: A review of 15 cases. *J Am Anim Hosp Assoc* 23:63-69, 1987.
36. Prasse KW, Winston SM: Cytology and histopathology of feline eosinophilic keratitis. *Vet Comp Ophthal* 6:74-81, 1996.
37. Nasisse MA, et al: Detection of feline herpesvirus 1 DNA in corneas of cats with eosinophilic keratitis or corneal sequestration. *Am J Vet Res* 59:856-858, 1998.
38. Ward DA, et al: Squamous cell carcinoma of the corneoscleral limbus in a dog. *J Am Vet Med Assoc* 200:1503-1506, 1992.
39. Schmidt GM, Prasse KW: Corneal epithelial inclusion cyst in a dog. *J Am Vet Med Assoc* 168:144, 1976.
40. Hazel SJ, et al: Laboratory evaluation of aqueous humor in the healthy dog, cat, horse, and cow. *Am J Vet Res* 46: 657-659, 1985.
41. Lappin MR, Black JC: *Bartonella* spp. infection as a possible cause of uveitis in a cat. *J Am Vet Med Assoc* 214:1205-1207, 1999.
42. Michau TM, et al: *Bartonella vinsonii* subspecies *berkhoffi* as a possible cause of anterior uveitis and choroiditis in a dog. *Vet Ophthalmol* 6:299-304, 2003.
43. Keller. In Gelatt KN: *Textbook of Veterinary Ophthalmology.* Philadelphia, Lea & Febiger, 1981, pp 375-389.
44. Davidson MG: Toxoplasmosis. *Vet Clin North Am Small Anim Pract* 30:1051-1062, 2000.
45. Carlton. In Peiffer RL Jr: *Comparative Ophthalmic Pathology.* Springfield, Ill Charles C Thomas, 1983, pp 289-298.
46. Schaffer EH, Gordon S: Das feline okular melanom. Klinische und pathologisch anatomische befund von 37 fallen. *Tierarztl Prax* 21:255-264, 1993.
47. Dubielzig and Lindley: The transition from iris freckle to diffuse iris melanoma of cats: a histopathologic study [abstract]. *Proceedings of the American College of Veterinary Ophthalmology,* Phoenix, 1993.
48. Grossniklaus HE: Fine-needle aspiration biopsy of the iris. *Arch Ophthalmol* 110:969-976, 1992.
49. Michau TM, et al: Intraocular extramedullary plasmacytoma in a cat. *Vet Ophthalmol* 6:177-181, 2003.
50. Peiffer RL Jr: In Peiffer RL Jr: *Comparative Ophthalmic Pathology.* Springfield, Ill Charles C Thomas, 1983, pp 183-212.
51. Miller, Dubielzig: In Withrow, Vail: *Small Animal Clinical Oncology,* ed 4, St. Louis, Saunders, 2007, pp 686-698.
52. Legendre AM, et al: Canine blastomycosis: a review of 47 clinical cases. *J Am Vet Med Assoc* 178:1163-1168, 1981.
53. Carlton. In Peiffer RL Jr: *Comparative Ophthalmic Pathology.* Springfield, Ill Charles C Thomas, 1983, pp 299-317.

54. Buyukmihci N, et al: Protothecosis with ocular involvement in a dog. *J Am Vet Med Assoc* 167:158-161, 1975.

55. Dubielzig RR: Ocular sarcoma following trauma in three cats. *J Am Vet Med Assoc* 184:578-581, 1984.

56. Dubielzig RR, et al: Clinical and morphologic features of post-traumatic ocular sarcomas in cats. *Vet Pathol* 27:62-65, 1990.

57. Zeiss CJ, et al: Feline intraocular tumors may arise from transformation of lens epithelium. *Vet Pathol* 40:355-362, 2003.

58. Heath S, et al: Primary ocular osteosarcoma in a dog. *Vet Ophthalmol* 6:85-87, 2003.

59. Grahn BH, et al: Exophthalmos associated with frontal sinus osteomyelitis in a puppy. *J Am Anim Hosp Assoc* 31:397-401, 1995.

60. Laus JL, et al: Orbital cellulitis associated with *Toxocara canis* in a dog. *Vet Ophthalmol* 6:333-336, 2003.

61. Gilger BC, et al: Orbital neoplasms in cats: 21 cases (1974-1990). *J Am Vet Med Assoc* 201:1083-1086, 1992.

62. Hanig CJ, Hornblass A: Treatment of postenucleation orbital cysts. *Ann Ophthalmol* 18:191-193, 1986.

63. Ramsey DT, et al: Ophthalmic manifestations and complications of dental disease in dogs and cats. *J Am Anim Hosp Assoc* 32:215-224, 1996.

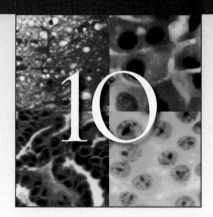

The External Ear Canal

P.K. Patten, R.L. Cowell, and R.D. Tyler

CHAPTER 10

CAUSES OF OTITIS

Otitis externa is commonly encountered in veterinary practice. It may be unilateral, bilateral, acute, or chronic. Otitis externa in some form is estimated to affect 15% of dogs and 4% of cats presented for veterinary care.[1] These animals generally show one or more of the following signs: head shaking, pain, pruritus, erythema, swelling, malodor, otic discharge, crusting, alopecia, excoriation, and pyotraumatic dermatitis.[1-3] Conformation, habits, skin diseases, organisms, tumors, and trauma are some of the factors thought to initiate, predispose, or perpetuate otitis externa (Boxes 10-1 and 10-2). Each is briefly addressed subsequently.[1-4]

Conformation

A long, relatively narrow ear canal tends to trap moisture, foreign debris, and glandular secretions. Excessive hair in the external ear canal inhibits ventilation and increases retention of cerumen. Also, dogs with pendulous ears have decreased ventilation, which increases humidity within the ear canal. Such a moist environment can destroy the protective barrier of the epidermis and allow opportunistic infection.[1,3,4]

Habits

Dogs housed outside and hunting dogs are more likely to have foreign bodies (such as grass awns, dirt, or twigs) lodge in the ear canal.[1,3] Dogs that swim or are frequently bathed may develop otitis externa, since frequent wetting of the ear canal may stimulate ceruminous gland activity resulting in overproduction of secretions. Moisture trapped in the ear canal may also affect the protective function of the epidermis.[2,4]

Skin Diseases

Generalized skin disease may affect the pinna and external ear canal epithelium (e.g., atopy, food allergy, contact hypersensitivity, autoimmune disease) or cause overproduction of cerumen (e.g., seborrhea, endocrinopathies). As many as 50% to 83% of atopic dogs reportedly have

signs of otitis. In a few of these cases, otitis may be the only clinical sign.[1,3-5]

Organisms

Bacteria, yeasts, and/or parasites are commonly involved in otic disorders. Small numbers of bacteria and *Malassezia* yeast are present in the ear canals of many clinically normal dogs and cats. These organisms can secondarily overgrow and infect the ear canal when predisposing conditions permit. Ear mites are one of the major primary causes of otitis externa in cats with a much lower prevalence in dogs.[1-6]

Tumors

Any cutaneous neoplasm can occur in the ear canal and may predispose the animal to otitis externa.[1,5,7,8]

Trauma

Traumatic use of cotton-tipped swabs or irritating solutions secondary to overzealous ear cleaning can damage the epithelial lining and allow organisms to colonize and infect the ear canal. Self-inflicted lacerations due to scratching may also predispose the animal to secondary infection.[1-4]

DIAGNOSIS

Most cases of acute otitis externa can be readily managed using the information gained from a thorough history, physical examination, otoscopic examination, and cytologic evaluation of ear canal secretions. Careful evaluation of the patient's skin is also important because ear disease is often associated with generalized skin disease. Foreign bodies, tissue masses, abnormal ear canal conformation, mites, ticks, and other abnormalities can be detected during otoscopic examination, and any microorganisms present can be identified cytologically. Serial cytologic evaluation is also useful to monitor the response to therapy.[1,3,4,6,9] The algorithm in Figure 10-1 can be used to aid in the evaluation of ear canal secretions. Additional diagnostic tests (such as culture, thyroid evaluation,

---

BOX 10-1

Predisposing Causes of Otitis Externa

Ear conformation
Pendulous ears
Long narrow ear canal
Excessive hair in canal

Habits
Frequent swimming/bathing
Animals housed outside with increased exposure to
    foreign objects

Trauma
Excessive ear cleaning
Scratching

Tumors
Benign or malignant neoplasia causing obstruction of
    the ear canal

BOX 10-2

Primary and Secondary Causes of Otitis Externa

Primary Causes
Foreign bodies
Plant material (especially grass awns), dirt, other debris
Ear mites
Otodectes cynotis (common)
Otobius megnini (found in southwest U.S.)
Demodex and other mites (rare)
Generalized skin diseases
Atopy
Contact hypersensitivity
Food allergy
Autoimmune disease
Seborrhea
Endocrinopathies, etc.

Secondary/Perpetuating Causes
Bacteria
    Bacterial cocci:
        Staphylococcus (common)
        Enterococcus (occasionally found)
        Streptococcus (occasionally found)
    Bacterial rods:
        Pseudomonas (common)
        Proteus (occasionally found)
        Escherichia coli (occasionally found)
Fungi
    Malassezia (common)

---

intradermal skin testing, and biopsy) are generally needed to determine the underlying cause of chronic or recurrent otitis externa.[1,3,6]

COLLECTION AND STAINING OF SAMPLES

Samples of ear canal secretions for cytologic evaluation are best collected with cotton-tipped swabs. Anesthesia may be required to obtain samples from uncooperative animals or animals with painful ears. Cytology samples are preferably obtained after performing otoscopic examination to evaluate the tympanic membrane, because the swab may compress debris in the horizontal canal and obscure the tympanum. Collection of cytology samples should be performed before any cleaning agents or medications are placed in the ear. Samples may be collected by passing a cotton-tipped swab through the cone of an otoscope (Figure 10-2). The use of a separate, clean otoscope cone for each ear is recommended to prevent cross-contamination. Sterile cones are required to obtain samples for culture. Passing a cotton-tipped swab through the cone of an otoscope allows the operator to visualize the horizontal ear canal and be sure the specimen is collected from that area. Collecting ear swabs from the horizontal ear canal is desirable because most bacterial ear infections begin in this area. Another method is to carefully pass a swab into the ear canal without the aid of an otoscope collecting samples from the junction of the vertical and horizontal ear canals. Further blind advancement of the swab into the horizontal ear canal is not recommended because injury could occur if the animal moves unexpectedly. Always collect samples from both ears because animals that appear to have unilateral otitis may also have mild, less apparent disease in the other ear.[1,3,6]

After ear canal secretions have been collected, the swab is gently rolled on a clean, dry, glass slide. The sample should be rolled onto the slide in a thin layer because thick smears are difficult to evaluate. Heat fixation of slides is not necessary.[10] Freshly made slides can be examined microscopically on low power for ear mites before the material has dried. After the material on the slide is allowed to air-dry, it is stained with any of the usual hematologic stains (e.g., Diff-Quik or Wright's stain). Some slides should always be stained and examined microscopically for organisms and inflammatory cells.[6] It is recommended to have two set of staining jars, one reserved for ear cytology and one reserved for other samples (e.g., blood smears, mass aspirates) because yeast and bacteria from ear cytologies can overgrow in the stain solutions and contaminate other slides.

CYTOLOGIC EXAMINATION

Smears of external ear canal secretions should be evaluated for different types and relative numbers of bacteria (rods, cocci), yeasts (*Malassezia* spp.), mites, neutrophils, cerumen, and neoplastic cells.

Bacteria

The ear canals of clinically normal dogs often contain small numbers of bacteria. The bacterial concentration typically is low enough that one sees only occasional or no bacteria on cytologic preparations (Figure 10-3). Many of these bacteria are potentially pathogenic and can colonize the ear canal

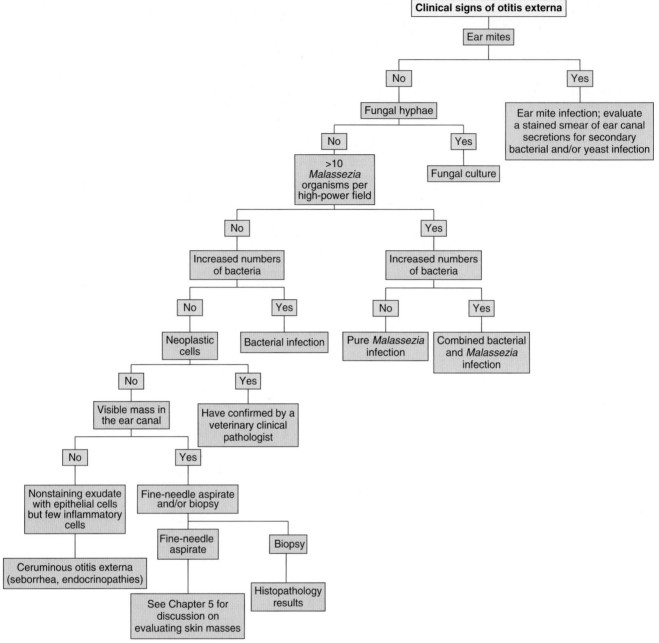

Figure 10-1 Flow chart for evaluation of smears of ear canal secretions.

when normal conditions are altered.[2-4,6] In animals with bacterial otitis, cytologic evaluation of ear canal secretions often reveals large numbers of bacteria free in the smear (Figure 10-4). Sometimes neutrophilic inflammation is also present, and bacteria may be observed phagocytized within neutrophils (Figure 10-5). Identifying whether the bacterial infection involves cocci or rods assists with initial selection of antibiotics since most cocci are gram positive and most rods are gram negative. A combination of rods and cocci may also be found. Infections involving cocci usually represent *Staphylococcus* or occasionally other species such as *Enterococcus* or *Streptococcus*. For infections containing bacterial rods, *Pseudomonas* is the most common species cultured but other species are occasionally found including *Proteus* and *Escherichia coli*.[2-6,9,11]

When routine therapy is ineffective, culture and sensitivity testing is indicated because of the high incidence of antimicrobial resistance associated with otitis externa.[11]

Fungi

Malassezia pachydermatis is by far the most common yeast associated with otitis externa in dogs and cats, but can be found in both normal and otic ears. Overgrowth occurs when predisposing factors provide a favorable environment. Pure *Malassezia* infections tend to develop copious, dark-brown exudate with a sweet odor. However, concurrent bacterial infections and *Malassezia* infections (see Figure 10-4) commonly occur.[1-6,9,11] *Malassezia* (Figure 10-6) is a broad-based budding, basophilic staining,

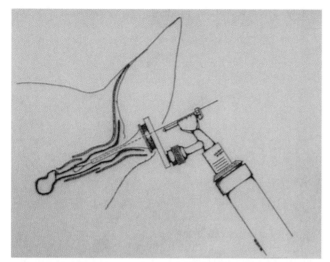

Figure 10-2 Smears of horizontal ear canal secretions may be collected by passing a cotton-tipped swab through the cone of an otoscope after otoscopic examination.

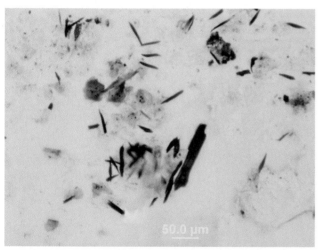

Figure 10-3 Ear swab from a normal dog shows some staining and nonstaining epithelial cells and debris. Note the absence of inflammatory cells and bacteria. (Wright's stain, original magnification 200×.)

oval yeast that has a characteristic peanut or footprint shape when observed budding. These yeast are fairly small, ranging from 2.0 μm × 4.0 μm up to 6.0 μm × 7.0 μm.[1,5,6] Finding >10 *Malassezia* organisms per high power field (40× objective) suggests yeast overgrowth. In this case, *Malassezia* should be considered as a contributing cause to the otitis externa.[12,13] Other fungi, such as *Candida* and *Microsporum*, have rarely been reported in cases of otitis externa.[2,14,15] When unidentified yeasts or hyphae are observed cytologically, culture is indicated for identification.

Mites

Ear mites are a primary cause of otitis externa and are especially common in cats. *Otodectes cynotis* reportedly accounts for 50% of feline and 5% to 10% of canine

cases of otitis externa (Figure 10-7).[1-2,5] In animals hypersensitized to mite antigens, clinical signs of otitis externa may develop with as few as two or three mites in the ear canal.[1,4-6] Typically, a dry, black, granular discharge is seen. Secondary bacterial and/or yeast infections often coexist and can cause the discharge to become moist.[2,3,6] Larval and nymph stages of the spinous ear tick, *Otobius megnini*, found in the southwest United States can cause acute otitis externa most commonly in dogs and infrequently in cats.[2,4] *Demodex canis* in dogs and *Demodex cati* in cats are rare causes of otitis externa, which may or may not be associated with lesions on other areas of the skin. In these rare cases, large numbers of adult Demodex mites were seen in cerumen smears.[2,4,16,17] *Sarcoptes scabiei*, *Notoedres cati*, and *Eutrombicula alfreddugesi* (chiggers) are other parasites that infrequently infest the ear canal and may be observed on cytology.[2,4,6]

Because small numbers of mites may not be visualized on otoscopic examination, careful cytologic evaluation of unstained exudate for eggs, larvae, or adult mites should be undertaken (see Figure 10-7). Both unstained and stained slides of ear canal secretions should be evaluated. Mites readily wash off slides during the staining process and are seldom seen on stained slides. Hence, unstained slides are best for finding mites, and stained slides are best for recognizing increased numbers of bacteria and/or yeast. Finding mites can be challenging, especially in hypersensitive patients with a low mite burden. Failure to find mites on cytologic examination should not definitively exclude the possibility of a mite infestation.

Neoplasia

The ear canal can potentially develop any of the tumors that occur on skin, as well as ceruminous gland tumors.[1,7] In one large study of ear canal tumors in dogs and cats, the most common benign neoplasms were polyps, papillomas, basal cell tumors, and ceruminous gland adenomas. The most common malignant neoplasms were ceruminous gland adenocarcinomas, squamous cell carcinoma, and carcinoma of undetermined origin[8] (Box 10-3). Unfortunately, neoplastic cells are rarely seen on cytologic evaluation of external ear canal secretions. Many tumors are covered by normal epithelium and their neoplastic cells are not available for collection by an ear swab. These tumors may alter the ear canal condition and allow secondary infection to develop.[4] Cytologically, inflammation may be all that is observed from an ear swab. If a mass is observed on otoscopic examination of the ear canal and cytologic examination of an ear swab does not establish the cause of the mass, fine-needle aspiration or biopsy should be performed to help identify the mass.[9] In cats, fine-needle aspirates have been shown to be useful in distinguishing inflammatory polyps from neoplasia. However, benign and malignant neoplasia may be difficult to distinguish on cytology, and histopathologic confirmation is recommended[18] (Figure 10-8). See earlier chapters for further discussion on the evaluation of cutaneous and subcutaneous masses.

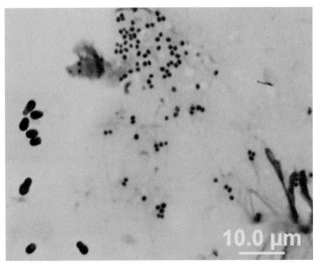

Figure 10-4 Mixed infection characterized by large numbers of bacterial cocci. Some *Malassezia* organisms are also present. (Wright's stain, original magnification 1000×.)

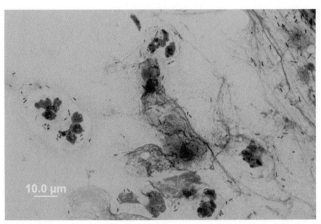

Figure 10-5 Ear swab from a cat with a bacterial infection. Numerous bacterial rods are present phagocytized within degenerate neutrophils and free in the background. (Wright's stain, original magnification 1000×.)

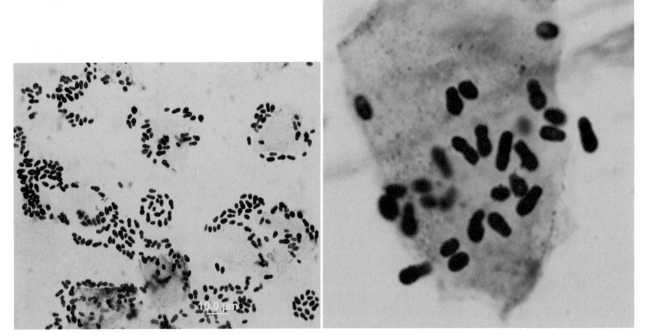

Figure 10-6 *Malassezia* infections are characterized by large numbers of broad-based, budding yeast organisms. Image on the right displays a magnified area. (Wright's stain, original magnification 1000×.)

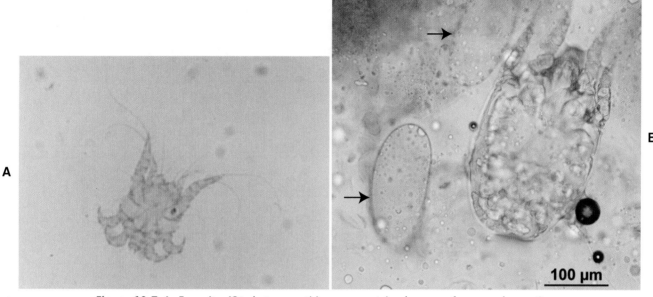

Figure 10-7 A, Ear mite *(Otodectes cynotis)* on an unstained smear of ear canal secretions. (Original magnification 25×.) **B,** Two mite eggs (arrows) and an ear mite *(O. cynotis)* embedded in debris from an unstained smear of ear canal secretions. (Original magnification 200×.)

BOX 10-3

Ear Canal Tumors in Dogs and Cats

Study of 145 cases[8]

Dogs

Benign tumors (n = 33)
  Benign polyps: 8
  Papillomas: 6
  Sebaceous gland adenomas: 5
  Basal cell tumor: 5
  Ceruminous gland adenoma: 4
  Histiocytoma: 2
  Plasmacytoma: 1
  Benign melanoma: 1
  Fibroma: 1

Malignant tumors (n = 48)
  Ceruminous gland adenocarcinoma: 23
  Carcinoma of undetermined origin: 9
  Squamous cell carcinoma: 8
  Round cell tumor: 3
  Sarcoma: 2
  Malignant melanoma: 2
  Hemangiosarcoma: 1

Cats

Benign tumors (n = 8)
  Benign polyp: 4
  Ceruminous gland adenoma: 3
  Papilloma: 1

Malignant tumors (n = 56)
  Ceruminous gland adenocarcinoma: 22
  Squamous cell carcinoma: 20
  Carcinoma of undetermined origin: 13
  Sebaceous gland adenocarcinoma: 1

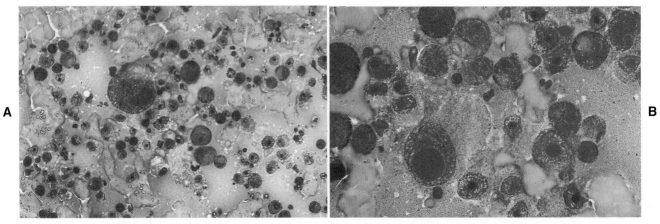

Figure 10-8 Fine-needle biopsy (aspiration technique) of a canine ear mass. **A,** Marked anisocytosis, anisokaryosis, and large, prominent nucleoli are shown. The mass was diagnosed as a carcinoma of undetermined origin by both cytology and histopathology. (Wright's stain, original magnification 100×.) **B,** Higher magnification of the same tumor. (Wright's stain, original magnification 400×.)

Miscellaneous

Ceruminous otitis externa is associated with some seborrheic diseases.[1,2] The characteristic oily, yellow discharge may grossly resemble purulent exudate. However, because these secretions contain very few inflammatory cells and cerumen fails to take stain, very little material may be visible on microscopic examination of the discharge.[6]

References

1. Scott DW, et al: *Muller & Kirk's Small Animal Dermatology,* ed 6, Philadelphia, W.B. Saunders, 2001, pp 1204-1235.
2. Rosser EJ Jr: Causes of otitis externa. *Vet Clin North Am Small Anim Pract* 34:459-468, 2004.
3. Greene CE: *Infectious Diseases of the Dog and Cat.* St. Louis, Saunders Elsevier, 2006, pp 815-818.
4. Logas DB: Diseases of the ear canal. *Vet Clin North Am Small Anim Pract* 24:905-919, 1994.
5. McKeever and Globus. In Bonagura JD: *Kirk's Current Veterinary Therapy XII.* Philadelphia, W.B. Saunders, 1995, pp 647-655.
6. Angus JC: Otic cytology in health and disease. *Vet Clin North Am Small Anim Pract* 34:411-424, 2004.
7. Fan TM, de Lorimier LP: Inflammatory polyps and aural neoplasia. *Vet Clin North Am Small* 34:489-509, 2004.
8. London CA, et al: Evaluation of dogs and cats with tumors of the ear canal: 145 cases: 1978-1992. *J Am Vet Med Assoc* 208:1413-1418, 1996.
9. Rosychuk RA: Management of otitis externa. *Vet Clin North Am Small Anim Pract* 24:921-952, 1994.
10. Toma S, et al: Comparison of 4 fixation and staining methods for the cytologic evaluation of ear canals with clinical evidence of ceruminous otitis externa. *Vet Clin Pathol* 35:194-198, 2006.
11. Graham-Mize CA, Rosser EJ Jr: Comparison of microbial isolates and susceptibility patterns from the external ear canal of dogs with otitis externa. *J Am Anim Hosp Assoc* 40:102-108, 2004.
12. Cafarchia C, et al: Occurrence and population size of *Malassezia* spp. in the external ear canal of dogs and cats both healthy and with otitis. *Mycopathologia* 160:143-149, 2005.
13. Rausch FD, Slinner GW: Incidence and treatment of budding yeasts in canine otitis externa. *Modern Vet Pract* 59:914-915, 1978.
14. Guedeja-Marron J, et al: A case of feline otitis externa due to *Microsporum canis. Med Mycol* 39:229-232, 2001.
15. Godfrey D: *Microsporum canis* associated with otitis externa in a Persian cat. *Vet Rec* 147:50-51, 2000.
16. Knottenbelt MK: Chronic otitis externa due to *Demodex canis* in a Tibetan spaniel. *Vet Rec* 135:409-410, 1994.
17. van Poucke S: Ceruminous otitis externa due to *Demodex cati* in a cat. *Vet Rec* 149:651-652, 2001.
18. de Lorenzi D, et al: Fine-needle biopsy of external ear canal masses in the cat: cytologic results and histologic correlations in 27 cases. *Vet Clin Pathol* 34:100-105, 2005.

The Lymph Nodes

J.B. Messick

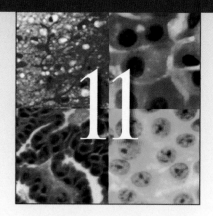

CHAPTER

11

ARCHITECTURE

When interpreting a cytological specimen of the lymph node, it is useful to keep in mind the histological structure and different cell types that are found in this tissue. The node is composed of a capsule, cortex, medulla, and sinuses (subcapsular, cortical, and medullary).[1] The cortex or more peripheral area of the node is divided into follicular and diffuse (parafollicular cortex or paracortex) regions, and the medulla or more central area, into the medullary cords and sinuses (Figure 11-1).

Within the parafollicular cortex are high endothelial venules through which both B- and T-lymphocytes from the blood enter the node. This region is also rich in interdigitating reticulum cells (IDCs), a specialized antigen-presenting cell. The initial immune response requires that the antigen presented by IDCs be recognized by T-lymphocytes and early B-lymphocytes in the parafollicular cortex, whereas the differentiation of B-lymphocytes in response to antigen occurs in the follicular cortex.

Follicles contain predominantly B-lineage lymphocytes. The primary follicles are composed of small, dark-staining lymphocytes. In contrast, secondary follicles have a peripheral rim or mantle zone of small dark lymphoid cells similar to those in primary follicles and a central germinal center. In the germinal center, specialized cells of the mononuclear phagocytic system (MPS), the follicular dendritic cells (FDCs) capture antigen on their surfaces to promote B-lymphocyte differentiation. Thus, small resting B-cells undergo mitosis and divide to become the larger, more irregular small-cleaved, intermediate and large blast cells in the germinal center of a reactive node (follicular hyperplasia). T-cells (mainly CD4+ helper cells) that play a role in stimulating B-cells are also found in the follicles. Surviving B-cells may eventually differentiate into plasma cells, migrating to the medullary cords or leaving the node.

The parafollicular zone of the lymph node gradually transforms into medullary cords that are populated by B-cells and plasma cells. Sinuses containing macrophages surround these cords. A reactive process in the lymph node may also result in hyperplasia of the parafollicular region, of sinus cells (sinus histiocytosis), or of plasma cells (plasma cell hyperplasia). These different types of hyperplasia may occur by themselves or in combination.

Lymph nodes are strategically located at sites throughout the body and are involved in a variety of local and systemic disease processes. Antigen reaches the node via the afferent lymphatics. The lymph percolates through the sinus and sinusoidal walls into the parenchyma (Figure 11-2), where foreign substances (antigens) are taken up and processed by specialized cells of the MPS. The sinuses (subcapsular, cortical and medullary) form a network of branching channels that converge at the hilus of the node to exit by the efferent lymphatics. The primary functions of the lymph nodes include filtering particles and microorganisms, exposing antigens to circulating lymphocytes, and activating B- and T-lymphocytes. The superficial, subcutaneous location of some lymph nodes (mandibular, superficial cervical, inguinal, and popliteal) allows easy detection of enlargement and access for fine-needle aspiration (FNA) cytology. It is appropriate to aspirate any node that is enlarged, and in the case of lymph nodes draining areas affected by neoplasia, even in the absence of enlagement, aspiration may be justified.[2]

GENERAL CONSIDERATIONS

Lymph node aspiration cytology has become a popular procedure in human medicine in recent years, because of its great convenience.[3] Similarly, this high-yield diagnostic technique is frequently used in veterinary medicine.[4-7] There are a few points to consider when obtaining nodal samples for cytological evaluation.

A normal lymph node is small and often difficult to aspirate. It is not uncommon for the cytology of a normal node to contain mostly perinodal adipose tissue and only a few or no lymphocytes. If multiple nodes are enlarged, then sampling from several nodes is recommended. Because the submandibular nodes drain the oral cavity, they often become enlarged, reactive, and/or inflamed. A confusing mixture of malignant, reactive, and inflammatory cells may limit the accuracy of cytologic diagnosis of lymphoma based on an FNA of these nodes. Thus, sampling of submandibular nodes should be avoided in cases where there

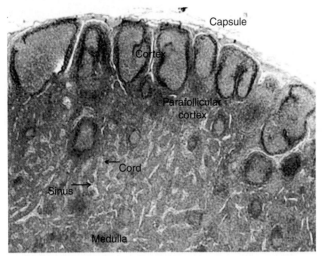

Figure 11-1 The lymph node has two basic parts, the cortex and the medulla. The cortex has both follicular and diffuse or parafollicular regions. The parafollicular region gradually transforms into medullary cords of B-lymphocytes and plasma cells, which are surround by sinuses containing macrophages attached to reticular fibers. Different populations of lymphyocytes in these areas and other cells are found in nodal aspirates. (H&E stain.)

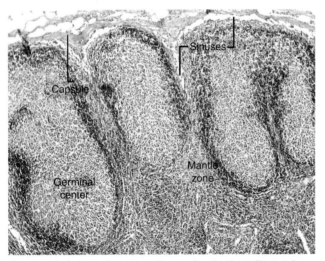

Figure 11-2 Lymph enters the node via the afferent lymphatics, percolating through subcapsular sinuses and sinusoids, where foreign substances (antigens) are taken up and processed. The secondary follicles in this node have a peripheral rim or mantle zone and a pale-staining, central germinal center. The differentiation of B-lymphocytes in response to antigen occurs in the germinal center of the follicular cortex. (H&E stain.)

is generalized lymph node enlargement. The prescapular and popliteal nodes are often a better choice. The mandibular salivary gland is not uncommonly mistaken for a node and aspirated. However the presence of large, foamy epithelial cells either individually or in clusters and mucus in the background allows the tissue to be easily identified.

Consideration also should be given to the size of the lymph node when deciding which node to aspirate — very large nodes may have areas of hemorrhage or necrosis. If

---

BOX 11-1

The Role of Fine-Needle Aspiration Cytology of Lymph Nodes

1. Diagnosis of infectious disease.
2. Diagnosis of hyperplasia or reactive lymphadenopathy and recognition of specific conditions (i.e., lymph node hyperplasia of young cats). If a cause for the change is not apparent and/or resolution does not occur, follow-up and subsequent biopsy is indicated.
3. Diagnosis of metastatic neoplasia and indication of possible primary site.
4. Diagnosis of lymphoma that is optimally followed by a biopsy for confirmation and accurate subtyping.
5. If known malignancy, such as lymphoma or a metastatic mast cell tumor, staging and monitoring for relapse or effects of chemotherapy.
6. Allows sampling of multiple sites as well as obtaining samples from surgically inaccessible sites or from medically unfit patients.
7. Obtaining material for clonality and research studies.

the node must be sampled, the needle should be directed tangentially, avoiding the more central portions.[8] Finally, when obtaining a sample for cytological evaluation, it is important to remember that the lymph node is a heterogenous tissue, and multiple areas within the node should be sampled to be certain that what you have obtained is representative. While keeping the needle in the node, repeatedly advance and withdraw the needle in multiple directions until a small amount of aspirate appears in the hub of the needle. This procedure can be done using a syringe to apply gentle suction or with only the needle. If the former technique is used, release the suction before removing the needle from the node. Overly vigorous aspiration of the lymph node can produce significant hemodilution and cells can rupture, limiting the interpretation of your sample. A large volume of aspirate is not required; the material within the hub of your needle is sufficient for making cytologic preparations. Because the lymphocytes are fragile, care also must be taken to apply only minimal pressure when making slide preparations to prevent excessive rupturing of cells. The slides are air-dried (not heat-fixed) and stained for evaluation.

FINE-NEEDLE ASPIRATION

FNA is a relatively safe and painless procedure, allowing for rapid and inexpensive sampling of peripheral lymph nodes. It does not require hospital admission or anesthesia of the pet. The role of this procedure is summarized in Box 11-1.

CYTOLOGIC FINDINGS

Normal Lymph Node

In the absence of architectural features that can be appreciated in a histologic section of a lymph node, the interpretation of cytology relies on proportions of different

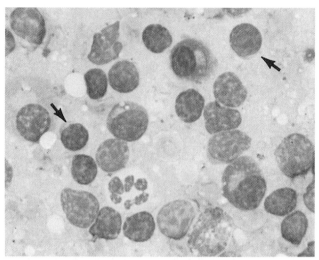

Figure 11-3 Aspirate from a hyperplastic lymph node. Small lymphocytes *(arrows)* and plasma cells characterize the reaction. Note that small lymphocytes are smaller than neutrophils and their nuclei are about the size of a red blood cell. Many free nuclei, identified by pink, homogeneous chromatin and an absence of cytoplasm, are evident. (Wright's stain.)

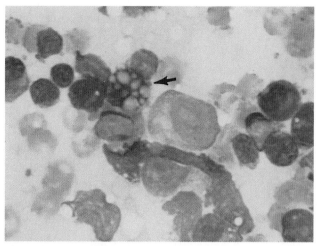

Figure 11-5 Plasma cells, small lymphocytes, and two large lymphocytes (lymphoblasts) characterize this aspirate from a hyperplastic lymph node. The plasma cell with the vacuolated cytoplasm is a Mott cell containing Russell bodies *(arrow).* The pink, amorphous structures are free nuclear material. (Wright's stain.)

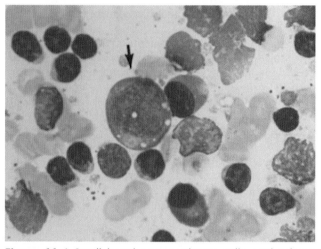

Figure 11-4 Small lymphocytes, plasma cells, and a large transformed lymphocyte *(arrow)* characterize this aspirate from a hyperplastic lymph node. Irregular, pink nuclei from lysed cells are seen. (Wright's stain.)

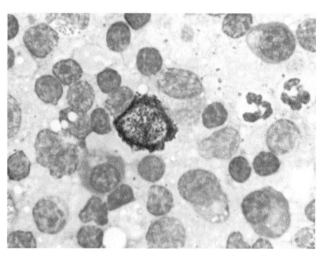

Figure 11-6 Small lymphocytes, plasma cells, neutrophils, and a single mast cell are present in this aspirate from a hyperplastic lymph node. (Wright's stain.)

cell types and an understanding of what proportions are normal versus abnormal for these cell types. Small, well-differentiated lymphocytes compose greater than 75% to 85% of the total nucleated cell population (Figures 11-3 through 11-7).[4-7] They have round nuclei that are about 1.0 to <1.5 times the size of a mature red blood cell (RBC) with an overall cell size that is smaller than that of a neutrophil. Their chromatin is densely clumped and nucleoli are not visible. The nuclear-to-cytoplasmic ratio is high with a narrow rim of basophilic cytoplasm. In addition to small lymphocytes, a normal node should have low numbers (<10% to 15%) of lymphocytes that are intermediate to large (often called *lymphoblasts*) in size; their nuclei are 1.5 to 3 times the size of an RBC with an overall size

ranging from about that of a neutrophil or larger to up to 4 times the size of an RBC (see Figure 11-5). Their chromatin is less clumped and nucleoli may be visible and even multiple and/or prominent. The cytoplasm is pale blue and more abundant than in small lymphocytes.

Plasma cells have small, round, eccentric nuclei with condensed chromatin (see Figures 11-3 through 11-6). Their abundant cytoplasm is deep blue and has a prominent, clear Golgi zone. Immature plasma cells (transformed B-lymphocytes) are larger and have less aggregated chromatin and a higher nuclear-to-cytoplasmic ratio (see Figure 11-4). Their very blue cytoplasm may contain discrete vacuoles. Plasma cells in various stages of development are seen in small numbers in normal lymph

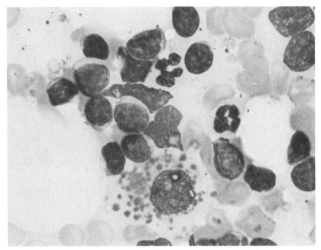

Figure 11-7 Seen among small and medium-sized lymphocytes is a large macrophage containing phagocytized debris. (Wright's stain.)

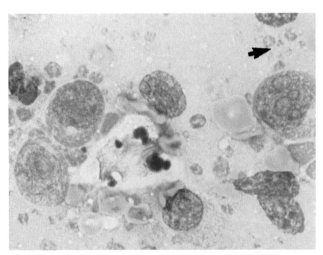

Figure 11-8 In this aspirate from a lymphomatous lymph node are large immature lymphocytes with prominent nucleoli, dispersed chromatin, and abundant blue cytoplasm. The large cell in the center with bluish cytoplasmic globules is a tingible-body macrophage. The small blue structures *(arrow)* are lymphoglandular bodies. (Wright's stain.)

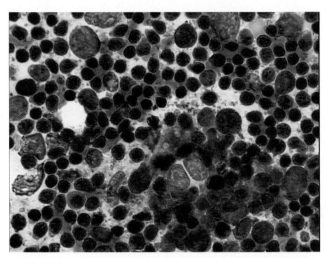

Figure 11-9 Several reticuloendothelial cells are seen in this lymph node aspiration cytology. Their nuclei are swollen, and they are devoid of cytoplasm. Small lymphocytes are the predominant cell type in this mildly hyperplastic node.

making this assessment. Reticular cells and endothelial cells are common in lymph nodes, but these tissue-bound cells are rarely aspirated intact. They usually appear as large swollen nuclei, often devoid of cytoplasm (Figure 11-9).

Because of the pressures of the aspiration technique, lymphocytes, which are very fragile, may rupture and release their nuclei. Free nuclei are swollen and uniformly pink in contrast to the blue blocky or granular pattern of intact lymphocyte nuclei (see Figures 11-3 through 11-5). Blue nucleoli are often exposed in the nuclear chromatin of ruptured cells. These free nuclei carry no diagnostic significance and should not be confused with large immature lymphocytes. Lymphoglandular bodies are cytoplasmic fragments and are highly characteristic of lymphoid tissue (see Figures 11-8 and 11-10). They are round, homogeneous, basophilic structures similar in size to platelets.

LYMPHADENOPATHY

One of the most common indications for performing aspiration cytology is enlargement of one or more lymph nodes. Three general processes cause lymph node enlargement: inflammation (lymphadenitis—suppurative, pyogranulomatous, granulomatous, and eosinophilic), immune stimulation (hyperplasia or reactive lymphadenopathy), and neoplasia (lymphoma or metastatic). The cytological evaluation of a sample obtained by FNA or touch imprint from the excised node usually allows differentiation of these processes. However, these processes are not mutually exclusive and may occur simultaneously.

Lymphadenitis

Lymphadenitis or inflammation of the node may be a primary (node itself is inflamed or necrotic) or secondary (node is draining an area of inflammation or

nodes, but typically represent <3% of the total nucleated cell population.

Macrophages, characterized by abundant cytoplasm often containing vacuoles and granular debris, also are found in small numbers (see Figure 11-7). Macrophages from areas of intense lymphopoiesis and cellular turnover may contain prominent basophilic nuclear debris (tingible bodies) (Figure 11-8). Occasionally, small numbers of neutrophils, eosinophils, and mast cells are observed in a normal node (see Figure 11-6). Each of these cell types should represent less than 1% of the cell populations in a normal node. It is important to consider the amount of blood contamination when

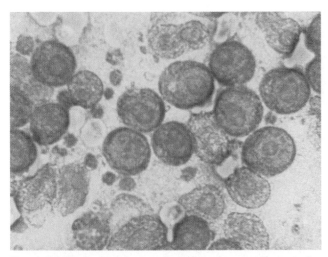

Figure 11-10 Immature, neoplastic lymphocytes characterize this smear from a dog with malignant lymphoma. Note that the cells are much larger than red blood cells. The pink structures lacking cytoplasm and containing prominent nucleoli are nuclei from lysed cells. Small blue lymphoglandular bodies are numerous. (Wright's stain.)

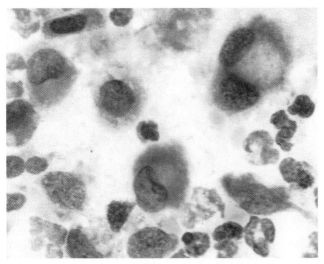

Figure 11-11 This aspirate from an animal with blastomycosis is characterized by pyogranulomatous inflammation. Neutrophils, epithelioid macrophages, and a single multinucleated giant cell are present. (Wright's stain)

necrosis) finding. This process is characterized cytologically by accumulation of inflammatory cells. Neutrophils, eosinophils, and macrophages occur singly or in combination. Inflammation is probably present when the population is >5% neutrophils or >3% eosinophils, provided there is no significant blood contamination. Macrophage numbers can increase in inflammation but also in hyperplasia and sometimes in neoplasia. Macrophages also may appear as epithelioid cells and multinucleated giant cells in granulomatous inflammation. Epithelioid macrophages are characterized by blue cytoplasm with minimal vacuolation and contain very little phagocytic debris (Figure 11-11). Organisms may, however, be present within the cytoplasm. These cells may occur in aggregates.

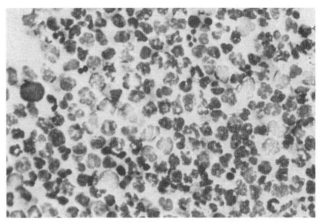

Figure 11-12 Purulent inflammation is characterized by the predominance of neutrophils. (Wright's stain.)

Inflammatory cells may represent only a small portion of the total cell population that otherwise suggests lymphoid hyperplasia, or they may completely replace the normal cell population.

Most bacterial infections elicit a neutrophilic or purulent response (Figure 11-12) but *Mycobacterium* spp. (Figure 11-13) can cause a granulomatous response. An eosinophilic exudate of varying degrees is common in lymph nodes draining allergic inflammations of the skin, respiratory tract, and digestive tract. Systemic fungal infections such as histoplasmosis (Figure 11-14), blastomycosis (Figure 11-15), coccidioidomycosis (Figure 11-16), and cryptococcosis (Figure 11-17); protozoal infections such as cytauxzoonosis (Figure 11-18), toxoplasmosis (Figure 11-19), and leishmaniasis (Figure 11-20); and algal infections such as prototothecosis (Figure 11-21) characteristically evoke a granulomatous or pyogranulomatous response (Figure 11-22) in lymph nodes. In salmon disease, there is lymphoid depletion and sinus macrophage hyperplasia or sinus histiocytosis (Figure 11-23).

Reactive or Hyperplastic Node

No clear line of separation exists between a normal and a hyperplastic lymph node based on cytology alone. Differentiation, however, is probably a moot point, because enlarged lymph nodes are reactive to some degree. Typically, a heterogeneous cell population is usually obtained as the needle is directed through follicular centers, paracortical area, medullary cords, and medullary sinuses. If the reactive pattern is principally follicular hyperplasia, intermediate and large lymphocytes from expanding germinal centers are found in increased numbers. These cells may constitute up to 15% to 25% or more of the total cell population (Figure 11-24).[4-7] However, small lymphocytes are still the predominant cell type in hyperplastic as well as normal lymph nodes. Plasma cell numbers may vary from none to >5% to 10% of the population in some areas of the smear. They occasionally are filled with vacuoles (Russell bodies) (see Figure 11-5). Immature plasma cells or transformed lymphocytes, which are medium to

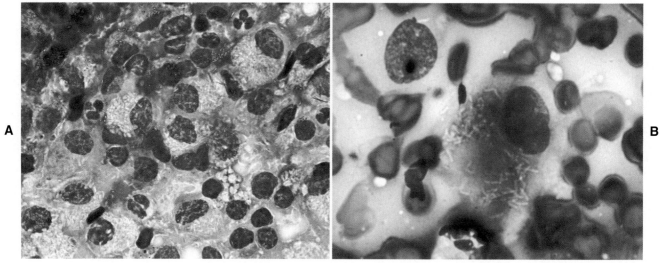

Figure 11-13 A, Lymph node aspirates showing a high number of macrophages containing nonstaining bacterial rods indicative of a *Mycobacterium* infection. **B,** Higher magnification of a single macrophage containing nonstaining bacterial rods identified as clear streaks through the cell. (Wright's stain.) *(Courtesy Dr. R.L. Cowell, IDEXX Laboratories.)*

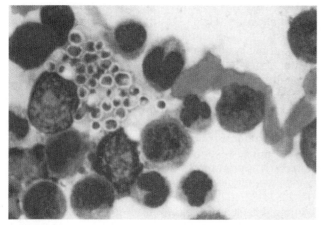

Figure 11-14 Macrophage containing numerous *Histoplasma* organisms. *Histoplasma* organisms are small, round to oval, yeast-like organisms that have a nucleus that stains dark purple and a thin clear halo. (Wright's stain.) *(Courtesy Oklahoma State University.)*

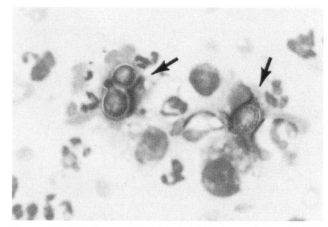

Figure 11-15 *Blastomyces dermatitidis (arrows)* is a bluish, spherical, thick-walled, yeast-like organism. Occasionally a single, broad-based bud may be present. (Wright's stain.)

large in size, also may be observed. Macrophages may on occasion represent >2% of the population, particularly with hyperplasia of sinus macrophages. An aspirate from a node with parafollicular hyperplasia is also heterogenous; however, immunoblasts are prominent in association with plasma cell hyperplasia, and tingible-body macrophages are lacking. The main cytological characteristics of the immunoblasts (parafollicular zone cells) are their medium size, fine chromatin, and large centrally located nucleolus. In reactive lymph nodes of dogs associated with mammary tumor lymphadenopathies, systemic lupus erythematosus, and leishmaniasis, these cells may be found in high numbers.[9] Any enlarged lymph node with the aforementioned cytologic findings should be considered hyperplastic, since a normal node should not be enlarged.

Hyperplasia occurs when antigens in high concentration reach the draining lymph node and stimulate the immune system. In some instances, these antigens also cause inflammation and attract inflammatory cells to the node (lymphadenitis). In many cases, reactions causing hyperplasia are localized, but they may be systemic and affect all nodes. Generalized lymphadenopathy with a hyperplastic cytologic picture may occur in feline leukemia virus infection (FeLV), feline immunodeficiency virus infection (FIV), bartonellosis, Rocky Mountain spotted fever, and ehrlichiosis. It can occasionally be especially difficult to distinguish reactive nodal hyperplasia from lymphoma in cats. In these cases, additional testing is needed, such as histopathology, immunophenotyping, and polymerase chain reaction (PCR) for the assessment of clonality.[10-15]

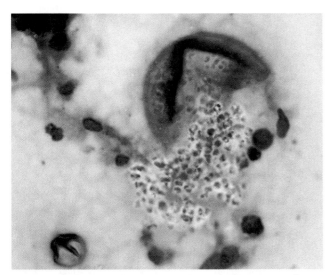

Figure 11-16 *Coccidioides immitis* organisms are large, double-contoured, clear to blue-staining, spherical bodies that range in size from 10 microns to greater than 100 microns. Occasionally endospores varying from 2 to 5 microns in diameter may be seen within some of the larger spherules. (Wright's stain.) *(Courtesy Dr. R.L. Cowell, IDEXX Laboratories.)*

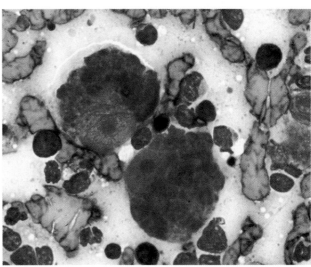

Figure 11-18 Lymph node aspirate from a cat showing two huge mononuclear cells with abundant cytoplasm, eccentric nuclei, and prominent nucleoli. These cells contain developing cytauxzoon merozoites, which appear as either small dark-staining bodies or larger irregularly defined clusters. (Wright's stain.) *(Courtesy Dr. R.L. Cowell, IDEXX Laboratories.)*

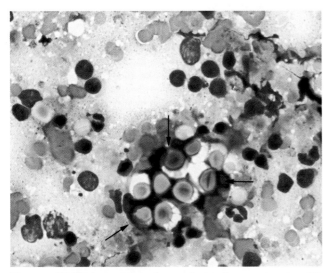

Figure 11-17 Lymph node aspirate from a cat with cryptococcosis. Scattered red blood cells, small lymphocytes, and a group of *Cryptococcus* organisms *(arrows)* are shown. *Cryptococcus* organisms stain eosinophilic to clear and may be the smooth form (large clear capsule) or rough form (small clear capsule) as shown here. (Wright's stain.) *(Courtesy Dr. R.L. Cowell, IDEXX Laboratories.)*

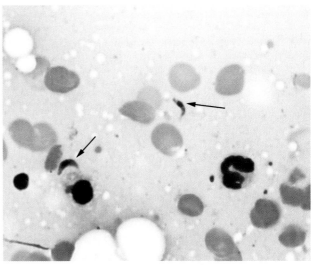

Figure 11-19 *Toxoplasma gondii* tachyzoites *(arrows)* appear as small, crescent-shaped bodies with a light blue cytoplasm and a dark-staining pericentral nucleus. (Wright's stain.) *(Courtesy Dr. R.L. Cowell, IDEXX Laboratories.)*

Malignant Lymphoma

FNA is often sufficient for establishing a diagnosis of lymphoma in dogs and cats. This is due to the predominance of monomorphic lymphoid cells that lack the polymorphism of a reactive population. Still the opportunity must not be missed at the outset of the disease process to also obtain nodal tissue for histologic, immunocytochemistry, and molecular evaluation. This will allow for the diagnosis to be confirmed and accurate subtyping performed as well as providing archival materials, which may be of use to further advances in diagnosis and/or treatment.

Malignant lymphoma is characterized by lymphocytes that eventually replace the entire normal cell population (Figures 11-25 and 11-26). However, not all lymphomas are the same; they are a diverse group of lymphoid neoplasms. Each of these neoplasms represents a clonal expansion of an anatomic or developmental

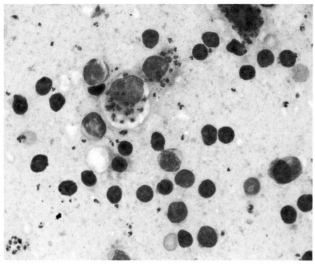

Figure 11-20 Lymph node aspirate from a dog showing many lymphocytes and two macrophages containing numerous *Leishmania donovani* organisms. *L. donovani* organisms are small, round to oval organisms with a clear to very light blue cytoplasm, an oval nucleus, and a small, dark, ventral kinetoplast. (Wright's stain.) *(Courtesy Dr. R.L. Cowell, IDEXX Laboratories.)*

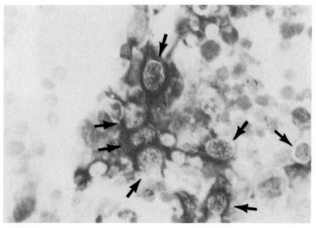

Figure 11-21 *Prototheca* organisms *(arrows)* are round to oval and have a granular basophilic cytoplasm and a clear cell wall. (Wright's stain.)

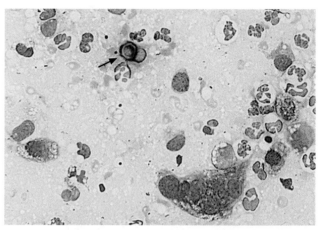

Figure 11-22 Pyogranulomatous inflammation from a dog with blastomycosis. A *Blastomyces dermatitidis* organism *(arrow)* is in the center of the field. Neutrophils, macrophages, and an inflammatory giant cell are present. (Wright's stain.)

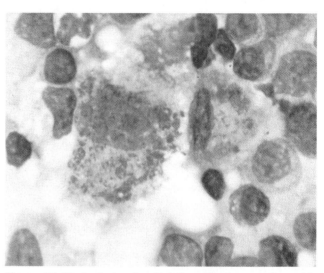

Figure 11-23 Aspirate of a lymph node from a dog with salmon disease. Large macrophages contain the causative agent, *Neorickettsia helminthoeca*. (Wright's stain.)

compartment of lymphoid cells in the node, which have distinct morphologic and immunophenotypic characteristics.[16-18] When immature cells compose >50% of the cell population, a diagnosis of malignant lymphoma can be reliably made, but smaller numbers may be present in early stages, making a diagnosis by cytologic examination alone more difficult. Usually these neoplastic lymphocytes are larger than neutrophils and have finely granular dispersed chromatin, nucleoli, a lower nuclear-to-cytoplasmic ratio, and basophilic cytoplasm. The lymphocytes are considered medium and large if their nuclei are 1.5 to 2 times or >2 to 3 times the size of RBCs, respectively. Frequently, the percentage of the medium to large lymphocytes exceeds 80%, making the diagnosis more certain. Mitoses may be more numerous than in hyperplasia and tingible-body macrophages may indicate intense lymphopoiesis and cell turnover (Figure 11-27), but neither alone is a reliable indicator of neoplasia. Lymphoglandular bodies are more numerous than in hyperplasia.

Occasionally, lymphoma is manifested as the small, well-differentiated lymphocyte type (Figure 11-28). Its diagnosis is based on recognizing a monotonous or restricted population of small, normal-appearing lymphoid cells in the FNA. Mitoses are extremely rare. This form is very difficult to distinguish from hyperplasia because small lymphocytes predominate in each. In some cases, small cell lymphoma is not diagnosed until there is significant blood involvement.

Alimentary lymphoma occasionally consists of neoplastic lymphocytes that contain magenta intracytoplasmic

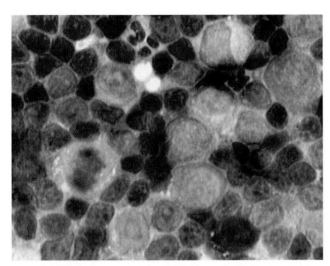

Figure 11-24 Intermediate and large lymphocytes from expanded germinal centers are found in increased numbers in this hyperplastic node (follicular hyperplasia). However, small lymphocytes are still the predominant cell type.

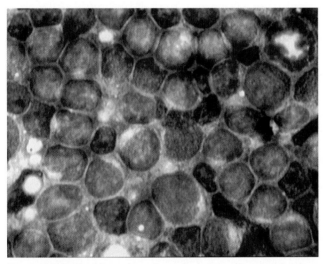

Figure 11-25 In this aspirate from an enlarged node of a dog, a monomorphic population of immature lymphocytes that are intermediate in size is seen. Some of the nuclei in these cells are indented (clefted) and uniformly have a fine diffuse chromatin pattern; however, nucleoli are inapparent. The mitotic rate is high. This is a high-grade, aggressive T-cell lymphoblastic lymphoma with an associated paraneoplastic hypercalcemia. The cells of B- and T-cell lymphoblastic lymphoma are not distinguishable by cytology alone, but are different morphologically from other high-grade lymphomas. Immunophenotyping was done to establish the T-cell type. (Wright's stain.)

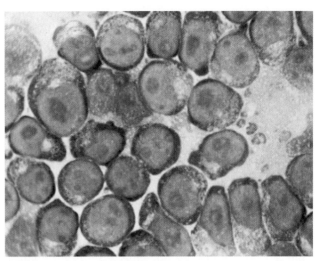

Figure 11-26 In this nodal aspirate from a cat, a monomorphic population of immature lymphocytes that are large in size is shown. These cells have a high nuclear-to-cytoplasmic ratio and often a single prominent nucleolus or several in a paracentral location. The cytoplasm is deeply basophilic. The histopathology showed a mitotic rate that was high with a diffuse nodal involvement. Although these high-grade lymphomas are often B-cell phenotype, the T-cell counterpart cannot be distinguished by morphology alone. (Wright's stain.)

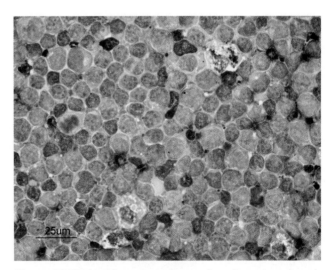

Figure 11-27 In this aspirate from a lymphomatous lymph node, there were many tingible-body macrophages, an indication of intense lymphopoiesis and cell turnover. (Wright's stain.)

granules and is referred to as large granular lymphoma. However, neither the granules nor lymphocytes are consistently large (Figure 11-29).

Several classification schemes have been adapted in an attempt to characterize canine and feline lymphomas.[16-21] The ultimate goals for classification are to correlate the variety of cell subtypes and architectural features of lymphoma to clinical behavior in terms of responsiveness to therapy and outlook for the patient. For the dog, cytomorphologic classification into low (small cell and low mitotic rate) or high (large cells and high mitotic rate) grades of lymphoma has been shown to have prognostic importance.[22-23] Although low-grade lymphomas permit long survivals, they are virtually incurable and may not

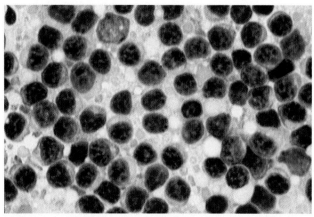

Figure 11-28 A monotonous population of small, well-differentiated lymphocytes is seen in this nodal aspirate from a dog. Mitoses are not observed. Their chromatin pattern is densely clumped, nucleoli are not visible, and mitotic figures are not observed. The presence of a generalized lymphadenopathy and monomorphic lymphoid cells that lack the polymorphism of a normal node or of a reactive population is a useful characteristic that supports this diagnosis. However, the effacement of normal nodal architecture by histopathology is needed to confirm this suspicion. The cells of B- and T-cell small cell lymphoma/chronic lymphocytic leukemia cannot be distinguished by morphology alone. The cells of this low-grade lymphoma are a T-cell type. (Wright's stain.)

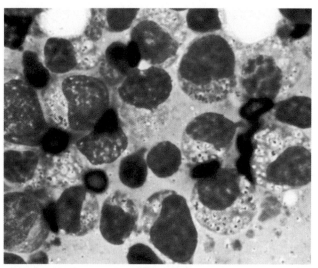

Figure 11-29 An aspirate from an alimentary lymph node in a cat with large granular lymphoma. Most of the lymphocytes are large and contain magenta intracytoplasmic granules. (Wright's stain.) *(Courtesy Dr. R.L. Cowell, IDEXX Laboratories.)*

be treated initially. On the other hand, the high-grade lymphomas initially respond well to chemotherapy, and disease remission is achieved; yet if left untreated they are rapidly progressive and deadly. There is a predominance of high-grade lymphomas in dogs and cats. Within the

high-grade lymphomas, lymphoblastic and Burkitt-type lymphomas in dogs have poorer prognoses.[22]

Immunohistochemistry of histologic preparations have been used to aid in classifying lymphomas. Approximately 70% to 80% of canine lymphomas are of B-cell origin. T-cell lymphomas in the dog that are high grade have a worse prognosis than B-cell lymphomas of the same grade.[22] Cytospin preparations from FNAs also have been used in immunophenotypic analysis of canine malignant lymphomas.[23] Assessment of the immunophenotype does not appear to be of prognostic significance in cats.[24]

If a diagnosis is equivocal, the entire lymph node should be removed with the capsule intact and fixed in 10% buffered formalin. A complete cross section is then examined to determine if a homogenous population of neoplastic cells has obliterated the normal nodal architecture. A confusing mixture of malignant and reactive elements may limit the accuracy of both the histologic and cytologic diagnoses of lymphoma. This may be due to partial nodal involvement and is intrinsic to some lymphomas such as Hodgkin's disease and T-cell rich B-cell lymphomas.[15,17] Ancillary techniques, including immunophenotypic assessment of smears and histologic sections,[14,15] quantitative immunophenotyping using flow cytometry,[18] and PCR to determine clonality and cell lineage, also can be used to confirm a diagnosis. To exclude the possibility of a primary leukemia that has infiltrated the node, a complete blood count should always be assessed concurrently as part of the routine workup.

Metastatic Neoplasia

The presence of cells not normally found in lymph nodes or an increase in numbers of certain cell types normally present (i.e., mast cells) may suggest metastatic neoplasia (see Figures 11-30, 11-31, 11-33, 11-34, and 11-36). Carcinomas frequently metastasize to lymph nodes. Metastatic epithelial cells (Figures 11-30 and 11-31) can occur singly or in groups. They are very large and bear no resemblance to cellular constituents of normal or hyperplastic nodes. Epithelial cells of any type in a lymph node aspirate indicate neoplasia, but these cells must be differentiated from epithelioid cells of granulomatous inflammation, described previously. Salivary epithelial cells (Figure 11-32) from the submandibular salivary gland may be accidentally aspirated. These cells are uniform in size and have round to oval nuclei and abundant blue foamy cytoplasm and should not be confused with carcinoma cells.

Malignant melanomas metastasize to lymph nodes. The melanocyte usually can be identified by its granular brown-black cytoplasmic pigment (Figure 11-33). Do not confuse pigment in melanocytes with that in melanophages that have phagocytized melanin originating from pigmented structures or lesions in the area drained by the node. Melanophages also phagocytize pigment released by melanocytes. Differentiation may be difficult, but melanocytes usually have more attenuated and less vacuolated cytoplasm. Hemosiderin, carbon, bile, and other pigments in macrophages must not be confused with melanin.

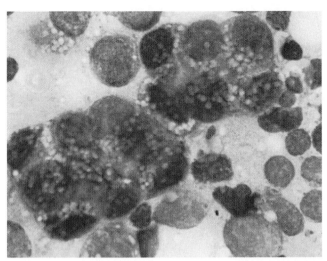

Figure 11-30 An epithelial cell cluster from a transitional cell carcinoma that metastized to a lymph node. (Wright's stain.)

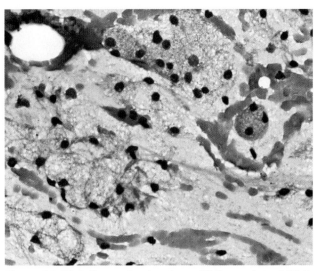

Figure 11-32 Salivary gland aspirate. High number of RBCs and foamy secretory cells from a normal salivary gland in a thick basophilic mucoprotein background. (Wright's stain.) *(Courtesy Dr. R.L. Cowell, IDEXX Laboratories.)*

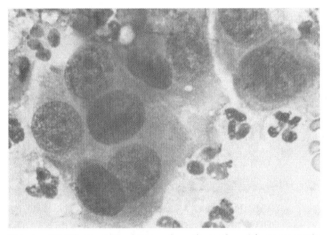

Figure 11-31 Aspirate from a lymph node with metastatic carcinoma. Several carcinoma cells and neutrophils are present. (Wright's stain.) *(Courtesy Dr. Duncan, University of Georgia.)*

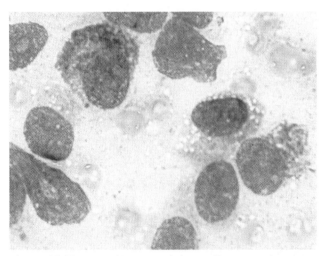

Figure 11-33 An aspirate containing malignant melanocytes that have metastasized to the lymph node. Greenish-black cytoplasmic granules characterize these cells. (Wright's stain.)

Although sarcomas do not metastasize to lymph nodes as frequently as carcinomas, spindle cells in significant numbers should suggest a sarcoma of some type. Malignant mast cell tumors can metastasize to lymph nodes (Figure 11-34). The tumor cells may be well differentiated and distinguished from normal mast cells only by the large number of cells present. More than 3% mast cells raise the suspicion of neoplasia. However, the presence of foci or nests of mast cells is more supportive of metastatic disease than mildly increased numbers of single cells. Undifferentiated mast cell tumors have larger cells with fewer, less prominent granules. The presence of matching internal tandem duplication of the c-kit gene may be a more sensitive method for confirming the presence of metastasis in the node.[25-26] Transmissible venereal tumors (Figure 11-35) may metastasize to lymph nodes.

In cases of neoplasia, one is usually specifically looking for metastatic neoplastic cells because the justification for lymph node aspiration was a malignant tumor identified in the area drained by the particular node. Tumor cells are usually obtained if metastasis has progressed to cause clinically evident enlarged nodes; however, small foci in normal-sized nodes may be missed on aspiration. Negative findings in palpably enlarged nodes should always be subordinate to clinical findings.[28] The sensitivity of detection of low numbers of metastatic cells may be increased by the use of immunocytochemical assessment of nodal preparations or by the use of molecular techniques to detect the presence of tumor antigen messenger RNA.[27,28]

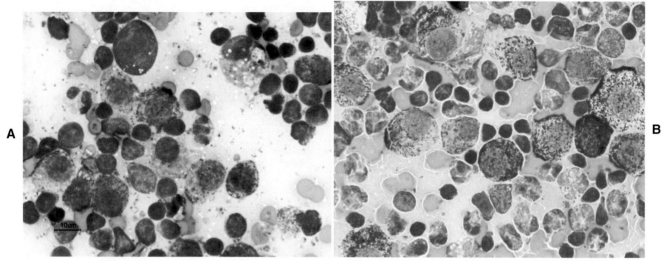

Figure 11-34 A, Among these small lymphocytes are a few eosinophils, a large reactive lymphoblast, and many mast cells. The presence of poorly differentiated mast cells, having fewer and less prominent granules, is supportive of metastatic disease. (Wright's stain.) **B,** Lymph node aspirate. Metastatic mast cell tumor with a high number of mast cells and many eosinophils along with the lymphoid cells. (Wright's stain.) *(Courtesy Dr. R.L. Cowell, IDEXX Laboratories.)*

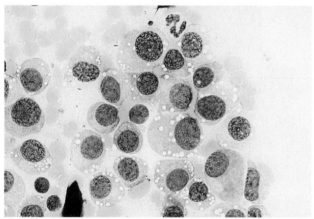

Figure 11-35 Aspirate from a transmissible venereal tumor (TVT). Numerous TVT cells with coarse chromatin and smoky gray vacuolated cytoplasm are shown. (Wright's stain.)

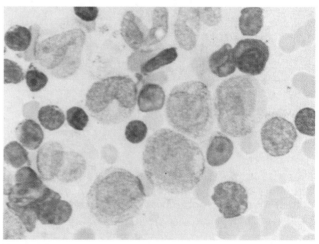

Figure 11-36 Among small lymphocytes and a plasma cell are very immature neutrophils. This lymph node aspirate is from an animal with granulocytic leukemia. (Wright's stain.)

Various myeloproliferative disorders may result in a leukemic hemogram and neoplastic cells in the sinuses of lymph nodes. Cytologic examination of a lymph node FNA reveals the cell population of a normal or hyperplastic node and a population of leukemic cells (Figure 11-36). In acute leukemias, blast cells compose the neoplastic cell population and may be difficult to differentiate from lymphoblasts. In chronic leukemias, various maturation stages are present. Extramedullary hematopoiesis can occur in lymph nodes and contribute to cytologic findings of various stages of erythroid and myeloid cells and megakaryocytes. It is a rare occurrence in chronic anemias.

In conclusion, FNA cytology of the lymph node is a valuable diagnostic tool. With some experience, one can usually determine the type of disease present and may even make a disease or etiologic diagnosis. This inexpensive, relatively painless and rapid technique may not only help in establishing a primary diagnosis, but is also a useful method for following up patients with known malignancies, and even guiding therapy. Figure 11-37 presents an algorithm for evaluation of lymph node aspirates or impression smears.

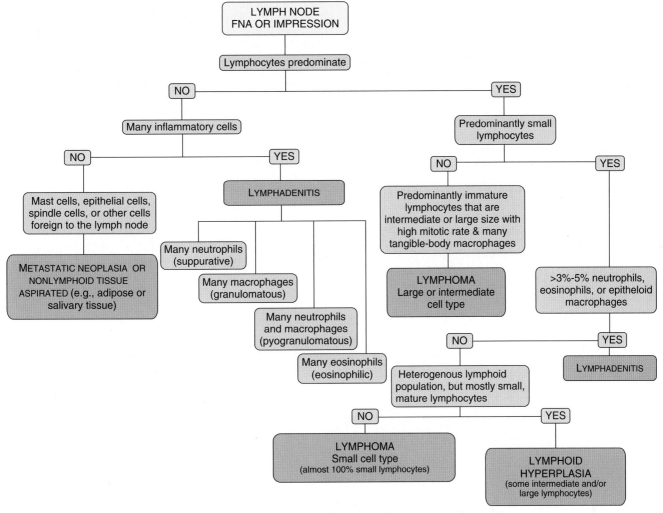

Figure 11-37 An algorithm for evaluation of lymph node aspirates or impression smears.

References

1. H.-Dieter: *Dellmann's Textbook of Veterinary Histology*, ed 6. Eurell J, Frappier BL: Ames, Iowa, Blackwell Publishing, 2006, pp 143-147.
2. Soderstrom: *Fine-Needle Aspiration Biopsy*. New York, Grune & Stratton, 1966.
3. Frable: Fine-needle aspiration biopsy: A review. *Human Pathol* 14:9-28, 1983.
4. Perman et al: *Cytology of the Dog and Cat*. Denver, American Animal Hospital Association, 1979.
5. Rebar: *Handbook of Veterinary Cytology*. St. Louis, Ralston Purina, 1980.
6. Thrall DE: Cytology of lymphoid tissue. *Comp Cont Educ Pract Vet* 9:104-111, 1987.
7. Raskin RE, Meyer D: *Atlas of Canine and Feline Cytology*. Philadelphia, Saunders, 2001.
8. Vernau W: Lymph node cytology of dogs and cats. In *50th Congresso Nazionale Multisala SCIVA, 2005*, Rimini, Italy.
9. Fournel C, et al: An original perifollicular zone cell in the canine reactive lymph node: A morphological, phenotypical and aetiological study. *J Comp Pathol*. 113(3):217-231, 1995.

10. Werner JA, et al: Characterization of feline immunoglobulin heavy chain variable region genes for the molecular diagnosis of B-cell neoplasia. *Vet Pathol* 42(5):596-607, 2005.
11. Moore PF, et al: Characterization of feline T cell receptor gamma (TCRG) variable region genes for the molecular diagnosis of feline intestinal T cell lymphoma. *Vet Immunol Immunopathol* 106(3-4):167-178, 2005.
12. Burnett RC, et al: Diagnosis of canine lymphoid neoplasia using clonal rearrangements of antigen receptor genes. *Vet Pathol* 40(1):32-341, 2003.
13. Lana SE, et al: Utility of polymerase chain reaction for analysis of antigen receptor rearrangement in staging and predicting prognosis in dogs with lymphoma. *J Vet Intern Med* 20(2):329-334, 2006.
14. Gabor LJ, et al: Immunophenotypic and histological characterisation of 109 cases of feline lymphosarcoma. *Aust Vet J* 77(7):436-441, 1999.
15. Fournel-Fleury C, et al: Cytohistological and immunological classification of canine malignant lymphomas: Comparison with human non-Hodgkin's lymphomas. *J Comp Pathol* 117(1):35-59, 1997.

16. Valli VEO, et al: Anatomic and histological classification of feline lymphoma using the National Cancer Institute Working Formulation. 9th *Annul Conf Vet Cancer Soc* 1989.

17. Valli VERM, et al: Tumors of lymphoid system. In Schulman YF (ed): *Histological Classification of Hematopoietic Tumors of Domestic Animals,* 2nd series, vol. 8, Washington, DC, Armed Forces Institute of Pathology, 2002.

18. Wilkerson MJ, et al: Lineage differentiation of canine lymphoma/leukemias and aberrant expression of CD molecules. *Vet Immunol Immunopathol* 106(3-4):179-96, 2005.

19. Carter RF, et al: The cytology, histology, and prevalence of cell types in canine lymphoma classified according to the National Cancer Institute Working Formulation. *Can J Vet Res* 50:154-164, 1986.

20. Greenlee PG, et al: Lymphomas in dogs: A morphologic, immunologic, and clinical study. *Cancer* 66(3):480-490, 1990.

21. Ponce F, et al: Prognostic significance of morphological subtypes in canine malignant lymphomas during chemotherapy. *Vet J* 167(2):158-166, 2004.

22. Fournel-Fleury C, et al: Canine T-cell lymphomas: A morphological, immunological, and clinical study of 46 new cases. *Vet Pathol* 39(1):92-109, 2002.

23. Caniatti M, et al: Canine lymphoma: immunocytochemical analysis of fine-needle aspiration biopsy. *Vet Pathol* 33: 204-212, 1996.

24. Patterson-Kane JC, et al: The possible prognostic significance of immunophenotype in feline alimentary lymphoma: A pilot study. *J Comp Pathol* 130(2-3):220-222, 2004.

25. Turin L, et al: Expression of c-kit proto-oncogene in canine mastocytoma: A kinetic study using real-time polymerase chain reaction. *J Vet Diagn Invest* 18(4):343-349, 2006.

26. Zavodovskaya R, et al: Use of kit internal tandem duplications to establish mast cell tumor clonality in 2 dogs. *J Vet Intern Med* 18(6):915-917, 2004.

27. Matos AJ, et al: Detection of lymph node micrometastases in malignant mammary tumours in dogs by cytokeratin immunostaining. *Vet Rec* 158(18):626-630, 2006.

28. Catchpole B, et al: Development of a multiple-marker polymerase chain reaction assay for detection of metastatic melanoma in lymph node aspirates of dogs. *Am J Vet Res* 64(5):544-549, 2003.

Synovial Fluid Analysis

P.J. Fernandes

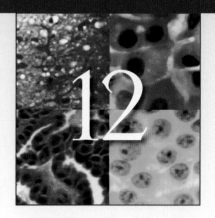

CHAPTER 12

Synovium is essentially a living ultrafiltration membrane with fenestrated capillaries just below an intimal surface containing no epithelial cells, no basement membrane, no cell junctions, and wide intercellular gaps. Fenestrated synovial capillaries, up to 50 times more permeable to water than continuous capillaries, allow water and small solutes into the subintima, but exclude varied proportions of albumin and most larger proteins, such as fibrinogen and clotting factors.

As fluid enters and leaves the joint cavity, its diffusion and composition is regulated by connective tissue of the subintima and cells of the intima or synovial lining. The intima has two major cell populations: macrophages (type A cell) and secretory fibroblast-related synoviocytes (type B cell). Type A are derived from blood-borne mononuclear cells and considered resident tissue macrophages, much like hepatic Kupffer cells. The type B cells secrete components for tissue interstitium and synovial fluid that include collagens, fibronectin, hyaluronan, and lubricin.

ARTHROCENTESIS

In the verification, localization, diagnosis, and management of arthritis, synovial fluid examination is a key component of an initial medical database that includes clinical history, physical examination, radiographs, complete blood count, biochemical profile, and urinalysis. See Boxes 12-1 and 12-2 for indications and contraindications for arthrocentesis.

RESTRAINT

As temperament under physical immobilization and tolerance for discomfort of each individual is different, the clinician must judge which method of restraint is appropriate to allow for controlled manipulation and centesis of the joint. Complications of inadequate restraint can include damage to blood vessels, nerves, synovial membrane, and articular cartilage surfaces, along with blood contamination and retrieving a diagnostically insufficient volume of synovial fluid.

ASEPSIS

Routine aseptic technique should be followed. Normal joint spaces are sterile.

EQUIPMENT

Sterile disposable 3-ml syringes and 1-inch, 22-gauge or 25-gauge (small dogs and cats), hypodermic needle are recommended. In large breed dogs sampling of the elbow or shoulder joints may require a 1½-inch needle and the hip joint may necessitate a 3-inch spinal needle. Microscope glass slides with frosted ends, red-top tubes, and ethylene-tetra-acetic acid (EDTA) blood tubes should be readied and labeled with the patient's name and the joint sampled. See Box 12-3 for a complete list of materials.

APPROACHES

In most cases arthrocentesis is performed with the patient in lateral recumbency and the joint to be sampled uppermost. Palpation of the joint during manual flexion and extension helps identify the space to be entered. In all cases the needle should be advanced gently toward and through the joint capsule to avoid damaging the articular cartilage. Once the needle is inside the joint space, the volume of fluid obtained depends on the particular joint and the disorder. Ordinarily, some synovial fluid is readily collected from the stifle joint, but it is most difficult to obtain from the carpal and tarsal joints. Obviously, when joint spaces are swollen, fluid is more easily aspirated. The plunger of the syringe should be released before the needle is removed from the joint space. This minimizes blood contamination of the sample as the needle is withdrawn.

Carpal Joint

Entry is obtained via the antibrachiocarpal joint or the middle carpal joint. In either case, the carpus is flexed to increase access to the joint's spaces. The needle is introduced from the dorsal aspect, just medial of center, then

---

BOX 12-1

Indications for Arthrocentesis

Fever of unknown origin
Unexplained lameness
Generalized pain
Joint swelling or effusion
Weakness
Acute monoarthropathy
Abnormal limb function or gait
Shifting leg lameness or polyarthropathy

BOX 12-2

Contraindications for Arthrocentesis

Absolute: Cellulitis or dermatitis over arthrocentesis site
Relative: Bacteremia or severe coagulopathy

---

inserted perpendicular to the joint. Landmarks for the antibrachiocarpal joint are the distal radius and the proximal radial carpal bone. The middle carpal joint is between the distal portion of the radial carpal bone and the second and third carpal bones.

Elbow Joint

The elbow is flexed to a 90-degree angle and the needle introduced just proximal to the olecranon and medial to the lateral epicondylar crest. The needle will be inserted parallel to the olecranon and the long axis of the ulna.

Shoulder Joint

Access is gained from the lateral aspect with the needle introduced distal to the acromion of the scapula and caudal to the greater tubercle of the humerus. The needle is directed medial to the greater tubercle and distal to the supraglenoid tubercle of the scapula.

Tarsal Joint

Access is gained via a cranial or lateral approach. In the cranial approach, the tarsus is slightly flexed and the needle is introduced at the space palpated between the tibia and talus (tibiotarsal) bones, just lateral to the tendon bundle. For the lateral approach, the needle can be inserted just distal to the lateral malleolus of the fibula with either a slightly cranial or plantar path.

Stifle Joint

The stifle is flexed and the needle introduced just lateral to the patellar ligament and distal to the patella. The needle is advanced in a medial and proximal direction pointing toward the medial condyle of the femur.

BOX 12-3

Materials for Arthrocentesis

1-inch, 25-gauge needles (small dogs and cats)
½-inch, 22-gauge needles (large to medium dogs)
3-ml syringes
3-ml EDTA blood tubes (lavender top)
3-ml no additive blood tubes (red top)
20-ml blood culture bottle (for 1 to 3 ml of fluid)
Glass slides
Clippers
Sterile gloves
Sterile scrub solution and alcohol

Hip Joint

The femur is abducted and the leg extended caudally. The needle is introduced cranial to the greater trochanter of the femur and inserted caudal and distal or ventral toward the joint.

SAMPLE HANDLING AND TEST PRIORITIES

Laboratory tests performed can be limited by volume of synovial fluid collected. While the sample is in the syringe, volume, color, and turbidity should be noted. Viscosity is then assessed as the sample is expelled onto a glass slide for direct smears. Direct smears are immediately made for subsequent cytologic examination, nucleated cell differential count, and subjective assessment of cellularity. See Tables 12-1 and 12-2 for specific volumes needed and sequence of testing. When larger volumes of fluid are collected, a total nucleated cell count, mucin clot test, and total protein estimation, in order of priority, can be added to the aforementioned procedures.

Normal synovial fluid does not clot. However with the possibility of incidental blood contamination, intraarticular hemorrhage, or protein exudation in various inflammatory diseases, it is best to put some portion into an EDTA anticoagulant blood tube. The smallest EDTA blood tube available should be used for storage or preservation of the synovial fluid retrieved, since gross mismatches by using large EDTA tubes can lead to erroneous test results. EDTA is preferred for cytologic examination, whereas heparin or a plain blood tube is recommended for the mucin clot test. Either anticoagulant (EDTA or heparin) is suitable for other routine tests.

When sufficient fluid is collected for cell counting, various types of preparations can be made in accordance with the sample's cellularity. When the nucleated cell count is <5000 cells/μl, cytologic examination is enhanced by cytocentrifuge concentration. About 5 minutes at 1000-1500 rpm in a cytocentrifuge is satisfactory. Fluids with nucleated cell counts >5000 cells/μl can be smeared directly onto glass slides. Although cytocentrifuge concentration is helpful, it is not essential to a good evaluation, and practitioners can get accurate results from direct smears only.

Cells in sediment smears and direct smears of fluid with the normally high viscosity may not spread out well on slides, making cell identification and differential cell count difficult.

TABLE 12-1

Test Priorities for 2 ml or More Synovial Fluid

Amount	Test	
1 drop	Cytology and WBC differential with viscosity estimate	Glass slide
0.5 to 1.0 ml	Total nucleated cell count	Lavender top or plain
1 to 3 ml	Bacterial culture and sensitivity	20-ml (pediatric) BD BBL Septi-Chek blood culture tube
or	or	or
0.5 to 1.0 ml	Bacterial culture and sensitivity	Sterile plain blood tube

TABLE 12-2

Test Priorities for Less than 1 ml of Synovial Fluid

Amount	Test	
1 drop	Cytology and WBC differential with total nucleated cell estimate and viscosity	Glass slide
2 or 3 drops	Bacterial culture and sensitivity	Culturette

If this problem is encountered, it can be overcome by mixing an equal volume of hyaluronidase at 150 IU/ml with the synovial fluid and incubating for at least 10 minutes.[1] The result is a fluid that facilitates better presentation of cell morphology and more complete cytologic evaluation.

A cytocentrifuge is a low-speed centrifuge that allows for concentration of poorly cellular fluids directly onto a glass slide with a minimum number of cells destroyed in the process. Samples with good to fair viscosity must be pretreated with hyaluronidase, otherwise the synovial fluid mucin clogs the cytocentrifuge filter paper and interferes with proper slide preparation. This technique is helpful and used by many commercial laboratories, but is not essential for an adequate evaluation in most cases, and the practicing veterinarian can obtain diagnostically useful information from a direct smear.

Slides can be stained with any Romanowsky-type stain for routine cytologic evaluation. It is advisable to make synovial fluid smears soon after collection. Delays of several hours, particularly at warm temperatures, can result in artificial vacuolation of macrophages along with pyknosis and karyorrhexis of nucleated cells.

Microbiologic evaluation of samples collected aseptically can be done if cytologic and clinical findings suggest an infectious agent is present. If possible, synovial fluid should be placed into a culture system immediately after collection. Use of an EDTA tube is undesirable because EDTA interferes with growth of some bacteria; a red-top tube is undesirable because it may not be sterile.

LABORATORY ANALYSIS AND REFERENCE VALUES

Volume

An approximate or subjective estimation of fluid volume collected should be recorded.

Synovial fluid volumes depend on patient size and which joint is being collected (within an individual there is variation from joint to joint). In normal animals, fluid volume can range from 1 drop to 1.0 ml in dogs and 1 drop to 0.25 ml in cats.[1-3] Clinical experience is an extremely valuable guide to detecting an articular effusion. This judgment is based on the degree of joint capsule distension, ease of fluid collection, and volume readily obtained. The aim of arthrocentesis for synovial fluid analysis is to collect some synovial fluid, but not to drain the joint space.

Color and Turbidity

Normal synovial fluid is transparent and colorless to very light yellow or straw-colored. Samples with increased cellularity exhibit variable discoloration and increased turbidity. When a fluid is blood tinged, hemarthrosis should be distinguished from iatrogenic contamination. In cases of hemarthrosis, the fluid is uniformly bloody throughout the time of collection. If the fluid was initially free of blood, but there is a subsequent admixture during the sampling procedure, contamination should be suspected. As an alternative and when the volume is sufficiently large for centrifugation, recent hemorrhage is associated with a sediment of red blood cells (RBCs) and a clear to straw-colored supernatant. The supernatant of fluids with chronic hemorrhage have a yellow to yellow-orange discoloration due to hemoglobin breakdown products.

Viscosity

Normal synovial fluid is very viscous because of its high concentration of hyaluronic acid. Viscosity can be measured using a viscometer; however, this is rarely done in small animal practice, but instead, is assessed subjectively. When slowly expressed from a needle attached to a syringe held horizontal, normal synovial fluid forms a long strand that is at least 2.5 cm before separating from the needle. When a drop of fluid is placed between the thumb and forefinger, a similar strand bridges the two digits as they are moved apart. Viscosity is usually recorded as normal, decreased, or markedly decreased.

Viscosity is easily assessed at the time of collection. However, if it must be evaluated after the sample is added to an anticoagulant, heparin is probably preferable to EDTA for sample preservation. EDTA tends to degrade hyaluronic acid and may decrease the sample's viscosity.[4]

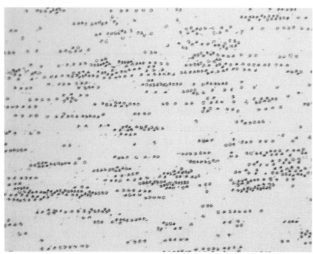

Figure 12-1 Direct smear of synovial fluid from a dog with acute suppurative arthritis. Note the markedly increased cell count and linear arrangement of cells. The latter, referred to as *windrowing*, suggests normal viscosity. (Wright's stain, original magnification 160×.) *(From Parry: In Pratt PW: Laboratory Procedures for Veterinary Technicians, ed 2. Goleta, Calif, American Veterinary Publications, 1992.)*

Viscosity can also be subjectively assessed when cytologically evaluating direct or sediment smears such that smears of fluids with normally high viscosity tend to have cells aligned in a linear pattern that is sometimes referred to as *windrowing* (Figure 12-1). In contrast, synovial fluid samples with decreased viscosity have cells more randomly arranged on the smear (Figure 12-2).

Mucin Quality

If sufficient sample remains following slide preparation and nucleated cell count, synovial fluid mucin quality or hyaluronic acid may be assessed using a mucin clot test. When there is the potential for clotting of joint fluid, heparin is recommended as an anticoagulant because EDTA interferes with the mucin clot test by degrading hyaluronic acid.[4]

One part synovial fluid is added to four parts 2.5% glacial acetic acid, which causes mucin to precipitate and sometimes agglutinate or clot. The test can be performed in test tubes when sufficient fluid is collected or on glass slides when only a drop is available for this test. The mixture is gently agitated and the nature of the clot observed. Assessment is enhanced by reading the test against a dark background. In inflammatory arthropathies, hyaluronic acid is degraded by proteases from neutrophils. This results in a decreased hyaluronic acid or hyaluronate concentration and decreased viscosity.

The following subjective classifications are commonly used: good (normal), when there is a compact, ropey clot in a clear solution; fair (slightly decreased), when there is a soft clot in a slightly turbid solution; poor, when there is a friable clot in a cloudy solution; and very poor, when there is no actual clot, just some large flecks in a very turbid solution. If clot quality is initially debatable, it can be reassessed after about 1 hour at room temperature. When the solutions are gently shaken during assessment, good clots remain ropey, and poor clots fragment.

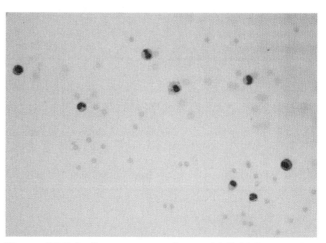

Figure 12-2 Sediment smear of synovial fluid from a dog with degenerative arthropathy. Note the normal (low) cell count and random distribution of cells. The latter suggests decreased viscosity. (May-Grünwald-Giemsa stain, original magnification 200×.)

Total Cell Counts

Nucleated cell counts in normal synovial fluid vary from joint to joint within an individual animal.[1] However, surveys have not shown these differences to be either statistically significant or clinically relevant. Various canine reference intervals have been reported (Table 12-3). As a generalization from these studies, most normal joints have nucleated cell counts <3000 cells/μl.

A recent study of synovial fluid samples from clinically normal cats, showed white blood cell (WBC) counts of 161 ± 209 cells/μl (mean ± SD) and median WBC of 91 cells/μl with a range of 2 to 1134 cells/μl.[3] Samples were excluded from this study when there was gross evidence of blood contamination, radiographic evidence of osteoarthritis, or histologic evidence of synovitis or if postmortem physical examination revealed abnormalities. As a generalization from this study, most normal joints have nucleated cell counts <1000 cells/μl (Table 12-4).

A comparison of manual hemacytometer and electronic, automatic, particle counting of nucleated cells in canine synovial fluid revealed that the mean electronic total nucleated cell count was statistically higher than the mean manual count.[5] Manual counting methods can demonstrate within-day and between-day analytical imprecision that is statistically higher than that of automated particle counting instruments.[6,7] In general, differences in mean cell counts and precision have not proven to be clinically relevant; therefore, the efficiency and speed of automatic particle counters offer an advantage over manual methods.

EDTA is preferred as an anticoagulant and preservative for cytologic examination and nucleated cell counts. In comparison of EDTA versus heparin anticoagulants as a preservative for synovial fluid, samples stored in heparin showed a 4-fold and 9-fold greater decrease in total nucleated cell counts over 24 hours and 48 hours at 4°C, respectively.[6] On the other hand, EDTA reportedly decreases synovial fluid mucin quality; therefore, total nucleated cell counts on fluid samples collected into EDTA may not be increased by hyaluronidase. Regardless of the anticoagulant/preservative used, synovial fluid should be pretreated with hyaluronidase when automated hematology analyzers are used for cell counts.[8,9]

Nucleated cell counts may also be performed using a hemocytometer. In clear or nonturbid specimens (i.e., specimens that appear to have a low total nucleated cell count) the sample may be counted undiluted. However, if the sample is turbid and the anticipated nucleated cell count is high, the specimen should be diluted. A WBC-diluting pipette and physiologic saline are suitable for this purpose. The BD Unopette brand test for manual WBC/platelets counts can also be used; however, the use of an acetic acid diluent should be avoided because it causes mucin to clot and invalidates the results.

Due to the lack of clinical application, RBC counts are not typically reported. Samples from normal patients contain very few RBCs and are a result of incidental blood contamination at the time of collection.

Total Protein Concentration

Comparatively few studies have reported baseline values for total protein concentration, which probably reflects the relatively low priority given to this value. Other tests are preferred because sample volume is usually insufficient to allow for protein measurement. Synovial fluid protein concentration is best measured by a quantitative biochemical assay because refractometry measures other solutes and protein. A study of normal stifle, shoulder, and carpal joints reported a total protein concentration reference interval of 1.8 to 4.8 g/dl, as measured by refractometer.[1] Normal synovial fluid does not clot in vitro because it is essentially free of fibrinogen and other clotting factors. Joint fluid can form a thixolabile gel if left undisturbed for several hours. Because clots are not thixotropic, normal fluid is distinguishable from clotting by gently shaking the sample to restore fluidity. If a specimen forms a clot after collection, this indicates intra-articular hemorrhage or inflammation with increased vascular permeability and protein exudation into the joint space.

CYTOLOGIC EXAMINATION

When only a few drops of fluid are collected, cytologic reports should include subjective assessments of the amount of blood present, total nucleated cell count, and sample viscosity. When a cell count and mucin clot test can be performed, incongruities with the subjective assessments should be reported.

Normal synovial fluid contains very few RBCs. Increased RBC numbers may result from hemorrhage associated with collection and trauma or inflammation involving the joint capsule. Generalizations regarding the cellularity of synovial fluid can be consistently made via freshly prepared direct smears. The body of the smear of normal specimens contains about 2 cells/field at 400× magnification (40× objective). Cellularity of direct smears are categorized as normal (see Figure 12-2), slightly increased, moderately increased (Figure 12-3), or markedly increased (see Figure 12-1). Due to unpredictable variation among processing techniques and instrumentation, such assessments are impractical with concentrated specimens (sediment and cytocentrifuge smears).

Because of the high viscosity of normal synovial fluid, cells of direct and centrifuged sediment smears tend to line up in rows (i.e., windrowing, see Figure 12-1). This characteristic arrangement can be used to comment on sample viscosity, when volume is not sufficient for viscosity and mucin clot tests. However, in smears from synovial fluid with low cell counts, windrowing may not be apparent, even though viscosity is normal.

Smears of normal, and sometimes abnormal, synovial fluid can have a pink granular proteinaceous background (see Figures 12-3 and 12-13) that must not be confused with bacteria.

Nucleated cells should be classified as neutrophils, large mononuclear cells, lymphocytes, or eosinophils. Classification as mononuclear cells encompasses those that are phagocytically active. These cells could be derived

TABLE 12-3

Reference Intervals for Synovial Fluid Total Nucleated Cell Counts in Healthy Dogs

Range (cells/µl)	Joints sampled
33-2495[1]	12 joints: stifle, shoulder, carpus
0-2900[2]	55 joints: hip, stifle, hock, elbow, shoulder, carpus
700-4400[10]	20 stifles
327-1450[11]	14 stifles
50-2725[12]	58 stifles
209-2070[5]	19 stifles

TABLE 12-4

Reference Intervals for Synovial Fluid in Healthy Dogs and Cats

Parameter	DOG[2]		CAT[3]	
	Range	Mean	Range	Mean
Volume (ml)	1 drop – 1.0	0.24	1 drop – 0.25	—
Nucleated cell count (cells/µl)	0 – 2900	430	2 – 1134	161
Neutrophils (%)	0 – 12	1.4	0 – 39	3.6
Mononuclear cells (%)	88 – 100	98.6	61 – 100	96.4

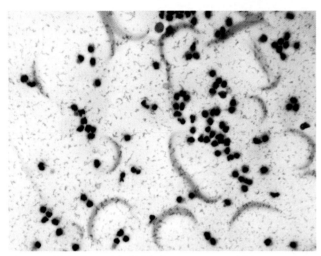

Figure 12-3 Synovial fluid from a cat with suppurative (neutrophilic) arthritis. Fluid protein is observed as pink granular or stippled material and crescents. (Wright's stain, original magnification 500×.)

from blood monocytes, tissues macrophages, or synovial lining cells. The origin of these cells has little practical importance regarding clinical diagnosis and therapy. The proportion of large mononuclear cells that have phagocytized debris, cells, or microorganisms should be recorded. On smears that are freshly made or from fluid not exposed to EDTA, the degree of vacuolated large mononuclear cells should be noted and reported as mild, moderate, or marked. Overall assessment of nucleated cell morphology ought to include comments on the degree of karyolysis, pyknosis, and karyorrhexis. Delayed processing can lead to nuclear degeneration and increased numbers of markedly vacuolated large mononuclear cells.[1] Synovial fluid nucleated cell differentials are reported as percentage values and are incorporated into the interpretation of a total nucleated cell count or subjective assessment of cellularity.

Reports of normal canine synovial fluid nucleated cell differentials indicate neutrophils can make up as much as 12% of nucleated cells, but frequently compose < 5% of all nucleated cells.[1,2,10,11] Eosinophils are absent.[1,2,10-12] Lymphocyte values can be quite variable, with studies reporting 0% to 100% (mean 44%) and 3% to 28% (mean 11%).[1,2] The balance of nucleated cells in normal joints are large mononuclear cells, ranging from 64% to 97% in one study, to 60% to 92% in another study. In samples of normal joints processed immediately by direct smear, the percentage of large mononuclear cells that were markedly vacuolated was about 9%.[1] As with delayed processing, pre-treatment of fluid with hyaluronidase can increased the percentage of large mononuclear cells that are markedly vacuolated to about 14% to 18%.

A study of normal feline synovial fluids reports that mononuclear cells predominate, ranging from 61% to 100% of all nucleated cells (mean 96.4%), with smaller proportions of neutrophils that vary from 0% to 39% of all nucleated cells (mean 3.6%).[3] Within the mononuclear cell component, lymphocytes or small mononuclear cells

make up 0% to 45% of all mononuclear cells (mean 9.1%) and large mononuclear cells include 0% to 100% of all mononuclear cells (mean 81%). Freshly prepared smears from these cats reveal that among mononuclear cells, 0% to 100% are vacuolated (mean 9.9%).

BACTERIOLOGIC CULTURE

Conventional agar-based or broth-type bacteriologic culture methods have been shown to lack sensitivity when compared with blood culture methods.[13-15] Liquid blood culture media offers several advantages, including culture of larger volumes compared with culture plates, resins that decrease the inhibitory affects of antibiotics and substances intrinsic to synovial fluid, and lytic agents that release microorganisms phagocytized by inflammatory cells. Because relatively small volumes are retrieved with

---

BOX 12-4

Classification of Arthropathies

Noninflammatory
- Degenerative
- Trauma
- Acute hemarthrosis

Inflammatory
- Chronic hemarthrosis
- Infectious
  - Bacterial
  - Viral
  - Rickettsial
  - Spirochetal
  - Fungal
  - Protozoal
  - Mycoplasmal
- Noninfectious or immune-mediated
  - Nonerosive
    - Idiopathic (type I)—no identified concurrent disease
    - Reactive (type II)—extra-articular infectious/inflammatory disease
    - Enteropathic (type III)—primary infectious/inflammatory gastrointestinal or hepatic disease
    - Malignancy-associated (type IV)—neoplasia distant from joint
    - Drug-associated
    - Vaccine reaction
    - Polyarthritis-meningitis syndrome
    - Polyarthritis-polymyositis syndrome
    - Systemic lupus erythematosus
    - Lymphoplasmacytic gonitis
    - Juvenile-onset polyarthritis of Akitas
    - Synovitis-amyloidosis of Shar-Peis
  - Erosive
    - Rheumatoid arthritis (idiopathic erosive polyarthritis)
    - Progressive feline polyarthritis

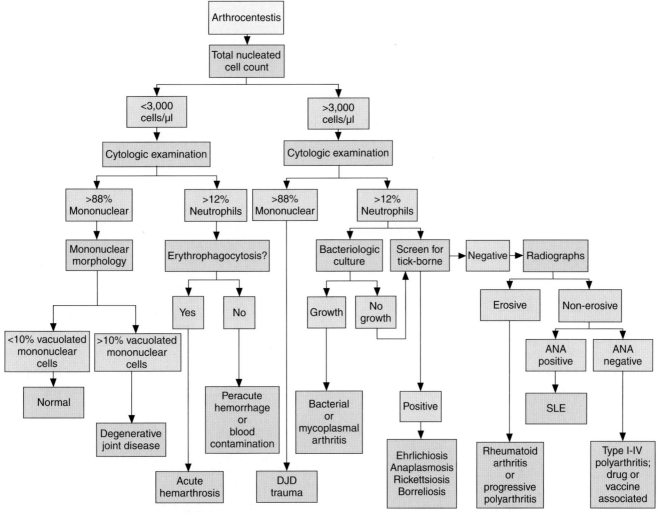

Figure 12-4 Diagnostic plan for cytologic evaluation of canine synovial fluid. *ANA,* Antinuclear antibodies; *SLE,* systemic lupus erythematosus; *DJD,* degenerative joint disease.

arthrocentesis of cats and dogs, pediatric blood culture bottles or tubes are most appropriate. Blood culture tubes or bottles should be inoculated at the time of fluid collection and incubated for 24 hours at 37°C, at which time the result is transferred to appropriate growth media.

It has been suggested that culturing a synovial membrane biopsy specimen may be superior to culture of synovial fluid, but this was not shown to be the case when stifle joints were experimentally infected with *Staphylococcus intermedius.*[15]

SYNOVIAL FLUID CHANGES IN DISEASED JOINTS

Because synovial fluid demonstrates a limited spectrum of response to diseases and distinction among subcategories of long-standing disease is difficult, arthropathies are initially classified by broad categories such as inflammatory or noninflammatory and infectious or immune-mediated (Box 12-4). More definitive classification of arthritis requires supporting diagnostics that include radiographs, microbial culture, serology, molecular diagnostics and a

minimum medical database incorporating history and physical examination, complete blood count, biochemical profile, and complete urinalysis (Figure 12-4).

NONINFLAMMATORY ARTHROPATHIES

Degenerative Arthropathies

Degenerative arthropathies are linked to trauma, congenital or genetic bone anomalies, acquired anatomic disorders that impose abnormal stresses on articular surfaces, metabolic disturbance, nutritional disorders, or neoplasia.[16] Orthopedic diseases that may cause degenerative arthropathies include primary osteoarthritis, osteochondritis dissecans, elbow dysplasia, avascular necrosis of the femoral head, hip dysplasia, chronic patellar dislocations, and joint instabilities caused by ligament damage (e.g., rupture of the cranial cruciate ligament).

General synovial fluid changes are outlined in Table 12-5. Cytologic findings may be abnormal before radiographic changes are readily apparent.[17] Cytologic examination of the effusion may reveal a number of changes.[2,16,17] The total nucleated cell count is usually normal to slightly

TABLE 12-5

Characteristics of Synovial Fluid Responses to Articular Injury

Category	Color	Turbidity	Viscosity	Mucin Clot	NUCLEATED CELL DENSITY		Causes
					Total	Differential	
Acute hemarthrosis	Red	Increased proportional to amount of blood	Mild to marked decrease	Fair to poor	Increased proportional to amount of blood	Differential may be similar to peripheral blood with platelets	Coagulopathies, like factor deficiency; severe blunt force trauma
Degenerative arthropathy	Normal	Usually normal	Normal to mildly decreased	Fair to poor	Likely increased	Mo: Normal to increased with vacuolation and phagocytic activity PMN: Increased	Osteoarthrosis or degenerative joint diseases; trauma; neoplasia
Inflammatory arthropathy	Yellow to off-white or red-brown	Increased in relation to the amount of inflammation and hemorrhage	Mildly to markedly decreased	Fair to very poor	Increased	Mo: normal to increased PMN: Increased	Infection; immune-mediated arthropathies

Mo, large mononuclear cells; *PMN,* neutrophils.

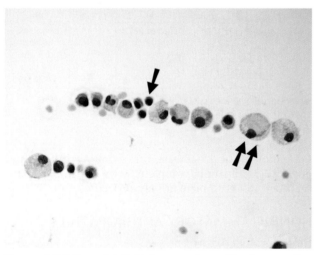

Figure 12-5 Synovial fluid from a dog with degenerative arthropathy, showing large mononuclear cells *(double arrow)* or macrophage-type cells mingled with lymphocytes *(arrow)*. (Wright's stain, original magnification 500×.)

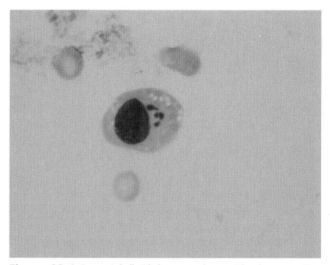

Figure 12-6 Synovial fluid from a dog with degenerative arthropathy. Note the leukophagocytic macrophage, indicating chronic inflammation. (May-Grünwald-Giemsa stain, original magnification 1250×.)

increased with a predominance of large mononuclear cells, of which >10% are moderately to markedly vacuolated or phagocytic (Figures 12-5 and 12-6). The percentage of neutrophils is typically within reference limits or they are absent, although in some cases the neutrophil percentage may be somewhat increased. The total protein concentration is frequently within the reference interval to slightly increased, and the fluid does not clot. Hemorrhage is marginal to absent; but in patients with capsular trauma, there may be superimposition of transient, mild inflammation

and hemorrhage. If damage to articular cartilage is severe enough, osteoclasts and chondrocytes may exfoliate into the fluid component (Figure 12-7).

Dogs with a partial rupture of the cruciate ligament may have synovial fluid with a moderate increase in cellularity, which is predominantly due to mononuclear cells, or in some patients, a slight increase in the percentage of neutrophils.[18,19] In contrast, cell counts in the synovial fluid of dogs with a complete rupture of the cruciate ligament were similar to those of normal dogs.[18] The

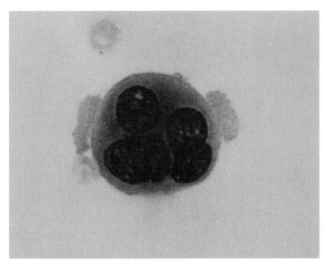

Figure 12-7 Synovial fluid from a dog with degenerative arthropathy. Note the osteoclast, which indicates articular cartilage erosion to subchondral bone. (May-Grünwald-Giemsa stain, original magnification 1250×.)

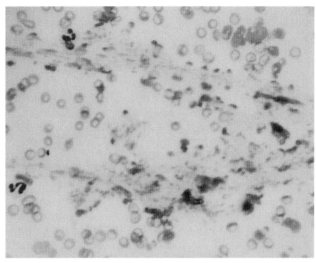

Figure 12-8 Direct smear of synovial fluid from a dog. Note the platelet clump, indicating recent hemorrhage. In this case, hemorrhage was due to iatrogenic contamination. (May-Grünwald-Giemsa stain, original magnification 500×.)

volume of fluid present may vary from slightly to markedly increased.

Acute Hemarthrosis

Differential diagnoses associated with hemarthrosis include accidental iatrogenic blood contamination or concurrent hemorrhage associated with inflammatory and noninflammatory joint effusions.

In acute hemarthrosis, arthrocentesis yields bloody fluid from the time the sample first flows through the needle. With hemodilution, turbidity will increase and fluid viscosity tends to decrease. Hemarthrosis elicits an inflammatory response, and within hours, erythrophagocytosis and a mildly increased neutrophil density is evident. Lameness caused by hemarthrosis usually has an acute onset. With long-standing intra-articular hemorrhage, the joint fluid may have a xanthochromic supernatant. Recurrent hemarthrosis and resulting lameness is the most common manifestation of canine hemophilia A.[20] Intra-articular hemorrhage, for periods as short as 4 days, can cause decreases in cartilage matrix proteoglycan content and synthesis, which can interfere with cartilage metabolism and repair and eventually result in degenerative joint disease.[21]

With iatrogenic hemorrhage, synovial fluid usually is not bloody at the beginning of the procedure. But as the arthrocentesis goes on, an admixture of blood may suddenly appear, signaling puncture or rupture of a blood vessel. As soon as iatrogenic hemorrhage is recognized, collection at that joint should be ended. Blood contamination can be reduced by using a minimum of negative pressure for retrieval of fluid and gently releasing negative pressure of the syringe before withdrawing the needle from the joint capsule. Cytologically, only a small amount of blood is present and often without erythrophagocytosis. Platelets may be observed with recent, peracute hemorrhage or iatrogenic blood contamination (Figure 12-8).

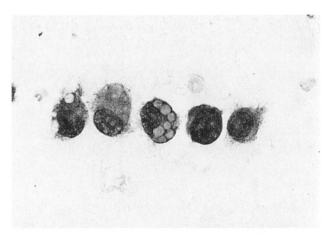

Figure 12-9 Synovial fluid from a dog with degenerative arthropathy. Note the erythrophagocytic macrophage, which indicates concurrent hemorrhage (i.e., not iatrogenic contamination). (Wright's stain, original magnification 1250×.)

Hemorrhage associated with degenerative and inflammatory arthropathies is usually mild when compared with true hemarthrosis. Cytologically, erythrophagocytosis appears in conjunction with changes characteristic of the underlying cause (Figure 12-9).

It is important to always send premade, direct smears, especially if the fluid sample is mailed to a laboratory because erythrophagocytosis, along with other cell changes, may occur in transit and interfere with interpretation. Submitting premade smears along with the fluid sample allows for identification of artifacts that developed in transit.

Neoplasia

Although uncommon, neoplasms can arise within joints, invade from adjacent tissues, or metastasize to joints. Neoplasms that may affect the joints include synovial cell sarcoma, chondrosarcoma, osteosarcoma, fibrosarcoma,

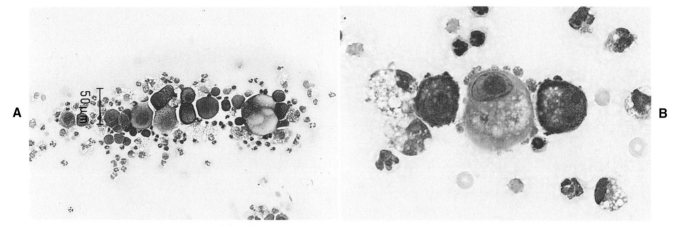

Figure 12-10 Synovial fluid from a dog with a metastatic bronchiolar-alveolar carcinoma. **A,** Low-magnification view showing a mixture of cells that includes metastatic carcinoma cells with many criteria of malignancy, including large prominent nucleoli. (Wright's stain, original magnification 100×.) **B,** Higher magnification showing metastatic carcinoma cells. (Wright's stain, original magnification 250×.)

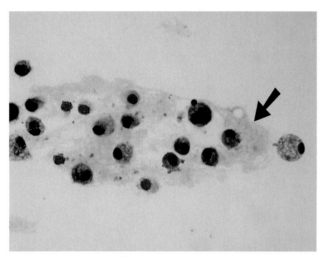

Figure 12-11 Synovial fluid from a dog with degenerative arthropathy. Note the large clump of fibrin with enmeshed cells *(arrow)*. This is more often seen in inflammatory arthropathies. (Wright's stain, original magnification, 500×.)

metastatic bronchial carcinoma, and lymphoma.[22-25] Diagnosis is made by obtaining a biopsy of the lesion for histopathologic examination. Cytologic examination of such biopsies is described in other chapters throughout this textbook. Synovial fluid changes are poorly described, but conceivably there would be characteristics of a degenerative or inflammatory arthropathy. Neoplastic cells are infrequently evident in these fluids (Figure 12-10).

INFLAMMATORY ARTHROPATHIES

Inflammatory arthropathies are either infectious or noninfectious and immune-mediated (see Box 12-4) and associated with an exudate showing increased neutrophil numbers and variable increases in the number of large mononuclear cells, which maybe vacuolated or have engulfed debris. Concurrent and often mild hemorrhagic diapedesis is common. Other findings are listed in Table 12-5.

Fundamentally, the greater the inflammatory reaction the more discolored and turbid the fluid, and the poorer the viscosity. Mucin clot test results often parallel sample viscosity. The total protein concentration is increased and the sample may readily clot. Fibrin strands often cause clumping of inflammatory cells in the smear. If not apparent on a routinely stained smear, fibrin strands may be demonstrated by staining with new methylene blue (Figure 12-11).

Infectious Arthritides

Infectious arthritis is an inflammatory arthropathy in which the causative infectious agent might be cultured or isolated from synovial membrane or joint fluid. This is not to be confused with infectious diseases remote from the joint that cause arthritis via a hypersensitivity disorder. Although infectious arthritides are uncommon among dogs and cats, bacteria are the most frequently isolated cause with far fewer cases attributed to rickettsiae, spirochetes, mycoplasma, fungus, virus, and protozoa. Clinical presentation and history can be quite helpful because most infectious arthritides of a mature animal are monoarticular, acute in onset, and often the result of a percutaneous penetrating or surgical wound. When polyarticular infectious arthritides do occur they are likely of hematogenous origin, as in omphalophlebitis of neonates or bacterial endocarditis in mature animals.

Bacterial Arthritides

Bacterial infectious arthritides demonstrate a markedly increased total nucleated cell count, usually greater than 50,000 cells/μl, with a predominance of neutrophils that are often > 75% of all nucleated cells.[26] Neutrophils are often intact and inconsistently show karyolysis or pyknosis and karyorrhexis (Figure 12-12). Karyolytic degeneration of cells suggests a septic process; however in many infected joints, degenerative leukocyte changes or microorganisms are not observed. When clinical observations and intuition dictate, joint fluid should be reflexively cultured.

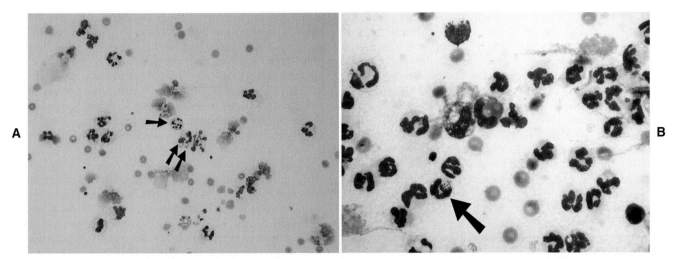

Figure 12-12 Synovial fluid from a dog with septic suppurative (neutrophilic) arthritis. **A,** Note nucleated cell with pyknotic nuclear material *(arrow)* and neutrophil with engulfed bacteria *(double arrow)*. Background contains other neutrophils with hydropic degeneration (degenerative neutrophils) along with nuclear debris and erythrocytes (Wright's stain, original magnification 500×.) **B,** Note neutrophil with engulfed bacteria *(arrow)*. (Wright's stain, original magnification 1000×.)

Organisms commonly cultured from dogs with an infected joint include *Staphylococcus intermedius, Staphylococcus aureus,* or beta-hemolytic *Streptococcus* spp.[27] Among cats with bacterial arthritis, hemolytic strains of *Escherichia coli* or *Pasteurella multocida* are most common.[28] Failure to isolate organisms on culture does not necessarily exclude a bacterial cause. The absence of bacteria on cytologic specimens may represent prior antibiotic therapy or an exuberant inflammatory response. Caution is warranted when attributing favorable clinical response to empiric antibiotic therapy with tetracyclines (e.g., doxycycline), because some of these drugs have immune modulatory, anti-inflammatory, and chondroprotective properties.[29,30]

Rickettsial Arthritides

Granulocytic morulae have been observed in joint fluid of dogs infected with *Ehrlichia ewingii.*[31] Polymerase chain reaction (PCR) amplification of *E. ewingii* DNA was used to differentiate it from infection with *Anaplasma phagocytophila,* formerly called *Ehrlichia equi.* Patients presented with fever, lameness, thrombocytopenia, and on occasion, central nervous system signs (i.e., proprioceptive deficits, neck pain, paraparesis, or ataxia). Neutrophilic polyarthritis was diagnosed in dogs with lameness and joint fluid contained a total nucleated cell count ranging from 16,000 to 125,000/µl, of which neutrophils made up 63% to 99%. As with other rickettsial infections, polyarthritis is likely caused by immune-complex–mediated disease or hemarthrosis.[32] Reports suggest that granulocytic morulae might be observed in 1% to 7% of neutrophils in synovial fluid and 0.1% to 26% of neutrophils in peripheral blood[33] (Figure 12-13).[34] Tentative identification of granulocytic morulae as *A. phagocytophila* can be based on geographic distribution because the tick vectors for this organism are found in Western United States and Canada and the upper Midwest and Northeast United States.[35]

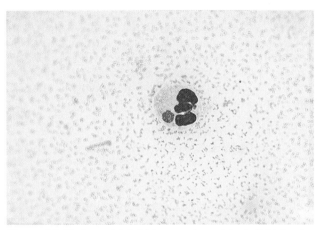

Figure 12-13 Synovial fluid from a dog with ehrlichial polyarthritis. Note the *Ehrlichia* morula in the neutrophil and the normal granular, eosinophilic proteinaceous background. (Wright's stain, original magnification 1250×.)

Spirochetal Arthritides

Arthritis is the most common clinical sign in dogs with Lyme disease, which is caused by the spirochete *Borrelia burgdorferi.* Joints closest to the infecting tick bite site are often involved in the first episodes of lameness and demonstrate the most extreme synovial fluid abnormalities. Although not observed on routine microscopy, live spirochetes are mostly frequently cultured from synovial membranes closest to the bite site.[36] Chronic oligoarthritis can be transient to persistent, and caused by wider migration of spirochetes or antibody-mediated and T-lymphocyte-driven responses.[37] Because acute Lyme arthritis presents with monoarthritis or oligoarthritis, synovial fluid changes can be varied from joint to joint within the same dog. Joints of limbs that demonstrate lameness can have total nucleated cell counts that range between 1400 and 76,200 cells/μl (median 12,700 cells/μl) with neutrophils composing up to 97% of all nucleated cells (median 54%). In the same dog with monoarthritis or oligoarthritis, other joints can be quite dissimilar with total nucleated cell counts that range between 100 and 3300 cells/μl (median 710 cells/μl) and sometimes include up to 19% neutrophils (median 0%). Dogs without lameness that are culture positive and seropositive for *B. burgdorferi* typically have total nucleated cell counts ranging between 100 and 3000 cells/μl (median 600 cells/μl), but do not contain more that 15% neutrophils (median 0%).[36]

Fungal Arthritides

Fungal arthritides are uncommon but have been reported as a sequela of osteomyelitis or disseminated infection by *Blastomyces dermatitidis*, *Cryptococcus neoformans*, *Aspergillus* spp., *Coccidioides immitis*, *Histoplasma capsulatum*, and *Sporothrix schenckii*.[38,39] On occasion, fungal elements might be visible in synovial fluid.

Mycoplasmal Arithritides

Mycoplasmal arthritis has been diagnosed as a few rare cases in dogs and cats. The inflammatory reaction is neutrophilic with good cell morphology. Organisms may be observed on Romanowsky-stained smears or on mycoplasmal culture. Erosive polyarthritis of young Greyhounds has been associated with *Mycoplasma spumans*.[40] *Mycoplasma gateae* and *Mycoplasma felis* have been isolated from synovial fluid of immuncompromised cats with polyarthritis.[28,41]

Protozoal Arthritides

Polyarthritis has been documented with canine visceral leishmaniasis that is caused by geographic variants of the *Leishmania donovani* complex, *L. donovani*, or *L. infantum*. Synovial fluid sometimes shows mononuclear inflammation and *Leishmania* spp. amastigotes in synovial fluid macrophages.[42,43]

Viral Arthritides

Feline calicivirus infection has been associated with lameness in kittens.[44] However, synovial fluid changes in experimental infections were minimal, with synovial fluid macrophage numbers subjectively increased to a moderate degree, and some leukophagocytosis exhibited.[45] Occasionally, cellularity may be markedly increased, but there will still be a predominance of macrophages with many exhibiting leukophagocytosis.[46]

IMMUNE-MEDIATED ARTHROPATHIES

Immune-mediated arthritides of dogs and cats are generally considered to be a type III hypersensitivity phenomenon.[47,48] Emerging evidence suggests concurrent cell-mediated or genetic mechanisms.[49,50] Arthritis is caused by immune complexes that are composed of circulating antigen and immunoglobulin G (IgG) or IgM antibody. Much like renal glomeruli, synovial capillaries ultrafilter plasma, and as a result immune complexes commonly deposit at these locations. Deposited immune

complexes activate inflammatory cells to secrete cytokines that increase vascular permeability, augmenting immune complex deposition, and further accelerating tissue and vessel damage via complement and Fc receptor–mediated pathways. Clinicopathologic features of immune-mediated arthritides are a reflection of immune complex predisposition for certain sites and are not determined by the primary source of the antigen. Because antibodies involved in immune-mediated arthropathies are not usually against fixed cell or tissue antigen, these immune complex–mediated diseases tend to have a systemic component, affecting multiple joints either concurrently or consecutively. Signals of systemic disease in patients with immune-mediated arthritis include fever, generalized stiffness, peripheral blood cytopenias, difficult to localize pain, neck or back pain, lymphadenopathy, or proteinuria.[51] Polyarthritis, associated with systemic immune-complex disease, is sometimes subclinical, and a patient may not demonstrate joint swelling or pain; therefore, four or more joints should be sampled with sufficient volume for complete fluid analysis[39,52]; see Boxes 12-5 and 12-6 for summaries of diagnostic features.

NONEROSIVE ARTHROPATHIES

Idiopathic (Type I) Polyarthritis

Idiopathic or immune-mediated polyarthritis is diagnosed by exclusion of other possible causes or specific disease and breed associations. Among canine immune-mediated arthritides, idiopathic type I polyarthritis is the most common.[47] Dogs frequently present with stiffness, pyrexia, lymphadenopathy, and inappetence. Clinical signs of joint inflammation are commonly observed in all limbs, or less often just the hind legs, with carpal, hock, or stifle joints typically affected.[53] It would not be unusual for the likelihood of type I polyarthritis to be overestimated due to limitations of a patient's medical workup; therefore this diagnosis and subsequent immunosuppressive therapy should be employed with caution. Reported cases indicate that synovial fluid total nucleated cell counts ranged from 3700 to 130,000 cells/μl (mean 41,900 cells/μl) and are composed of approximately 20% to 98% neutrophils.[53]

Reactive (Type II) Polyarthritis

Reactive polyarthritis is defined as an aseptic inflammatory joint disease associated with extra-articular sites of infection, such as urogenital tracts, respiratory tract, and skin.[39,54] Research suggests that difficult to culture bacteria may persist within the articular cavity, evading complete removal by the immune system through antigenic modulation, intracellular localization, molecular mimicry, and Th1/Th2 imbalances.[55] Because the evasion is incomplete, intra-articular inflammation can be caused by persistent bacterial antigens such as lipopolysaccharides and portions of free bacterial DNA.[55] Reactive polyarthritis has been linked to various tick-transmitted diseases including bartonellosis, borreliosis, Rocky Mountain spotted fever, canine and feline ehrlichiosis, and canine and feline anaplasmosis.[31,56-61]

BOX 12-5

Diagnostic Features of Nonerosive, Immune-Mediated Arthritides

Idiopathic polyarthritides for which other causes of inflammatory arthropathy have been ruled out

Type I – no evidence of types II, III, or IV.

Type II – Concurrent inflammatory process distant from joint (i.e., respiratory, urogential, or integumentary systems).

Type III – Associated with gastroenteritis of various causes or hepatopathy.

Type IV – Polyarthritis associated with malignancy remote from joint.

Drug-associated reaction

Arthritis develops in association with drug administration.

Previous exposure or long-term therapy.

Most commonly antibiotics such as potentiated sulfonamides, penicillins, and cephalosporins.

Signs resolve within 7 days of discontinuation.

Vaccine reaction

5 to 7 days after first dose of primary immunization.

Self-limiting, lasting 1 to 3 days.

Noted with feline calicivirus and canine polyvalent modified live virus vaccines.

Polyarthritis-meningitis syndrome

Concurrent signs of polyarthritis and neck pain.

Cerebrospinal fluid pleocytosis.

Reported with Bernese Mountain dog, Boxers, Corgi, German shorthair pointer, Newfoundland, or Weimaraner.

Negative antinuclear antibody test.

Polyarthritis-polymyositis syndrome

Exercise intolerance and stiffness.

Myositis diagnosed in at least two muscle biopsies.

Systemic lupus erythematosis

Positive antinuclear antibody test.

Diagnosis of multisystemic immune-mediated disease (three of the following, serially or concurrently):

- Polyarthritis
- Mucosal/cutaneous lesions
- Anemia, leukopenia, or thrombocytopenia
- Glomerulonephritis or persistent proteinuria
- Polymyositis
- Serositis

Lymphoplasmacytic gonitis

Linked to subset of dogs with cranial cruciate ligament rupture.

Juvenile-onset polyarthritis of Akitas

Clinical signs before 8 months of age, most before 1-year-old.

Neutrophilic arthritis noted with:

- Cyclical pain
- Generalized lymphadenopathy
- Nonregenerative anemia
- Rarely concurrent meningitis

Synovitis-amyloidosis of Shar-pei dogs

Swollen joints with recurrent fever.

Glomerular disease from amyloidosis (proteinuria).

Enteropathic (Type III) Polyarthritis

Enteropathic arthritis is associated with inflammatory bowel diseases. The specific pathogenesis is unknown, but current hypothesis suggests an impaired barrier function of intestinal mucosa to bacterial antigens and defective local immune regulation. Clinical signs of polyarthritis are occasionally noted in dogs with colitis and only rarely observed in cats and dogs with idiopathic inflammatory bowel diseases.[62] Hepatopathic arthropathy, considered a variant of enteropathic polyarthritis, has been observed in dogs with chronic active hepatitis and cirrhosis.[47]

Malignancy-Associated (Type IV) Polyarthritis

Polyarthritis linked to extra-articular neoplasms has been reported with canine tumors such as mammary adenocarcinoma, squamous cell carcinoma, chemoreceptor neoplasia (heart base tumor), leiomyoma and feline myeloproliferative disease.[39]

Polyarthritis-Meningitis Syndrome

Polyarthritis-meningitis syndrome is observed in both cats and dogs, among which cases are reported in the Bernese Mountain dog, Boxer, Corgi, German short-haired pointer, Newfoundland, and Weimaraner.[39] This condition has been called polyarteritis nodosa.[47] Polyarthritis and meningitis have shared clinical signs such as fever, cervical rigidity, and stiff gait. Therefore, patients diagnosed with nonerosive, nonseptic polyarthritis and spinal pain could benefit from cerebrospinal fluid analysis because untreated meningitis can result in permanent neurologic deficits. Reports indicated that dogs diagnosed with concurrent steroid-responsive meningitis-arteritis and polyarthritis did not have lameness or joint swelling.[63] Among these patients, 25% to 100% of joints sampled demonstrated inflammation that was typically neutrophilic, or sometimes, mixed inflammation.

BOX 12-6

Diagnostic Features of Erosive, Immune-Mediated, Arthritides

Canine and Feline Rheumatoid Arthritis (Idiopathic erosive polyarthritis)

- Seropositive for rheumatoid factor
- Joint tenderness, pain, or swelling (one or more joints)
- Additional joints affected with 3 months of first joint
- Eventual symmetrical joint swelling
- Inflammatory joint fluid, often neutrophilic
- Subcutaneous nodules
- Radiographic evidence of perichondral/subchondral osteolysis, cyst formation, and erosion
- Lesions confirmed via histopathologic examination of synovial membrane or subcutaneous nodules

Progressive Feline Polyarthritis

- More common among young adult male cats
- Concurrent infection with feline leukemia and foamy viruses
- Periosteal proliferative bone lesions (common type)
  - Neutrophilic inflammatory joint fluid
- Erosive bone lesions
  - Variable joint fluid; normal to neutrophilic or mixed and mononuclear inflammation

---

Polyarthritis-Polymyositis Syndrome

Polyarthritis-polymyositis syndrome is of unknown etiology. Dogs diagnosed with this syndrome have symmetrical nonerosive neutrophilic polyarthritis, inflammatory myopathy found in two or more individual muscles ($\geq$ 6 individual muscles sampled per patient), and systemic lupus erythematosus (SLE), rheumatoid arthritis, or bacterial endocarditis are excluded. In some patients, plasma creatine phosphokinase (CPK) and plasma aldolase are increased above the reference intervals; however, the increases are inconsistent and should not be relied on to rule out the presence of polymyositis. The syndrome is assumed to have an immune-mediated component due to the absence of a detectible infectious cause and favorable response to immunosuppressive therapy.[64]

Drug-Associated Polyarthritis

Drug-associated polyarthritis is most commonly linked to antibiotics such as sulfonamides, and to a lesser degree, cephalosporins, penicillins, erythromycin, orlincomycin.[47] Doberman pinchers, Miniature Schnauzers, and Samoyeds are especially prone to systemic hypersensitivity reactions associated with sulfonamides and their potentiated formulations.[65] Unlike Doberman pinchers, among which all reported cases have polyarthritis, Miniature Schnauzers and Samoyeds less frequently demonstrate an associated arthropathy. More common abnormalities include fever, thrombocytopenia, hepatopathy (i.e., necrosis and cholestasis), transient neutropenia, keratoconjunctivitis sicca, and hemolysis. Among patients with a sulfonamide hypersensitivity reaction, those with an associated thrombocytopenia or hepatopathy are less likely to recover.[65]

Vaccine-Associated Polyarthritis

Vaccine-associated polyarthritis is reported in dogs and cats. Polyarthritis and radiographic lesions or clinical signs similar to hypertrophic osteodystrophy have been reported in young Weimaraners. Clinical signs typically appear within 7 days of polyvalent modified-live virus vaccine. All Weimaraners have a low serum immunoglobulin concentration that includes IgG or IgM and infrequently IgA.[66,67] Cats vaccinated against or infected with feline calicivirus have been reported to develop polyarthritis, which is often transitory and completely resolving within 48 hours.[68]

Systemic Lupus Erythematosus

Polyarthritis is the most consistent pathologic finding among dogs with SLE with carpal and tarsal joints more severely affected than elbow and stifle joints.[47] Cats with SLE can have arthritis, although less frequently than dogs, and some cats may not demonstrate lameness. Detection of antinuclear antibodies (ANA) is paramount to the diagnosis of SLE, but there are no universally accepted criteria for further classification. In addition to polyarthritis, dogs will demonstrate one or two systemic manifestations involving the kidneys, skin, or peripheral blood cytopenias, such as anemia and thrombocytopenia. Feline SLE is most commonly diagnosed by a characteristic dermatopathy or glomerulonephritis, and with lower frequency, polyarthritis, anemia, or central nervous system dysfunction.[69] Patients with SLE have a dysregulated immune system and are more likely to form autoantibodies, which can result in a type II hypersensitivity reaction against RBCs, platelets, or coagulation proteins.[47] Lupus erythematosus (LE) cells are rarely seen in synovial fluid, but when present are diagnostic for SLE (Figure 12-14).[47] LE cells can be confused with leukophagocytic macrophages (see Figure 12-6) or neutrophils containing particulate nucleic acid (Figure 12-15), which are erroneously referred to as ragocytes. The term *ragocyte* refers to a neutrophil with numerous, small, dark intracytoplasmic granules observed on unstained wet preparations, not on stained smears. The granules in ragocytes are phagocytized immunoglobulin and complement. To avoid confusing terminology, consider describing the neutrophils' contents observed on a stained smear. The LE cell preparation test detects serum antibodies to DNA histone complexes and has been used to diagnose SLE, but because of difficulties with test interpretation and poor performance characteristics, LE preps have been replaced by ANA testing. Low ANA titers can be detected with neoplastic, inflammatory, or infectious diseases and sometimes, clinically normal animals.[70]

Lymphoplasmacytic Gonitis

Lymphoplasmacytic gonitis has been linked to a small proportion of dogs that eventually develop or are currently diagnosed with a cranial cruciate ligament rupture.[47]

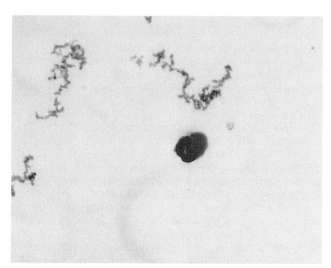

Figure 12-14 Synovial fluid from a dog with systemic lupus erythematosus and resultant immune-mediated polyarthritis. Note the lupus erythematosus cell. (Wright's stain, original magnification 1650×.)

Although the etiology or sequence of lesions is unclear, there is evidence that suggests a primary immune-mediated disease.[19]

Juvenile-Onset Polyarthritis of Akitas

Clinical signs of polyarthritis syndrome in Akitas typically appear before 8 months of age and include neutrophilic arthritis, cyclical pain, generalized lymphadenopathy, and nonregenerative anemia. Rarely dogs have concurrent meningitis, have positive ANA tests, or are positive for rheumatoid factor.[71] There is speculation this may be a canine overlap syndrome, in which patients have concurrent SLE and rheumatoid arthritis.

Polyarthritis-Amyloidosis of Shar-Pei Dogs

Unlike other breeds affected by amyloidosis, Chinese Shar-Pei dogs with familial amyloidosis can have swollen joints and recurrent fever that precedes glomerular disease.[72] Lameness and arthritis can be monoarticular and sometimes pauciarticular, which typically affects tarsal joints and less often, carpal joints.[73]

EROSIVE ARTHROPATHIES
Rheumatoid Arthritis (Idiopathic Erosive Polyarthritis)

Rheumatoid factor is IgM, and occasionally IgG or IgA that reacts to the constant region of the heavy chain of autologous IgG. The significance of rheumatoid factor in the pathogenesis of rheumatoid arthritis is currently unknown. Immune complexes involving rheumatoid factor are in part a cause of polyarthritis, and patients are often seropositive for rheumatoid factor. Other criteria for the diagnosis of rheumatoid arthritis include joint pain, tenderness, and swelling that can involve additional joints within 3 months, eventually leading to symmetrical joint swelling. Radiographic lesions include perichondral and

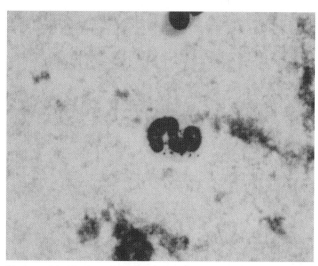

Figure 12-15 Synovial fluid from a dog with immune-mediated polyarthritis. Note the neutrophil containing phagocytosed material, probably nucleic acid. This material must be distinguished from bacteria. This dog was negative on a lupus erythematosus preparation and positive on antinuclear antibody assay and rheumatoid factor assay. Culture of synovial membrane and fluid was unproductive. Stain precipitate is present in the right of the photograph. (May-Grünwald-Giemsa stain, original magnification 1250×.)

subchondral osteolysis, cyst formation, and erosion with transition to destruction of bone. Eventually there can be narrowing of the joint space and varying degrees of joint subluxation or luxation.[74] Obtaining biopsies of synovial membranes and subcutaneous nodules are needed for histopathologic confirmation of lesions that are consistent with rheumatoid arthritis. Synovial fluid analysis reveals inflammation with a predominance of neutrophils, among which many have karyorrhetic and pyknotic nuclei.[75] On occasion patients may have a low positive, or sometimes transient, ANA titer.

Progressive Feline Polyarthritis

There are two types of progressive feline polyarthritis that include an erosive form, clinically similar to canine erosive arthritis, and a more commonly diagnosed periosteal proliferative form. This disease most frequently affects young adult male cats. Feline foamy (syncytium-forming) virus infection is consistently isolated from cats with chronic progressive polyarthritis, among which a majority are co-infected with feline leukemia virus.[76] Synovial fluid analysis reveals an inflammatory arthropathy with a predominance of neutrophils. Cats with the erosive form may have total nucleated cell counts within the reference interval or more prominent fractions of lymphocytes and large mononuclear cells.

References

1. Fernandez FR, Grindem CB, Lipowitz AJ: Synovial fluid analysis: Preparation of smears for cytologic examination of canine synovial fluid. *J Am Anim Hosp Assoc* 19:727-734, 1983.
2. Sawyer DC: Synovial fluid analysis of canine joints. *J Am Vet Med Assoc* 143:609-612, 1963.

3. Pacchiana PD, et al: Absolute and relative cell counts for synovial fluid from clinically normal shoulder and stifle joints in cats. *J Am Vet Med Assoc* 225(12):1866-1870, 2004.

4. Ogston AG, Sherman TF: Degradation of the hyaluronic acid complex of synovial fluid by proteolytic enzymes and by ethylenediaminetetra-acetic acid. *Biochem J* 72(2):301-305, 1959.

5. Atilola MA, Lumsden JH, Rooke F: A comparison of manual and electronic counting for total nucleated cell counts on synovial fluid from canine stifle joints. *Can J Vet Res* 50(2):282-284, 1986.

6. Salinas M, et al: Comparison of manual and automated cell counts in EDTA preserved synovial fluids: Storage has little influence on the results. *Ann Rheum Dis* 56(10):622-626, 1997.

7. de Jonge R, et al: Automated counting of white blood cells in synovial fluid. *Rheumatology* (Oxford) 43(2):170-173, Epub Oct 1, 2003.

8. Sugiuchi H, et al: Measurement of total and differential white blood cell counts in synovial fluid by means of an automated hematology analyzer. *J Lab Clin Med* 146(1):36-42, 2005.

9. Aulesa C, et al: Use of the Advia 120 hematology analyzer in the differential cytologic analysis of biological fluids (cerebrospinal, peritoneal, pleural, pericardial, synovial, and others). *Lab Hematol* 9(4):214-224, 2003.

10. Atilola MA, et al: Intra-articular tissue response to analytical grade metrizamide in dogs. *Am J Vet Res* 45(12):2651-2657, 1984.

11. Warren CF, Bennett GA, Bauer W: The significance of the cellular variations occurring in normal synovial fluid. *Am J Path* 11:953-968, 1935.

12. McCarty DJ Jr, Phelps P, Pyenson J: Crystal-induced inflammation in canine joints. I. An experimental model with quantification of the host response. *J Exp Med* 124(1):99-114, 1966.

13. MacWilliams PS, Friedrichs KR: Laboratory evaluation and interpretation of synovial fluid. *Vet Clin North Am Small Anim Pract* 33(1):153-178, 2003.

14. Shirtliff ME, Mader JT: Acute septic arthritis. *Clin Microbiol Rev* 15(4):527-544, 2002.

15. Montgomery RD, et al: Comparison of aerobic culturette, synovial membrane biopsy, and blood culture medium in detection of canine bacterial arthritis. *Vet Surg* 18(4):300-303, 1989.

16. Johnson KA, Watson ADJ: Skeletal diseases. In Ettinger SJ, Feldman EC (eds): *Textbook of Veterinary Internal Medicine: Diseases of the Dog and Cat*, ed 6. St. Louis, Saunders, 2005, pp 1965-1991.

17. Lewis DD, et al: A comparison of diagnostic methods used in the evaluation of early degenerative joint disease in the dog. *J Am Anim Hosp Assoc* 23:305-315, 1987.

18. Griffen DW, Vasseur PB: Synovial fluid analysis in dogs with cranial cruciate ligament rupture. *J Am Anim Hosp Assoc* 28:277-280, 1992.

19. Hayashi K, Manley PA, Muir P: Cranial cruciate ligament pathophysiology in dogs with cruciate disease: A review. *J Am Anim Hosp Assoc* 40(5):385-390, 2004.

20. Mansell P: Hemophilia A and B. In Giger U (ed): *Schalm's Veterinary Hematology*, ed 5. Baltimore, Lippincott Williams and Wilkins, 2000, pp 1026-1029.

21. Hooiveld M, et al: Blood-induced joint damage: long term effects in vitro and in vivo. *J Rheumatol* 30(2):339-344, 2003.

22. Pool RR, Thompson KG: Tumors of joints. In Meuten DJ (ed): *Tumors in Domestic Animals*, ed 4. Ames, Iowa, Iowa State Press, 2002, pp 199-243.

23. Thompson KG, Pool RR: Tumors of bones. In Meuten DJ (ed): *Tumors in Domestic Animals*, ed 4. Ames, Iowa, Iowa State Press, 2002, pp 245-317.

24. Wilson DW, Dungworth DL: Tumors of The respiratory tract. In Meuten DJ (ed): *Tumors in Domestic Animals*, ed 4. Ames, Iowa, Iowa State Press, 2002, pp 365-399.

25. Lahmers SM, et al: Synovial T-cell lymphoma of the stifle in a dog. *J Am Anim Hosp Assoc* 38(2):165-168, 2002.

26. Marchevsky AM, Read RA: Bacterial septic arthritis in 19 dogs. *Aust Vet J* 77(4):233-237, 1999.

27. Clements DN, et al: Retrospective study of bacterial infective arthritis in 31 dogs. *J Small Anim Pract* 46(4):171-171, 2005.

28. Liehmann L, et al: *Mycoplasma felis* arthritis in two cats. *J Small Anim Pract* 47(8):476-479, 2006.

29. Jauernig S, et al: The effects of doxycycline on nitric oxide and stromelysin production in dogs with cranial cruciate ligament rupture. *Vet Surg* 30(2):132-139, 2001.

30. Greene CE, Watson ADJ: Antibacterial chemotherapy. In Greene CE (ed): *Infectious Disease of the Dog and Cat*, ed 3. St. Louis, Saunders, 2006, pp 274-301.

31. Goodman RA, et al: Molecular identification of *Ehrlichia ewingii* infection in dogs: 15 cases (1997-2001). *J Am Vet Med Assoc* 222(8):1102-1107, 2003.

32. Greene CE, Budsberg SC: Musculoskeletal infections. In Greene CE (ed): *Infectious Diseases of the Dog and Cat*, ed 3. Saunders, 2006, pp 823-841.

33. Goldman EE, et al: Granulocytic ehrlichiosis in dogs from North Carolina and Virginia. *J Vet Intern Med* 12(2):61-70, 1998.

34. Stockham SL, et al: Evaluation of granulocytic ehrlichiosis in dogs of Missouri, including serologic status to *Ehrlichia canis*, *Ehrlichia equi* and *Borrelia burgdorferi*. *Am J Vet Res* 53(1):63-68, 1992.

35. Poitout FM, et al: Genetic variants of *Anaplasma phagocytophilum* infecting dogs in Western Washington State. *J Clin Microbiol* 43(2):796-801, 2005.

36. Straubinger RK, et al: *Borrelia burgdorferi* migrates into joint capsules and causes an up-regulation of interleukin-8 in synovial membranes of dogs experimentally infected with ticks. *Infect Immun* 65(4):1273-1285, 1997.

37. Straubinger RK, et al: *Borrelia burgdorferi* induces the production and release of proinflammatory cytokines in canine synovial explant cultures. *Infect Immun* 66(1):247-247, 1998.

38. Huss B, et al: Polyarthropathy and chorioretinitis with retinal detachment in a dog with systemic histoplasmosis. *J Am Anim Hosp Assoc* 30:217-224, 1994.

39. Bennett D: Immune-mediated and infective arthritis. In Ettinger SJ, Feldman EC (ed): *Textbook of Veterinary Internal Medicine: Diseases of the Dog and Cat*, ed 6. St. Louis, Saunders, 2005, pp 1958-1965.

40. Barton MD, et al: Isolation of *Mycoplasma spumans* from polyarthritis in a greyhound. *Aust Vet J* 62(6):206-207, 1985.

41. Moise NS, et al: *Mycoplasma gateae* arthritis and tenosynovitis in cats: case report and experimental reproduction of the disease. *Am J Vet Res* 44(1):16-21, 1983.

42. Gaskin AA, et al: Visceral leishmaniasis in a New York foxhound kennel. *J Vet Intern Med* 16(1):34-44, 2002.

43. Agut A, et al: Clinical and radiographic study of bone and joint lesions in 26 dogs with leishmaniasis. *Vet Rec* 153(21):648-652, 2003.

44. TerWee J, et al: Comparison of the primary signs induced by experimental exposure to either a pneumotrophic or a 'limping' strain of feline calicivirus. *Vet Microbiol* 56(1-2):33-45, 1997.

45. Pedersen NC, Laliberte L, Ekman S: A transient febrile limping syndrome of kittens caused by two different strains of feline calicivirus. *Feline Pract* 13:26-35, 1983.

46. Levy JK, Marsh A: Isolation of calicivirus from the joint of a kitten with arthritis. *J Am Vet Med Assoc* 201(5):753-735, 1992.

47. Pedersen NC: A review of immunologic diseases of the dog. *Vet Immunol Immunopathol* 69(2-4):251-342, 1999.

48. Bennett D: Immune-based non-erosive inflammatory joint disease of the dog. III. Canine idiopathic polyarthritis. *J Small Anim Pract* 28:909-928, 1987.

49. Ollier WE, et al: Dog MHC alleles containing the human RA shared epitope confer susceptibility to canine rheumatoid arthritis. *Immunogenetics* 53(8):669-673, 2001. Epub Oct 13, 2001.

50. Hewicker-Trautwein M, et al: Immunocytochemical demonstration of lymphocyte subsets and MHC class II antigen expression in synovial membranes from dogs with rheumatoid arthritis and degenerative joint disease. *Vet Immunol Immunopathol* 67(4):341-357, 1999.

51. Goldstein RE: Swollen joints and lameness. In Ettinger SJ, Feldman EC (eds): *Textbook of Veterinary Internal Medicine: Diseases of the Dog and Cat*, ed 6. St. Louis, Saunders, 2005, pp 83-87.

52. Center SA: Fluid accumulation disorders. In Willard MD, Tvedten H, Turnwald GH, (eds): *Small Animal Clinical Diagnosis by Laboratory Methods*, ed 4. St. Louis, Saunders, 2004, pp 263-266.

53. Clements DN, et al: Type I immune-mediated polyarthritis in dogs: 39 cases (1997-2002). *J Am Vet Med Assoc* 224(8):1323-1327, 2004.

54. Rondeau MP, et al: Suppurative, nonseptic polyarthropathy in dogs. *J Vet Intern Med* 19(5):654-662, 2005.

55. Sibilia J, Limbach FX: Reactive arthritis or chronic infectious arthritis? *Ann Rheum Dis* 61(7):580-587, 2002.

56. MacDonald KA, et al: A prospective study of canine infective endocarditis in northern California (1999-2001): Emergence of *Bartonella* as a prevalent etiologic agent. *J Vet Intern Med* 18(1):56-64, 2004.

57. Goodman RA, Breitschwerdt EB: Clinicopathologic findings in dogs seroreactive to *Bartonella henselae* antigens. *Am J Vet Res* 66(12):2060-2064, 2005.

58. Summers BA, et al: Histopathological studies of experimental lyme disease in the dog. *J Comp Pathol* 133(1):1-13, 2005.

59. Greene CE, Breitschwerdt EB: Rocky Mountain spotted fever, murine typhuslike disease, rickettsial pox, typhus, and Q fever. In Greene CE (ed): *Infectious Diseases of The Dog and Cat*, ed 3. St. Louis, Saunders, 2006, pp 232-245.

60. Breitschwerdt EB: Obligate Intracellular bacterial pathogens. In Ettinger SJ, Feldman EC, (eds): *Textbook of Veterinary Internal Medicine*. St. Louis, Saunders, 2005, pp 631-636.

61. Tarello W: Microscopic and clinical evidence for *Anaplasma (Ehrlichia) phagocytophilum* infection in Italian cats. *Vet Rec* 156(24):772-774, 2005.

62. Guilford WG: Idiopathic inflammatory bowel diseases. In Guilford WG, et al (eds): *Strombeck's Small Animal Gastroenterology*, ed 3. Philadelphia, Saunders, 1996, pp 451-486.

63. Webb AA, Taylor SM, Muir GD: Steroid-responsive meningitis-arteritis in dogs with noninfectious, nonerosive, idiopathic, immune-mediated polyarthritis. *J Vet Intern Med* 16(3):269-273, 2002.

64. Bennett D, Kelly DF: Immune-based non-erosive inflammatory joint disease of the dog. II. Polyarthritis/ polymyositis syndrome. *J Small Anim Pract* 28:891-908, 1987.

65. Trepanier LA, et al: Clinical findings in 40 dogs with hypersensitivity associated with administration of potentiated sulfonamides. *J Vet Intern Med* 17(5):647-652, 2003.

66. Couto CG, et al: In vitro immunologic features of Weimaraner dogs with neutrophil abnormalities and recurrent infections. *Vet Immunol Immunopathol* 23(1-2):103-112, 1989.

67. Foale RD, Herrtage ME, Day MJ: Retrospective study of 25 young Weimaraners with low serum immunoglobulin concentrations and inflammatory disease. *Vet Rec* 153(18):553-558, 2003.

68. Gaskell RM, Dawson S, Radford AW: Feline respiratory disease. In Greene CE, (eds): *Infectious Diseases of the Dog and Cat*, ed 3. St. Louis, Saunders, 2006, pp 145-154.

69. Stone M: Systemic lupus erythematosus. In Ettinger SJ, Feldman EC (eds): *Textbook of Veterinary Internal Medicine*, ed 6. St. Louis, Saunders, 2005, pp 1952-1957.

70. Monier JC, et al: Canine systemic lupus erythematosus. II. Antinuclear antibodies. *Lupus* 1(5):287-293, 1992.

71. Dougherty SA, et al: Juvenile-onset polyarthritis syndrome in Akitas. *J Am Vet Med Assoc* 198(5):849-856, 1991.

72. Vaden SL: Glomerular disease. In Ettinger SJ, Feldman EC , (eds): *Textbook of Veterinary Internal Medicine*, ed 6. St. Louis, Saunders, 2005, pp 1786-1800.

73. May C, Hammill J, Bennett D: Chinese Shar Pei fever syndrome: A preliminary report. *Vet Rec* 131(25-26):586-587, 1992.

74. Allan G: Radiographic signs of joint disease. In Thrall DE (ed): *Textbook of Veterinary Diagnostic Radiology*, ed 4. Philadelphia, Saunders, 2002, pp 187-207.

75. Bennett D: Immune-based erosive inflammatory joint disease of the dog: Canine rheumatoid arthritis. I. Clinical, radiological and laboratory investigations. *J Small Anim Pract* 28:779-797, 1987.

76. Pedersen NC, Pool RR, O'Brien T: Feline chronic progressive polyarthritis. *Am J Vet Res* 41(4):522-535, 1980.

The Musculoskeletal System

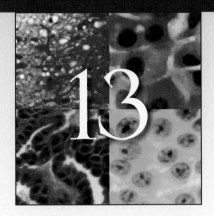

S.E. Fielder and E.A. Mahaffey

CHAPTER 13

Although cytologic techniques have not been used extensively in evaluating diseases of the musculoskeletal system, they can be valuable aids in the diagnosis of certain important diseases affecting this system. One would perhaps suspect that muscle, being a soft tissue, would be a more productive tissue for cytologic examination than bone. In fact, the opposite is true. Diseases of bone yield diagnostic cytology specimens more often than do diseases of muscle. The following are several reasons for this difference:

- Inflammatory and neoplastic lesions lend themselves to cytologic diagnosis, but degenerative diseases do not. There are relatively few clinically important inflammatory and neoplastic diseases of muscle compared with those of bone.
- Aspirates and imprints of muscle tissue typically yield only blood. Striated muscle cells do not exfoliate readily, and inflammatory diseases of muscle, when they do occur, are often characterized by modest infiltration of inflammatory cells.
- Although healthy bone tissue is difficult to sample and contains few cells and abundant matrix, both inflammatory and neoplastic bone diseases are usually accompanied by bone lysis and increased cellularity. Both lytic and proliferative bone lesions are often easily aspirated.

SAMPLE COLLECTION

Collection of material from bone lesions for cytologic examination can be complicated by the hardness of cortical bone. Lesions that have a major soft tissue component can be aspirated by techniques similar to those for any soft tissue mass (see Chapter 1). Even heavily mineralized masses can often be aspirated with a fine needle by careful palpation and exploration of the lesion surface. Examination of radiographs may reveal portions of the lesion that are less heavily mineralized and more likely to produce useful aspirates. Some lesions in which the cortical bone remains intact will not yield to fine-needle aspiration. In such instances, the best way to obtain diagnostic material is to use a trephine to obtain a core biopsy specimen. Imprints can be made for cytologic evaluation

before the specimen is fixed in formalin for histologic processing. Remember it is important to keep cytology smears away from formalin fumes because these will inactivate cellular enzymes and interfere with cytologic staining and evaluation.

Cytologic specimens from skeletal muscle lesions can be collected by methods similar to those used for dermal and subcutaneous masses that are described in Chapter 5.

INFLAMMATORY DISEASES

Inflammatory lesions of the skeleton are important causes of disease in domestic animals, and cytology can be a valuable diagnostic tool in identifying certain lesions. Cytologic specimens from inflammatory lesions of bone are generally similar to exudates from other organs. Neutrophils typically predominate in specimens from animals with osteomyelitis, although activated macrophages and multinucleate giant cells are a significant component of some exudates. Inflammatory lesions that are accompanied by new bone proliferation may yield cytologic specimens that also contain small numbers of osteoblasts, which typically range from plump and ovoid to fusiform with round to ovoid eccentric nuclei and dark blue cytoplasm. They differ from neoplastic osteoblasts in that they are smaller and more uniform and lack nuclear manifestations of malignancy (see Chapter 2).

Osteoclasts may also be found in small numbers in specimens from inflammatory lesions. These cells resemble multinucleate giant cells and arise from precursor cells of the monocyte/macrophage cell line. They are very large and irregularly shaped with variable numbers (typically 6 to 10) of uniform, round nuclei arranged randomly throughout the cell and the abundant, light blue cytoplasm (Figure 13-1).

Some specific infectious agents that cause osteomyelitis may be identified in cytologic preparations. *Actinomyces* spp. occasionally cause osteomyelitis in dogs. These organisms appear as branching, filamentous rods that cannot be distinguished from *Nocardia* spp. on Romanowsky-type stains. Neutrophils predominate in aspirates from actinomycotic lesions as well as in aspirates from other

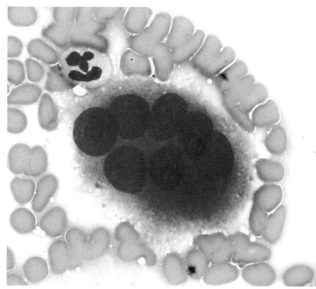

Figure 13-1 Osteoclast with multiple, relatively uniform nuclei and abundant cytoplasm from a lytic bone lesion. (Wright's stain.)

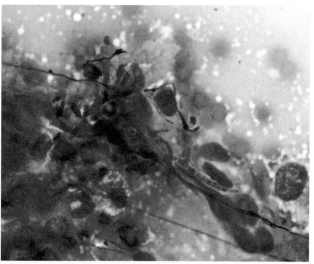

Figure 13-2 Fungal hyphae from lytic bone lesion in a dog. *Aspergillus* was cultured from this lesion. (Wright's stain.)

types of bacterial osteomyelitis. Bacterial cocci in such aspirates are indicative of infection by staphylococci or streptococci, and bipolar rods are typical of infection by gram-negative organisms.[1,2]

Osteomyelitis is also a relatively common manifestation of coccidioidomycosis and the organisms may be detected in the exudate. The exudate in *Coccidioides immitis* infections is typically more mixed than that in bacterial infections and often contains a much larger component of activated macrophages and multinucleate giant cells. Other fungal organisms, including *Blastomyces dermatitidis* and *Histoplasma capsulatum,* may produce osteomyelitis with a similar exudates.[3] Hyphating fungal organisms such as *Aspergillus* spp. can also be seen and appear as staining or nonstaining fungal hyphae (Figures 13-2 and 13-3).

NEOPLASTIC DISEASES

Tumors of Bone

Neoplasms of bone are relatively common in domestic animals, and cytologic examination is useful in establishing the diagnosis in some of these diseases. As with the interpretation of histologic sections of bone, evaluation of cytologic specimens from bone requires knowledge of the clinical and radiographic features of a specific lesion. Cytology is probably more useful in distinguishing inflammatory bone disease from neoplasia than in identifying specific bone tumors; however, osteosarcomas and chondrosarcomas do have characteristic cytologic features that can aid in diagnosis.

Osteosarcoma: Osteosarcoma is the most common primary bone tumor, and the appendicular skeleton is more commonly affected. In the dog, osteosarcoma occurs more commonly in the front limbs with the distal radius and

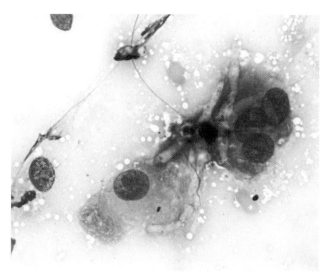

Figure 13-3 Nonstaining fungal hyphae from a lytic bone lesion. (Wright's stain.)

proximal humerus as the most common sites.[4] Aspirates of osteosarcomas are often more highly cellular than aspirates of soft tissue sarcomas. Cells may occur singly or in clusters. One characteristic feature that may be evident on low-power examination of the slide is the presence of islands of osteoid surrounded by tumor cells.[5,6] Osteoid (Figure 13-4) appears as a somewhat fibrillar, bright pink material on Wright's-stained slides. These structures are not found in most aspirates from osteosarcomas; however, when found, their presence provides strong evidence that a tumor is of bone origin. Individual tumor cells vary from round to plump to fusiform, and often vary greatly in size (Figure 13-5). They often have many of the classic cytologic features of malignancy, such as karyomegaly, anisokaryosis, large nucleoli, and multiple nucleoli that differ in size (see Chapter 2). Cytoplasm is typically dark blue

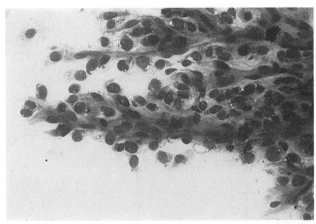

Figure 13-4 Osteoblasts interspersed with pink-staining intercellular matrix (osteoid) from an osteosarcoma. (Wright's stain.)

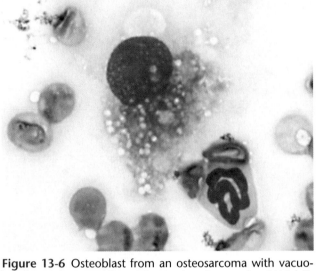

Figure 13-6 Osteoblast from an osteosarcoma with vacuolated cytoplasm and fine pink cytoplasmic granules. (Wright's stain.)

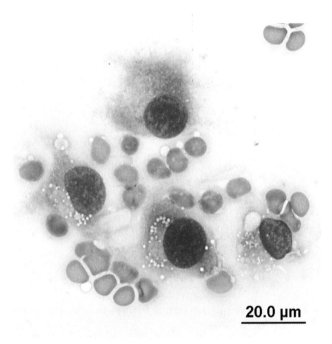

20.0 μm

Figure 13-5 Aspirate of an osteosarcoma showing marked variation in cell size and shape. (Wright's stain.)

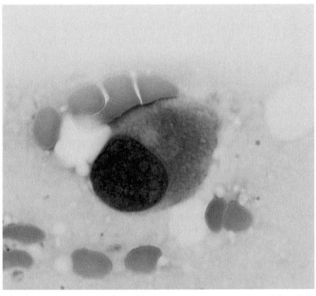

Figure 13-7 Osteoblast from an osteosarcoma with pink cytoplasmic granules. (Wright's stain.)

and may contain several clear vacuoles (Figure 13-6). A proportion of the cells from most osteosarcomas contain scattered, pink cytoplasmic granules (Figure 13-7). These granules are not specific to osteosarcomas; similar granules may also occur in cells from chondrosarcomas and, less commonly, from fibrosarcomas. Cells from more differentiated osteosarcomas (Figure 13-8) are more uniform and may be difficult to distinguish from normal osteoblasts. Small numbers of inflammatory cells, nonneoplastic osteoblasts, and osteoclasts similar to those described in the previous section on inflammation may also be found in aspirates from osteosarcomas.

Chondrosarcoma: These tumors are the second most common sarcomas of bone. The ribs, turbinates, and pelvis are the most common sites for chondrosarcomas of dogs, and the scapulae, vertebrae, and ribs are more common sites in cats.[7] One useful cytologic feature of chondrosarcomas that may be evident on low-power examination of aspirates is the presence of lakes of bright pink, smooth or slightly granular material, in which cells may be embedded (Figure 13-9). This material is the intercellular matrix of cartilage and has been called *chondroid*.[6] Although the presence of this material suggests the possibility of a cartilaginous origin of a tumor, it is not a consistent finding in aspirates of chondrosarcomas.

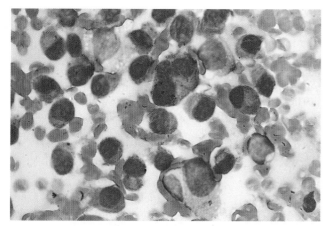

Figure 13-8 Relatively well-differentiated osteoblasts with eccentric nuclei and deeply basophilic cytoplasm from an osteosarcoma. (Wright's stain.)

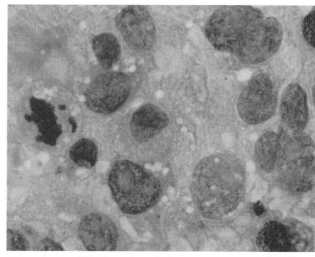

Figure 13-10 Aspirate of a chondrosarcoma with pleomorphic connective tissue cells, including one cell in mitosis. (Wright's stain.)

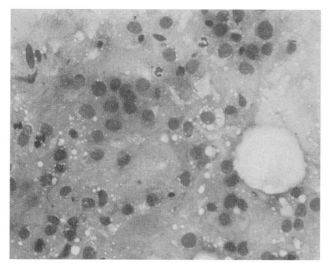

Figure 13-9 Low-power view of an aspirate from a chondrosarcoma showing tumor cells surrounded by pink matrix material resembling mucus. (Wright's stain.)

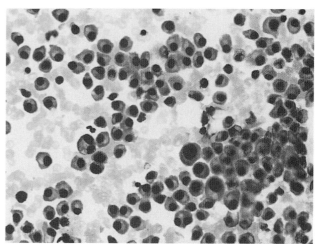

Figure 13-11 Sheets of neoplastic plasma cells from a lytic bone lesion in a dog with plasma cell myeloma. (Wright's stain.)

Individual chondroblasts from chondrosarcomas have cytologic features that are similar to those of osteosarcoma cells. They vary from round to fusiform with large nuclei and dark blue cytoplasm (Figure 13-10). Anisokaryosis is prominent, and multinucleate tumor cells may be found. The cytoplasm often contains several small, clear vacuoles, and cells may occasionally contain fine pink cytoplasmic granules similar to those in cells from osteosarcomas. If a tumor is causing bone lysis, osteoclasts may also be found in cytologic specimens. Even though it is often not possible to distinguish chondrosarcomas from osteosarcomas in cytologic specimens, characterization of the lesion as neoplastic often provides clinically important information.

Other Bone Neoplasms: Fibrosarcomas and hemangiosarcomas are among the other neoplasms that arise with some frequency in bone. Cytologic features of these tumors are similar to those of the same tumors

when they occur in soft tissues. Metastatic tumors may also present clinically as bone tumors; carcinomas exhibit this behavior most commonly. The cytologic features of metastatic neoplastic cells are similar to those of the soft tissue tumors from which they originated. Most hematopoietic neoplasms that involve bone marrow do not present clinically as bone tumors. One major exception is the plasma cell myeloma (Figure 13-11), which may have radiographic manifestations of bone lysis. Aspirates of lytic lesions may yield sheets of neoplastic plasma cells. These cells often appear atypical with several nuclear criteria of malignancy, but may also be well differentiated and exhibit only mild pleomorphism.[8] Bone marrow aspirates from nonlytic areas often yield increased numbers of plasma cells, but do not provide sufficient evidence for a definitive diagnosis of plasma cell myeloma.

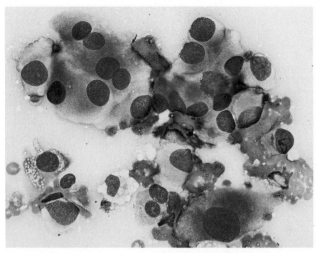

Figure 13-12 Aspirate of a rhabdomyosarcoma showing criteria of malignancy such as anisocytosis, anisokaryosis, and prominent nucleoli. (Wright's stain.)

SKELETAL MUSCLE TUMORS

Primary skeletal muscle tumors, rhabdomyomas and rhabdomyosarcomas, rarely occur. Canine rhabdomyomas have been primarily reported in the larynx, whereas canine rhabdomyosarcomas have been reported in numerous sites including the myocardium, urinary bladder, vagina, tongue, larynx, scapular muscle region, and triceps muscle.[9,10] On cytology, both rhabdomyomas and rhabdomyosarcomas consist of individualized polygonally shaped cells that contain a large amount of granular eosinophilic cytoplasm and resemble oncocytes[11]. These cells have also been reported to sometimes have vacuolated cytoplasm and contain intracytoplasmic invaginations.[12,13] Elongated cells with cross-striations, "strap cells" are rarely seen on cytology of either lesion.[14] A second population of smaller reserve cells may be seen in aspirates from rhabdomyomas.[10] Differentiation between a rhabdomyoma and rhabdomyosarcoma on cytology is difficult, but if sufficient criteria of malignancy are present, a rhabdomyosarcoma should be suspected. Rhabdomyosarcomas often display increased pleomorphism, including spindle and ovoid shaped cells, with marked anisocytosis and anisokaryosis and multiple nucleoli of varying size within a single nucleus (Figure 13-12).[15,16] Rhabdomyosarcomas may also contain several multinucleate cells.[17,18] Histopathology with special stains and immunohistochemistry are usually required for a definitive diagnosis of rhabdomyoma or rhabdomyosarcoma.[11-13]

Lipomas, fibrosarcomas, and malignant fibrous histiocytomas are among the more common tumors presenting clinically as skeletal muscle tumors. Although most of these tumors probably arise in the subcutis, they may infiltrate underlying muscle so extensively that they appear as muscle tumors on presentation. Their cytologic features are described in Chapter 5.

References

1. Emmerson TD, Pead MJ: Pathologic fracture of the femur secondary to haematogenous osteomyelitis in a Weimaraner. *J Small Anim Pract* 40(5):233-2335, 1999.
2. Dehghani SN, Hajighahramani S: Eosinophilia due to osteomyelitis in a dog. *J Vet Sci* 6(3):255-257, 2005.
3. Wolf AM: *Histoplasma capsulatum* osteomyelitis in the cat. *J Vet Intern Med* 1(4):158-162, 1987.
4. Thompson and Pool. In Mueten (ed): *Tumors in Domestic Animals*. Ames, Iowa, Iowa State Press, 2002, pp 266-283.
5. Rebar AH. In Rebar: *Handbook of Veterinary Cytology*. St Louis, Ralston Purina, 1978, pp 37-50.
6. Willems. In Linsk and Franzen: *Clinical Aspiration Cytology*. New York, Lippincott, 1983, pp 349-359.
7. Pool. In Moulton: *Tumors in Domestic Animals*. Berkeley, Calif, University of Calif Press, 1978, pp 89-149.
8. Patel PT, et al: Multiple myeloma in 16 cats: A retrospective study. *Vet Clin Pathol* 34(4):341-352, 2005.
9. Ueno H, et al: Perianal rhabdomyosarcoma in a dog. *J Small Anim Pract* 43:217-220, 2002.
10. Akkoc A: et al: Cardiac metastasizing rhabdomyosarcoma in a great dane. *Vet Rec* 158:803-804, 2006.
11. Barnhart K, Lewis B: Laryngopharyngeal mass in a dog with upper airway obstruction. *Vet Clin Pathol* 29(2):47-50, 2000.
12. Liggett AD: et al: Canine laryngopharyngeal rhabdomyoma resembling an oncocytoma: Light microscopic ultrastructural and comparative studies. *Vet Pathol* 22:526-532, 1985.
13. Rivera RY: Carlton WW: Lingual rhabdomyoma in a dog. *J Comp Pathol* 106:83-87, 1992.
14. Meuten DJ: et al: Canine laryngeal rhabdomyoma. *Vet Pathol* 22:533-539, 1985.
15. Ginel PJ: et al: Skeletal muscle rhabdomyosarcoma in a dog. *Vet Rec* 151:736-738, 2002.
16. Suzuki K: et al: Vaginal rhabdomyosarcoma in a dog. *Vet Pathol* 43:(2), 186-188, 2006.
17. Brockus CW, Myers RK: Multifocal rhabdomyosarcoma within the tongue and oral cavity of a dog. *Vet Pathol* 41:273-274, 2004.
18. Fallin CW, et al: What is your diagnosis? A 12-month-old dog with multiple soft tissue masses. *Vet Clin Pathol* 24(3):80, 1995.

Cerebrospinal Fluid Analysis

M. Desnoyers, C. Bédard, J.H. Meinkoth, and M.A. Crystal

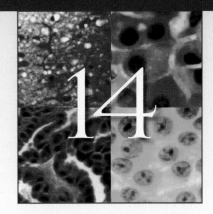

CHAPTER 14

Cytology of the cerebrospinal fluid (CSF) may be an important component of the diagnostic evaluation of patients with neurologic diseases. It may also be useful in patients with neck or limb pain and/or fever of unknown origin. As we will see in this chapter, it is important to emphasize that different pathologies may result in similar CSF changes due to the narrow range of inflammatory response in the central nervous system (CNS). Moreover, the absence of changes in the CSF does not eliminate the possibility of a process affecting the central nervous system. Therefore, in most instances a final diagnosis can be reached only with a combination of clinical history, physical findings, medical imaging, CSF findings, and other tests such as a complete blood count (CBC), biochemistry panel as well as serology, polymerase chain reaction (PCR), and histopathology.

COLLECTION TECHNIQUES

CSF collection is performed while the patient is under anesthesia. Atlantooccipital puncture is performed using a 3.8-cm (1½-inch), 22-gauge spinal needle (occasionally, a 5-cm [2-inch] needle may be needed for dogs over 25 kg or for smaller dogs that are obese). For cats and dogs weighing less than 6 to 8 kg, a 1.2-cm (½-inch), 21-gauge butterfly catheter may be used. Lumbar puncture is performed using a 3.8-cm (1½-in) or 5.4-cm (2⅛-in), 22-gauge spinal needle. Other materials needed for CSF collection include clippers, supplies for sterile preparation of the site, sterile surgical gloves, and ethylene-tetra-acetic acid (EDTA) (purple top) and a sterile evacuated (red top) tubes in which to catch and submit the fluid. The laboratory should be notified before the collection is performed because rapid processing of the sample is important in achieving accurate results.

Before CSF collection, the patient should be assessed for clinical signs that might suggest an increase in intracranial pressure. Signs of increased intracranial pressure are variable, but may include cranial nerve signs (such as anisocoria or mydriatic/nonresponsive pupils), dull mentation/altered state of consciousness, rigid paresis, altered respiratory patterns and heart rhythms (bradycardia), and coma. If these are present, CSF collection should be postponed and appropriate therapy instituted. If CSF collection cannot be postponed, mannitol (2 g/kg, intravenously [IV]) should be given over 30 minutes, 1 hour before induction, and furosemide (2 mg/kg, IV) and either dexamethasone sodium phosphate (1 mg/kg, IV) or prednisolone sodium succinate (20 mg/kg, IV [slowly]) should be given 10 to 15 minutes before induction. Additionally, the patient should be positively hyperventilated for 5 minutes before the start of the procedure.

The location for CSF collection is selected based on the neurologic localization of the lesion. For lesions above the foramen magnum and of the extreme craniocervical spinal cord, CSF is collected from the atlantooccipital space (cerebellomedullary cistern). For lesions below the craniocervical spinal cord, CSF is collected from the lumbar subarachnoid space between lumbar vertebrae 5 and 6 (L5-6). Approximately 0.2 ml/kg of CSF can be safely collected.

For atlantooccipital collection, an area extending 3 to 4 cm from midline in each lateral direction from just cranial to the occipital protuberance to just caudal to the dorsal spinous process of the axis is clipped and sterilely prepared. The patient is then placed in lateral recumbency (right lateral for right-handed individuals), the nose is positioned parallel to the table, and the head is flexed ventrally to maximally open the atlantooccipital space. With sterile gloves, the clinician inserts the needle (bevel facing cranial for lesions cranial to the foramen magnum or caudal for extremely craniocervical lesions) on the midline just in front of the dorsal spinous process of the axis in the caudal area of a triangle formed by the cranial aspects of the wings of the atlas and the occipital protuberance. The needle should be aimed toward the tip of the nose. Usually, a popping sensation can be felt when the needle penetrates the dura mater. The stylet is then removed from the needle and, avoiding the first drop to minimize sample contamination, CSF fluid is allowed to drip into the collection tubes (the EDTA tube is of greater importance and thus should be used first).

If a popping sensation is not felt, and the needle has been advanced enough to potentially be through the dura mater, the stylet should be removed and 2 to 3 seconds allowed for CSF flow. If flow is not detected, the stylet can be replaced and the needle advanced farther. This technique is repeated until CSF flow occurs. It is always best to remove the stylet to check for CSF flow every 2 to 3 mm if the needle-tip position is uncertain because penetration of the medulla oblongata can result in death by cardiorespiratory arrest.

If the needle strikes bone during insertion, slight cranial or caudal redirection can be attempted to enter the atlantooccipital space. In this case, success is usually achieved only by withdrawing the needle, reassessing landmarks, and repeating the procedure. If the CSF drips at an extraordinarily slow rate, bilateral jugular vein compression can be attempted to hasten flow. Once fluid has been collected, the needle is removed and any fluid remaining in the needle is allowed to drip into one of the collection tubes. If a butterfly catheter is used, the needle is inserted as described previously and slowly advanced until fluid is seen entering the clear tubing attached to the needle.

For lumbar puncture, an area extending 3 to 4 cm from midline in each lateral direction from just caudal to the wings of the ileum to the dorsal spinous process of L4 is clipped and sterilely prepared. The patient is then placed in lateral recumbency (right lateral for right-handed individuals) and the lumbosacral area is flexed by bringing the hind limbs forward. With sterile gloves, the clinician inserts the needle on the midline, perpendicular to the spine at the cranial border of the dorsal spinous process of L6. Occasionally, the hind limbs will flinch, indicating penetration of the dura. The stylet is then removed from the needle and, avoiding the first drop to minimize sample contamination, CSF fluid is allowed to drip into the collection tubes. If fluid is not obtained, the stylet is replaced, and the needle is advanced to the floor of the spinal canal. The stylet is then removed and the needle is slowly withdrawn until CSF flow is observed. If the needle strikes bone during insertion, slight cranial or caudal redirection can be attempted, but withdrawing the needle, reassessing landmarks, and repeating the procedure are usually required for success.

Hemorrhage noted during CSF collection is usually a result of needle penetration into a blood vessel or the vertebral sinus and is rarely a result of hemorrhage into the subarachnoid space from a true disease process. If hemorrhage is noted, the needle should be withdrawn and discarded, and the procedure should be repeated with a new needle. An initial hemorrhagic tap does not necessarily lead to blood contamination on subsequent CSF collection attempts.

As mentioned earlier, it is important to emphasize that fluid obtained caudally to the lesion has more chances to be representative of the lesion rather than a fluid taken cranially to that lesion.[1]

SAMPLE PROCESSING

Because total protein and nucleated cell count are usually low compared with whole blood, a sample collected in a red-top (serum) tube is adequate for the great majority of CSF samples[2] without risk of sample clotting. The cerebrospinal fluid is a fairly labile substance and, unless a stabilizing agent is added, is stable under refrigerated conditions for about 4 to 8 hours but, preferably should be analyzed within 30 minutes to 1 hour.[2] Samples with higher protein content (> 50 mg/dl) are stable for a longer period than samples with lower protein content (< 50 mg/dl).[3] A recent study[3] showed a change in the percentage of large mononuclear cells after 2 hours, in small mononuclear cells after 12 hours, and in neutrophils after 24 hours in samples with no added stabilizing agents. Interestingly, the *total* cell count in those samples did not change significantly over a 24-hour period.[3]

Therefore, if a CSF sample cannot be analyzed within 1 hour of collection, the following procedure should be followed if there is sufficient sample (> 1 ml): the CSF should be separated into two aliquots: (1) one aliquot (unaltered) should be used for total protein and nucleated/red blood cell (RBC) count determination and (2) an aliquot containing 20% (volume:volume) fetal calf serum (FCS) or 10% (volume:volume) autologous serum should be used to perform the differential cell count. If the CSF sample is small (< 0.5 ml), adding hetastarch at a ratio of 1:1 should be done and all tests can be performed on the sample because adding hetastarch does not influence total protein. Keep in mind to correct the total cell count due to the dilution effect of the hetastarch.[3,4]

Cell Count

Usually, the CSF cell count is too low to be analyzed by automated machines such as the Cell-Dyn or Advia. Therefore, a cell count using a hemacytometer is still the gold standard for nucleated and red cell count.[2] Some clinical pathologists prefer to stain the cells with new methylene blue (NMB) prior to counting, whereas others count unstained cells.

One technique to stain cells with NMB is to draw NMB into an unheparinized capillary tube until the capillary tube is about one-third full. Then, the stain is emptied from the tube and excess stain is blotted from the tip of the tube. The tube is then filled with CSF. The NMB adhered to the side of the tube stains the cells sufficiently to reveal cellular morphology. Due to the small amount of stain that is retained within the tube, this method does not influence cell count.[3]

Another technique is to draw a small amount of NMB into a capillary tube. The tube is tilted to allow the small amount of NMB to migrate to the middle of the tube, leaving an air pocket on either side of the NMB. A small amount of CSF is then drawn into the tube. The two liquids do not touch each other due to the presence of the air pocket. The capillary tube is then rocked back and forth several times so that the two columns of liquid move side to side, without touching. The tube is then allowed to sit for 10 minutes. The presence of the air pocket prevents the CSF and NMB from mixing together. Therefore, this technique does not influence the cell count.[5]

Cell counts (both nucleated and red cells) are performed by counting all cells (each cell type separately) in the nine large chambers of the hemacytometer. Both sides of the hemacytometer are counted and an average count is obtained by dividing the total of both sides by 2. Because the total area of one side of the hemacytometer is 0.9 mm^3, multiplying the cell count by 1.1 gives the number of cells/μl². Experience may be needed to differentiate small nucleated cells from RBCs: usually nucleated cells have a granular appearance, whereas RBCs have a smooth appearance or may be crenated. If NMB is used, leukocytes will have a blue appearance, whereas RBCs will be unstained (Figure 14-1).

Total Protein Determination

CSF fluid protein concentration is too low to be measured accurately by conventional biochemistry total protein techniques such as biuret or refractometer method. Instead, CSF total protein concentration is measured by using a Coomasie blue or pyrogallol red assay (Fisher Scientific, St-Laurent, QC). A crude method to determine the presence of excess protein in the clinical setting is to use urine chemstrip dipsticks (e.g., Multistix, Bayer Corporation, Elkhart, Ind.; Chemstrip 9, Roche Diagnostics, Laval, QC): the presence of a positive reaction indicates the presence of albumin because globulins are not detected by the dipsticks. Trace to 1+ protein is considered normal.[6]

The Pandy test is a screening test for the presence of immunoglobulin. It is performed by adding 2 or 3 drops of CSF to 1 ml of a 10% carbolic acid solution (10 mg of carbolic acid in 100 ml of distilled water[2]). Turbidity indicates the presence of globulins. The test is fairly sensitive with a sensitivity of approximately 50 mg/dl.[5,7] Agarose gel protein electrophoresis can also be performed on CSF.[8]

Cytologic Slide Preparation

Because CSF is almost always poorly cellular, concentration techniques are required. In a university or private laboratory setting, the use of a cytocentrifuge is the preferred method of preparation. At the University of Montreal, we typically use 200 μl of CSF for slide preparation and prepare between two and four slides (if enough sample is available) in order to get an adequate number of cells. This results in the presence of an adequate number of evenly distributed cells that can be readily recognized. Slides are routinely stained with a modified Wright's stain with some slides retained unstained if special stains are required.

In a private clinic setting, preparation of adequately cellular slides is more problematic. Sometimes, laboratories at local human hospitals can be used to prepare concentrated slides using a cytocentrifuge. These slides can then be examined in-house or mailed off for evaluation. If this is not available, a sedimentation technique is probably the most practical method. One such technique can be found in reference 2 and utilizes the barrel of a tuberculin syringe (the end where the needle is normally attached has been cut off). A hole that is slightly larger than the inside diameter of the syringe barrel, but less than the outside diameter is punched on a piece of filter paper, which is used to absorb excess fluid. The filter paper is placed on top of a clean glass slide, with the hole centered on the slide. The syringe barrel is placed, cut side up, on top of the filter paper so that the hole of the syringe barrel aligns with the hole of the filter paper. The flanged portion of the syringe barrel must then be clamped to the slide to remain steady during the sedimentation process. A sample of CSF is placed within the barrel of the syringe and allowed to sit for 30 to 60 minutes. At the end of the sedimentation period, excess fluid is aspirated or wicked off, and the slide is dried and then stained. Cell recovery is acceptable and representative of the CSF, but this technique is more time consuming.

NORMAL CSF

Normal CSF is a clear, colorless, water-like fluid. The presence of any color or turbidity must be considered abnormal (Table 14-1).

Cell Count

A. Dogs: cell count varies depending on the site of the CSF collection.
   1. Cisternal tap: reference values vary between 1.5 and 5 cells/μl[9,10]
   2. Lumbar taps: reference values vary between 0.5 and 5 cells/μl[9,10]
B. Cats:
   1. Cisternal and lumbar taps: reference values vary between 2 and 8 cells/uL.[10-12]

Total Protein

A. Dogs:
   1. Cisternal tap: reference values vary between 14 and 30 mg/dl[9,10]
   2. Lumbar tap: reference values vary between 30 and 45 mg/dl[9,10]
B. Cats
   1. Cisternal taps: reference values between 18 and 36 mg/dl[11]
   2. Lumbar taps: reference values between 40 and 46 mg/dl[11]

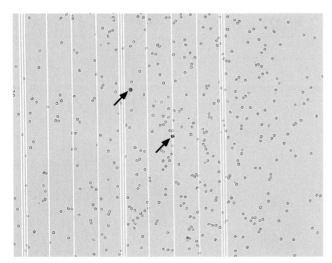

Figure 14-1 Numerous erythrocytes and two leukocytes present on a hemacytometer. The two nuclei of the two leukocytes in the center of the field stain dark purple *(arrows)*. (NBM, original magnification 50×.)

TABLE 14-1

Reference Values for Canine and Feline Cerebrospinal Fluid

Species	Nucleated Cell Count (/µl)	Cell Population	Total Protein (mg/dl)
Canine (cisternal)	1.5-5[9-10]	Predominance of mononuclear cells	14-30[9-10]
		Usually less than 10% neutrophils but sometimes up to 25%[2]	
Canine (lumbar)	0.5-5.0[9-10]	Similar to cisternal	30-45[9-10]
Feline (cisternal)	2-8[10-12]	Similar to dogs	18-36[11]
Feline (lumbar)	2-8[10-12]	Similar to dogs	40-46[11]

Superscripts refer to references in the text.

Type of Cells

The great majority of cells in the CSF are mononuclear in nature with a mixture of small (Figures 14-2 and 14-3) and large (Figures 14-4 and 14-5) mononuclear cells. The presence of less than 10% nondegenerate neutrophils is considered normal by most authors[12,13]. Some studies have found up to 25% nondegenerate neutrophils in normal CSF.[2] The term macrophage should be restricted to mononuclear cells showing evidence of material ingestion in their cytoplasm[13] (Figure 14-6). If contamination from skin occurs, a few anucleate superficial keratinized cells may also be present (Figure 14-7).

Other Parameters

1) *Glucose:* the CSF glucose concentration is usually 60% to 80% that of the blood glucose concentration in both dogs and cats.[2]
2) *Albumin quota:* this value is easily obtained by dividing CSF albumin by serum albumin (CSF albumin/serum albumin). In dogs, the normal value varies between 0.17 and 0.3. An increase of the albumin quota indicates a blood-brain barrier disturbance.[8]
3) *Protein electrophoresis:* if total protein is increased in the CSF, agarose electrophoresis is possible and as little as 10 µl is required for this test. Increased values of immunoglobulins in the CSF associated with a normal albumin quota indicate intrathecal production of immunoglobulins.[8]

INTERPRETATION OF ABNORMAL CSF

CSF cytology can be abnormal even though the cell count is within reference range.[14] Therefore, even when CSF cell count and total protein values are within reference limits, a cytologic examination can be of value.

Blood Contamination and Hemorrhage

Due to the sometimes difficult nature of CSF collection, blood contamination is possible. For instance, in human medicine, one in five lumbar punctures are contaminated

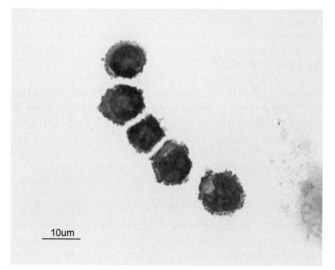

Figure 14-2 Small mononuclear cells in a cerebrospinal fluid sample. (Wright-Giemsa stain.)

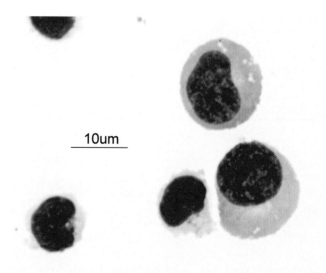

Figure 14-3 Small mononuclear cell in a cerebrospinal fluid sample. The two cells to the left have slightly increased amounts of cytoplasm. (Wright-Giemsa stain.)

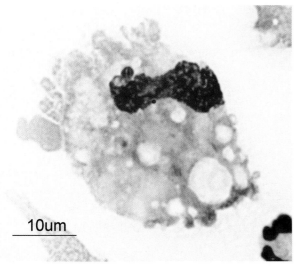

Figure 14-4 Large mononuclear cell with cytoplasmic vacuolation in a cerebrospinal fluid sample. (Wright-Giemsa stain.)

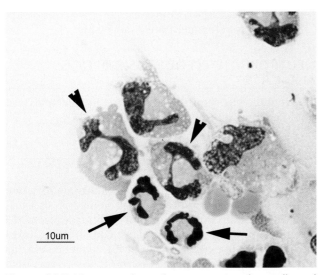

Figure 14-5 Numerous large foamy mononuclear cells and two neutrophils *(arrows)* in a sample of cerebrospinal fluid. Large mononuclear cells may have nuclei that are similar in shape to band cells or neutrophils, only larger *(arrowheads)*. (Wright-Giemsa stain.)

with blood.[15] This blood contamination may result in a pink to frankly reddish appearance. When blood is present, the first thing to determine is if the blood present is contamination (iatrogenic) or secondary to hemorrhage in the CNS (Figure 14-8). If hemorrhage is older than 12 hours, evidence of erythrophagia by macrophages will be seen on cytology. Theoretically, the presence of fresh blood contamination should result in a combination of RBCs without erythrophagia and presence of platelets but, from our own experience, platelets may be difficult to visualize. Also, if hemorrhage of several days' duration is present, the CSF supernatant should be xanthochromic (have a yellow to

yellow-orange discoloration). However, some recent human studies suggest that the human eye cannot reliably detect xanthochromia in CSF. This means that hemoglobin breakdown products may be present in the CSF, but not detectable by the naked eye.[16-17] Therefore, subarachnoid hemorrhage may be present in some instances, but a CSF discoloration will not be recognized. It can also be difficult to differentiate xanthochromia from icterus: a recent human study showed that about 80% of CSF samples with a significant amount of bilirubin appeared red instead of yellow macroscopically.[17] Only spectrophotometry can differentiate xanthochromia from icterus adequately.

Effect of Blood Contamination on Total and Differential Cell Counts and Total Protein Concentration

The influence of blood contamination on total and differential cell counts and total protein concentration depends on the degree of blood contamination (Table 14-2). Some studies have shown that blood contamination yielding RBC counts of up to 15,000 RBC/μl does not influence either nucleated cell count or total protein concentration.[18,19] Another study, however, found that an increase of 1 white blood cell (WBC)/100 RBCs could be found in some cases of blood contamination.[13] Therefore, if the observed WBC count is higher than the predicted increase of 1 WBC/100 RBCs, the increased WBC count is likely real (i.e., it cannot be attributed to blood contamination alone). However, if the CSF WBC count is less than or equal to the predicted blood contamination value, the increase in WBCs might be real or might be secondary to blood contamination. If blood contamination of CSF appears likely from its gross appearance, the best approach is to try to repeat the CSF tap. As a general rule, RBC count > 3000/μl warrants collection of another sample (J. Parent, neurologist, Université de Montréal, Canada, personal communication).

Use of Formulas to Establish Reliable Leukocyte Differential Counts in Cases of Blood Contamination

Several studies in human and veterinary medicine[18,20,21] have shown that correction formulas do not reliably estimate "uncontaminated" WBC values in CSF. This is probably due to the fact that contamination of CSF samples by blood usually results from small meningial or spinal cord vessels that do not have the same proportion of WBCs/RBCs as large peripheral veins.[18]

CHANGES IN THE PERCENTAGE OF LEUKOCYTES WITHOUT PLEOCYTOSIS

Neutrophils

The presence of an increased percentage of neutrophils (10% to 20%) without a pleocytosis can be seen in several conditions (Figure 14-9). Acute trauma to the spinal cord, intravertebral disease,[5] low-grade inflammation secondary to neoplasia, and thiamine deficiency (in cats)[22] can result in an increased percentage of neutrophils without a pleocytosis.

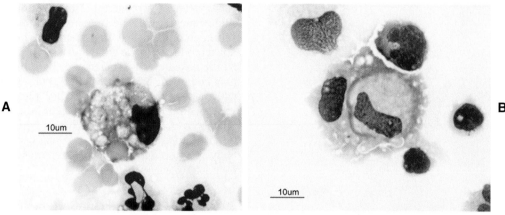

Figure 14-6 Macrophages in cerebrospinal fluid showing evidence of **(A)** erythrophagia and **(B)** cytophagia. (Wright-Giemsa stain.)

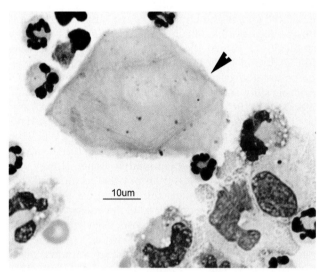

Figure 14-7 CSF sample from a dog. A single large keratinized epithelial cell is present *(arrowhead)*. Squamous epithelial cells represent cutaneous contamination. (Wright-Giemsa stain.)

Eosinophils

It is extremely rare to find eosinophils in CSF from normal dogs and cats. An increased percentage of eosinophils without pleocytosis has been reported in some cases of parasite migration and protozoal diseases[5].

ABNORMAL FINDINGS ASSOCIATED WITH INCREASED CELL COUNT (PLEOCYTOSIS)

Pleocytosis refers to an elevated nucleated cell count in the CSF. The magnitude of the pleocytosis and the type of cells present are both important in recognizing certain disease processes. For the purposes of this discussion, *mild* will refer to counts higher than reference limits but less than 25 cells/µl, *moderate* will refer to cell counts between 26 and 100 cells/µl, and *marked* will refer to cell counts in excess of 100 cells/µl.[5]

    A *neutrophilic* pleocytosis is defined as >50% neutrophils

    A *mixed* pleocytosis as >20% of two or more cell types (e.g., neutrophils, lymphocytes, and mononuclear cells)
    Mononuclear as >75% mononuclear cells
    Lymphocytic as >75% lymphocytes
    Eosinophilic as >20% eosinophils
    References for aforementioned ranges:[22,23]

NEUTROPHILIC PLEOCYTOSIS IN DOGS AND CATS

Neutrophilic pleocytosis can be caused by infectious and noninfectious conditions.

INFECTIOUS/SEPTIC CONDITIONS

Bacterial Meningoencephalitis

Bacterial meningoencephalitis is an uncommon cause of neutrophilic pleocytosis in small animals.[24] In small animals, noninfectious causes of meningoencephalitis are more common than infectious ones (Figures 14-10 and 14-11).[25] Bacteria involved with septic meningitis include *Staphylococcus* spp., *Escherichia coli*, *Pasteurella*, *Bacteroides*, *Fusobacterium*, *Peptostreptococcus*, *Eubacterium*, *Proprionobacterium*, and *Streptococcus*.[24] Bacterial meningoencephalitis usually occurs in one of three ways: (1) direct access, (2) local spread, or (3) hematogenous route.[24] Clinical signs are quite variable depending on the anatomic location and severity of the inflammation[24] but frequently include ataxia and pain. Neck and limb rigidity, paresis, seizures, and cranial nerve dysfunction may be present. Even though the process is septic, fever is not always present.[26]

    CSF analysis usually reveals severe pleocytosis (>100 cells/µl) with marked predominance of neutrophils. Neutrophils may be nondegenerate or degenerate depending on the bacteria present (Figure 14-12). The presence of degenerate neutrophils should push the cytologist to look very carefully for the presence of microorganisms.[5] The protein level is usually elevated in cases of septic meningoencephalitis. The number of bacteria seen on cytology may vary greatly: in some instances, bacteria are readily visible (see Figure 14-12), whereas in other cases bacteria are not found and culture can be negative.[26] For example, a case of inflammatory polyp of the middle ear in a cat resulted in a severe

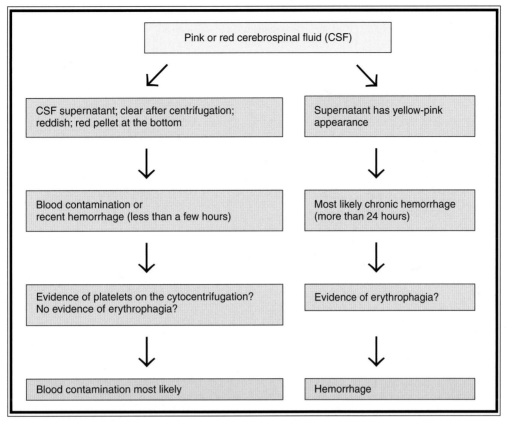

Figure 14-8 Hemorrhage versus blood contamination.

TABLE 14-2

Influence of Blood Contamination on Nucleated Cell Count and Total Protein

Red Blood Cell Count	Influence on Total Protein	Influence on Nucleated Cell Count
Less than 15,000/μl	No[18,19]	No[18,19]
Greater than 15,000/μl	Yes: overestimate[18,19]	Yes: overestimate[18,19]

neutrophilic pleocytosis with absence of bacteria on both the CSF and CSF culture. However, computed tomography scan revealed the presence of a thickened right tympanic bulla: material from the bulla yielded bacterial growth[27].

Acute Distemper in Dogs

Due to widespread vaccination, distemper is now an uncommon disease. In cases of acute distemper infection, neurologic signs associated with a neutrophilic pleocytosis in the CSF may be present. Distemper is caused by a *Morbillivirus* (*Paramyxoviridae* family). Acute encephalitis occurs mostly in younger dogs (less than 1 year old) or in adult dogs that are unable to mount an adequate immune response to the virus.[28] In those cases, other clinical signs are present in addition to the neurologic signs: these signs include nasal discharge, coughing, vomiting, hyperkeratosis, and diarrhea. Neurologic signs include seizures, "chewing-gum fits" (rhythmic contraction of the masticatory muscles), circling, and visual impairment.[28]

CSF analysis usually reveals a mild to moderate pleocytosis with a mixture of nondegenerate neutrophils and mononuclear cells. Protein levels are usually only slightly elevated.

This contrasts with *chronic* cases of distemper where the pleocytosis is usually mononuclear in nature and the protein level is moderately increased. Detection of the virus through nested polymerase chain reaction (RT-PCR)[29] or by detection of antibodies to the virus are the best tools for the final diagnosis of distemper.[28]

Cryptococcosis in Dogs

Cryptococcus neoformans, the agent responsible for crytococcosis, has a predilection for the CNS in dogs and cats.[30] This fungus is most commonly isolated from soil contaminated with pigeon droppings.[28] Most cases are secondary to inhalation of the encapsulated form of the fungus. Dogs are usually younger than 4 years of age. *Cryptococcus* locates itself in the cerebrum, particularly the olfactory bulb,

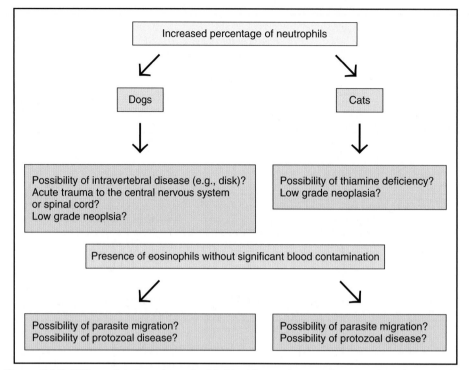

Figure 14-9 Differential of cerebrospinal fluid without pleocytosis, normal total protein but abnormal differential in dogs and cats.

and induces clinical signs such as seizures, ataxia, head tilt, obtundation, and cranial nerve deficits.[30] A thorough eye examination may reveal granulomatous chorioretinitis.[30]

CSF examination usually reveals the presence of yeast forms of the fungus (Figures 14-13 and 14-14). In one study, organisms were visualized in more than 90% of the CSF samples.[31] CSF analysis can be variable and may show either a neutrophilic[32] mononuclear, mixed, or eosinophilic pleocytosis.[32] Total protein is usually elevated. Culturing the organism may be done in dogs but is not as rewarding as in people.[30] Latex agglutination can be performed in either serum or CSF to identify capsular antigen. Sensitivity varies between 91% and 98% and specificity was reported at 98%.[30]

Cryptococcosis in Cats

Cryptococcosis is more common in cats than in dogs and is reported to be the most common systemic fungal disease in cats.[30] There does not seem to be a sex predilection for this disease. Surprisingly, outdoor cats seem only slightly more susceptible than indoor cats to development of cryptococcosis.[34] Clinical signs as well as changes in the CSF are similar to those seen in dogs.

Coccidioidomycosis

Coccidioides immitis is found in the soil in the Lower Sonoran life zone of California, Arizona, and Texas, as well as in Mexico and Central and South America.[35] Infection is usually secondary to inhalation of airborne arthrospores, resulting in pulmonary infection. In dogs with poor immune systems or subjected to an overwhelming exposure, infection to regional lymph nodes and CNS may occur.[35] If the CNS is involved, clinical signs may

include persistent or fluctuating fever, seizures, ataxia, circling, behavioral changes, and possible coma.[35]

CSF changes include a neutrophilic or mixed neutrophilic/mononuclear pleocytosis, increased total protein and globulins.[28] Microorganisms are rarely found on cytology. Serology (complement fixation, immunodiffusion, or enzyme-linked immunosorbent assay [ELISA]) can be useful for a final diagnosis.[36]

Compared with dogs, cats seem to be relatively resistant to coccidioidomycosis.[36] There is no obvious age, breed, or sex predilection, and CNS involvement seems to be very rare.[36]

Phaeohyphomycosis

This is a very rare cause of neutrophilic pleocytosis in the dog and cat. Phaeohyphomycosis refers to infection by pigmented fungi[37] that comprise several genera. Rare cases are found in the literature[37] with animals showing signs of seizures, ataxia, and altered mental state. CSF usually reveals a neutrophilic pleocytosis (sometimes > 100 cells/µl, between 45% and 75% nondegenerate neutrophils) with increased protein, but in some cases, cell count is only slightly increased.[38] Visualization of the fungus is uncommon[39] and culture of the CSF can be negative. Diagnosis therefore may require histopathology.[40] Prognosis for phaeohyphomycosis is usually poor and neurosurgical resection of cerebral lesions is thought to be the most important factor for survival.[30]

Rocky Mountain Spotted Fever

Rocky Mountain spotted fever (RMSF) is caused by *Rickettsia rickettsii* and is transmitted by the wood tick (*Dermacentor andersoni*) in the western part of the United

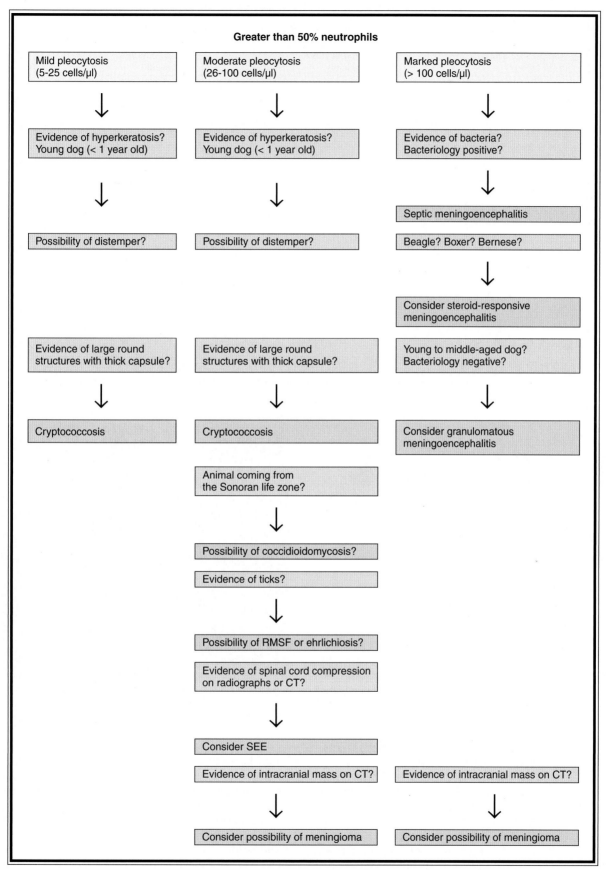

Figure 14-10 Differential diagnosis for neutrophilic pleocytosis in dogs.

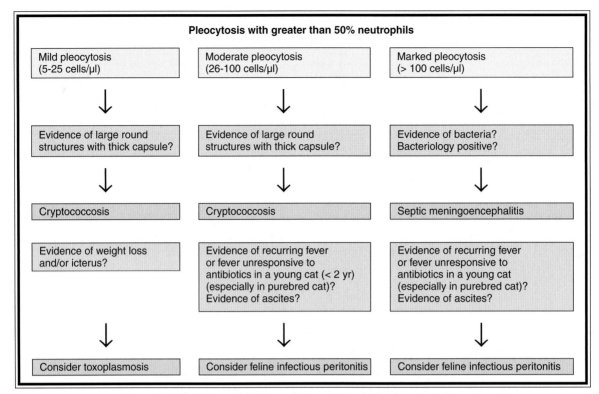

Figure 14-11 Differential diagnosis for neutrophilic pleocytosis in cats.

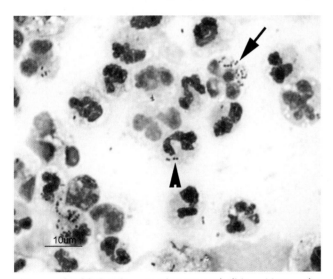

Figure 14-12 Septic meningoencephalitis. Note the degenerate neutrophils and the presence of bacteria *(arrow)*. (Wright-Giemsa stain.)

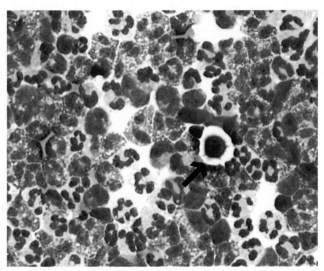

Figure 14-13 Cryptococcosis. Note the presence of *Cryptococcus (arrow)* and the presence of numerous eosinophils. (Modified Wright's stain, 500x.)

States and, in the eastern part of the United States, is transmitted by the American dog tick *(Dermacentor variabilis)*. Recently, it has been shown that the common brown tick *(Rhipicephalus sanguineus)* can also transmit *R. rickettsii* in Arizona.[41] Neurologic signs can be present in up to 43% of dogs with RMSF. Neurologic signs include paraparesis, tetraparesis, seizures, hyperesthesia, stupor, coma, and vestibular dysfunction.[42] Dogs are frequently younger than 5 years old and most cases are seen during the summer.[42] Clinicopathologic findings may include thrombocytopenia, hypoalbuminemia, and leukocytosis.

CSF analysis often reveals moderate pleocytosis (cell count between 25 and 40 cells/μl) with a predominance of either nondegenerate neutrophils, mononuclear cells, or a combination of both.[42] Total protein is often high, with levels of 100 mg/dl or more frequently seen.[42]

Final diagnosis is made by a combination of clinical signs, clinicopathologic findings, CSF findings, and determination of indirect fluorescent antibody (IFA). A titer of ≥ 1:512 is indicative of active infection according to some authors, whereas others suggest a titer ≥1:1024 to indicate active disease.[42]

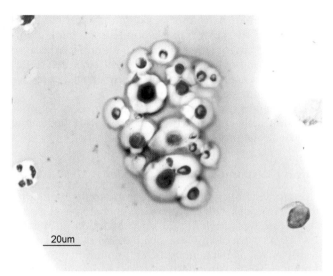

20um

Figure 14-14 Cryptococcosis. Numerous yeasts show a thick clear capsule. Narrow-based budding is also evident. (Wright-Giemsa stain.)

Feline Infectious Peritonitis

Even though feline infectious peritonitis (FIP) has an overall low prevalence in the cat population (about 1% to 2%), it continues to be a clinically important disease.[43] Cats affected by FIP are more likely to be young, purebred, sexually intact males.[43] Abyssinians, Bengals, Birmans, Himalayans, Ragdolls, and Rexes appear to be more susceptible to FIP than other breeds.[44] Clinical signs can be quite variable and often depend on the affected organs.[45] Neurologic signs may include abnormal behavior, seizures, nystagmus, photophobia, and gait abnormalities.[22]

CSF changes can vary greatly. Nucleated cell count can vary from slightly (6 to 50 cells/μl) to markedly increased (>1000 cells/μl). The pleocytosis can vary from suppurative to mixed (neutrophilic/mononuclear) to mononuclear.[22] Total protein concentration is usually elevated but, as with cell count and type, can vary greatly. Total protein concentrations from 30 mg/dl to greater than 2000 mg/dl[22] have been reported. CSF total protein concentration has been found to be within reference limits[22] in rare cases of FIP.

Toxoplasmosis and Neosporosis

Toxoplasma gondii is the agent responsible for toxoplasmosis. Domestic cats and other *Felidae* are the definitive hosts,[46] whereas other species (including humans) are, intermediate hosts. Infection with *Toxoplasma* usually occurs via three modes: (1) congenital infection, (2) ingestion of infected tissues, or (3) ingestion of water or food contaminated with oocysts.[46]

Neospora caninum has been recognized since 1988 as a distinct agent to *T. gondii*.[46] Prior to that time, neosporosis was often misdiagnosed as toxoplasmosis because

both organisms cause similar clinical signs and look similar cytologically.[47] The mode of transmission is similar to *Toxoplasma*. Chronic, subclinical infections can be reactivated by immunosuppressive treatment.[28]

Type and severity of infection depends on both the degree and site of tissue injury.[46] Clinical signs often include persistent or intermittent fever, weight loss, anorexia, icterus (if the liver is affected), and neuromuscular signs.[46] In a study looking at 100 cats with toxoplasmosis, pulmonary (97.7%), CNS (96.4%), hepatic (93.3%), pancreatic (84.4%), cardiac (86.4%), and ocular (81.5%) tissues were the most commonly affected histologically.[46]

CSF changes vary, with either a neutrophilic or mixed inflammation occurring. Total protein concentration is usually mildly increased. However, in some instances, CSF results may be normal. Toxoplasma or Neospora tachyzoites are rarely found in CSF samples.[5]

Spinal Epidural Empyema in Dogs

Spinal epidural empyema (SEE) is also referred to as spinal epidural abcess[48] and is an infection due to either a hematogenous spread of bacteria or direct local extension. Clinical signs may include spinal pain, anorexia, paresis, paralysis, and incontinence.[48]

CSF findings include a mild to moderate neutrophilic or, less commonly, a mixed neutrophilic/mononuclear pleocytosis (5 to 30 cells/μl) and slightly increased protein (31 to 44 mg/dl). In a recent study of SEE, no bacteria were seen on cytologic examination of the CSF.[48]

NONINFECTIOUS/NONSEPTIC CONDITIONS (see Figures 14-10 and 14-11)

Steroid-Responsive Meningitis

Beagles, Boxers, and Bernese Mountain dogs seem to be predisposed to this disease. In a retrospective study, two of these breeds (Boxers and Bernese Mountain dogs) represented approximately 30% of cases each.[49] Fever is a common finding as well as hyperesthesia.[49] Other clinical signs include decreased mental status, gait abnormalities, and cranial nerve/proprioception deficits.[50] These clinical signs may wax and wane.[49]

CSF examination frequently reveals a pleocytosis that is usually neutrophilic or can be mixed (neutrophils/mononuclear cells) (Figure 14-15). The degree of pleocytosis can be marked, varying between 14 and 10,000 cells/μl.[50] Total protein concentration is usually elevated with values often around 100 mg/dl.[50] High levels of IgA and α-2 globulins in both serum and CSF are common in this disease as well.[49,50]

Recurrence or worsening of clinical signs is possible despite steroid therapy. However, clinical signs will disappear in a large proportion of animals with a marked decrease in CSF cell count. An increase in the cell count may occur during relapses of the disease. Therefore, monitoring of CSF cell count in dogs with this disease seems to be a sensitive indicator of success of treatment.[51]

Steroid-responsive meningoencephalitis is also possible in cats but is less frequent than in dogs. Clinical signs may include seizures, circling, and ataxia.[22] CSF cell counts can be moderately to markedly elevated (varying

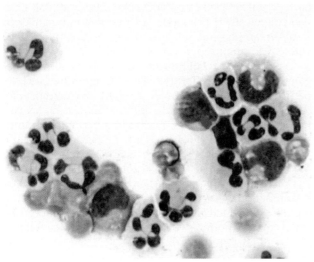

Figure 14-15 Steroid-responsive meningitis in a Bernese Mountain dog. Mixed inflammation with nondegenerate neutrophils and mononuclear cells. (Modified Wright's stain, 500x.)

between 600 to 2960 cells/µl in one study).[22] Total protein is also elevated in cases with high cell counts. Inflammation seems to be either mixed (nondegenerate neutrophils and mononuclear cells) or mononuclear. Clinical signs, as well as CSF changes, can mimic feline infectious peritonitis.[22]

Fibrocartilaginous Emboli in Dogs and Cats

Fibrocartilaginous emboli (FCE) are mostly seen in large and giant breed dogs but can also be present in smaller breeds such as the Miniature Schnauzer.[52] This condition is also present, albeit less frequently, in cats. The FCE is histochemically similar to the nucleus pulposus of intervertebral disks.[53] In dogs, clinical signs are often related to trauma or exercise and occur rapidly (matter of hours) following the event. Clinical signs may include loss of nociception (pain perception) and lower motor neuron dysfunction.[53] In a retrospective study of 36 dogs with FCE, about half had abnormal CSF findings with either increased protein and/or pleocytosis (values for protein concentration and total and differential cell counts were not given).[53] In another study reviewing 75 cases of FCE, CSF analysis was within reference limits in the majority of cases.[54]

In cats with FCE, CSF findings can be normal but, in contrast with dogs, a mild to moderate neutrophilic pleocytosis may be present, with cell counts varying between 10 and 495 cells/µl and > 50% nondegenerate neutrophils. Total protein is frequently within reference limits.[55,56]

MIXED, MONONUCLEAR, OR LYMPHOCYTIC INFECTIOUS/SEPTIC CONDITIONS

Rabies

Rabies is present almost worldwide, and estimates suggest that 50,000 people or more die from the disease annually, mostly in the Indian subcontinent.[57] Dogs with rabies tend to be young and live outdoors. In North America, racoons, skunks, bats, and foxes are the most common reservoir for the virus.[58] Bite wounds from wildlife animals may be absent when the animal is examined because the wounds either healed or are too small to be detected.[28] Clinical signs are highly variable but dysphagia, excessive salivation, and ataxia are common.[28]

CSF analysis usually reveals a mild to moderate mononuclear (usually lymphocytic) pleocytosis with moderately increased total protein (Figures 14-16 and 14-17).[59]

Chronic Distemper

Chronic distemper occurs more commonly in mature dogs. Many dogs with chronic distemper are vaccinated[28]. Neurologic signs include sudden contraction of muscles (myoclonus) involving the head or limbs and cranial nerves as well as gait deficits. Fever, respiratory signs, conjunctivitis, and gastrointestinal signs (vomiting and diarrhea) were also common in 38 dogs with the chronic form of the disease.[49]

CSF may be normal or have moderate mononuclear pleocytosis (compared with neutrophilic or mixed neutrophilic/mononuclear in cases of acute distemper) and mildly elevated protein concentration.[49] Final diagnosis is made by detection of antibodies to canine distemper in the CSF or by in situ hybridization.[28,49]

Ehrlichiosis

Ehrlichiosis caused by *Ehrlichia canis*, *Ehrlichia ewingii*, or *Anaplasma phagocytophalum* (formerly known as *Ehrlichia equi*) infrequently results in CNS signs such as seizures or neck pain.[60,61] In two reported cases, the animals with CNS signs also had nonregenerative anemia and thrombocytopenia. In both cases, nucleated cell counts were moderately elevated (32 cells/µl in one case and 34 cells/µl in the other) with either a mononuclear or mixed (neutrophil/mononuclear) nucleated cell population. Total protein was reported in only one case[60] and was increased (80 mg/dL). In both cases, *Ehrlichia* morulae were found in either neutrophils or mononuclear cells (Figure 14-18). Ehrlichiosis should be included in the differential diagnosis of CSN signs in endemic areas, especially if hematologic (e.g., nonregenerative anemia, thrombocytopenia) and clinical signs (e.g., presence or known exposure to ticks, lameness, fever) are found as well.

Fungal Infections

The fungi discussed in the previous neutrophilic pleocytosis section can also cause mixed, mononuclear, or lymphocytic pleocytosis. See section on neutrophilic pleocytosis for further discussion of the organisms, incidence, clinical signs, and so on.

Feline Infectious Peritonitis

FIP peritonitis can cause mixed mixed, mononuclear, or lymphocytic pleocytosis, as well as neutrophilic pleocytosis (discussed previously). See section on FIP in neutrophilic pleocytosis for further discussion of FIP.

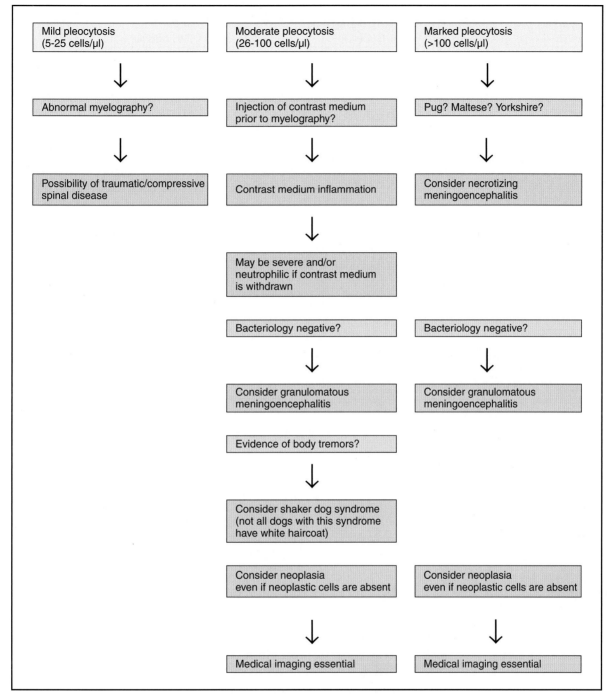

Figure 14-16 Pleocytosis with mixed (neutrophil/monouclear) or mononuclear cells in dogs.

NONINFECTIOUS/NONSEPTIC CONDITIONS

Traumatic/Compressive Spinal Disease

Compressive diseases of the cervical or thoracolumbar spinal cord (e.g., intervertebral disk [IVD] disease, cervical spondylomyelopathy [wobbler syndrome], and fractures) are common causes of paresis and paralysis in small animals. CSF evaluation is commonly performed before myelography in such patients to rule out the presence of primary inflammatory diseases; however, compressive spinal cord disease alone can effect changes in CSF protein and total nucleated cell count. CSF changes associated with compressive disorders have been reviewed, and in many cases, the CSF analysis is within reference limits.[5] If present, common abnormalities are increased protein concentration and/or mild pleocytosis. Changes in CSF depend on the site, severity, and duration of the lesion, as well as the site of CSF collection. Abnormalities

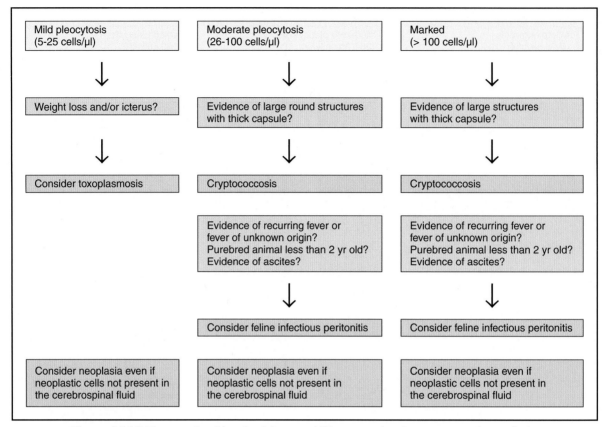

Figure 14-17 Pleocytosis with mixed (neutrophil/mononuclerar) or mononuclear cells in cats.

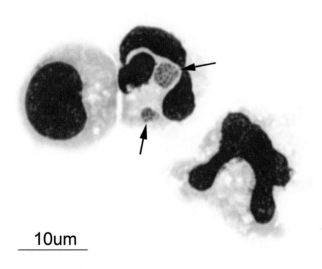

10um

Figure 14-18 Cerebrospinal fluid from a dog with ehrlichiosis. Two *Ehrlichia* morulae are evident in the central cell *(arrows)*.

are more often present and pronounced in samples collected caudal to the lesion. Also, abnormalities are more commonly seen when the clinical disease is acute and clinically severe.

Pleocytosis, when it occurs, is almost always mild, regardless of the site of the lesion or sample collection. In most cases, pleocytosis comprises >90% mononuclear cells; however,

a significant percentage of neutrophils (>30%) is present in some acute, clinically severe lesions as a result of trauma-induced inflammation. In one study, pleocytosis was present in 12.5% of cerebellomedullary cistern (CMC) samples from dogs with thoracolumbar IVD disease compared with 39% of lumbar space (LS) samples. Protein content of the CSF is also increased more often in LS samples than in CMC samples. In thoracolumbar disease, the protein concentration increases seen in CMC samples tend to be mild (<50 mg/dl), whereas protein concentration in LS samples is often >100 mg/dl. Therefore the presence of elevated CSF protein concentration and mild pleocytosis should not preclude myelography in patients suspected to have compressive disorders.

Contrast Medium

Nonionic contrast medium drugs are commonly used for myelography. These drugs are not as irritating to the CNS as iodine-based mediums[62] but still can cause changes in the CSF. In animals in which the contrast medium was not removed post-myelography, a mild to moderate mixed or rarely neutrophilic pleocytosis may be seen as well as a slight increase in total protein (usually <50 mg/dl). In animals in which the contrast medium is removed following the myelography, pleocytosis may be greater than in animals without the withdrawal, with nucleated cell count >100/µl possible. Total protein can also be higher with values >350 mg/dl possible.[62] It is important to note that the contrast material will cause a false-positive Pandy test.[62]

Necrotizing Meningoencephalitis (Pug Dog Encephalitis)

This type of inflammation can occur in Maltese and Yorkshire Terrier dogs, as well as Pugs.[63,64] Affected dogs are usually young, but older animals can be affected as well (6 months to 7 years). Clinical signs may be acute or chronic. In acute cases, seizures are extremely common and are frequently accompanied by abnormal behaviour, ataxia, neck pain, and blindness.[28] Progression of the disease is usually quick. In chronic cases, recurrent seizures are common.

CSF analysis shows a moderate to marked increase in nucleated cells (70 to 600 cells/µl) and elevated protein concentrations (often greater than 100 mg/dl) (Figure 14-19). One study reported a predominance of large granular lymphocytes (LGL) in the CSF of a 3-year-old miniature poodle with a final diagnosis of necrotizing meningoencephalitis.[65]

Although some patients improve temporarily with steroids, long-term prognosis is poor.

Granulomatous Meningoencephalitis

Granulomatous meningoencephalitis (GME) is a nonseptic inflammatory disease of the central nervous system.[66] It generally affects young to middle-aged small breed female dogs, but dogs of any age, sex, or breed can be affected.[66] The etiology and pathogenesis of this disease are unknown. The rapidity of clinical signs vary. Some animals develop signs in a matter of days, whereas others develop signs over a period of several months. Clinical signs include proprioception deficits, cranial nerve deficits, gait abnormalities, decreased mental status, changes in behavior, and hyporeflexia.[49]

CSF often reveals a mild to marked pleocytosis. In a study of 22 dogs with GME, total nucleated cell counts varied from 9 to >5000 cells/µl in cisternal CSF and from

12 to 1600 cells/µl in lumbar CSF.[67] Total protein varied from 13 to >1000 mg/dl for cisternal CSF and from 111 to 244 mg/dl in lumbar CSF.[67] Another study looking at 20 dogs revealed cell counts varying between 13 and 5000 cells/µl.[66] Total protein in that study was reported only as either a positive or negative Pandy test. Sixteen of the dogs had positive Pandy test results and four had negative Pandy test results. Two of the four dogs with negative Pandy test results were being treated with steroids when the CSF was samples were collected.[66] Differential cell counts can vary greatly, with some animals having an almost pure mononuclear population, whereas others may show a mixed population with up to 50% neutrophils[66] (Figures 14-20 and 14-21). Mixed pleocytosis seems to be more common in acute cases.

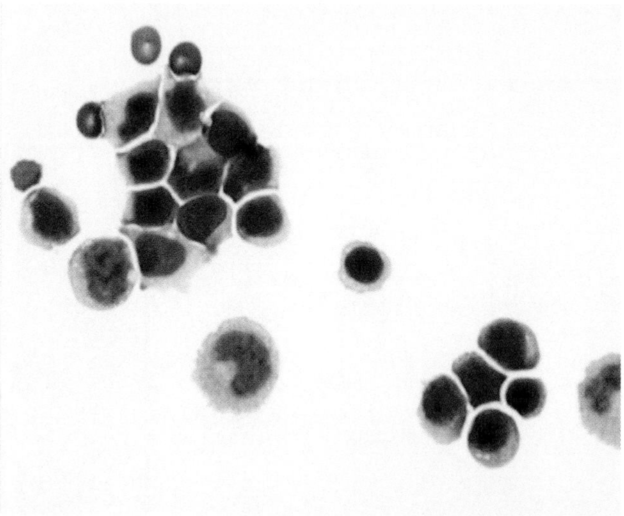

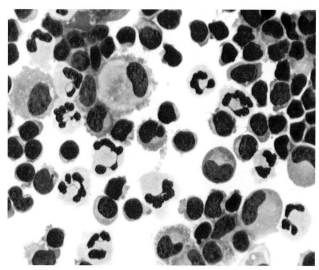

Figure 14-20 Granulomatous meningoencephalitis. Mixed mononuclear and neutrophilic inflammation. (Modified Wright's stain, 500x.)

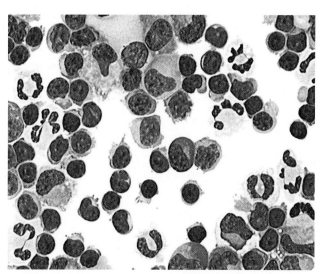

Figure 14-21 Granulomatous meningoencephalitis. Mixed mononuclear and neutrophilic inflammation. Note the presence of a plasma cell in the center. (Modified Wright's stain, 500x.)

Figure 14-19 Necrotizing meningoencephalitis in a pug. Mixed mononuclear inflammation. (Modified Wright's stain, 500x.)

Shaker Dog Disease (White Shaker Syndrome)

This syndrome occurs in dogs between the ages of 5 months and 3 years and was first reported in white-haired small dogs such as Maltese and West Highland White Terrier, thus the name *white shaker syndrome (WSS)*. However, WSS can be found in several sized and colored dogs, including Shih Tzu, Beagles, Yorkshire Terriers, Australian Silky Terriers, and Miniature Pinscher dogs.[68] Because animals with hair color other than white can be affected, the term *shaker dog disease* is now used.[68] Clinical signs are characterized by body tremors that often worsen day by day and spread to the whole body. These signs can improve with treatment of corticosteroids and benzodiazepines.[68]

Reports of CSF findings in this syndrome are rare. One report mentions a moderate pleocytosis of 68 cells/µl with a mixed population of neutrophils and mononuclear cells, a total protein of 44 mg/dl, and a positive Pandy test,[68] whereas another showed an absence of or slight pleocytosis (average of 3 cells/µl) and normal protein level (average of 16 mg/dl).[69]

Eosinophilic Meningoencephalitis

Eosinophilic meningoencephalitis may be idiopathic or infectious. Among infectious causes, protozoa such as *Toxoplasma* and *Neospora*, fungi such as *Cryptococcus*, and larval migrations (e.g., *Dirofilaria* spp., *Baylisascaris* spp.) must be considered.[5] Except for *Cryptococcus*, microorganisms may be difficult to visualize.

Idiopathic eosinophilic meningoencephalitis has been rarely reported in the veterinary literature. Six cases, three of which were Golden Retrievers, were reported in one report,[70] whereas three cases in Rottweilers were reported in another.[71] Clinical signs may include ataxia, change of behavior, neck pain, and depression.[71] Interestingly, all reported cases are males. Etiology for this disease remains unknown but the presence of numerous eosinophils and response to glucocorticoid therapy suggests an immune-mediated disease, even though an undiagnosed infectious agent cannot be ruled out.[71]

Cell counts in the CSF varied from 11 to 5500 cells/µl and the percentage of eosinophils varied from 21% to 98% (Figures 14-22 and 14-23). In Rottweilers, all cases had >90% eosinophils.[71] Total protein was frequently (but not always) elevated with values >1000 mg/dl sometimes present.[70,71]

NEOPLASIA

Lymphoma in the Dog

CNS involvement of lymphoma may be primary or secondary to metastasis from other sites. Usually, the only way to differentiate primary from secondary CNS lymphoma is by exclusion of any other organ's involvement by the lymphoma.[72] Clinical signs will depend on the degree of CNS involvement and may include paresis, cranial nerve deficit, seizures, and loss of vision.[23,73]

Even though neoplastic lymphocytes tend to exfoliate fairly well, not all CSF samples will demonstrate their presence. In some cases, there will be absence of a pleocytosis, but in most cases, total protein will be elevated (often >100 mg/dl). If pleocytosis is present, there can be a mixed inflammation of nondegenerate neutrophils, mononuclear cells with small lymphocytes,[23,73] or small lymphocytes only.[23] If neoplastic cells are present, they will present features similar to other lymphoma cells (Figure 14-24).

Lymphoma in the Cat

Lymphoma is the most common feline neoplasm, but CNS involvement is not common.[74] Clinical signs are often acute and include asymmetric paraparesis, focal hyperesthesia, head tilt, and progressive ataxia.[22,74] These signs usually progress rapidly. This type of lymphoma seems to mostly affect young cats (often less than 3 years of age).[74]

As with dogs, not all cases of feline lymphoma involving the CNS results in neoplastic cells in the CSF. Therefore,

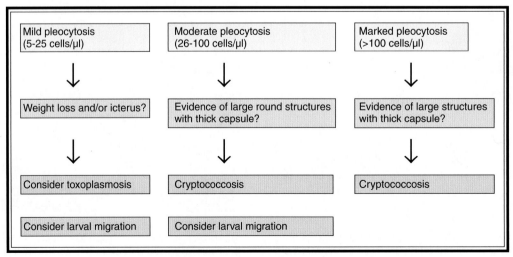

Figure 14-22 Pleocytosis with greater than 20% eosinophils in cats.

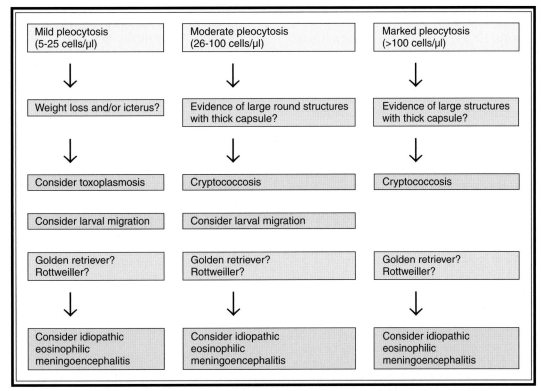

Figure 14-23 Pleocytosis with greater than 20% eosinophils in dogs.

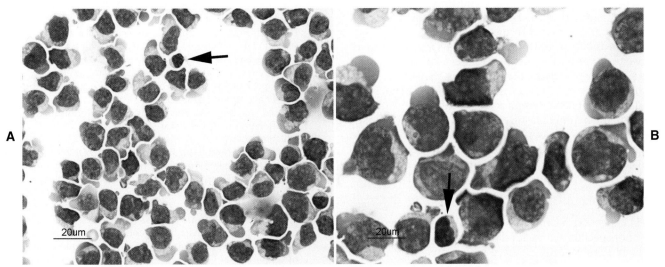

Figure 14-24 CSF samples from a dog with CNS lymphoma. **A,** Low magnification shows a cellular slide consisting almost entirely of large, pleomorphic lymphoid cells. A mature lymphocyte with condensed, mature chromatin is present *(arrow).* **B,** Higher magnification of the same slide. Lymphoid cells are large with pleomorphic nuclei and immature chromatin. Some cells have distinct nucleoli. A mature lymphocyte with condensed chromatin is present *(arrow).* (Wright-Giemsa stain.)

negative CSF results do not rule out CNS neoplasia. In a retrospective study of 23 cats with CNS lymphoma, the great majority had a pleocytosis (mean of 140 cells/µl; range 0 to 1625 cells/µl) and elevated total protein concentration (mean of 140.7 mg/dl, range of 12 to 405 mg/dl), but neoplastic cells were present in only one third of the animals.[74] In other animals the character of pleocytosis varied, with neutrophils predominating in some cases and mixed pleocytosis in other cases.[74] However, another study looking at six cats with CNS lymphoma reported neoplastic cells in the CSF in five of the six animals.[22] All cats in that study had a pleocytosis (range, 6 to 1144 cells/µl). Protein levels were either normal or elevated (range, 31 to 1000 mg/dl).

Meningioma in the Dog

Meningioma is the most common intracranial tumor in the dog.[23,75] Dogs with meningiomas tend to be old, with a mean age of 11 years.[23] Golden Retrievers, as well as Boxers, seem to be at greater risk for intracranial neoplasia, including meningioma.[23] The most common clinical signs include seizures, circling, ataxia, and head tilt.[76]

It is often reported that meningiomas result in neutrophilic pleocytosis with cell counts often >50 cells/μl and more than 50% nondegenerate neutrophils.[77] However, a recent study that reviewed 56 cases of intracranial meningiomas revealed that more than 70% of dogs had a nucleated cell count of less than 5/μl and less than 20% of dogs had a neutrophilic pleocytosis. The authors of this report concluded that neutrophilic pleocytosis may not be present in cases of meningiomas, especially meningiomas located within the middle or rostral portion of the cranial fossa.[78]

Nephroblastoma

Nephroblastoma (also known as embryonal nephroma) is a rare tumor of dogs and cats. Animals between the ages of 6 months and 3 years are most commonly affected.[79] In dogs, nephroblastomas usually involve one kidney or the spinal cord, but rarely both.[79] Clinical signs will depend on the location of the tumor. In dogs with spinal nephroblastoma, neurologic signs involving the spinal cord between the third thoracic and third lumbar spinal cord segments occur and may include paraparesis, as well as urinary and fecal incontinence.[79]

CSF is usually unrewarding and results may be normal. However, in rare cases, neoplastic cells may be present in the CSF.[80] These cells are usually in clusters. The cytologic characteristics of nephroblastoma cells in CSF may be similar to neoplastic lymphocytes.[79] Therefore caution is warranted when neoplastic cells with features of neoplastic lymphocytes are found in young animals with a single mass in the spinal canal and nephroblastoma should be considered, especially if the cells appear to be cohesive.

Other Tumors

CSF changes with other intracranial neoplasia are generally nonspecific. Often total protein concentration and cell count are slightly elevated with a mixed population of inflammatory cells.[23]

References

1. Thompson CE, Kornegay JN, Stevens JB: Analysis of cerebrospinal fluid from the cerebellomedullary and lumbar cisterns of dogs with focal neurologic disease. *J Am Vet Med Assoc* 196(11):1841-1844, 1990.
2. Cook JR, DeNicola DB: Cerebrospinal fluid. *Vet Clin North Am Small Anim Pract* 18:475-500, 1988.
3. Fry MM, et al: Effects of time, initial composition, and stabilizing agents on the results of canine cerebrospinal fluid analysis. *Vet Clin Pathol* 35:72-77, 2006.
4. Bienzle D, McDonnell JJ, Stanton JB: Analysis of cerebrospinal fluid from dogs and cats after 24 and 48 hours of storage. *J Am Vet Med Assoc* 216:1761-1764, 2000.
5. Meinkoth JH, Crystal MA: Cerebrospinal fluid analysis. In Cowell RL, Tyler RD, Meinkoth JH (eds): *Diagnostic Cytology and Hematology of the Dog and Cat.* St. Louis, Mosby, 1999, pp 125-141.
6. Jacobs RM, Cochrane SM, Lumsden JH: Relationship of cerebrospinal fluid protein concentration determination by dye-binding and urinary dipstick methods. *Can Vet J* 31: 587-588, 1990.
7. Jamison EM, Lumsden JH: Cerebrospinal fluid analysis in the dog: Methodology and interpretation. *Semin Vet Med Surg Small Anim* 3:122-132, 1988.
8. Sorjonen DC: Total protein, albumin quota, and electrophoretic patterns in cerebrospinal fluid of dogs with central nervous system disorders. *Am J Vet Res* 48(2):301-305, 1987.
9. Bailey CS, Higgins RJ: Comparison of total white cell count and total protein content of lumbar and cisternal cerebrospinal fluid of healthy dogs. *Am J Vet Res* 46: 1162-1165, 1985.
10. Freeman KP, Raskin RE: Cytology of the central nervous system. In Raskin RE, Meyer DJ (eds): *Atlas of Canine and Feline Cytology.* Philadelphia, Saunders, 2001, pp 325-366.
11. Rand JS: The analysis of cerebrospinal fluids in cats. In Kirk RW, Bonagura JD (eds): *Current Veterinary Therapy XII: Small Animal Practice.* Philadelphia, Saunders, 1995.
12. Baker B, Lumsden JH: Cerebrospinal fluid. In Baker R, Lumsden JH (eds): *Color Atlas of Cytology of the Dogs and Cat.* St. Louis, Mosby, 2000, pp 95-116.
13. Rand JS, et al: Reference intervals for feline cerebrospinal fluid: Cell count and cytologic features. *Am J Vet Res* 51:1044-1054, 1990.
14. Christopher MM, Perman V, Hardy RM: Reassessment of cytologic values in canine cerebrospinal fluid by use of cytocentrifugation. *J AM Vet Med Assoc* 192:1726-1729, 1988.
15. Jenson HB, Baltimore RS: *Pediatric Infectious Diseases: Principles and Practices.* ed 2. Philadelphia, Saunders, 2002.
16. Sidman R, et al: Xanthochromia? By what methods? A comparison of visual and spectrophotometric xanthochromia. *Ann Emerg Med* 46:51-55, 2005.
17. Petzold A, Keir G, Sharpe LT: Spectralphotometry for xanthochromia. *N Eng J Med* 351:1695-1696, 2004.
18. Wilson JW, Stevens JB: Effects of blood contamination on cerebrospinal fluid. *J Am Vet Med Assoc* 71:256-258, 1977.
19. Hurtt AE, Smith EO: Effects of iatrogenic blood contamination on results of cerebrospinal fluid analysis in clinically normal dogs and dogs with neurological disease. *J Am Vet Med Assoc* 211:866-867, 1997.
20. Sweeney CR, Russell GE: Difference in total protein concentration, nucleated cell count, and red blood cell count among sequential samples of cerebrospinal samples of cerebrospinal fluid form horses. *J Am Vet Med Assoc* 217: 54-57, 2000.
21. Bonsu BK, Harper MB: Correction for leukocytes and percent of neutrophils do not match observations in blood-contaminated cerebrospinal fluid and have no value over uncorrected cells for diagnosis. *Ped Infect Dis J* 25: 8-11, 2006.
22. Singh M, et al: Inflammatory cerebrospinal fluid analysis in cats: Clinical diagnosis and outcome. *J Feline Med Surg* 7: 77-93, 2005.
23. Snyder JM, Shofer FS, Van Winkle TJ, Massicotte C: Canine intracranial primary neoplasia: 173 cases (1986-2003). *J Vet Intern Med* 20:669-675, 2006.
24. Irwin PJ, Parry BW: Streptococcal meningoencephalitis in a dog. *J Am Anim Hosp Assoc* 35:417-422, 1999.
25. Meric SM: Canine meningitis, a changing emphasis. *J Vet Intern Med* 2:26-35, 1988.

26. Radaelli ST, Platt SR: Bacterial meningoencephalitis in dogs: A retrospective study of 23 cases (1990-1999). *J Vet Intern Med* 16:159-163, 2002.

27. Cook LB, et al: Inflammatory polyp in the middle ear with secondary suppurative meningoencephalitis in a cat. *Vet Radiol Ultrasound* 44:648-651, 2003.

28. Thomas WB: Inflammatory diseases of the central nervous system in dogs. *Clin Tech Small Anim Pract* 13:167-178, 1998.

29. Jozwik A, Frymus T: Comparison of the immunofluorescence assay with RT-PCR and nested PCR in the diagnosis of canine distemper. *Vet Res Commun* 29:347-359, 2005.

30. Lavely J, Lipitz D: Fungal infections of the central nervous system in the dog and cat. *Clin Tech Small Anim Pract* 20: 212-219, 2005.

31. Berthelin CF, Legrendre AM, et al: Cryptoccosis of the nervous system in dogs. II. Diagnosis, treatment, monitoring, and prognosis. *Progr Vet Neurol* 5:136-146, 1994.

32. Jergens AE, Wheeler CA, Collier LL: Cryptococcosis involving the eye and central nervous system of a dog. *J Am Vet Med Assoc* 189:302-304, 1986.

33. Sutton RH: Cryptococcosis in dogs: A report of 6 cases. *Aust Vet J* 57:558-564, 1981.

34. Gerds-Grogan S, Daryell-Hart B: Feline cryptococcosis: A retrospective evaluation. *J Am Anim Hosp Assoc* 33:118-122, 1997.

35. Greene RT: Coccidiomycosis. In Greene CE (ed): *Infectious Diseases the Dog and Cat*, ed 2. Philadelphia, Saunders, 1998, pp 391-398.

36. Kerl ME: Update on canine and feline fungal diseases. *Vet Clin North Am Small Anim Pract* 33:721-747, 2003.

37. Mariani CL, et al: Cerebral phaeohyphomycosis caused by *Cladosporium* spp. in two domestic shorthair cats. *J Am Anim Hosp Assoc* 38:225-230, 2002.

38. Anor S, et al: Systemic phaeohyphomycosis *(Cladophialophora bantiana)* in a dog—clinical diagnosis with stereotactic computed tomographic-guided brain biopsy. *J Vet Intern Med* 15:257-261, 2001.

39. Shroeder H, Jardine JE, Davis V: Systemic phaeohyphomycosis caused by *Xylohypha bantiana* in a dog. *J South Afr Vet Assoc* 65:175-178, 1994.

40. Janovsky M, et al: Phaeohyphomycosis in a snow leopard (Unciauncia) due to *Cladophialophora banttiana*. *J Com Pathol* 134(2):245-248, 2006.

41. Demma LJ, et al: Rocky Mountain spotted fever from an unexpected tick vector in Arizona. *N Engl J Med* 353(6): 587-594, 2005.

42. Milkszewski JS, Vite CH: Central nervous system dysfunction associated with Rocky Mountain spotted fever infection in five dogs. *J Am Hosp Assoc* 41:259-266, 2005.

43. Rohrbach BW, et al: Epidemiology of feline infectious peritonitis among cats examined at veterinary medical teaching hospitals. *J Am Vet Med Assoc* 218(7):1111-1115, 2001.

44. Pesteanu-Somogyi LD, Radzai C, Pressler BM: Prevalence of feline infectious peritonitis in specific cat breeds. *J Feline Med Surg* 8(1):1-5, 2006.

45. Desnoyers M, Overvelde S: Feline infectious peritonitis: A review. *Med Vet Quebec* 33(4):165-169, 2003.

46. Dubey JP, Lappin MR: Toxoplasmosis and Neosporosis. In Greene CE (ed): *Infectious Diseases of the Dog and Cat*, ed 2. Philadelphia, Saunders, 1998, pp 493-501.

47. Dubey JP, et al: Newly recognized fatal protozoan disease of dogs. *J Am Vet Med Assoc* 192:1269-1285, 1998.

48. Lavely JA, et al: Spinal epidural empyema in seven dogs. *Vet Surg* 35:176-185, 2006.

49. Tipold A: Diagnosis of inflammatory and infectious diseases of the central nervous system in dogs: A retrospective study. *J Vet Intern Med* 9:304-314, 1995.

50. Behr S, Cauzinille L: Aseptic suppurative meningitis in juvenile Boxer dogs: Retrospective study of 12 cases. *J Am Anim Hosp Assoc* 42(4):277-282, 2006.

51. Cinizauskas S, Jaggy A, Tiplod A: Long-term treatment of dogs with steroid-responsive meningitis-arteritis: Clinical, laboratory and therapeutic results. *J Small Anim Pract* 41(7):295-301, 2000.

52. Hawthorne JC, et al: Fibrocartilaginous emboli myelopathy in miniature Schnauzers. *J Am Anim Hosp Assoc* 37: 374-383, 2001.

53. Cazinille L, Kornegay JN: Fibrocartilaginous embolism of the spinal cord in dogs: Review of 36 histologically confirmed cases and retrospective study of 26 suspected cases. *J Vet Intern Med* 10(4):241-245, 1996.

54. Gandini G, et al: Fibrocartilaginous embolism in 75 dogs: Clinical findings and factors influencing the recovery rate. *J Small Anim Pract* 44(2):76-80, 2003.

55. Mikszewski JS, Van Winkle TJ, Troxel MT: Fibrocartilaginous emboli myelopathy in five cats. *J Am Anim Hosp Assoc* 42: 226-233, 2006.

56. Abramson CJ, Platt SR, Stedman NL: Tetraparesis in a cat with fibrocartilaginous emboli. *J Am Anim Hosp Assoc* 38:153-156, 2002.

57. Public Health Agency of Canada, May 2005.

58. Woldehitz Z: Clinical laboratory advances in the detection of rabies virus. *Clin Chim Acta* 351:49-63, 2005.

59. Barnes HL, et al: Clinical evaluation of rabies virus meningoencephalitis in a dog. *J Am Anim Hosp Assoc* 39(6):547-550, 2003.

60. Meinkoth JH, et al: Ehrlichiosis in a dog with seizures and non regenerative anemia. *J Am Vet Med Assoc* 195:1754-1755, 1989.

61. Maretzki CH, Fisher DJ, Greene CE: Granulocytic ehrlichiosis and meningitis in a dog. *J Am Vet Med Assoc* 205:1554-1556, 1994.

62. Widner WR, et al: Cerebrospinal fluid response following metrizamide myelography in normal dogs: Effect of routine myelography and postmyelography removal of contrast medium. *Vet Clin Pathol* 19:66-76, 1990.

63. Cordy DR, Holliday TA: A necrotizing meningoencephalitis of pug dogs. *Vet Pathol* 26:191-194, 1989.

64. Stalis IH, et al: Necrotizing meningoencephalitis of Maltese dogs. *Vet Pathol* 32:230-235, 1995.

65. Garma-Avina A, Tyler JW: Large granular lymphocyte pleocytosis in the cerebrospinal fluid of a dog with necrotizing meningoencephalitis. *J Comp Pathol* 121:83-87, 1999.

66. Demierre S, et al: Correlation between the clinical course of granulomatous encephalitis in dogs and the extent of mast cell infiltration. *Vet Rec* 148:467-472, 2001.

67. Bailey CS, Higgins RJ: Characteristics of cerebrospinal fluid associated with canine granulomatous meningoencephalitis: A retrospective study. *J Am Vet Med Assoc* 188(4): 418-421, 1986.

68. Yamaya Y, et al: A case of shaker dog disease in a Miniature Daschund. *J Vet Med Sci* 66(9):1159-1160, 2004.

69. Wagner SO, Podell M, Fenner WR: Generalized tremors in dogs: 24 cases (1984-1995). *J Am Vet Med Assoc* 211:731-735, 1997.

70. Smith-Maxie LL, et al: Cerebrospinal fluid analysis and clinical outcome of eight dogs with eosinophilic meningoencephalitis. *J Vet Intern Med* 3(3):167-174, 1989.

71. Bennett PF, et al: Idiopathic eosinophilic meningoencephalitis in Rottweiler dogs: Three cases (1992-1997). *Aust Vet J* 75(11):786-789, 1997.

72. Vernau KM, et al: Primary canine and feline nervous system tumors: Intraoperative diagnosis using the smear technique. *Vet Pathol* 38:47-57, 2001.

73. Bush WW, et al: Intravascular lymphoma involving the central and peripheral nervous systems in a dog. *J Am Anim Hosp Assoc* 39:90-96, 2003.

74. Lane SB, et al: Feline spinal lymphosarcoma: A retrospective evaluation of 23 cats. *J Vet Intern Med* 8:99-104, 1994.

75. Meada H, et al: A case of anaplastic meningioma in a dog. *J Vet Med Sci* 67:1177-1180, 2005.

76. Bagley RS, et al: Clinical signs associated with brain tumors in dogs: 97 cases (1992-1997). *J Am Vet Med Assoc* 215: 818-819, 1999.

77. Bailey CS, Higgins RJ: Characteristics of cisternal cerebrospinal fluid associated with primary brain tumors in the dog: A retrospective study. *J Am Vet Med Assoc* 188:414-417, 1986.

78. Dickinson PJ, et al: Characteristics of cisternal cerebrospinal fluid associated with intracranial meningiomas in dogs. *J Am Vet Med Assoc* 228:564-567, 2006.

79. Gasser AM, et al: Extradural spinal bone marrow, and renal nephroblastoma. *J Am Anim Hosp Assoc* 39:80-85, 2003.

80. Vaughan-Scott T, Glodin J, Nesbit JW: Spinal nephroblastoma in an Irish wolfhound. *J South Afr Vet Assoc* 70:25-28, 1999.

Effusions: Abdominal, Thoracic, and Pericardial

T.E. Rizzi, R.L. Cowell, R.D. Tyler, and J.H. Meinkoth

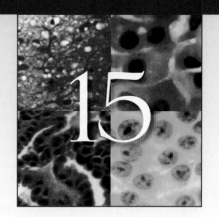

CHAPTER 15

Abdominal viscera, thoracic viscera, and the heart are bathed in and lubricated by a small amount of fluid, which is essentially an ultrafiltrate of blood. The amount of lubricating fluid in the cavity is determined by the amount of fluid entering the cavity minus the amount exiting the cavity. Therefore the amount of fluid increases when more enters the cavity than is removed from it. Ectopic sources of fluid in the abdomen, such as rupture of the urinary bladder and hemorrhage into body cavities, are discussed in this chapter.

ABDOMINAL AND THORACIC EFFUSIONS

Most effusions are not noticed by pet owners until they become severe. Dogs and cats with pathologic thoracic effusions often show dyspnea as the most common clinical sign.[1,2] Other clinical signs include a crouched, sternal recumbent position with extension of the head and neck; open-mouth breathing; tachypnea; and forceful abdominal respiration. Cyanosis may be present. With milder effusions, lethargy and lack of stamina may be the only clinical signs. Animals, especially cats, with mildly to moderately severe effusions often adapt by decreasing their activity, thus concealing their illness until it is severe. With chronic pleural effusion, dogs and cats may present with coughing as the only clinical sign.[1]

Physical findings with pleural effusion depend on the amount of fluid present, but include muffled heart and lung sounds. Other physical findings such as distended jugular veins, often give clues as to the cause of the effusion.

Dogs and cats with abdominal effusions may be presented for lethargy, weakness, and abdominal distension. Owners may mistake the abdominal distension for weight gain, gas, or ingesta.

Physical findings in abdominal effusions include a fluid wave in high-volume effusions and pain if peritonitis is present.

PERICARDIAL EFFUSIONS

Pericardial effusions are less common in cats than dogs. In cats, pericardial effusion is generally related to congestive heart failure (CHF) or feline infectious peritonitis (FIP), but can be caused by primary cardiac neoplasia such as lymphoma.[3] The most common causes of pericardial effusion in dogs include cardiac neoplasia and idiopathic pericardial effusion (IPE).[4,5] Hemangiosarcoma is the most common cardiac neoplasm reported, but other reported neoplasms include chemodectoma, lymphoma, and thyroid carcinoma.[4]

Other less common causes include cardiac disease, inflammatory/infectious, trauma, coagulopathy, and congenital defects. Clinical signs include weakness, lethargy, exercise intolerance, collapse, and coughing. Physical findings of dogs with pericardial effusion vary with the volume of fluid present but include muffled heart sounds, weak pulses, and pallor. With careful palpation by an experienced clinician, pulsus paradoxus can occasionally be detected. This is an alteration in pulse quality that is associated with respiration. Cardiac tamponade refers to significant cardiac compression due to accumulating pericardial fluid.

Increased amounts of fluid in the abdominal cavity, thoracic cavity, or pericardium is not a disease in itself, but rather an indication of a pathologic process in the fluid production and/or removal system or an accumulation from an ectopic source. Fluid analysis, including cytologic evaluation and classification, is a quick, easy, inexpensive, and relatively safe way to obtain useful information for diagnosis, prognosis, and treatment of diseases resulting in abdominal, thoracic, and/or pericardial fluid accumulations.

COLLECTION TECHNIQUES

Thoracentesis

Pleural effusions are typically abundant and bilateral but may be mild, unilateral, and/or compartmentalized. Radiographs help determine the extent and location of the effusion. If the effusion is compartmentalized, radiographs can help establish the fluid's location and guide thoracentesis. If the fluid is not compartmentalized, thoracentesis is done approximately two-thirds down the chest, near the costochondral junction at the sixth, seventh, or eighth intercostal space.

The animal is restrained in sternal recumbency or standing. The site of needle insertion is shaved and aseptically prepared. Tranquilization and/or local anesthesia are generally not necessary for collecting a small sample for analysis, but may be needed if a large amount of fluid must be drained from the chest. Large dogs may require a 1½-inch, 18- to 20-gauge needle or over-the-needle catheter, but a ⅞-inch, 19- or 21-gauge. butterfly needle is preferred for cats and small dogs. The catheter unit allows the needle to be withdrawn after the catheter is introduced into the thoracic cavity, decreasing the chance of injury to intrathoracic organs.

The needle should be inserted next to the cranial surface of the rib to minimize the risk of lacerating the vessels on the rib's caudal border. As long as the needle or catheter is below the fluid line, air will not be aspirated into the thoracic cavity. If only a single syringe of fluid is to be collected, the syringe may be attached to the catheter, the fluid aspirated, and the catheter withdrawn with the syringe attached. If a larger volume of fluid is to be removed or the syringe is to be repeatedly filled, extension tubing and a three-way stopcock should be attached (Figure 15-1).

A sample of the effusion should be collected in an ethylene-tetra-acetic acid (EDTA) (lavender-top) tube to be used for a total nucleated cell count (TNCC), total protein (TP) determination, and cytologic examination. Other samples should be collected in a serum (red-top) tube if any biochemical analyses (e.g., cholesterol or triglyceride) are to be performed and in a culture-transport medium if culture is planned.

Abdominocentesis

Many techniques have been described for collecting abdominal fluid from dogs and cats. Some of those techniques are discussed subsequently.

The ventral midline of the abdomen, 1 to 2 cm caudal to the umbilicus, is the usual site of needle insertion. This site avoids the falciform fat, which can readily block the needle barrel. The urinary bladder is emptied to help avoid accidental cystocentesis. The site of needle insertion is shaved and aseptically prepared. Neither local nor general anesthesia is usually needed. With the animal in lateral recumbency, a ventral midline puncture is made using a 1- to 1½-inch, 20- to 22-gauge needle, or a 20- to 16-gauge, 1½- to 2-inch plain or fenestrated over-the-needle catheter without the syringe attached. Free-flowing fluid should be collected into appropriate collection tubes. The needle can be rotated if fluid is not visible in the needle hub or a syringe can be attached and gentle negative pressure applied.[6] If a previous surgical incision is present, the needle should be inserted at least 1.5 cm away from the site to avoid abdominal viscera that may have adhered to the abdominal wall in the area of the scar. The fluid is collected into an EDTA tube for cytologic examination, TP determination, and TNCC. A serum tube of fluid also is collected if any biochemical tests (e.g., creatinine, bilirubin) are to be performed, and fluid is collected in a culture-transport medium if culture is planned. To enhance fluid collection, abdominal compression may be applied when an over-the-needle catheter is used after the stylet has been removed, leaving only the catheter in the abdominal cavity.

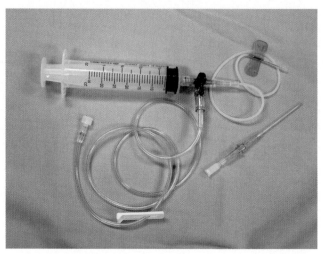

Figure 15-1 Basic equipment for thoracentsis, abdominocentesis, or pericardiocentesis: Syringe, three-way stopcock, extension tubing, butterfly catheter, and over-the-needle catheter.

Although the catheter may kink, sufficient fluid can usually be collected for analysis.

If the technique just described fails to yield fluid, a four quadrant paracentesis or diagnostic peritoneal lavage (DPL) can be performed. In the four quadrant paracentesis the umbilicus serves as a central point and a paracentesis, as previously described, is performed in the right and left cranial and caudal quadrants.[7] If DPL is performed, the animal is placed in dorsal recumbency, the area clipped and aseptically prepared, and a small 2-cm incision caudal to the umbilicus is made. Bleeders should be ligated to prevent blood contamination of the collected fluid. A peritoneal lavage catheter without the trocar is inserted into the abdominal cavity and directed caudally into the pelvis. A syringe is attached and gentle suction applied. If no fluid is obtained, warm sterile saline 20 ml/kg can be infused into the abdominal cavity. The patient is then rolled from side to side. The fluid can be collected via gravity drainage.[6,7]

Pericardiocentesis

Pericardiocentesis can be performed with the animal standing, in sternal or left lateral recumbency. Adequate restraint is needed to avoid cardiac puncture, coronary artery laceration, or pulmonary laceration. Sedation is used as necessary. Electrocardiogram (ECG) monitoring during pericardiocentesis is recommended, but not essential. Cardiac contact with the catheter or needle usually causes an arrhythmia. A large area of the right hemithorax from the third to the eighth rib is shaved and aseptically prepared. Local anesthesia including infiltration of the pleura with lidocaine can be used to minimize discomfort associated with pleura penetration. Puncture is generally between the fourth and fifth intercostal spaces at the costochondral junction. The needle is attached to a three-way stopcock, extension tubing, and syringe and gentle negative pressure is applied.[5,8]

A sample of the effusion should be collected in an EDTA tube to be used for a TNCC, packed cell volume

TABLE 15-1

Indications and Complications

Procedure	Abdominocentesis	Thoracentesis	Pericardiocentesis
Indications	Diagnostic evaluation	Diagnostic evaluation	Diagnostic evaluation
	Relieve intra-abdominal pressure	Relieve respiratory distress	Stabilization of patient with cardiac tamponade
Complications	Laceration of abdominal organs (liver, spleen)	Laceration of lung	Arrhythmia
	Laceration of tumor	Bacterial contamination	Cardiac puncture
	Bacterial contamination		Coronary artery laceration
			Pulmonary laceration
			Bacterial contamination

(PCV), and TP determination, and cytologic examination. Other samples should be collected in a serum tube if any biochemical analyses are to be performed and in a culture-transport medium if culture is planned (Table 15-1).

SLIDE PREPARATION AND STAINING

Preparation of the sample for cytologic evaluation depends on the character and quantity of the fluid, the type of stain used, and whether the cytologic evaluation will be performed in-hospital or sent to a consultant.

The character of the fluid (turbid or clear) usually indicates the process(es) that may be occurring and the probable nucleated cell concentration. Clear, colorless fluids are usually transudates and of low cellularity. Although fluids of low cellularity are the most difficult to prepare, diagnostic-quality smears can be made from most low-cellularity fluids by using sediment or line smear techniques. Amber, clear to mildly opaque fluids are often modified transudates of low to moderate cellularity. Moderately to markedly opaque fluids, however, are usually exudates of moderate to very high cellularity. Slide preparation techniques for various types of fluids are briefly presented later. Chapter 1 contains a detailed discussion and illustrations.

Sediment smears should be made on all nonturbid fluid specimens. This is done by centrifuging the fluid for 5 minutes at 165 to 360 G. This can be achieved in a centrifuge with a radial arm length of 14.6 cm by centrifuging the fluid at 1000 to 1500 rpm. After centrifugation, nearly all of the supernatant is poured off, leaving only about 0.5 ml of fluid with the pellet in the bottom of the test tube. The supernatant may be used for refractometric TP determination and, if the supernatant was not collected from an EDTA tube, other chemical analyses. The pellet is then resuspended in the remaining 0.5 ml of fluid by gentle agitation, a drop of the suspension is placed on a glass slide, and a routine pull smear or squash prep is made (see Chapter 1). The smear is air-dried and then stained with any hematologic stain.

If it is not possible to centrifuge the fluid, line smears should be made from fresh, well-mixed fluid. Also, line smears are useful when making smears from the sediment of very low-cellularity fluids. Line smears are made by placing a drop of fluid on a glass slide and starting to make a pull smear. Instead of continuing until the fluid

makes a feathered edge, go only a short distance, stop, and lift the pull slide directly up. Cells concentrate in the fluid following the pull slide, creating a line of increased cellularity where the pull slide is lifted (see Chapter 1).

Opaque fluids may need only a direct smear because high cell concentrations are likely present. Direct smears may be made by making either pull smears or squash preps on well-mixed, uncentrifuged fluid.

When submitting samples to an outside laboratory for cytologic examination, it is best to request instructions for sample preparation from the person who will be examining the preparations. However, the following instructions generally suffice. Include direct smears and stained (optional) and unstained air-dried smears and prepared as described previously, along with an EDTA tube of the fluid. If premade, air-dried slides are not submitted and the fluid is delayed, the cellular constituents will begin to deteriorate, become hypersegmented and pyknotic, and cell morphology will be difficult if not impossible to evaluate. Even if the cells in the EDTA tube have become pyknotic, a TNCC and refractometric TP determination can be performed.[10]

Many acceptable stains are available. Diff-Quik (Harleco, Gibbstown, NJ) is one of the easiest to use. It stains cellular elements well and has little precipitate to confuse with bacteria. Some other commonly used hematologic stains are Wright's stain and new methylene blue (NMB). Gram stain and acid-fast procedures may be used to classify bacteria, but are much less sensitive than hematologic stains for finding bacteria. Also, care must be given to procedure when performing a Gram stain because the cellular elements, proteins, and other constituents in septic fluids can affect the staining.[10]

LABORATORY DATA

Cell Counts and Counting Techniques

A TNCC, which is a count of all nucleated cells present in the fluid, may be done by automated or manual methods. The automated cell counters may count debris, so only relatively clear fluids should be used. The Unopette (Becton Dickinson Rutherford, NJ) procedure is a good in-house method and is performed the same as for peripheral blood leukocyte counts. Cell clumping, cell fragmentation, and noncellular debris can cause counting errors with both the automated and manual techniques.[10]

TABLE 15-2

Biochemical Analysis of Effusion Fluid

Biochemical Test	Sample	Indications	Interpretation
Bilirubin	Effusion fluid and concurrent serum	Suspected bile peritonitis	Two-fold or greater concentration in effusion fluid than serum expected in bile peritonitis
Creatinine	Effusion fluid and concurrent serum	Suspected uroperitoneum	Two-fold or greater concentration in effusion fluid than serum expected in uroperitoneum
Triglyceride	Effusion fluid and concurrent serum	Suspected chylous effusion	Two-fold or greater concentration in effusion fluid expected in chylous effusion
Cholesterol	Effusion fluid and concurrent serum	Suspected pseudochylous effusion	Two-fold or greater concentration in effusion fluid expected in pseudo-chylous effusion

Red blood cell (RBC) counts offer little if any additional information over visual assessment and a PCV measurement on the effusion. Therefore RBC counts are seldom performed unless the TNCC is done on an automated instrument that automatically counts RBCs. Noting the presence of RBCs in effusions is important because they indicate blood contamination of the fluid during collection, hemorrhage into the cavity, or increased capillary permeability with diapedesis of RBCs into the cavity.[10]

Total Protein Measurement and Techniques

Effusion fluid protein concentration is used, with the TNCC, to classify effusions (transudates, modified transudates, exudates) and to estimate the severity of inflammation. The TP content may be determined biochemically or estimated by refractometry. The method of choice for determining TP concentration in peritoneal, pericardial, and pleural fluid is refractometry.[11] If the fluid is opaque, it is best to determine the refractive index of the supernatant after centrifuging the fluid. Otherwise, refraction of light by suspended nonprotein particles (i.e., lipoproteins, urea, cholesterol, and glucose) may result in an erroneously high TP reading.[10,11] Chylous or lipemic fluids often do not separate sufficiently to allow TP to be estimated by refractometry or chemical methods.

Biochemical Analysis

See Table 15-2.

Other Tests

The pH testing of pericardial fluid initially was thought to assist in differentiating neoplastic from nonneoplastic effusions.[12] A later study conducted on 42 client-owned dogs found the pH of pericardial fluid from dogs with neoplasia was higher than pericardial fluid from dogs with nonneoplastic etiologies; however, there was significant overlap between the two groups. Because of this overlap it was determined the use of pH testing is not useful in differentiating neoplastic from nonneoplastic conditions.[13] In a more recent study by de Laforcade et al,[14] pericardial effusion samples were collected on 41 client-owned dogs with pericardial effusions for biochemical analysis. Results of pH testing of the effusion fluid differed from previous studies in that the pH of dogs with neoplasia was lower than nonneoplastic conditions; however, again the degree of overlap of the two populations limited the usage of pH testing to differentiate neoplastic from nonneoplastic conditions.[14] The differences in pH values between the studies may have been due to differences in methodologies used in determining the pH of the effusions.

MICROBIOLOGIC CULTURES

Not all effusions need to be cultured (e.g., true transudates). If cytologic evaluation of the fluid suggests infection, the fluid should be cultured for both aerobic and anaerobic bacteria. Fluid samples for aerobic and anaerobic cultures can be collected into a syringe, taking care to exclude air from the sample. The needle should be capped and the syringe containing the sample taken immediately to the laboratory for culture. For optimal results or if a delay is anticipated, the fluid should be placed in a transport system that supports both aerobic and anaerobic bacteria. Chapter 1 contains a further discussion of culturing.

CELLS AND STRUCTURES SEEN IN EFFUSIONS

Neutrophils

Neutrophils are present to some degree in most effusions and tend to predominate in effusions associated with inflammation. Cytologically, there are two general classifications of neutrophils: degenerate and nondegenerate. When evaluating neutrophil morphology, only neutrophils in the area of the slide corresponding to the monolayer of a blood slide should be evaluated. Neutrophils close to the feathered edge may appear degenerate because of the mechanical stresses of smear preparation.

Degenerate neutrophils are neutrophils that have undergone hydropic degeneration. This is a morphologic

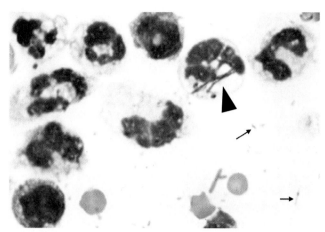

Figure 15-2 Numerous degenerate neutrophils. The nuclear chromatin is swollen. Phagocytized bacterial rods *(arrowhead)* and extracellular bacteria in the background *(arrows)*.

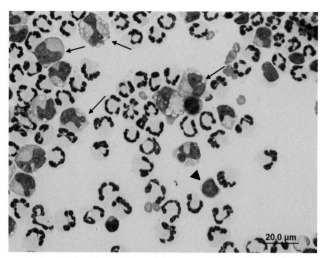

Figure 15-3 Abdominal fluid from a cat. Numerous nondegenerate neutrophils. The chromatin is clumped and segmented. Also present are macrophages *(arrows)* and a small lymphocyte *(arrowhead)*.

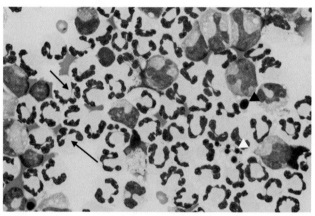

Figure 15-4 Abdominal fluid from same cat as Figure 15-3. Numerous nondegenerate neutrophils. Some neutrophils are hypersegmented with only thin chromatin strands connecting the segments *(small arrows)*. Pyknotic nuclei *(arrowheads)*, are also present.

change that occurs in tissue or effusions because bacterial toxins alter cell membrane permeability. This allows water to diffuse into the cell and through the nuclear pores, causing the nucleus to swell, fill more of the cytoplasm, and stain homogeneously eosinophilic. This swollen, loose, homogeneous eosinophilic nuclear chromatin pattern characterizes the degenerate neutrophil (Figure 15-2). Although all cell types are exposed to the same toxin, degenerative change is evaluated only in neutrophils.

Nondegenerate neutrophils, such as peripheral blood neutrophils, are those with tightly clumped, basophilic nuclear chromatin (Figure 15-3). Some neutrophils in effusions may be hypersegmented. Hypersegmentation is an age-related change; the nuclear chromatin condenses and eventually breaks into round, tightly clumped spheres (pyknosis) (Figure 15-4). These aged neutrophils are often seen phagocytized by macrophages (cytophagia) (Figure 15-5). The presence of nondegenerate neutrophils suggests that the fluid is not septic; however, bacteria that are not strong toxin producers, such as *Actinomyces* spp., may be associated with nondegenerate neutrophils. Also, nonbacterial infectious agents (e.g., *Ehrlichia* and *Toxoplasma* spp. and various fungi) may be associated with nondegenerate neutrophils.

Effusions may also contain toxic neutrophils. Toxic changes (e.g., Dohle bodies, toxic granulation, diffuse cytoplasmic basophilia, foamy cytoplasm) develop in the bone marrow in response to accelerated granulopoiesis due to inflammation. Toxic neutrophils in the peripheral blood migrate into the body cavity and are observed in effusions of the cavity.[10] Although foamy cytoplasm is considered a toxic change, cytoplasmic vacuolation may be seen in neutrophils of peritoneal/thoracic fluid smears because of age-related change or EDTA-induced artifact.

Mesothelial/Macrophage-Type Cells

Mesothelial cells line the pleural, peritoneal, and pericardial cavities as well as visceral surfaces, and are present in variable numbers in most effusions (Figures 15-6 and 15-7). They are large cells that may be present singly or in clusters or rafts. They generally contain a single

round to oval nucleus but may be multinucleated. The nuclear chromatin has a fine reticular pattern. Nucleoli may be present in activated mesothelial cells. Activated mesothelial cells may have morphologic characteristics similar to cells from malignant neoplasms, but should not be confused with neoplastic cells. Mesotheliomas are rare in small animals and difficult to diagnose cytologically. Their cytoplasm is slightly basophilic and may contain phagocytic debris, because activated mesothelial cells may become phagocytic. A blue or red corona may be present around nucleated cells within effusions, especially mesothelial cells, as an artifact of slow drying and is of no diagnostic significance.

Peritoneal macrophages generally have a single oval to bean-shaped nucleus; however, multinucleation and variable nuclear shape may be present (Figures 15-8 and 15-9). Their nuclear chromatin is lacy and their cytoplasm is frequently vacuolated and may contain phagocytic debris.

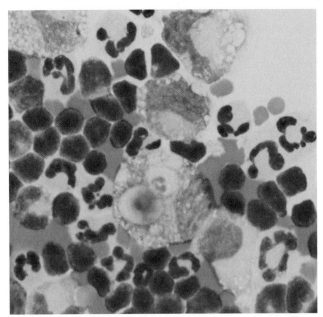

Figure 15-5 Abdominal fluid from a cat. There is a large macrophage in the center with a phagocytized remnant of a neutrophil. Numerous small lymphocytes and macrophages are present.

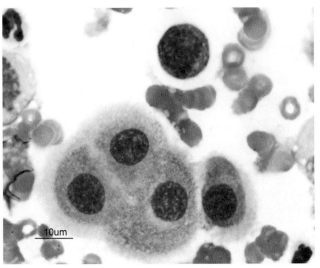

Figure 15-7 A small cluster of mesothelial cells.

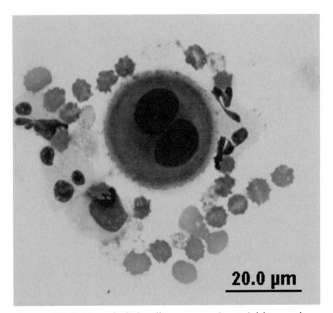

Figure 15-6 Mesothelial cells are seen in variable numbers in effusions. A binucleate mesothelial cell, with deeply basophilic cytoplasm with an eosinophilic encircling calyx, is also present.

Determining whether some cells are mesothelial cells or macrophages may be difficult. Differentiating these cells is seldom of diagnostic significance.

Lymphocytes

Lymphocytes are present in many effusions and may be the predominant cell type in chylous and lymphomatous effusions. With lymphoma, neoplastic lymphocytes

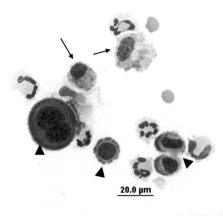

Figure 15-8 Macrophages *(arrows),* mesothelial cells *(arrowheads),* and nondegenerate neutrophils.

frequently—but not always—exfoliate into the fluid and are present in large numbers. Chylous effusions primarily consist of small lymphocytes (Figure 15-10), whereas lymphomatous effusions primarily consist of lymphoblasts (Figures 15-11 and 15-12). The small lymphocytes seen in chylous effusions have a small amount of clear to blue cytoplasm, an oval to bean-shaped nucleus, clumpy nuclear chromatin, and no visible nucleoli. These cells are typically smaller than neutrophils. Reactive lymphocytes (Figure 15-13) may be seen in inflammatory effusions. These lymphocytes are slightly larger than small lymphocytes, have a small to moderate amount of very blue cytoplasm, and may become plasmacytoid.

Care must be taken not to confuse reactive lymphocytes in inflammatory conditions with neoplastic lymphocytes. Neoplastic lymphocytes are usually lymphoblasts and have a moderate amount of clear to blue cytoplasm, variably shaped nuclei, finely stippled nuclear chromatin,

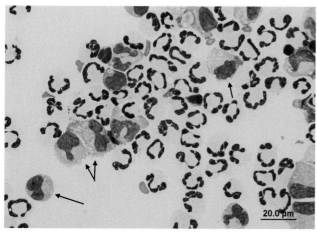

Figure 15-9 Numerous nondegenerate neutrophils and macrophages with variable nuclear morphologies *(arrows).*

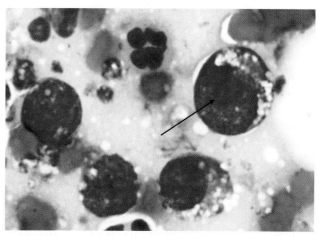

Figure 15-11 Lymphoblast with visible nucleolus *(arrow).* There are small vacuoles in the cytoplasm.

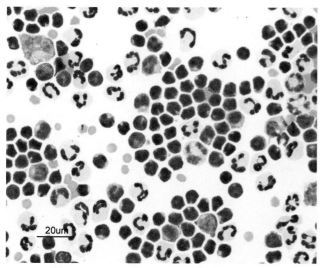

Figure 15-10 Chylous effusion from a cat. Small lymphocytes are the predominant cells. The small lymphocytes are typically smaller than neutrophils. They have round or indented nuclei and a small amount of cytoplasm.

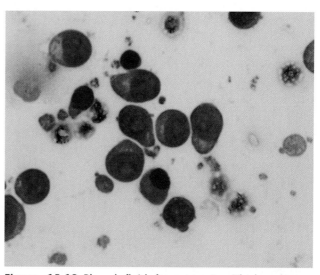

Figure 15-12 Pleural fluid from a cat with lymphoma. Numerous lymphoblasts with visible nucleoli are present.

and nucleoli (often irregular in shape and size) and are larger than neutrophils.

Eosinophils

Eosinophils (Figure 15-14) may be present in effusions and are readily recognized by their rod-shaped (in cats) or variably sized round (in dogs), orange granules. Moderate to large numbers of eosinophils (Figure 15-15) may be seen in effusions secondary to mast cell tumors,[15] heartworm disease, allergic reactions, hypersensitivity, and paraneoplastic response. Concomitant peripheral eosinophilia may or may not be present.

Mast Cells

Mast cells (Figure 15-16) are readily identified by their red-purple granules. Mast cell tumors within body cavities may be associated with effusions and frequently

exfoliate large numbers of mast cells into the effusion. Visceral forms of mast cell neoplasia are rare in the dog.[15,16] Visceral forms of mast cell tumors are more common in cats than dogs and are either spleen associated or an intestinal type.[16]

Mast cells (Figure 15-17) are commonly observed in small numbers in effusions from dogs and cats with many different inflammatory disorders.

Erythrocytes

Erythrocytes may be seen cytologically within effusions secondary to overt hemorrhage or contamination with peripheral blood. It is important to differentiate iatrogenic cause from true intracavity hemorrhage, based on clinical signs and the presence or absence of erythrophagia and platelets in the effusion, as described in the discussion of hemorrhagic effusions later in this chapter.

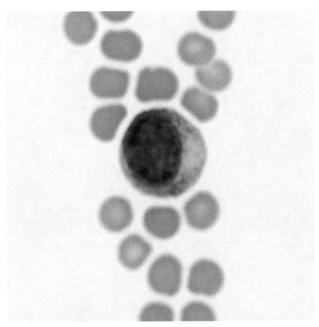

Figure 15-13 Reactive lymphocyte.

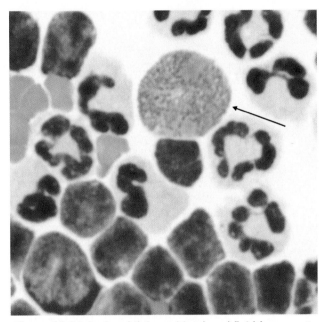

Figure 15-14 Eosinophil *(arrow)* in pleural fluid from a cat.

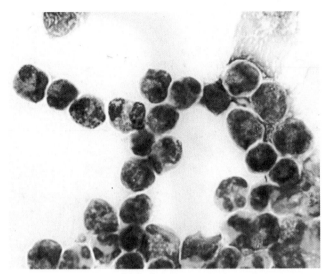

Figure 15-15 Numerous eosinophils.

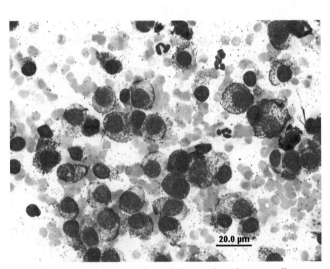

Figure 15-16 Many heavily granulated mast cells.

Neoplastic Cells

Neoplastic cells may be observed in effusions with many different types of neoplasia. Various carcinomas and adenocarcinomas (epithelial cell tumors), lymphoma and mast cell tumors (discrete cell tumors), hemangiosarcomas (vascular endothelial-derived neoplasia), and mesotheliomas may exfoliate neoplastic cells into the pleural, peritoneal, or pericardial cavity. Identification of the neoplastic cells depends upon the viewer's ability to recognize the cell type and signs of malignancy. (See the discussion of neoplasia later in this chapter and the general criteria of malignancy in Chapter 1.)

Miscellaneous Findings

Glove Powder: Cornstarch (glove powder) may be seen on slides made from effusion fluid (Figure 15-18). Typically, it is a clear-staining, large, round to hexagonal structure with a central fissure. Glove powder is an incidental finding and should not be confused with an organism or cell.

Microfilariae: Microfilariae are occasionally seen within hemorrhagic effusions from dogs. These are generally *Dirofilaria* or *Dipetalonema* larvae that have entered the cavity with the peripheral blood.

Basket Cells: Basket cells are ruptured nucleated cells. The nuclear chromatin spreads out and stains eosinophilic. Nucleated cells may rupture because of the stresses induced in slide preparation; however, certain effusions (i.e., chylous effusions and septic exudates) cause increased cell fragility, and basket cells are often seen.

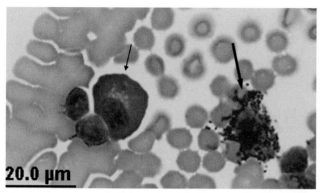

Figure 15-17 Mast cell *(arrow)*, plasma cell *(small arrow)*, and three small lymphocytes in abdominal fluid from a dog.

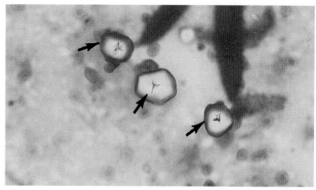

Figure 15-18 Glove powder artifact *(arrows)*.

CLASSIFICATION OF EFFUSIONS

In the following discussions, abdominal, thoracic, and pericardial fluid accumulations are classified as transudates, modified transudates, or exudates, based solely on their TNCC and TP concentration (Figure 15-19). Classifying the effusion can help determine the general mechanism of fluid accumulation. Occasionally, there is some overlap in these classifications (i.e., a fluid may have a TNCC in the transudate range and a TP in the modified transudate range). If a disparity exists, TP is the more important criterion in separating transudates from modified transudates, and cellularity is more important in separating modified transudates from exudates. Although evaluation of an effusion may be diagnostic for such conditions as neoplasia or infection, many effusions simply indicate a process. Historical, physical, and clinical information and imaging studies may aid in achieving a definitive diagnosis.

Transudates

Transudates are clear, colorless effusions of low protein concentrations (<2.5 g/dl) and low TNCC (<1500 cells/μl). Most transudates have protein concentrations <1.5 g/dl; however, 2.5 g/dl is used as the cutoff point because it is the lowest protein concentration at which refractometry is reliable. It is important to remember that effusions occasionally classified as transudates with a total protein concentration >2.0 g/dl may be the result of processes that typically produce modified transudates.

Transudative effusions primarily consist of mononuclear cells (macrophages and small lymphocytes), mesothelial cells, and few nondegenerate neutrophils. They generally occur because of a loss of oncotic pressure due to hypoalbuminemia from such conditions as renal glomerular disease, hepatic insufficiency, and protein-losing enteropathy. Decreased osmotic pressure allows fluid to accumulate in the third space. Transudative effusions occurring, because of hypoalbuminemia alone generally require serum albumin concentration to be <1.0 g/dl. If increased vascular hydrostatic pressure is also occurring, transudative effusions may occur with serum albumin concentrations up to 1.5 g/dl. Rarely, leakage of low-protein lymph from intestinal lymphatics, typically secondary to obstruction of intestinal lymph flow (e.g., masses), may

cause transudative ascites. Also, ectopic causes of fluid accumulation, such as ruptured urinary bladder and resultant uroperitoneum, can result in a low-cellularity, low-protein fluid. Therefore classifying an effusion as a transudate narrows the differential diagnoses (rule out hypoalbuminemia first) and eliminates consideration of exudative disease (Figure 15-20).

Modified Transudates

Most modified transudates occur as a result of fluid leakage from lymphatics carrying high-protein lymph or blood vessels. Such leakage is caused by increases in hydrostatic pressure or permeability. Both of these conditions allow high-protein ultrafiltrate fluid to pass into the cavity. Neither of these conditions results in chemotactants in the cavity; therefore large numbers of inflammatory cells do not migrate into the fluid. Hence, high-protein, low to moderately cellular fluid develops.

Modified transudates have moderate cellularity (1000 to 7000 cells/μl) and protein concentration (2.5 to 7.5 g/dl). The TNCC of the modified transudate overlaps that of the transudate. Modified transudates vary in color from amber to white to red and are frequently slightly turbid to turbid. Nondegenerate neutrophils, mesothelial/macrophage cell types, small lymphocytes, or neoplastic cells may predominate, depending on the cause of the effusion.

Modified transudates often are the least specific from a diagnostic standpoint. In general, they are caused by conditions that produce an increase in vascular hydrostatic pressure and/or permeability within capillaries or lymphatics. There are many reported causes that include cardiac disease, liver disease, space-occupying lesions (i.e., granulomas), and neoplasia. An underlying cause may not be found, especially if the effusion is scant. Cytologic examination of the fluid may yield a more specific diagnosis in some instances. For example, neoplastic and chylous effusions are often readily recognized cytologically. When the cytologic picture is that of a nonspecific mixture of leukocytes and mesothelial cells, some of the more common causes of modified transudates must be pursued with other diagnostic procedures (Figure 15-21).

Cardiovascular disease (right-sided or biventricular failure) is one of the more common causes of modified

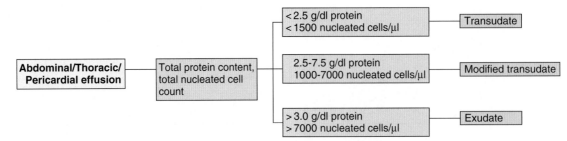

Figure 15-19 An algorithm to classify effusions as transudates, modified transudates, or exudates, based on TP content and TNCC.

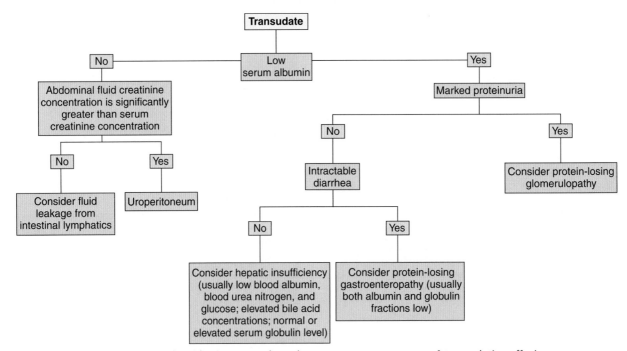

Figure 15-20 An algorithmic approach to the more common causes of transudative effusions.

transudates in dogs and cats. Either abdominal or thoracic effusion may develop; however, ascites is more common in dogs, and pleural effusion is typical in cats. The pleural effusion in cats is often chylous. Physical examination findings, thoracic radiographs, and echocardiography can often confirm functional abnormalities.

Neoplastic disease may result in a modified transudate, presumably by obstruction of lymphatics. Neoplastic cells may or may not be present in the effusion. Cytologic examination of effusion is most likely to be diagnostic in animals with lymphoma or carcinoma; mesenchymal tumors rarely exfoliate recognizable cells into an effusion. Nonexfoliating neoplasia should be strongly considered in an animal with a hemorrhagic (or serosanguinous) modified transudate when there is no history of trauma or coagulopathy.

Feline infectious peritonitis (FIP) is a common cause of abdominal or thoracic effusion and occasionally pericardial effusion in cats. Although FIP may produce an exudative effusion, modified transudates are also common. In most cases, the fluid has a very high protein concentration (>4.0 g/dl). Unfortunately, there is no conclusive cytologic feature in any effusion that is diagnostic of FIP. Other

physical examination or laboratory findings consistent with FIP (e.g., serum hyperglobulinemia, serum albumin-to-globulin ratio (A:G) < 0.8 g/dl, ocular lesions, neurologic abnormalities, nonregenerative anemia) may strengthen a clinical suspicion, but a histologic examination of affected tissues is the most reliable diagnostic modality.

Rupture of the urinary bladder is sometimes reported as causing an exudate. The fluid is most commonly a transudate or modified transudate at the time of diagnosis because the amount of fluid released into the peritoneal cavity dilutes out accumulated cells and protein. See the section on the uroperitoneum later in this chapter for further discussion.

Chylous effusions are usually easily recognized by their milky appearance and predominance of small lymphocytes; however, in some cases recognition is not so clear-cut. The cytology of such effusions can be variable, with neutrophils predominating in some instances, especially if previous centesis procedures have resulted in inflammation. Also, the fluid may appear opaque rather than milky white in animals that are anorectic and not ingesting lipids. In such instances, comparing serum and fluid levels of triglycerides and cholesterol may help

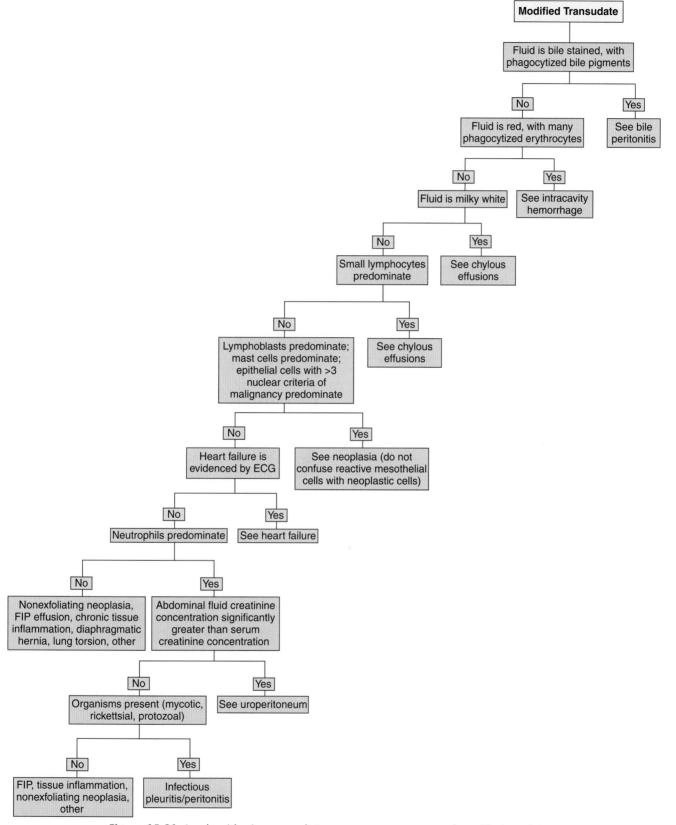

Figure 15-21 An algorithmic approach to some common causes of modified exudates.

determine the nature of the fluid. See the section on chylous/pseudochylous effusions later in this chapter for further discussion.

Effusions containing peripheral blood, as a result of either intracavitary hemorrhage or blood contamination during collection, are often classified as modified transudates because of added cells and serum proteins. Such effusions are easily recognized by their reddish appearance and the presence of numerous erythrocytes on cytologic examination. The presence of erythrophagocytosis or macrophages containing RBC-breakdown products hemosiderin and hematoidin helps differentiate true intracavitary hemorrhage from blood contamination. See the section on hemorrhagic effusions later in this chapter for further discussion.

Hepatic disease is a common cause of ascites and may also cause pleural effusion. If the serum albumin is significantly decreased due to hepatic disease and lack of production, a transudate secondary to hypoalbuminemia with loss of oncotic pressure can occur. If mild to moderate hypoalbuminemia is complicated with systemic venous hypertension or portal hypertension, it may produce a modified transudate.

Other miscellaneous causes of modified transudates include lung lobe torsion, diaphragmatic hernia, hyperthyroidism, and glomerulonephritis. The etiology of many of these effusions is multifactorial and the nature of the effusion is variable, depending upon the circumstances present in each individual case.

Exudates

Because this discussion classifies fluids based solely on their TNCC and TP, the exudate classification contains some fluids not typically thought of as true exudates (e.g., urine from ruptured urinary bladder and neoplastic effusions). However, their inclusion allows an easier, more complete diagnostic approach (Figure 15-22).

Exudates vary from amber to white to red and are turbid to cloudy fluids. Exudates have high protein concentrations (>3.0 g/dl) and a high TNCC (>7000 cells/μl). The protein concentration of an exudate overlaps that of a modified transudate. Exudates occur most commonly because of chemotactants in the cavity due to an inflammatory process. Therefore neutrophils are the predominant cell type in most inflammatory exudates. If the inflammation is due to bacterial infection, degenerate neutrophils generally predominate, unless the bacteria produce only weak or small amounts of toxin. Occasionally, an exudate develops because of abundant exfoliation of cells from a tumor or secondary to a chylous effusion, in which case neoplastic cells or small lymphocytes, respectively, may predominate. In these instances, the effusions are generally called *neoplastic* or *chylous effusions* rather than *exudate* to reflect the cytologic findings.

The term *septic* denotes the presence of bacteria, and *nonseptic* denotes the absence of bacteria. In septic exudates, intracellular and/or extracellular bacteria are generally seen cytologically, but in nonseptic exudates, bacteria are not observed cytologically, and culture is negative. Septic exudates typically consist primarily of degenerate neutrophils, but in nonseptic exudates the predominant cell type is variable and may be the nondegenerate neutrophil (inflammation), small lymphocytes (chylous), or neoplastic cells (carcinoma or lymphoma). When degenerate neutrophils are present, a thorough search for bacteria should be performed; however, not finding organisms cytologically does not totally rule out an infectious cause. Also, because not all bacteria produce strong or large amounts of toxin, the lack of degenerate neutrophils does not rule out the possibility of bacterial infection.

Sepsis may result from spread (hematogenous or lymphatic) of systemic sepsis or of an adjacent organ (e.g., pneumonia with pleural spread, intestinal perforation), or by introduction of organisms via penetration (i.e., trauma, foreign body, surgery, prior centesis). If organisms are not seen in an exudate, sepsis cannot be proven. Cultures should be obtained before a fluid is considered nonseptic, because organisms may be present in numbers low enough to escape detection. Causes of truly nonseptic exudates include disorders such as bile peritonitis, uroperitoneum, acute pancreatitis (may cause pleural effusion as well as abdominal effusion), necrosis associated with intracavitary neoplasia, and sterile exudate secondary to inflammation of an intracavitary organ (i.e., pleural exudate secondary to pneumonia).

EFFUSIONS IN SELECTED DISORDERS

Infections

Inflammation of the pleural cavity (pleuritis), peritoneal cavity (peritonitis), and pericardial space (pericarditis) is associated with chemotactants and vasoactive substances within the respective cavities. The chemotactants cause increased neutrophil and monocyte/macrophage numbers, and the vasoactive substances cause an influx of high-protein fluid. This results in an exudative effusion because of increased capillary permeability, with a massive outpouring of peripheral blood neutrophils and high-protein plasma filtrate into the cavity. Neutrophils, typically degenerate neutrophils, predominate in bacterial infections (Figure 15-23); organisms are seen intracellularly and/or extracellulary (Figures 15-24 and 15-25). The presence of long, slender, filamentous rods is suggestive of *Actinomyces* and *Nocardia* spp., and/or *Fusobacterium* spp. (Figure 15-26). Spirochetes are occasionally seen in association with bacterial peritonitis and pleuritis, especially secondary to bite wounds. Although bacterial infections are the most common, mycotic (Figures 15-27 and 15-28), protozoal (Figure 15-29), and rickettsial peritonitis and/or pleuritis are recognized. The FIP virus is discussed later as a specific entity.

Tissue Inflammation

Inflammation of an intracavity organ (e.g., liver, pancreas, lungs) or a walled-off abscess may cause an effusion. Inflammatory processes release chemotactants that cause influx of neutrophils and monocytes into the area of inflammation and vasoactive products that increase vascular permeability, causing an influx of high-protein

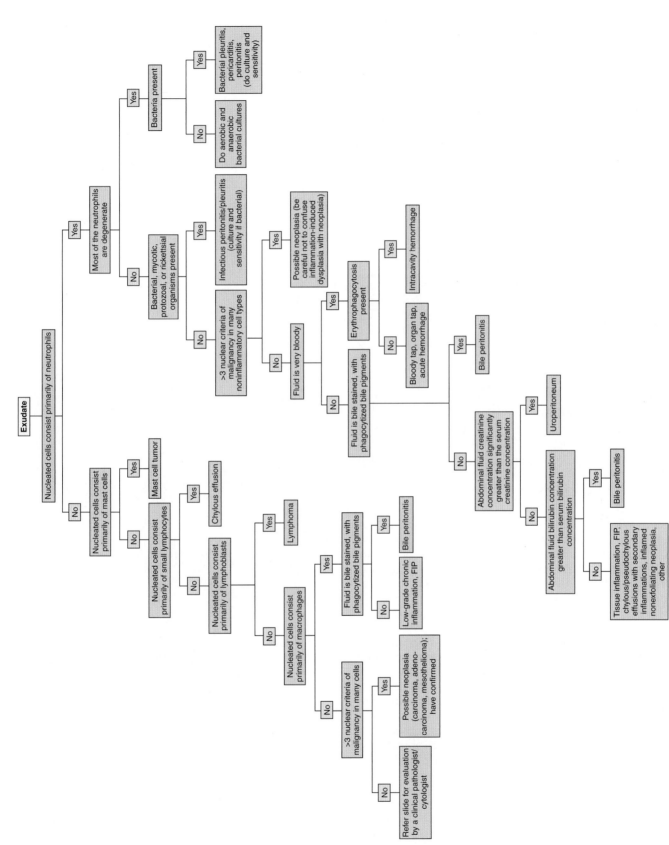

Figure 15-22 An algorithmic approach to the more common causes of exudate effusions.

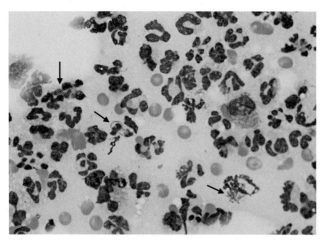

Figure 15-23 Septic exudates showing degenerate neutrophils and phagocytized bacteria *(arrow).*

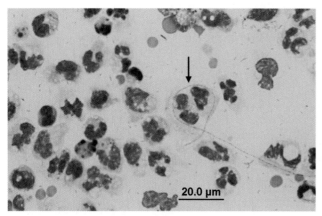

Figure 15-24 Extracellular bacteria *(arrow).*

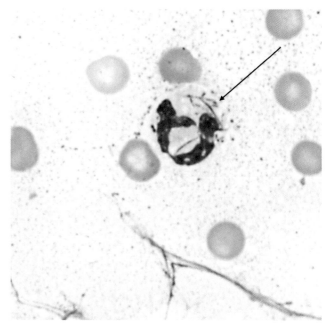

Figure 15-25 Phagocytized filamentous bacterial rod *(arrow).*

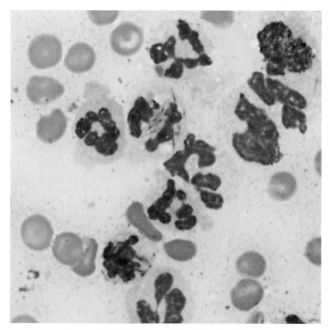

Figure 15-26 Filamentous bacterial rods.

fluid. When the inflammatory process extends into the cavity or inflammatory products are released into it, the cavity becomes inflamed and inflammatory cells tend to accumulate in large numbers. Therefore many factors, including duration and whether an accompanying pleuritis, peritonitis, or pericarditis has occurred, determine whether the effusion is in the modified transudate or exudate classification.

In effusions subsequent to tissue inflammation, nondegenerate neutrophils generally predominate, but macrophages, mesothelial cells, and some lymphocytes are also present. Macrophages, however, may become the predominant cell type in some chronic inflammatory processes. Cytologic evaluation of these effusions readily identifies the process but is typically nondiagnostic as to etiology and must be correlated with physical findings, history, and other diagnostic test results.

Feline Infectious Peritonitis

Clinical FIP can occur in cats of all ages, but in a recent study the proportion of cats with FIP between the ages of 6 months and 2 years was significantly higher than the control cats in similar age groups.[12] In effusive FIP, fluid may accumulate in the abdomen, thorax, and/or pericardium. Evaluation of the fluid is an easy way to obtain a presumptive diagnosis of FIP. The effusion is an odorless, straw-colored to golden, tenacious fluid that may contain flecks or fibrin strands. Bacteriologic cultures are typically negative, although the effusion usually has a high protein (>4.0 g/dl) concentration and a low to moderate cell count (2000 to 6000 cells/μl). Because of the high protein content, the effusion foams when shaken.

Cytologically, the typical FIP effusion has a precipitous eosinophilic background (Figure 15-30) because of the high protein content and consists primarily (60% to 80%) of nondegenerate to mildly degenerate neutrophils

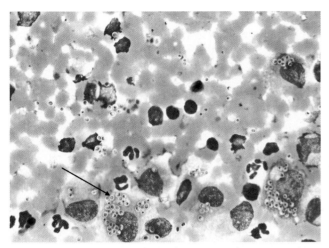

Figure 15-27 Numerous *Histoplasma capsulatum* organisms *(arrow)*. There are numerous organisms both phagocytized by macrophages and present extracellularly.

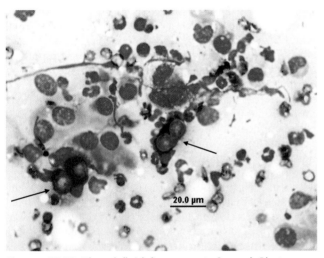

Figure 15-28 Pleural fluid from a cat. Several *Blastomyces* spp. organisms *(arrows)* are present.

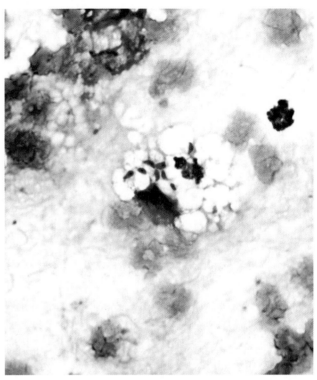

Figure 15-29 *Toxoplasma* organisms within a macrophage. *(Courtesy Susan Fielder, Oklahoma State University.)*

and lesser numbers of macrophages, small lymphocytes, and occasionally plasma cells. Effusions consisting primarily of neutrophils but with large numbers of macrophages are referred to as *pyogranulomatous*. Although these findings are not diagnostic of FIP, when associated with clinical findings, a presumptive diagnosis of FIP can be made. In many cases making a definitive diagnosis of FIP antemortem can be difficult. Other diagnostic tests are often used collaboratively to rule in or rule out FIP. These include determining the A:G in serum and fluid. Serum A:G less than 0.8 g/dl and effusion A:G less than 0.9 g/dl are often present with FIP. Antifeline corona virus (FCoV) antibodies in serum should be interpreted with caution because many healthy cats are FCoV antibody positive.[17,18] In a study by Hartmann et al,[18] low to medium titers (1:25, 1:100, 1:400) of FCoV antibodies were of no diagnostic value in determining FIP infection; however, antibody titers of 1:1600 increased the probability of FIP.[18] A negative test does not rule out

the possibility of FIP infection. In this study, the anti-FCoV antibody test was negative in 10% of the cats that did in fact have FIP.[18] Tests that show promise include reverse transcriptase-polymerase chain reaction (RT-PCR) performed on effusion fluids and an RT-PCR for the detection of FCoV messenger RNA (mRNA) in peripheral blood mononuclear cells. Thus far, histologic examination of tissue samples remains the gold standard for diagnosing FIP.

Bile Peritonitis

Release of bile into the abdominal cavity secondary to gallbladder or bile duct rupture produces peritonitis. Rupture may occur secondary to bile duct obstruction, as a consequence of biliary tract inflammation, trauma, mucoceles, and percutaneous biopsy of the liver. Bile in the peritoneal cavity causes a chemical peritonitis that is typically exudative. The effusion fluid color is typically greenish to yellow-orange and should cause the clinician or pathologist to consider bile peritonitis. Phagocytized, blue-green to yellow-green bile pigment can be seen within macrophages (Figure 15-31). These pigments may be difficult for the beginner to cytologically differentiate from hemosiderin pigment seen in hemorrhagic effusions. Occasionally, amorphous extracellular bile may be seen. When bile peritonitis is suspected because of the color of the abdominal fluid and/or cytologic presence of bile, the bilirubin concentration should be measured in the abdominal fluid and serum. Bile peritonitis typically has abdominal fluid bilirubin levels at least two-fold greater than concurrent serum bilirubin levels.

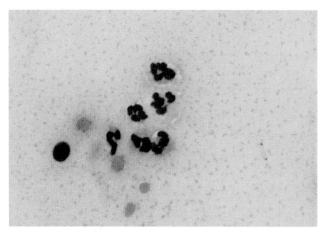

Figure 15-30 Abdominal fluid from a cat with effusive FIP. Note the nondegenerate neutrophils, red blood cells, and small lymphocyte in a granular eosinophilic background. (Wright's stain, original magnification 250×.)

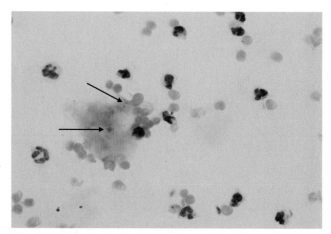

Figure 15-31 Abdominal fluid from a dog. Extracellular bile pigment *(arrows)* and many nondegenerate neutrophils.

A mucocele (mucinous cystic hyperplasia) of biliary and gallbladder epithelial cells can occur secondary to inflammation and cholelithiasis, although often the cause is unknown. In one retrospective study of 30 dogs, the histologic findings suggested mucoceles resulted from dysfunction of mucus-secreting cells within the gallbladder mucosa.[19] Rupture of a biliary mucocele can cause cytologically atypical bile peritonitis. The effusion fluid color may be yellow or red. The cellularity is typically in the exudative range and is composed of high numbers of nondegenerate to mildly degenerate neutrophils and low to moderate numbers of macrophages and reactive mesothelial cells. Varying amounts of mostly extracellular amorphous, basophilic material is seen. This material has been termed *white bile,* although this mucinous material does not contain bile constituents (Figure 15-32). In these cases, abdominal fluid bilirubin concentrations are typically, but not always, higher than serum bilirubin concentrations.[20]

Uroperitoneum

Uroperitoneum may result from leakage of urine from the kidney, ureter, urinary bladder, or urethra. These effusions may have varying numbers of inflammatory cells depending on the duration and dilutional effect of urine, but TNCCs are typically less than 4000/µl. The TP content is generally low (< 3.0 g/dl and often < 2.5 g/dl) due to the dilutional effect of urine volume. An animal with an abdominal effusion that has a moderate TNCC and low TP should raise the suspicion of uroperitoneum. Measuring creatinine levels of abdominal fluid and blood collected simultaneously helps diagnose uroperitoneum. With uroperitoneum, the creatinine concentration of the abdominal fluid is greater than that of serum. The urea nitrogen (UN) concentration in the abdominal fluid may or may not be significantly greater than the serum UN concentration because urea equilibrates between the cavity and blood more rapidly than creatinine. The measurement of creatinine levels in effusion fluid and serum is more reliable than the measurement of the UN level.

Heart Disease

Cats may develop a thoracic effusion secondary to cardiac insufficiency. These effusions are clear yellow to milky white and typically consist of > 50% (often > 80%) small lymphocytes (see the section on chylous/pseudochylous effusions later in this chapter). However, the proportion of neutrophils increases with repeated drainage of the effusion. The increase in neutrophil numbers is likely due to inflammation caused by thoracentesis and also possibly a proportional increase because of lymphopenia associated with lymphocyte loss.

Dogs can develop abdominal effusion secondary to right-sided heart failure. This effusion develops secondary to increased intrahepatic pressure and congestion with leakage of high-protein hepatic lymph. Most of the nucleated cells consist of a mixture of mesothelial/macrophage-type cells, nondegenerate neutrophils, and lymphocytes. There is no cytologic finding in these effusions that is pathognomonic for heart failure. Clinical signs, radiographs, echocardiography, and electrocardiographic examinations are usually necessary to establish a diagnosis of heart failure. An abdominal effusion in the modified transudate range with a diagnosis of heart failure suggests the effusion is secondary to cardiovascular disease.

Chylous Effusions

A chylous effusion contains the chylomicron-rich lymph fluid that is present in lymphatics that drain the intestinal tract and pass through the thoracic duct. Chylomicrons are triglyceride-rich lipoproteins absorbed from the intestines after the ingestion of food containing lipids. Lymphatics originating cranial to the diaphragm do not contain chyle. Chylous effusions in dogs and cats occur most frequently as bilateral thoracic effusions, but chylous ascites occurs less frequently.[21] The classic description of a chylous effusion is a milky effusion that does not clear after centrifugation. Cytologically, it contains mostly small lymphocytes.

Chyle normally drains from the thoracic duct into the venous system. Chylous effusions form when there is an obstruction (physical or functional) of lymphatic flow

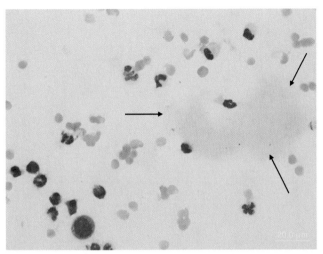

Figure 15-32 Abdominal fluid from a dog. Extracellular homogenous basophilic material, or "white bile" *(arrows)*, is shown.

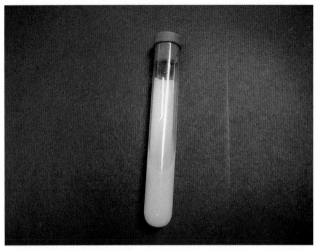

Figure 15-33 Milky white pleural fluid (chylous effusion) from a cat.

resulting in increased pressure within lymphatics and dilation of the thoracic duct (lymphangiectasia). Rupture of the thoracic duct (e.g., postsurgical, blunt trauma) is a rare cause of chylous effusion in veterinary medicine[21] and is usually self-limiting.[2,21] Physical obstructions of the thoracic duct may result from neoplasms, granulomas, or inflammatory reactions in the mediastinum that compress the thoracic duct or the vessels into which it drains or secondary to obstruction of intra-lymphatic flow with neoplastic cells. Functional obstructions may occur with cardiovascular disease due to increased central venous pressure (right-sided heart failure) or increased lymphatic flow due to increased hepatic lymph production that exceeds drainage capability.[21,22] Cardiovascular disease (e.g., cardiomyopathy, heartworm disease, pericardial effusions) that results in poor venous flow may also result in a chylous effusion.

Many other miscellaneous causes of chylous effusion have been reported, including coughing and vomiting,[22] diaphragmatic herniation, congenital defects, trauma, and thrombosis of the thoracic duct. Often, no underlying cause can be determined despite extensive testing (idiopathic).[2,21,22]

Although most milky effusions are true chylous effusions, they may rarely be pseudochylous. Pseudochylous effusions are milky effusions that do not contain chyle; their white color is classically thought to be the result of cellular debris, lecithin globulin complex, and/or cholesterol rather than chylomicrons. Pseudochylous effusions described in humans are most commonly the result of long-standing pleural effusions due to tuberculosis, rheumatoid pleuritis, and malignant effusions, with resultant cell breakdown within the fluid. Despite much discussion about differentiating these two types of fluids, pseudochylous effusions are not well described in veterinary medicine and are rare in dogs and cats.[2,21] Milky effusions caused by feline heart disease had previously been classified as pseudochylous because no thoracic duct rupture was demonstrated. They are now thought to be the result of lymphatic leakage without rupture, however, and are classified as true chylous effusions.[21]

Chylous effusions are odorless and vary in color from milky white (Figure 15-33) to yellow to pink, depending on diet (i.e., animals that are anorectic and not ingesting lipids may not have the characteristic opaque white fluid) and the number of RBCs in the fluid. Although small lymphocytes are typically thought of as the predominant cell type, chylous effusions can occur with neutrophils and/or lipid-containing macrophages (Figure 15-34) predominating.[19,22] Increased neutrophils occur secondary to inflammation induced by repeated thoracentesis and the presence of chyle in the pleural cavity. Chyle is considered a nonirritant, but it often causes an inflammatory reaction in some dogs and in most cats that can lead to pleural fibrosis.[19,22] Bacterial infection in chylous effusions is uncommon because of the bacteriostatic effect of the fatty acids in chyle,[2,21,22] but can occur as a result of repeated thoracentesis.

Because some chylous effusions are not milky nor predominantly made up of small lymphocytes, they are best identified by measuring triglyceride and cholesterol concentrations in both the effusion and the peripheral blood.[2,21,22] With chylous effusions, the triglyceride concentration is higher in the effusion than in the serum, and the cholesterol concentration is higher in the serum than in the effusion.[2,21,22] The reverse is true for nonchylous effusions.[2,21] Identifying fat droplets cytologically on Sudan III–stained smears of the effusion confirms a diagnosis of chylous effusion,[2,22] but is often unnecessary. Chylous effusions often form a top "cream" layer if the fluid is left standing.[21] Rarely, an effusion is white because of the large number of white blood cells present. These effusions are generally due to infectious causes, and degenerate neutrophils and bacteria are found cytologically. These effusions are clumpy (like curdled milk) rather than smooth (milky), as with chylous effusions.

Hemorrhagic Effusions

Hemorrhagic effusions occur with many different disorders. Hemostatic defects, trauma, heartworm infection, and neoplasia are some of the more common causes.

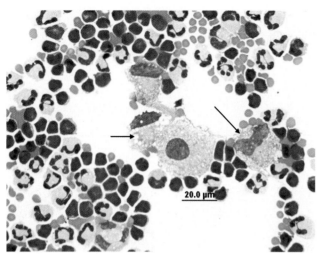

Figure 15-34 Numerous small lymphocytes and several macrophages containing small, distinct clear cytoplasmic vacuoles *(arrows)*.

Often, pericardial effusions are hemorrhagic to serosanguinous. Differentiating hemorrhagic effusions from iatrogenic blood contamination or inadvertent aspiration of an organ (e.g., liver, spleen) is of diagnostic importance. Unfortunately, differentiating blood contamination from acute hemorrhage can be difficult; however, if acute hemorrhage is severe, clinical signs indicating severe blood loss should be evident.

Hemorrhage of more than 1 day duration or chronic persistent hemorrhage can be differentiated from blood contamination by evaluating the smear for erythrophagocytosis (Figure 15-35) and the presence or absence of platelets or other RBC breakdown product, hemosiderin (Figures 15-36 and 15-37), and hematoidin (Figure 15-38). When blood enters a body cavity, the platelets quickly aggregate, degranulate, and disappear. Also, RBCs are phagocytized and digested by macrophages. Therefore, the absence of erythrophagocytosis and the presence of platelets suggest either peracute hemorrhage or iatrogenic blood contamination. The presence of both erythrophagocytosis and platelets suggests either chronic persistent hemorrhage or previous hemorrhage and iatrogenic contamination. The presence of erythrophagocytosis and the absence of platelets suggests chronic or previous hemorrhage.

Grossly bloody fluid is occasionally collected. In these instances, a splenic aspirate, a major vessel puncture, or intracavity hemorrhage should be considered. With a major vessel or splenic aspirate, the PCV of the fluid is generally equal to (vessel puncture) or greater than (splenic aspirate) the peripheral blood PCV. With severe intracavity hemorrhage, clinical signs of rapid blood loss should be evident.

Neoplasia

Effusions can occur secondary to neoplasia. If neoplastic cells are exfoliated into the effusion, a diagnosis can be made cytologically. In one study, the sensitivity of cytologic examination of effusions to detect malignant neoplasms

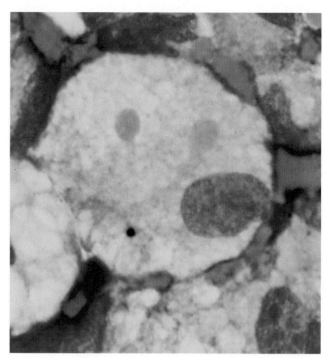

Figure 15-35 Erythrophagocytosis.

was 64% in dogs and 61% in cats.[24] Most effusions caused by tumors not exfoliating neoplastic cells are in the modified transudate range. However, most effusions caused by tumors that are exfoliating cells into the cavity and are secondarily inflamed are in the exudate category. Recognizing neoplastic cells is much more difficult if inflammation is present because cell dysplasia is readily induced by inflammation. Also, care must be taken not to confuse normal or reactive mesothelial cells with neoplastic cells.

Lymphoma, mast cell tumor, mesothelioma, and various carcinomas, adenocarcinomas, and rarely sarcomas have been diagnosed by cytologic evaluation of effusions. Lymphoma is diagnosed by large numbers of immature lymphocytes (lymphoblasts) in the effusion (Figure 15-39). Lymphoblasts have a moderate amount of clear to blue cytoplasm, variably shaped nuclei, finely stippled nuclear chromatin, and nucleoli (often irregular in shape and size); lymphoblasts are larger than neutrophils.

Mast cell tumors within body cavities may cause effusions and frequently exfoliate large numbers of mast cells into the effusion. Mast cells are readily identified by their red-purple granules. In effusions, mast cells tend to have their granules grouped to one side. Because the granules have a high affinity for stain, the nucleus may stain poorly or not at all. Diff-Quik stain does not undergo the metachromatic reaction and, therefore often does not stain mast cell granules well. Eosinophils are usually also present. Neutrophils, mesothelial cells, and macrophages may be present in variable numbers.

Sarcomas are rarely diagnosed cytologically in effusions. They are recognized by a characteristic spindle appearance and malignant criteria (see Chapter 2).

Mesotheliomas are uncommon tumors that are difficult to diagnose cytologically because of the variability

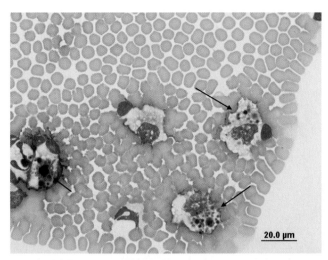

Figure 15-36 Numerous macrophages containing hemosiderin pigment *(arrows).*

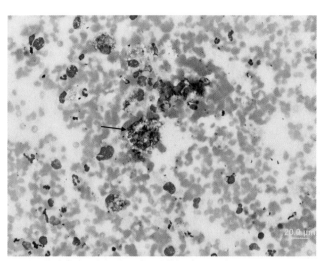

Figure 15-38 Hemorrhagic pericardial fluid and a macrophage containing hematoidin crystals *(arrow).*

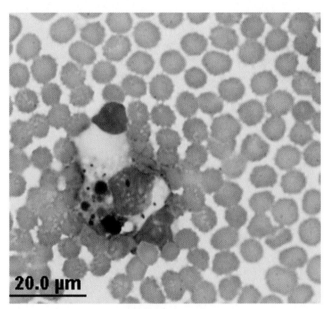

Figure 15-37 Macrophage containing hemosiderin pigment and numerous RBCs.

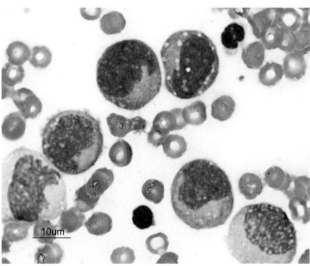

Figure 15-39 Pericardial fluid from a dog with lymphoma. Large lymphoblasts predominate. *(Courtesy James Meinkoth, Oklahoma State University.)*

of reactive mesothelial cells. Cytologically, the neoplastic cells resemble epithelium and are present both in clusters and individually. Their cytoplasm is generally clear to light blue and vacuolated, and they have well-defined cell borders. Multinucleation, giant forms, and multiple prominent angular nucleoli may be present. When mesothelioma cells are anaplastic enough to be recognized as malignant, they cannot be easily differentiated cytologically from carcinoma cells.

Carcinomas and adenocarcinomas are sometimes diagnosed by cytologic evaluation of effusions and can elicit an inflammatory response (Figure 15-40). These epithelial cell tumors are identified on the basis of their nuclear criteria of malignancy. Cytoplasmic aberrations are supportive but not diagnostic. Some of the criteria

of malignancy include anisokaryosis; nuclear gigantism; coarse nuclear chromatin; large, bizarre, or angular nucleoli; multiple nucleoli; nuclear molding; high nuclear-to-cytoplasmic ratios; numerous mitotic figures; anisocytosis; basophilic cytoplasm; and abnormal cytoplasmic vacuolation (Figures 15-41 and 15-42). Also, cluster formation is relatively common with epithelial tumors (carcinoma). Chapter 2 contains a detailed discussion of malignant criteria.

Because many tumors do not exfoliate neoplastic cells, the absence of neoplastic cells within effusions does not rule out neoplasia. Also, differentiating neoplastic cells from reactive mesothelial cells and/or activated macrophages may be difficult. Therefore unless the examiner is experienced in evaluating cytologic samples for neoplasia, samples interpreted as neoplastic or suspected of being

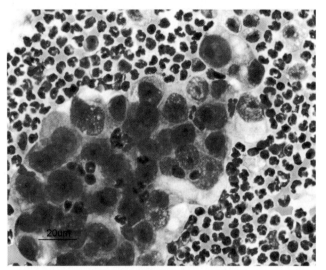

Figure 15-40 Pleural fluid from a dog with adenocarcinoma. There are a cluster of atypical cells and numerous nondegenerate neutrophils. *(Courtesy James Meinkoth, Oklahoma State University.)*

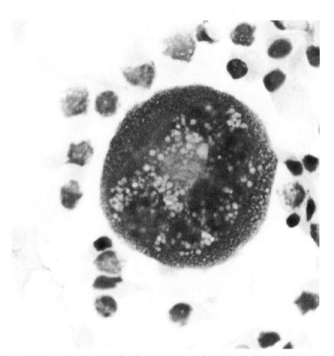

Figure 15-41 Note the large atypical multinucleated cell in pleural fluid from a dog with carcinoma.

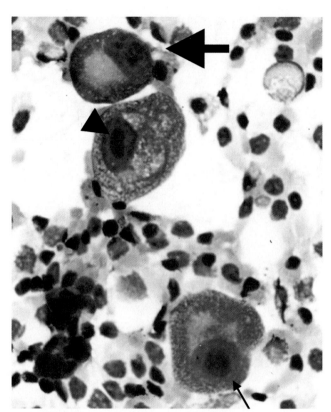

Figure 15-42 Several large atypical cells with large *(small arrow)*, angular *(arrowhead)*, and multiple *(large arrow)* nucleoli.

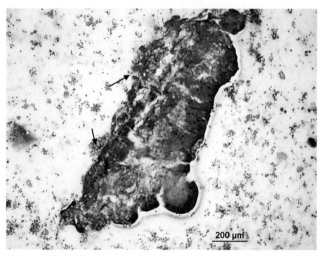

Figure 15-43 Remnant of metacestode. Note the size of the red blood cells and inflammatory cells in the background. The clear, nonstaining structures are calcareous corpuscles *(arrows).*

neoplastic should be confirmed by a veterinary clinical pathologist or other experienced cytologist.

Parasitic Effusion

Abdominal effusion due to aberrant larval migration of tapeworm *Mesocestoides* spp. is uncommon. Cases of canine infection are reported in northwestern United States, particularly in California, with fewer cases in Washington.[25] Clinical signs may include anorexia, vomiting, weight loss, depression, and abdominal distension.

Gross appearance of the fluid contains small opaque flecks which are the metacestodes.[25] Analysis of the aspirated fluid is in the exudative range. Cytologic features includes numerous inflammatory cells, partial to intact metacestodes, and numerous round to angular, clear to pink refractile calcareous corpuscles (Figures 15-43 and 15-44).

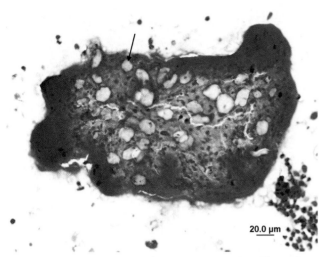

Figure 15-44 Remnant of a metacestode. The clear, nonstaining structures are calcareous corpuscles *(arrow)*.

References

1. Nelson OL: Pleural effusion. In Ettinger SJ, Feldman EC (eds): *Textbook of Veterinary Internal Medicine*. Philadelphia, Saunders, 2005, pp 204-207.
2. Fossum TW: Surgery of the lower respiratory system: pleural cavity and diaphragm. In Fossum TW (ed): *Small Animal Surgery*. St Louis, Mosby, 2005, pp 788-820.
3. Zoia A, Hughes D, Connolly DJ: Pericardial effusion and cardiac tamponade in a cat with extranodal lymphoma. *J Small Anim Pract* 45:467-471, 2004.
4. Tobias AH: Pericardial disorders. In Ettinger SJ, Feldman EC (eds): *Textbook of Veterinary Internal Medicine*. Philadelphia, Saunders, 2005, pp 1107-111.
5. Gidlewski J, Petrie JP: Therapeutic pericardiocentesis in the dog and cat. *Clin Tech Small Anim Pract* 20:151-155, 2005.
6. Fossum TW: Surgery of the abdominal cavity. In Fossum TW (ed): *Small Animal Surgery*. St Louis, Mosby, 2002, pp 271-272.
7. Walters JM: Abdominal paracentesis and diagnostic peritoneal lavage. *Clin Tech Small Anim Pract* 18(1):32-38, 2003.
8. D'Urso L: Thoracic and pericardial taps and drains. In Ettinger SJ, Feldman EC (eds): *Textbook of Veterinary Internal Medicine*. Philadelphia, Saunders, 2005, pp 380-831.
9. Johnson MS, et al: A retrospective study of clinical findings, treatment and outcome in 143 dogs with pericardial effusion. *J Small Anim Pract* 45:546-552, 2004.
10. Cowell R, et al: Collection and evaluation of equine peritoneal and pleural effusions. *Vet Clin North Am (Equine Pract)* 3:543-561, 1987.
11. George JW: The usefulness and limitations of hand-held refractometers in veterinary laboratory medicine: An historical and technical review. *Vet Clin Path* 30(4):201-210, 2001.
12. Edwards NJ: The diagnostic value of pericardial fluid pH determinations. *J Am Hosp Assoc* 32:63-67, 1996.
13. Fine DM, Tobias AH, Jacob KA: Use of pericardial fluid pH to distinguish between idiopathic and neoplastic effusions. *J Vet Intern Med* 17:525-529, 2003.
14. de Laforcade AM, et al: Biochemical analysis of pericardial fluid and whole blood in dogs with pericardial effusion. *J Vet Intl Med* 19:833-836, 2005.
15. Cowgill E, Neel J: Pleural fluid from a dog with marked eosinophilia. *Vet Clin Pathol* 32(4):147-149, 2003.
16. Takahashi T, et al: Visceral mast cell tumors in dogs: 10 cases (1982-1997). *J Am Vet Assoc* 216(2):222-226, 2000.
17. Rohrbach BW, et al Epidemiology of feline infectious peritonitis among cats examined at veterinary medical teaching hospitals. *J Am Vet Assoc* 218(7):1111-1115, 2001.
18. Hartmann K, et al: Comparison of different tests to diagnose feline infectious peritonitis. *J Vet Intern Med* 17:781-790, 2003.
19. Pike FS, et al: Gallbladder mucocele in dogs: 30 cases (2000-2002). *J Am Vet Assoc* 224(10):1615-1622, 2004.
20. Owens SD, et al: Three cases of canine bile peritonitis with mucinous material in abdominal fluid as the prominent cytologic finding. *Vet Clin Pathol* 32(3):114-120, 2003.
21. Meadows RL, MacWilliams PS: Chylous effusions revisited. *Vet Clin Pathol* 23:54-62, 1994.
22. Mertens MM, Fossum TW, Pleural and extrapleural diseases. In Fossum TW (ed): *Small Animal Surgery:* St Louis, Mosby, 2002, pp 1281-1282.
23. Harpster NK: Chylothorax. In Kirk RW (ed): *Current Veterinary Therapy* IX. Philadelphia, Saunders, 1986, pp 295-303.
24. Hirschberger J, et al: Sensitivity and specificity of cytologic evaluation in the diagnosis of neoplasia in body fluids from dogs and cats. *Vet Clin Path* 28(4):142-146, 1999.
25. Caruso KH, et al: Cytologic diagnosis of peritonel cestodiasis in dogs caused by *Mesocestoides* sp. *Vet Clin Pathol* 32(2): 50-60, 2003.

Transtracheal and Bronchoalveolar Washes

K. English, R.L. Cowell, R.D. Tyler, and J.H. Meinkoth

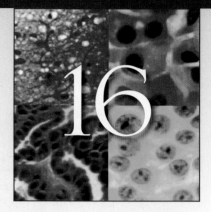

CHAPTER 16

Respiratory flush/washes sample the contents of the airways, the trachea, bronchi, and alveolar spaces. These samples can frequently provide clinically useful information of the pulmonary disease process, and may also provide definitive diagnosis in some patients. Pulmonary disease is frequently defined by the area that it affects (e.g., bronchitis) or by the changes that may occur as a result of the disease process (e.g., bronchiectasis); however, the underlying pathology may be variable with these disease presentations, and cytology and culture of a lower respiratory tract sample may be helpful in determining the etiology.[1,2,3] In pathologies that solely involve abnormal structure or function of the airways, or in diseases that do not have direct airway involvement, which may include some primary or metastatic neoplasias, the information obtained from a flush/wash sample may be limited.[4]

Tracheal wash/bronchoalveolar lavage (TW/BAL) samples are quick, easy, and inexpensive ways to obtain diagnostic samples from the respiratory tree. Although complications are uncommon, subcutaneous emphysema, pneumomediastinum, hemorrhage, resultant hypoxia, needle tract infection, transient hemoptysis, bronchoconstriction, and other complications have been reported.[5-7]

It is frequently helpful to perform radiography in conjunction with the wash procedure, although radiographic changes may not always be apparent in the early stages of respiratory disease.[8,9] Radiography prior to a flush/wash procedure may be invaluable if the disease is focal because this will indicate which lung lobe is most likely to provide a diagnostic yield and allow selective sampling, particularly if bronchoscope guided lavage is used. If the disease is diffuse then sampling of any area of the lung may be representative, although sampling from multiple sites is more likely to provide a diagnostic yield.[10]

The cell types noted in the sample may be variable depending on the site of sampling (Tables 16-1 and 16-2).

TECHNIQUE OF TRACHEAL WASH AND BRONCHOALVEOLAR LAVAGE

Approach to the lower respiratory tract may be transtracheal or endotracheal. If endotracheal, then sampling may be performed by bronchoscopic or nonbronchoscopic (blind) methods.

The advantage of the bronchoscope is that observation of the mucosa lining the airways and quantification of mucus or secretions present may provide additional patient assessment. More directed sampling of the individual lobes may also be performed. Nonbronchoscopic sampling, however, does not require expensive equipment and so may be more widely available in first opinion practice.

There are a number of reviews of the sampling techniques[11-14]; however, a brief summary is outlined here.

Transtracheal Sampling

The transtracheal or percutaneous method is optimal for patients who are a high anesthetic risk because it may be performed with local anaesthesia only, or with additional sedation if required. This technique may also be less prone to oropharyngeal contamination and therefore may be preferred if obtaining a sample for culture. Small amounts of fluid are instilled, and a cough reflex is essential for fluid recovery.

- The skin over the cranioventral larynx is clipped and the site is prepared as for aseptic surgery. Surgical gloves should be worn.
- A small amount of 1% to 2% lidocaine is infiltrated into the subcutaneous tissue. Very light sedation may be helpful in cats and small dogs[5]; intravenous ketamine has been recommended for sedation of cats.[6]
- The animal is restrained in a sitting position or sternal recumbency with the neck extended. Overextension of the neck, however, may result in increased oropharyngeal contamination (one author's observation).
- A small, triangular depression is digitally palpated just cranial to the ridge of the cricoid cartilage. This is the location of the cricothyroid ligament and of needle insertion (Figure 16-1). Alternatively, the catheter may be inserted between two tracheal rings 1 to 3 cm below the larynx (e.g., C2 to C3, or C3 to C4).[15]
- Using a large commercial intravenous catheter set, "through the needle," or intravascular catheter and a 3.5-French polyethylene urinary catheter,[6] with the

needle directed slightly caudad, the skin, subcutaneous tissue, and cricothyroid ligament of the larynx, or ligament between the tracheal rings, are penetrated. Smaller catheters are suggested for cats and very small dogs.

- Once in the tracheal lumen, the needle is positioned parallel to the trachea and the catheter is advanced through the needle and down the lumen of the trachea to a level just above the carina. Insertion of the needle and passage of the catheter induces coughing in most animals.[5,6]
- The catheter should pass easily; if it does not, it may have become embedded in the dorsal tracheal wall or failed to enter the trachea and may be embedded in the peritracheal tissue.[16] In either case, the needle and the entire catheter should be withdrawn, and the procedure repeated. Also, the catheter may bend, causing it to advance toward the oropharynx, resulting in the washing of the oropharynx, not the bronchial tree.
- Once the catheter is properly placed, the needle is withdrawn leaving the catheter in place. With some severe pulmonary diseases, a sample can be obtained by simply aspirating after positioning the catheter. However, the infusion of saline into the bronchial tree is usually necessary before aspiration to obtain an adequate sample. A 12-ml or larger syringe containing 1 to 2 ml of nonbacteriostatic, sterile, buffered saline for every 5 kg of body weight is attached to the catheter. The saline is injected into the bronchial lumen until either the animal starts to cough or all of the fluid is injected.
- The animal will typically start coughing before all of the saline is injected, at which time aspiration must start.

Only a small portion of the injected fluid will be retrieved. The injected fluid remaining in the tracheobronchial tree will be rapidly absorbed and is no cause for concern.[5]

- The operator aspirates for only a few seconds and then stops. Aspiration for a prolonged time results in more fluid being collected, but the chance of a contaminated wash is greatly increased because the animal will cough fluid into the oropharyngeal area and reaspirate the fluid, which now contains cellular and bacterial contaminants.

Maintaining gentle pressure on the puncture site for a few minutes generally inhibits the formation of subcutaneous emphysema.[15] Applying mild pressure to the puncture site with a gauze wrap for 12 to 24 hours also helps eliminate the formation of subcutaneous emphysema.

Endotracheal Tube Technique

Alternatively, samples are collected through an endotracheal tube (Figure 16-2). This procedure requires general anesthesia. This technique may be used to obtain either a tracheal sample or bronchoalveolar lavage. For a tracheal sample, the sample catheter extends beyond the end of the endotracheal tube, but does not extend past the carina. The location of the carina is externally assessed as approximately the level of the fourth intercostal space.[10] For a blind bronchoalveolar lavage, a sample tube of appropriate size for the patient (e.g., a 16-French polyvinyl chloride stomach tube in a medium- to large-sized dog,[17] and

TABLE 16-1

Lining Cells of the Lower Respiratory Tract that May Be Noted on TW/BAL Sampling

Airway	Lining cell[76]
Large airway, trachea, and bronchi	Ciliated columnar epithelium, goblet cell
Bronchiole	Columnar to cuboidal epithelium, ciliated to nonciliated Alveoli
Alveolus	Type I pneumocyte (not commonly observed on BAL cytology)

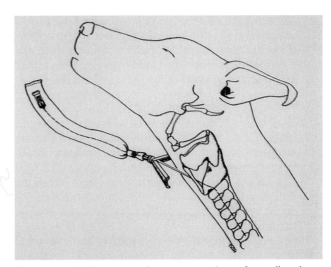

Figure 16-1 Diagrammatic representation of needle placement through the cricothyroid ligament of the larynx.

TABLE 16-2

Average of Mean Percentage Cell Differential of Nonepithelial Populations from a Number of Studies of BAL Samples from Healthy Dogs and Cats

	Macrophage	Neutrophil	Eosinophil	Lymphocyte	Mast Cell
Dog	71%	5%	5%	17%	2%
Cat	70%	6%	18%	4%	1%

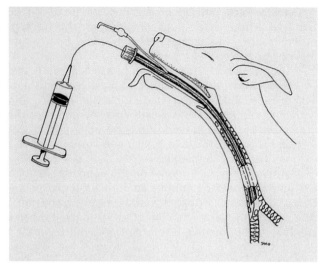

Figure 16-2 Diagrammatic representation of catheter placement and TW/BAL collection through an endotracheal tube.

a 5-French polypropylene urinary catheter in a cat[18]) was shown to consistently maintain a snug fit between the external land marks of the seventh and eleventh ribs, so the sample tubing should be a minimum length to reach the level of the eleventh rib.[17] Sterile tubing should be used.

- Once the patient has reached a suitable plane of anesthesia, an endotracheal tube should be carefully placed with as minimal contact with the oropharynx and larynx as may be achieved.
- Preoxygenation is recommended. Fitting of a T or Y piece to the endotracheal tube will allow delivery of oxygen and anesthetic gas throughout the procedure. If the leakage of gas is a particular concern to the veterinary staff then anesthesia may be maintained by injectable anesthetic agents administered via an intravenous (IV) catheter.
- The patient is placed in sternal or lateral recumbency; if lateral, then it is preferable to place the most affected side down.[14] In some cases use of a foam wedge to elevate the cranial part of the thorax above that of the caudal part has been recommended.[19]
- A bronchoscope, tube, or catheter through which the sample will be obtained is introduced through the endotracheal tube, ensuring this does not contact the oropharynx.

The canine bronchial tree is irregularly branching and has been reviewed in detail.[20] From this, briefly, when the patient is orientated in sternal recumbency the entrance to the right principal bronchus appears as almost a direct continuation of the trachea, with the left principal bronchus noted at a more acute angle. The first lobar bronchus on the right is the right cranial lung lobe, in the lateral wall of the bronchus opposite the carina. The next lobar bronchus is the right middle lung lobe, in the ventral floor, usually between the 6 and 8 o'clock positions. The right accessory lobe is located in the ventromedial to medial aspect of the right principal bronchus, just beyond the origin of the middle lobe bronchus, extending in a ventromedial direction. Beyond this bronchus is the lobar bronchus for the right caudal lung lobe. On the left the left cranial lung lobe is accessed ventrolateral to the lateral aspect of the left cranial bronchus. Beyond this, the left principal bronchus becomes the left caudal lung lobe bronchus.

- If the patient is in lateral recumbency the orientation and access to the lung for sampling may be altered.[21]
- When the desired level has been reached for TW or BAL (see previous), then fluid may be introduced. In order to optimize recovery of fluid from a BAL, the bronchoscope or tube should be wedged into the bronchi. This may be determined visually on a bronchoscope. If performing a blind BAL, then the tube should be advanced gently until it stops; it should then be withdrawn a few centimeters, rotated gently, and readvanced until resistance is felt at a consistent level.[17]
- Once a snug fit has been achieved, a syringe with an appropriate volume of fluid and an additional 5-ml of air to ensure complete delivery of the fluid is attached to the top of the sample tube. Volumes used may vary; however, a suitable volume in cats is reported to be aliquots of 5-ml/kg,[22] and this was found to provide adequate cellular yield in dogs.[23] Repeat aliquots may be administered until there is sufficient fluid retrieval; however, no more than three aliquots are generally used.
- Fluid recovery may be affected by the tightness of the fit of the bronchoscope or sample tubing in the airway. A double catheter technique has been described in which the catheter to collect the sample is a few centimeters above the level of the catheter delivering the fluid aliquot, with the authors reporting good fluid recovery without the need for a snug fit.[24]

Other measures that may increase fluid retrieval is tilting the head of the patient downward, or rotating the patient with the lavaged lung area uppermost to encourage fluid drainage.[25] This may be complicated in larger patients, and the risk of gastric dilation of the volvulus in large, deep-chested dogs may also be a concern with rotation of these patients.

Retrieved fluid should appear foamy if the sampling has been adequate, reported to reflect the presence of surfactant.[14]

Other techniques that have been reported via bronchoscopic sampling are bronchial brushings and biopsy.[15] One study suggests that in some instances bronchial brushing may be a more sensitive test to assess for inflammation, although in one patient BAL was the more sensitive test[26]; however, the criteria to determine what constitutes inflammation from these types of samples alone is not clearly defined.

Bronchoscopy may also be used for treatment, as in the removal of tracheobronchial foreign bodies.[27] Therapeutic bronchoalveolar lavage has also been described in one dog affected by pulmonary alveolar proteinosis.[28]

SAMPLE SUBMISSION

Several studies in healthy patients have shown that there are no significant differences between different lobes of the lung lavaged either in overall cell numbers or differential counts.[19,29] Therefore increases of cells will be interpreted similarly no matter which area of the lung the samples are derived from. The first aliquot is reported to have fewer epithelial cells and higher numbers of polymorphonuclear cells, and some authors recommend discarding the first aliquot, although if combined with subsequent aliquots it is unlikely to significantly affect clinical interpretation.[22]

It is recommended to prepare fresh smears at the time of sample collection, within 30 minutes[29] because cell morphology is not well preserved in TW/BAL samples. A direct smear of turbid fluid, or if mucous flecks are noted grossly, a smear of mucus material and additional cytocentrifuged preparations are likely to provide the most information from the sample. Cytocentrifugation has been reported to affect the cell populations, particularly reducing the number of small lymphocytes present.[30]

Recommendations for samples submitted to the laboratory are noted in Box 16-1. Guidelines for preparing smears from fluids are presented in Chapter 1.

If the TW/BAL is deemed unacceptable because of oropharyngeal contamination (or for any other reason) and is to be repeated, it should be repeated either immediately or after 48 hours. Even though a sterile saline solution is used for the wash, it induces a neutrophilic response that peaks about 24 hours after washing. If a TW/BAL is performed the next day (i.e., 24 hours after the first wash), an inflammatory response will be present and it may be difficult to tell whether it is secondary to the prior wash or because of an inflammatory lung disease.[31-33] However, there may be no significant difference in samples collected 48 hours apart.[23,31,33] If a contaminated wash is obtained, waiting at least 48 hours to re-collect a TW/BAL is ideal because it allows the lungs time to clear the oropharyngeal contaminants. Sometimes, however, such a delay is not practical. Although some contaminants from the previous wash may be collected, if the TW/BAL is repeated immediately, the amount of oropharyngeal contamination should be minimal, and this may be preferable to waiting 48 hours.

CELL COUNTS

Cell counts are difficult to perform on TW/BAL fluids because of the mucous content, and the dilution factor may be variable.[34] The method of obtaining cell counts is also varied in many studies of TW/BAL in dogs and cats, so values may not be directly comparable, and diagnostic significance is often difficult to determine. Cell counts are recommended by some authors to determine whether an adequate sample has been obtained and to assess whether resampling is necessary. However, this may not be easily applicable in the practice setting. Qualitative estimates (normal or increased) of cellularity can be done on stained sediment smears and may be useful.

CYTOLOGIC EVALUATION

Mucus

A small amount of mucus may be present in TW/BAL from clinically normal dogs and cats. Mucus appears as amorphous sheets ranging from blue to pink or as homogeneous strands that are frequently twisted or whorled[5,25] (Figure 16-3; see also Figures 16-6, 16-11, 16-12, 16-16, and 16-17). A granular appearance of the mucus is frequently associated with increased cellularity.[5] Inflammation, irritation, or upper airway damage, which may be a result of chronic airway disease, may result in increased numbers of goblet cells, and an increased amount of mucous is generally present, possibly with altered mucous properties.[5,31,35] In inflammatory conditions, mucus usually stains eosinophilic because of the incorporation of inflammatory proteins and material from lysed cells.[5]

Curschmann's spirals (see Figure 16-3) are mucous casts of small bronchioles that appear as spiral, twisted masses of mucus that may have perpendicular radiations, giving them a test tube-brush-like appearance.[4] They may be seen in TW/BAL from patients with any disorder that results in chronic, excessive production of mucous and are an indication of bronchiolar obstruction.

Cell Types

Many different types of cells (e.g., ciliated and nonciliated columnar cells, ciliated and nonciliated cuboidal cells, alveolar macrophages, neutrophils, eosinophils,

---

BOX 16-1

Samples for Submission to the Pathology Laboratory

Smears prepared from the flush/wash sample within 30 minutes of obtaining the sample

Ethylene-tetra-acetic acid sample for further cytology preparations

Plain sterile sample for culture

Optional specific media preparations (e.g., for mycoplasma culture); contact laboratory before sampling

---

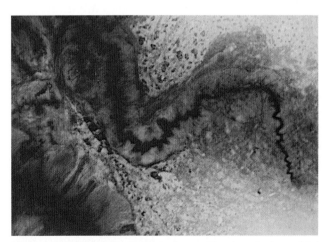

Figure 16-3 TW/BAL from a dog with chronic bronchial disease. A large Curschmann's spiral and scattered alveolar macrophages are present in an eosinophilic mucous background. (Wright's stain, original magnification 50×.)

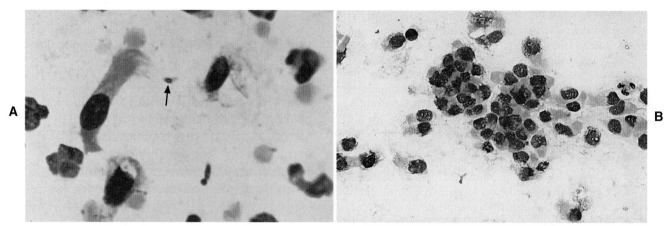

Figure 16-4 A, TW/BAL from a dog with toxoplasmosis. A ciliated columnar cell, RBCs, scattered neutrophils, and an extracellular *Toxoplasma gondii* organism *(arrow)* are shown. (Wright's stain, original magnification 250×.) **B,** Ciliated columnar cells are present both individually and in a cluster. The morphology of the cells in the cluster cannot be discerned. Cilia are evident on the cells that are well spread out. Many of the cells are traumatized as evidenced by their irregular nuclear outlines. (Wright's stain, original magnification 160×.)

lymphocytes, mast cells, erythrocytes, and dysplastic and neoplastic cells) may be seen with TW/BAL (see Tables 16-1 and 16-2). Ciliated and nonciliated columnar and cuboidal cells and alveolar macrophages are the cell types seen in washings from normal dogs and cats. They are also seen in many disease states unless the washed area is filled with exudative secretions or the disease process has obliterated normal lung parenchyma.

Columnar and Cuboidal Cells: Ciliated columnar cells (Figures 16-4 and 16-5) have an elongated or cone shape, with cilia on their flattened apical ends. The nucleus, which is generally round to oval with a finely granular chromatin pattern, is present in the basal end of the cells, which often terminate in a thin tail.[4] The ciliated cuboidal cells look similar to the ciliated columnar cells except that the cuboidal cells are as wide as they are tall. Nonciliated columnar and cuboidal cells look identical to their ciliated counterparts, except for the absence of cilia. These cell types are normal findings in TW/BAL. If these cell types are predominant in a sample, the washing procedure probably sampled mainly bronchi and bronchioles (as opposed to alveolar spaces).

Cuboidal and columnar epithelial cells may be present individually or in clusters (see Figure 16-4, *B*). Depending on the orientation of the cell on the slide (especially with cells in clusters), the cuboidal/columnar nature of the cells and cilia may be difficult to visualize. This is of little clinical significance, but these cells must not be interpreted as abnormal cell types.[4] Also, the majority of the columnar cells may be poorly preserved in many washes (see Figure 16-4, *B*) as a result of the low protein fluid in which they are collected. Cells traumatized during slide preparation may show irregular nuclear outlines or be overtly ruptured (e.g., smudge cells).

Goblet Cells: Goblet cells (see Figure 16-5) are mucus-producing bronchial cells that are generally elongated (i.e., columnar) with a basally placed nucleus and round granules of mucin, which frequently distend the cytoplasm.[4] Occasionally, the cytoplasm is so distended that the cell appears round. The granules stain from red to blue to clear with Romanowsky (e.g., Giemsa-Wright) stains. Free granules from ruptured goblet cells may be seen in the smear (see Figure 16-5, *B*). The shape of the cells and the large size of the granules are helpful in differentiating these cells from mast cells (see Figure 16-5, *C*). Goblet cells are not commonly seen; however, any chronic pulmonary irritant may result in increased numbers of goblet cells.

Macrophages: Alveolar macrophages (Figure 16-6) (see also Figures 16-8, 16-12, and 16-17) are readily found and are often the predominant cell type in TW/BAL from clinically normal animals. They are present in samples that have adequately washed the alveolar spaces and therefore are a useful indicator of sample adequacy. The nucleus is round to bean-shaped and eccentrically positioned. A binucleate alveolar macrophage is rarely seen in clinically normal animals. Alveolar macrophages have abundant blue-gray granular cytoplasm. When they become activated, their cytoplasm becomes more abundant and vacuolated (i.e., foamy) and may contain phagocytized material (see Figure 16-6, *B*).[29]

Neutrophils: TW/BAL neutrophils look like peripheral blood neutrophils (see Figures 16-10 and 16-11), although degenerative changes may be present. Increased numbers of neutrophils indicate inflammation; see the discussion on inflammation later in this chapter.

Eosinophils: Eosinophils (Figures 16-7 to 16-9) are polymorphonuclear granulocytes that contain intracytoplasmic granules, many of which have an affinity for the acid dye, eosin (i.e., eosinophilic), which stains them red with Romanowsky stains.[36] Increased numbers of eosinophils indicate a hypersensitivity reaction that is either allergic or parasitic[5]; see discussion on hypersensitivity later in this chapter.

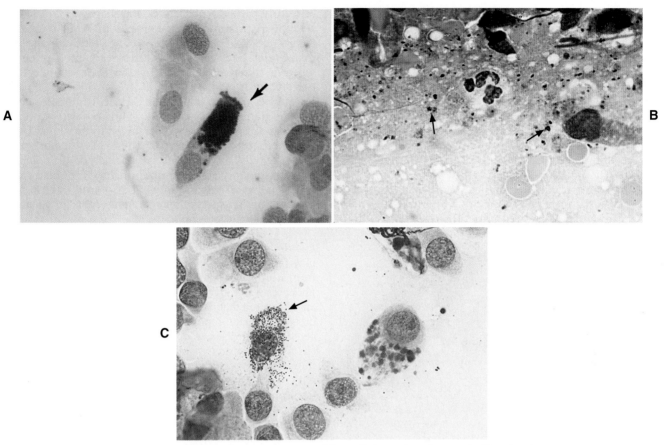

Figure 16-5 A, TW/BAL from a dog. A goblet cell *(arrow)* and several ciliated columnar cells are present. (Wright's stain, original magnification 250×). **B,** Granules from ruptured goblet cells are shown extracellularly *(arrows)* and must not be confused with bacterial cocci. (Wright's stain, original magnification 330×.) **C,** Goblet cells can be differentiated from mast cells *(arrow)*, which have smaller granules.

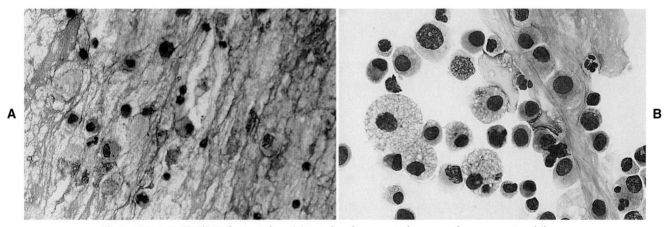

Figure 16-6 A, TW/BAL from a dog. Many alveolar macrophages and some neutrophils are present in an eosinophilic mucous background. (Wright's stain, original magnification 132×.) **B,** TW/BAL from a dog. Numerous stimulated and unstimulated alveolar macrophages and scattered granulocytes and lymphocytes are present in strands of mucus. (Wright's stain, original magnification 250×.)

Careful examination is required to distinguish eosinophils from neutrophils in some wash specimens. In thick areas where the cells are not well spread out, individual granules may be hard to see. If normal neutrophils are present, the contrast in cytoplasmic color is usually evident; however, caution must be used because the cytoplasm of neutrophils, especially in exudative samples, sometimes stains a diffuse, uneven, eosinophilic color. When differentiating these two cells, it is best to search for well-spread-out cells with definitive cytoplasmic granules instead of diffuse eosinophilic coloration. Individual granules are most readily observed in partially ruptured cells that are spreading out and are also free in the background of the smear (see Figure 16-8, *B*). In cats, eosinophils can be difficult to recognize because they tend to

be tightly packed with slender, rod-shaped granules that are not as pronounced in color as those in dogs (see Figure 16-8, *A*). Eosinophils tend to be slightly larger than neutrophils, and their nuclei are less segmented (often bilobed or trilobed), which can aid in their identification (see Figures 16-8, *A*, and 16-9, *B*).

Another distinct population of cells containing cytoplasmic granules similar to eosinophils, but with round to oval, eccentric nuclei, have been seen in bronchial wash specimens (see Figure 16-9, *B*).[29] These cells resemble globule leukocytes, a type of cell of uncertain origin reported in the respiratory and gastrointestinal tracts of many animals. The atypical, eosinophilic cells found in BAL fluid in dogs contain specific microgranules that are a feature of mammalian eosinophils.[37]

Lymphocytes/Plasma Cells: Lymphocytes (Figure 16-12) may represent a small percentage of the cells in TW/BAL from normal dogs and cats. Increased numbers of lymphocytes generally denote nonspecific inflammation and are of limited diagnostic value. Mildly increased numbers of lymphocytes reportedly occur with airway hyperreactivity, viral diseases of the tracheobronchial tree, and chronic infections.[5,38] Marked increases in lymphocyte numbers, especially lymphoblasts, may suggest pulmonary lymphoma. Lymphocytes become activated with immune stimulation; their cytoplasm becomes more abundant and stains a deep blue because of increased protein synthesis. Some lymphocytes also transform into plasma cells.

Mast Cells: Mast cells (see Figure 16-5, *C*), which are occasionally observed in TW/BAL from dogs and cats with many different inflammatory lung disorders, are usually present in low numbers and are of little diagnostic significance. They are readily identified by their small redpurple, intracytoplasmic granules, which are frequently

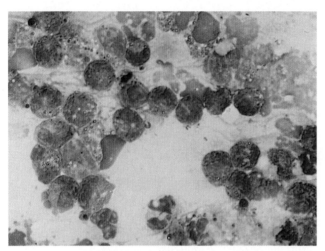

Figure 16-7 TW/BAL from a dog. Mucus, scattered neutrophils, and a large number of eosinophils are shown. Some extracellular bacterial rods, probably from oropharyngeal contamination, are also present. (Wright's stain, original magnification 330×.)

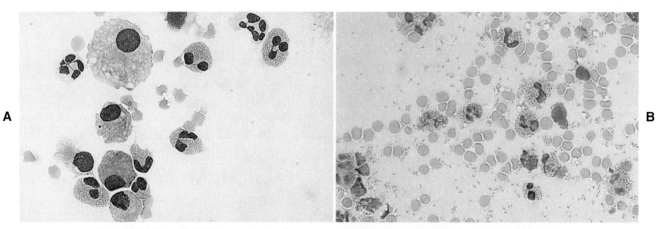

A

B

Figure 16-8 A, TW/BAL specimen from a cat with a hypersensitivity reaction. Several eosinophils with bilobed and trilobed nuclei, scattered alveolar macrophages, two neutrophils with mutilobulated nuclei, and a ciliated columnar epithelial cell are shown. The granules of the eosinophils are tightly packed, slender rods that can be easily overlooked. Note that the eosinophils are somewhat larger than the neutrophils and have less segmented nuclei. (Wright's stain, original magnification 250×.) **B,** Feline eosinophils. Granules are seen more easily in cells that are well spread out or partially ruptured. Many free eosinophil granules are seen in the background. (Wright's stain, original magnification 250×.)

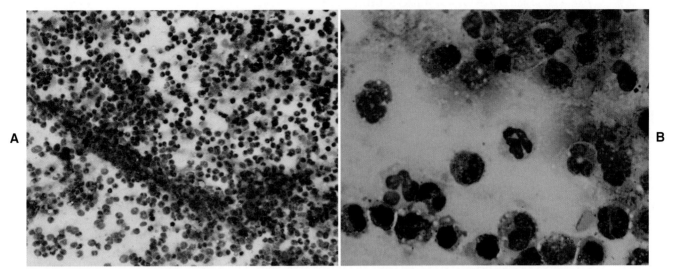

Figure 16-9 BAL from a dog with a hypersensitivity reaction. **A,** Note the abundant brightly staining eosinophils, in conjunction with less prominently staining cells. (Wright's stain, original magnification 200×.) **B,** Higher magnification of slide shown in **A.** Note the central neutrophil with pale eosinophilic staining cytoplasm and multilobulated nucleus. The eosinophils possess brightly staining eosinophilic granules, to the left an unlobulated nucleus, presumptive globule leukocyte, and to the right a trilobed nucleus, typical of eosinophils. (Wright's stain, original magnification, 1000×.)

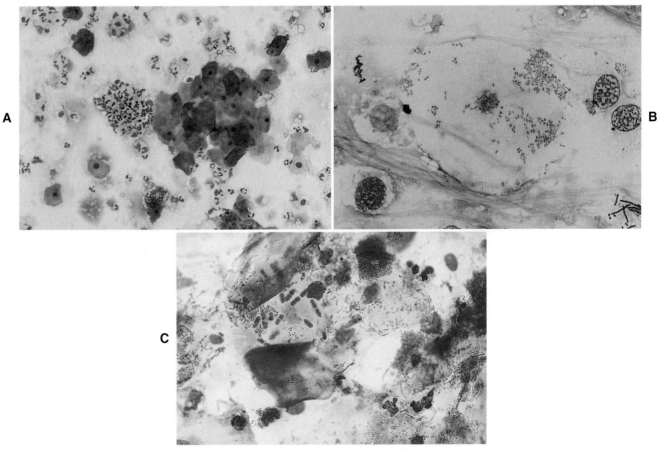

Figure 16-10 **A,** TW/BAL from a dog. Superficial squamous cells, which denote oropharyngeal contamination, and neutrophils are shown. (Wright's stain, original magnification 50×.) **B,** Oropharyngeal contamination in a TW/BAL from a dog. Mucus, alveolar macrophages, and a large superficial squamous cell (with bacteria adhering to its surface) are present. Bacteria are also scattered throughout the slide. (Wright's stain, original magnification 250×.) **C,** TW/BAL from a cat. High numbers of bacteria, including some *Simonsiella* spp., are adhering to the surface of the squamous epithelial cells. *Simonsiella* spp. are normal inhabitants of the oropharynx and indicate that the wash from this area is contaminated. (Wright's stain, original magnification 250×.)

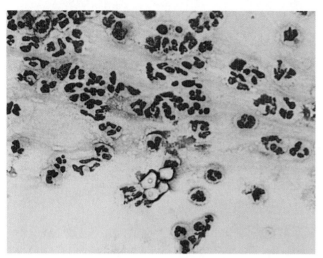

Figure 16-11 TW/BAL from a dog. High numbers of neutrophils, an alveolar macrophage, and a cluster of four granules of cornstarch (glove powder) are present in an eosinophilic mucous background. (Wright's stain, original magnification 165×.)

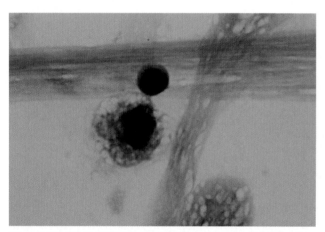

Figure 16-12 Small lymphocyte with scant cytoplasm trapped within mucin, and macrophage with vacuolated cytoplasm noted below. (Wright's stain, original magnification, 1000×.)

present in high numbers and may obscure the nucleus. Free, scattered granules from ruptured mast cells may be present on the slide and must not be confused with bacteria. A mild increase in mast cell numbers has been reported to occur with airway hyperreactivity.[38]

Superficial Squamous Cells: Superficial squamous cells are large epithelial cells with abundant, angular cytoplasm and small, round nuclei. Their presence in a TW/BAL indicates oropharyngeal contamination (see Figure 16-10). See the discussion of oropharyngeal contamination later in this chapter.

Erythrocytes: Erythrocytes may be present within macrophages or free on the slide. Erythrophagocytosis (see Figure 16-18) indicates intrapulmonary hemorrhage, or diapedesis. See the discussion of hemorrhage later in this chapter.

Atypical Cell Types

Atypical cells may be seen with pulmonary metaplasia, dysplasia, or neoplasia (primary or metastatic). Mild dysplasia of the respiratory epithelium may be seen whenever inflammation is present. Anticancer therapy (i.e., irradiation and chemotherapy) may result in such severe atypia of the cells of the tracheobronchial epithelium, the terminal bronchial epithelium, and the alveolar epithelium that differentiation from neoplasia is not reliable.[4] When atypical cells are observed cytologically, they should be evaluated for malignant criteria (see Chapter 2). TW/BAL collected after cancer therapy should be interpreted with caution.

Metaplasia: Metaplasia is an adaptive response of epithelial cells to chronic irritation.[4] Replacement of normal pulmonary epithelial cells of the trachea, bronchi, and bronchioles with stratified squamous epithelium (i.e., squamous metaplasia) is an example of pulmonary metaplasia.[39] These metaplastic cells mimic maturing squamous epithelium and must not be confused with neoplasia.

Dysplasia: Dysplasia is, by definition, a nonneoplastic change; however, severely dysplastic changes are sometimes referred to as carcinoma in situ.[39] Dysplastic changes include variation in cell size and shape, darker-staining cells, and increased nuclear-to-cytoplasmic ratio and numbers of immature cells.[39] These changes can be difficult to differentiate from neoplasia and may progress to neoplasia.[39]

Neoplastic Cells: Neoplastic cells are not often seen on cytologic evaluation of TW/BAL. Unless the neoplasm has invaded the tracheobronchial tree and the invaded bronchiole is not blocked by a mucous plug, they are not accessible for collection by a TW/BAL. Neoplastic cells, when observed, are generally from lymphoma or a carcinoma. High numbers of lymphoblasts may be seen in animals with lymphoma involving the respiratory system (see Figure 16-27). Carcinoma cells are large epithelial cells that may be present in clusters or as single cells (see Figure 16-26). Their cytoplasm is generally basophilic and vacuolated, and they show marked variation in cellular and nuclear size, often with grossly enlarged nuclei. They have a high nuclear-to-cytoplasmic ratio, coarse nuclear chromatin, and prominent nucleoli that are frequently large and angular. Care must be taken not to confuse inflammation-induced cell dysplasia with neoplasia.

Miscellaneous Findings

Corn Starch: Corn starch (glove powder) is occasionally seen cytologically on slides from TW/BAL. It is typically a large, round to hexagonal structure that stains clear or blue and has a central fissure (see Figure 16-11). Corn starch is an incidental finding and should not be confused with an organism or cell.

Plant Pollen: Plant pollen or plant cells may occasionally be present in TW/BAL and should not be confused with infectious organisms or cells.

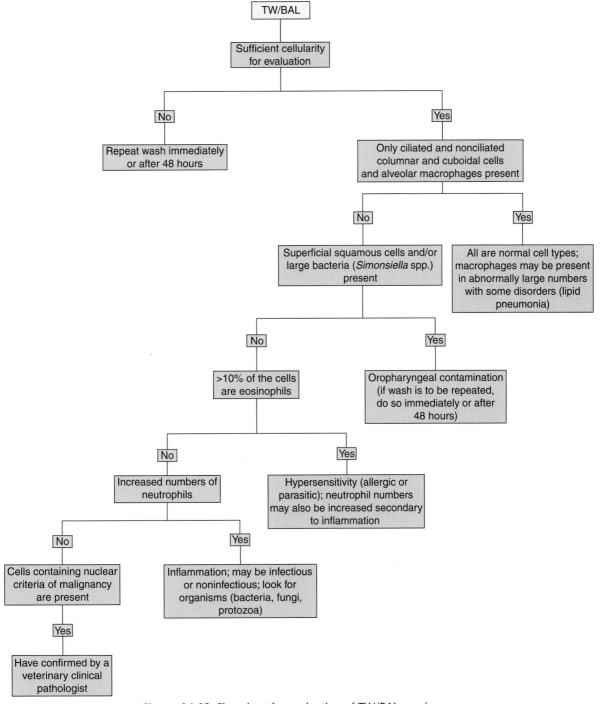

Figure 16-13 Flowchart for evaluation of TW/BAL specimens.

Barium Sulfate: aspirated barium sulfate has been reported to occur as greenish granular refractile material, most commonly noted in macrophages.[40]

CYTOLOGIC INTERPRETATION

Figure 16-13 presents an algorithm to aid in the evaluation of TW/BAL. Integrating historical, physical, and radiographic findings with the results of other diagnostic tests may allow for further diagnostic refinement. TW/BAL are interpreted according to the type,

quantity, and proportion of cells recovered. Cell proportions often differ between transtracheal aspirates and BALs.

Cellular patterns can generally be categorized as follows:

- Insufficient sample — no cells or an inadequate number of cells for evaluation
- Oropharyngeal contamination — superficial squamous cells and/or *Simonsiella* spp. of bacteria (see discussion of oropharyngeal contamination later in this chapter)

- Eosinophilic infiltrate — increased numbers of eosinophils (see discussion of hypersensitivity later in this chapter)
- Neutrophilic infiltrate — increased numbers of neutrophils (see discussion of inflammation later in this chapter)
- Macrophage (histiocytic or granulomatous) infiltrate — very cellular sample of primarily macrophages (see discussion of inflammation later in this chapter)
- Presence of atypical cells — evaluation for criteria of malignancy (see discussion of neoplasia later in this chapter)

These categories, aside from insufficient samples, are not mutually exclusive. Classification of TW/BAL into one or more of these categories may allow the process or processes to be identified.

Insufficient Sample

The absence of cells on a smear or concentrated preparation may indicate that this sample is not truly representative of the cytology of the respiratory tract. Additionally, when assessing a BAL sample in which columnar respiratory epithelial cells only are noted, the absence of macrophages would indicate that only the airways and not the alveolar space had effectively been sampled.

Oropharyngeal Contamination

Oropharyngeal contamination is much more likely to occur when a TW/BAL is collected by passing a catheter through an endotracheal tube than when a transtracheal sample is taken and the oropharyngeal area is bypassed. Regardless of the procedure used, careful attention must be paid to technique to avoid oropharyngeal contamination.

Superficial squamous cells and certain large bacteria (e.g., *Simonsiella* spp.[41]) are the hallmark of oropharyngeal contamination (see Figure 16-10). Superficial squamous cells are large epithelial cells with abundant, angular cytoplasm and small, round nuclei. Many bacteria may adhere to the surface of squamous epithelial cells (see Figure 16-10, *B* and *C*). *Simonsiella* spp. (see Figure 16-10, *C*) are bacteria that divide lengthwise, therefore lining up in parallel rows that give the impression of a single large bacterium. These are nonpathogenic organisms that may adhere to superficial squamous cell surfaces or be free in smears. When superficial squamous cells or *Simonsiella* spp. are present, indicating oropharyngeal contamination, whatever cellular constituents and bacterial organisms were present in the oropharyngeal area may also be present in a contaminated wash. Therefore a variety of bacterial rods and cocci may be present in a contaminated wash (see Figure 16-10, *B*). Bacteria are generally present without neutrophils when the wash primarily consists of oropharyngeal contaminants. Neutrophils may occur in a TW/BAL secondary to oropharyngeal contamination if the animal has a purulent or ulcerative oropharyngeal lesion. Therefore oropharyngeal contamination can significantly alter the cytologic evaluation and culture results.

Hypersensitivity

Increased numbers of eosinophils in a TW/BAL specimen indicate a hypersensitivity response. Normal animals of most species, including dogs, generally have very low numbers of eosinophils (<5%) in bronchial wash specimens, but clinically normal cats may have significantly higher numbers of eosinophils than other species.[22,42,43] In some studies, eosinophils compose an average of 20% to 25% of the cells present in bronchial wash specimens from asymptomatic cats with no evidence of pulmonary disease or parasitism. In a few of these animals, eosinophils were the predominant cell type present. Whether these findings are truly normal or merely represent a subclinical hypersensitivity response is not known, but these animals were asymptomatic throughout the observation periods; thus the clinical significance of a cytologic diagnosis of hypersensitivity reaction, when based on relatively low numbers of eosinophils (10% to 25% of cells present), may depend on the clinical and radiographic findings of the case.

Clinically normal dogs typically have wash specimens of less than 5% eosinophils.[29,44,45] Many of the studies describing normal BAL cytology were done using dogs reared in closed environments. In fact, one study showed that random source dogs had significantly higher percentages of eosinophils (24%) than dogs reared in an isolated environment with routine prophylactic anthelminthic treatment (<5%).[46] It was suggested that previously heavy parasitic burdens may be responsible for the high numbers of eosinophils in these animals; however, other studies have also found increased eosinophil percentages in apparently healthy dogs.[47,48] The authors' experience suggests that such a significant percentage of eosinophils is unusual in most clinically normal dogs. Specimens composed of more than 10% eosinophils are indicative of a significant hypersensitivity component of the disease process.

Increased numbers of neutrophils and/or macrophages may be seen along with increased numbers of eosinophils if tissue irritation is sufficient to induce an inflammatory response. Cells are not always evenly distributed throughout wash specimens, especially if thick mucous strands are present. Eosinophils, trapped in strands of mucous, often predominate in certain areas of the slides, whereas other areas may be predominantly neutrophilic. A careful examination of the entire slide is necessary for an accurate evaluation.

Allergic bronchitis/pneumonitis, feline asthma, lungworms, heartworms, and eosinophilic bronchopneumopathy (previously pulmonary infiltrates with eosinophils [PIE]) are some of the disorders that frequently cause the hypersensitivity responses seen in TW/BAL specimens. Specimens should be scanned on low power (10× objective) for parasitic larvae or ova (Figure 16-14). If present, parasitic larvae (e.g., *Filaroides* spp., *Aelurostrongylus abstrusus*, *Angiostrongylus vasorum*, and *Crenosoma vulpis*) and ova (e.g., *Capillaria aerophila* and *Paragonimus* spp.) are large and readily identified, but sometimes only an eosinophilic exudate is present. Multiple fecal examinations (including Baermann and zinc sulfate flotation techniques) may be helpful in identifying infestations. Even when not found in wash specimens, larvae can sometimes

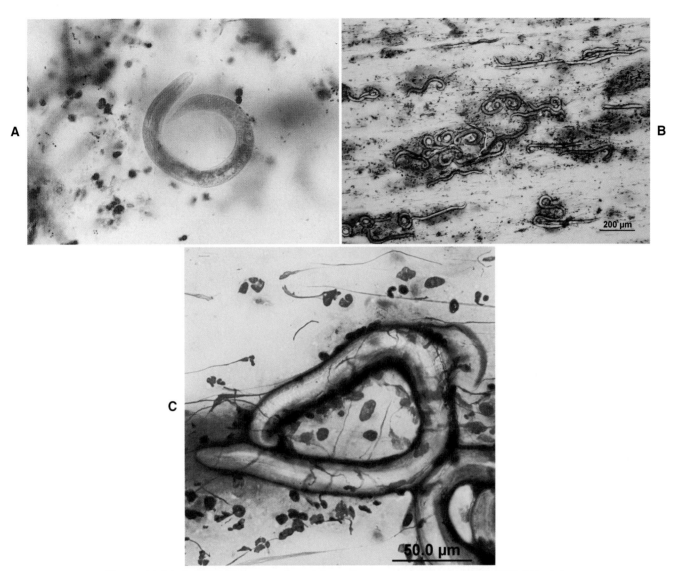

Figure 16-14 A, TW/BAL from a dog. A large lungworm larva is present. (Wright's stain, original magnification, 100×.) **B,** TW/BAL from a cat. Low-power magnification showing large numbers of lungworm larvae (*Aelurostrongylus* spp.). (Wright's stain.) **C,** Higher magnification from the same case shown in **B**. Lungworm larvae (*Aelurostrongylus* spp.) and scattered inflammatory cells are shown. (Wright's stain.) *(B and C courtesy Dr. T. Rizzi.)*

be identified in brushings or biopsies of parasitic nodules visible in the bronchi of affected animals.

Free eosinophil granules, which stain eosinophilic and should not be confused with bacteria, may be seen secondary to cell rupture in the smear. These granules may coalesce into a large crystal known as a Charcot-Leyden crystal (Figure 16-15), which can occur in any condition that causes large numbers of eosinophils to accumulate.

Inflammation

Neutrophils are present only in very low numbers (generally <5%) in TW/BAL from normal dogs and cats.[5,29] Cytologically, neutrophils in bronchial mucus look like peripheral blood neutrophils, but they may show degenerative changes because of bacterial toxins or be smudged (ruptured) secondary to trauma from collection

and preparation. An influx of neutrophils occurs early in an inflammatory response, making neutrophils from TW/BAL a sensitive indicator of inflammation.[31] Even very mild insults, such as sterile saline TW/BAL, result in marked influxes of neutrophils. As a result, neutrophil numbers are increased in nearly all conditions (infectious and noninfectious) that cause inflammation. Infectious disorders include bacterial (Figure 16-16), mycotic (see Figure 16-23), viral, or protozoal (see Figure 16-25) diseases. Noninfectious disorders include tissue irritation or necrosis secondary to inhalation of a toxic substance (e.g., smoke), as well as neoplasia that has outgrown its blood supply and developed a necrotic center. Whenever neutrophil numbers are increased, one should look closely (and, especially, intracellularly) for bacteria and other microorganisms (see Figure 16-16). Organisms can be found cytologically in most bacterial infections, but

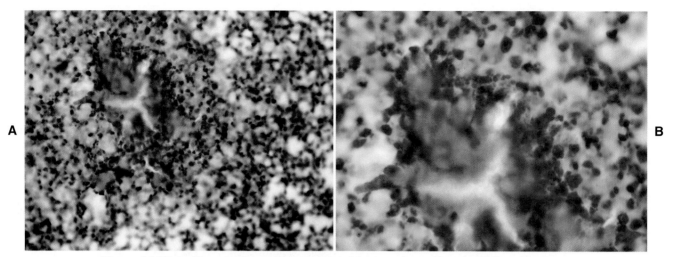

Figure 16-15 A, Fine-needle aspirate showing high numbers of eosinophils and a large eosinophilic crystal thought to be a Charcot-Leyden crystal. **B,** Higher magnification of same slide. (Wright's stain.) *(Courtesy Dr. Peter Fernandes.)*

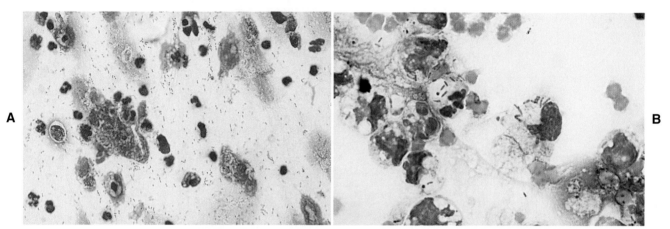

Figure 16-16 A, TW/BAL from a dog with bacterial tracheobronchitis. Many neutrophils and some mucous strands are shown. High numbers of bacterial rods are present, mostly extracellularly. (Wright's stain, original magnification 250×.) **B,** TW/BAL from a dog with bacterial pneumonia. A mixed population of bacteria is present; some bacteria are phagocytized within neutrophils. (Wright's stain, original magnification 400×.)

noninfectious inflammation is typified by the absence of microorganisms.

Increased numbers of macrophages are seen with many subacute and chronic lung disorders (e.g., congestive heart failure, granulomatous and lipid pneumonia). Alveolar macrophage numbers frequently increase with chronic persistent inflammation.[31] Binucleate and multinucleate giant cell macrophages (Figure 16-17) may be seen in conditions that produce chronic lung disease.[4] Large, lipid-containing vacuoles may be present within macrophages in lipid pneumonia.[4] Dark or black granules (anthracotic pigment) may be present within macrophages from clinically normal animals living in large cities or other areas with polluted air. Phagocytized erythrocytes (i.e., erythrophagia) and erythrocyte-breakdown products (e.g., hematoidin or hemosiderin) may be seen within macrophage cytoplasm in conditions that cause pulmonary hemorrhage or red cell diapedesis (Figure 16-18). Macrophages are also important to defend against

microorganisms, and phagocytized microorganisms (e.g., mycotic, protozoal, or bacterial) may be seen.

Hemorrhage

Erythrocytes may be seen in TW/BAL washes from dogs and cats with disorders that cause vascular damage or erythrocyte diapedesis in the lung. Iatrogenic hemorrhage (i.e., hemorrhage caused by the sampling procedure) may also result in erythrocytes noted on the smear. In order to demonstrate that the hemorrhage is a result of pulmonary pathology (intrapulmonary hemorrhage), erythrophagocytosis, hemosiderophages, or hem-pigment should be identified on the smears. Hemosiderophages have been referred to as "heart failure cells"; however, in one recent study in cats, in which the presence of hemosiderophages was specifically assessed with Prussian blue staining to identify the presence of iron, hemosiderosis was not a consistent feature in the tracheal wash specimens of cats with cardiac

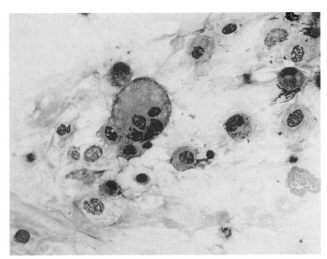

Figure 16-17 TW/BAL from a dog with chronic lung disease. Many alveolar macrophages, two neutrophils, and one multinucleated giant cell macrophage are present in an eosinophilic mucous background. (Wright's stain, original magnification 132×.)

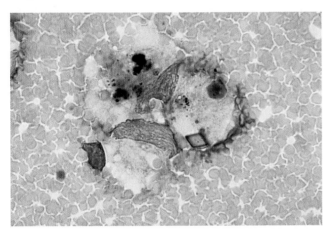

Figure 16-18 TW/BAL from a dog. Many RBCs and three macrophages that contain phagocytized RBCs and RBC breakdown products (dark-staining hemosiderin and golden hematoidin crystals) are present. This finding indicates intrapulmonary hemorrhage or diapedesis of erythrocytes. (Wright's stain, original magnification 330×.)

disease. Hemosiderosis was noted in cats with feline asthma, neoplasia (primary and metastatic), pneumonia (bacterial, parasites) secondary to inhaled irritants, bleeding diathesis, trauma, spontaneous pneumothorax, collapsed trachea, neurologic disease, and uncomplicated rhinitis.[49] Other causes of intrapulmonary hemorrhage that may be considered include other infectious agents (such as fungi), pulmonary embolism, and lung lobe torsion.

INFECTIOUS AGENTS

Bacteria

The culture of bacteria from a lower respiratory tract specimen should be assessed in conjunction with the clinical presentation because the tracheobronchial tree may not be regarded as sterile even in healthy individuals.[50,51] A number of studies have reported Gram-negative rods as the most

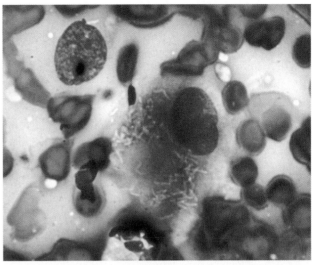

Figure 16-19 Fine-needle aspirate showing many RBCs and a large macrophage. The macrophage contains many, small, nonstaining, bacterial rods indicative of *Mycobacterium* spp. (Wright's stain.) *(Courtesy Dr. R.L. Cowell, IDEXX Laboratories.)*

common type of bacterial infectious agent.[52-55] Greater than 60% of dogs with lower respiratory tract disease are reported to have a single agent only isolated.[53] Quantitative assessment of both the culture results and cytologic examination of a BAL may provide increased diagnostic specificity.[53] A wide variety of bacteria have been reported as a cause of bacterial (septic) pneumonia, more than may be covered adequately here; organisms discussed later are highlighted with regard to specific culture requirements or concerns over identification. See chapter 3 for more pictures of infectious agents.

Mycobacteria: These bacteria do not readily take up Romanowsky stain and on the majority of preparations appear as negative-staining rods (Figure 16-19). Bacteria are generally located within macrophages, but may also be noted in neutrophils. These bacteria may be particularly hard to identify on flush/wash samples, and staining with a specific stain (e.g., Ziehl-Neelsen [acid-fast stain]) is recommended to assess for these bacteria. The bacteria stain red with beaded appearance with Ziehl-Neelsen stain. Calcospherite-like bodies, concentrically laminated crystalline structures, have been reported in a single case of canine tuberculosis.[56] Mycobacterial culture may be prolonged, generally at least 3 weeks, particularly if attempting to phenotype. If submitting unfixed material, it should be clearly labeled because the organism has zoonotic potential. It is necessary to specifically request culture for these bacteria on submission and is recommended to contact the laboratory prior to submission because not all laboratories will have appropriate containment facilities to culture the organism.

Mycoplasma: These small bacteria may have a variable appearance, from coccoid to coccobacilli.[57] These organisms have been associated with respiratory tract disease in both dogs[51,58] and cats.[59] Specific conditions are required for culture of these organisms, and culture for these organisms should be requested by the submitting clinician if there is a clinical suspicion. Additionally, many laboratories will supply culture medium for submission of specimens. The laboratory should be contacted prior to obtaining the sample for advice on submission and to allow time for media to be supplied if appropriate.

Fungi

TW/BAL sampling may provide definitive diagnosis in mycotic infections. The systemic mycotic infections blastomycosis, histoplasmosis, and coccidiomycosis frequently

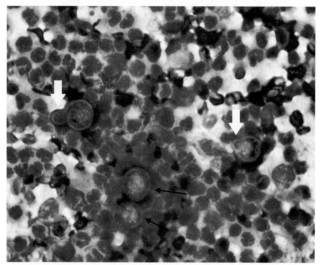

Figure 16-20 Four *Blastomyces dermatitidis* organisms *(arrows)* surrounded by high numbers of neutrophils, scattered macrophages, and some RBCs. *Blastomyces* organisms are spherical, thick-walled, yeast-like organisms that stain basophilic. The organisms are 5 to 20 microns in diameter and occasionally, a single, broad-based bud may be present *(broad arrows)*. (Wright's stain.) *(Courtesy Dr. R.L. Cowell, IDEXX Laboratories.)*

involve the lungs, and *Aspergillus* and *Cryptococcus* may also be observed. One study suggests that lavage of multiple lung lobes is most likely to obtain a diagnosis of mycotic infection, and that BAL may be more sensitive than TW.[10]

Aspergillus: This organism is uncommonly noted in the lung. The appearance of the organism is branching septate hyphae. In other species, calcium oxalate crystals have also been noted in the BAL sample with *Aspergillus* infections.[60] This organism is a frequent environmental contaminant and if cultured from a lower respiratory specimen, careful patient assessment is required to determine whether this is a likely etiologic agent.

Blastomyces: This fungal organism appears as blue, round, medium-sized (5 to 20 μm diameter), thick-walled yeasts. Occasional broad-based budding may be observed (Figure 16-20). In one review of cases, 85% of the dogs affected had lung involvement.[61] Although aspiration of other lesions may provide a diagnosis, BAL may also be helpful.[10]

Coccidioides: In vivo there are two forms noted, the thick-walled, blue-staining, spherical sporangia that range from 10 to greater than 100 μm in diameter and the smaller endospores that may be observed in some of the larger sporangia. The endospores are 2 to 5 μm in diameter and may also be noticed individually, released from ruptured sporangia (Figure 16-21). These highly infectious organisms may take 1 to 2 weeks to culture, and submission of the sample should be discussed with the laboratory because alternative diagnostic methods are always preferable with this organism.[62]

Cryptococcus: These yeast organisms are extremely variable in size but are generally 4 to 15 μm in diameter without their capsule and 8 to 40 μm with their capsule

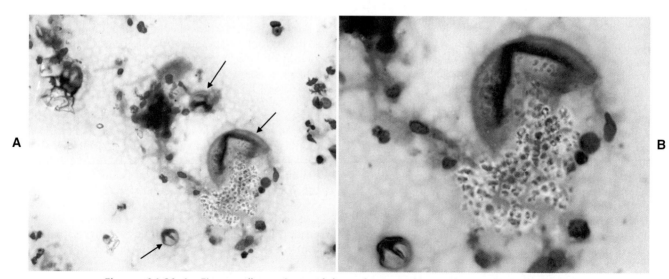

Figure 16-21 A, Fine-needle aspirate of lung from a dog with coccidioidomycosis. *Coccidioides immitis* organisms *(arrows)* are large, double-contoured, clear to blue-staining, spherical bodies that range in size from 10 microns to greater than 100 microns. Occasionally endospores varying from 2 to 5 microns in diameter may be seen within some of the larger spherules. **B,** Higher magnification of larger spherule containing endospores. (Wright's stain.) *(Courtesy Dr. R.L. Cowell, IDEXX Laboratories.)*

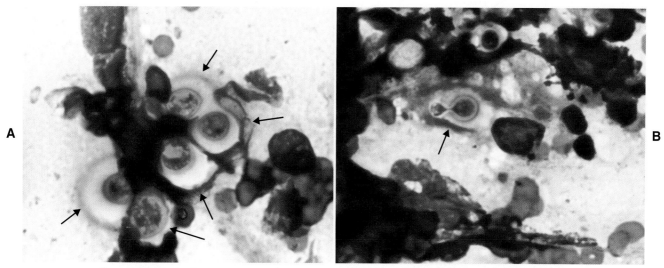

Figure 16-22 A, *Cryptococcus neoformans* is a spherical, yeast-like organism that frequently has a thick, clear-staining, mucoid capsule. Five *Cryptococcus* organisms *(arrows)* with nonstaining capsules are shown. **B,** *Cryptococcus* organism with a single narrow-based bud *(arrow)*. (Wright's stain.) *(Courtesy Dr. R.L. Cowell, IDEXX Laboratories.)*

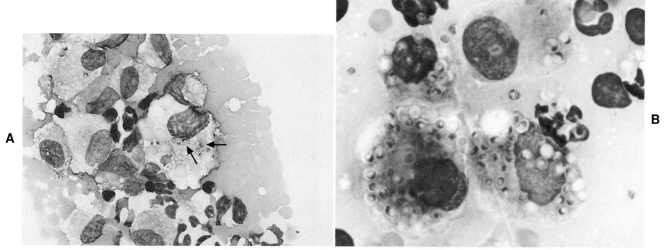

Figure 16-23 A, TW/BAL from a cat with pulmonary histoplasmosis. Many macrophages, some of which show the yeast phase of *Histoplasma capsulatum (arrows)*; scattered neutrophils and lymphocytes; and RBCs are seen. A macrophage also displays erythrophagocytosis. (Wright's stain, original magnification 250×.) **B,** Fine-needle aspirate of lung showing large macrophages containing numerous *H. capsulatum* organisms. *Histoplasma* organisms are small (1 to 4 microns in diameter), round to oval, yeast-like organisms that have a dark blue to purple staining nucleus. The organism is often surrounded by a thin, clear halo. (Wright's stain.) *(Courtesy Dr. R.L. Cowell, IDEXX Laboratories.)*

(smooth form of *Cryptococcus*). The yeast stains pink to blue-purple and may be slightly granular. The capsule is usually clear (nonstaining) and homogenous (Figure 16-22). Also, nonencapsulated forms of *Cryptococcus* may be observed (rough form of *Cryptococcus*). These appear similar but have a thin clear capsule. Occasional organisms showing narrow-based budding may be found. A case report in a cat demonstrated organisms 3 to 15 μm diameter with a thick nonstaining wall in the BAL, although the organisms from the lymph node of the patient were reported as 8 to 12 μm in size with a 1 to 6 μm nonstaining capsule.[9]

Histoplasma: Organisms may be more likely to be noted in BAL in the acute presentation of the disease, compared with a more chronic presentation. These organisms are most commonly noted intracellularly, but extracellular organisms may be observed on smears due to cell rupturing.

Histoplasma organisms are small (approximately 2 to 4 μm diameter) with a thin, clear halo surrounding a darker staining round to oval, yeast-like organism (Figure 16-23).[63]

Pneumocystis: This opportunistic fungal pulmonary pathogen that may be observed in either cyst (5 to 10 μm diameter with up to eight intracystic bodies)

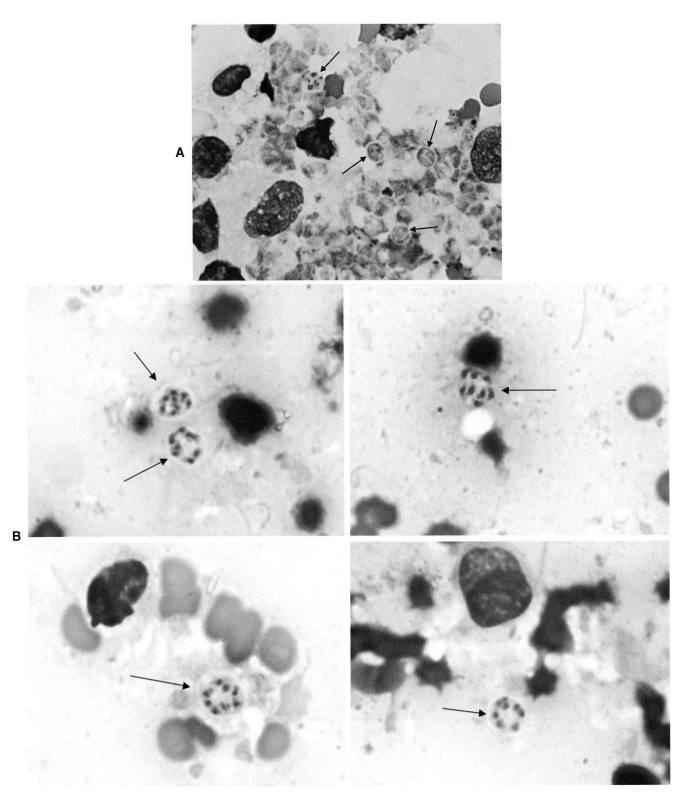

Figure 16-24 **A**, TTW from a dog with pneumocystosis. High numbers of *Pneumocystis carinii* cysts *(arrows)* are present. *P. carinii* cysts are 5 to 10 microns in diameter and usually contain four to eight intracystic bodies that are 1 to 2 microns in diameter. **B**, Composite showing high-magnification pictures of *P. carinii* cysts. (Wright's stain.) *(Courtesy Dr. R.L. Cowell, IDEXX Laboratories.)*

TABLE 16-3

Overview of the Nematode and Trematode Parasites of the Dog and Cat Lung[77-84]

Nematode Parasite	Host	Location in Lung	Stage in Lung Commonly Observed by Flush/Wash Sample
Aelurostrongylus abstrusus	Cat	Terminal and respiratory bronchioles and alveolar ducts	Ova and larvae Ova 70-80 μm by 50-75 μm, with thin shell, embryonated L1, 360-400 μm, short thick larvae with dorsal spine on tail, granular contents L3, 460-530 μm
Angiostrongylus vasorum	Dog	Pulmonary arteries and right heart	L1 310-400 μm length, cephalic button on anterior end
Capillaria aerophila	Dog and cat	Trachea and bronchi (nasal)	Ova Bipolar thick-walled, pigmented golden brown 60-74 μm length, 35-40 μm width
Crenosoma vulpis	Dog	Bronchioles to bronchi	L3, 458-549 μm length Slightly curved tail, no kink Adult worms, observed grossly, stout, white, ~1cm length
Filaroides hirthi	Dog	Respiratory bronchioles and alveoli	Embryonated ova and larvae Larvae ~10-14 μm width, slightly kinked tail Adults ~30-100 μm width, both stages have prominent basophilic granules internally
Oslerus osleri	Dog	Trachea and bronchial nodules	Ova and larvae practically identical to *Filaroides hirthi*
Trematode Parasite			
Paragonimus	Dog and cat	Primarily right caudal lung lobe	Ova 80-118 μm length, 48-60 μm width Ovoid with single flattened operculum, golden brown

(Figure 16-24) or troph form (1 to 2 μm).[64] Cytologically it may appear morphologically similar to a protozoal organism, and this originally led to misclassification. Particular breeds have been overrepresented in the literature—the Miniature Dachshund in the southern hemisphere[65] and the Cavalier King Charles Spaniel in the northern hemisphere[66]—however, this is likely to relate to the underlying immunodeficiencies that are reported in these breeds, because any breed may be affected. It is not possible to culture these organisms on media.

Parasites

When considering parasites of the lungs, nematodes (see Figure 16-14) and occasionally trematodes are most commonly considered, although *Toxoplasma* (Figure 16-25), a protozoal agent, is also classified as a parasitic organism.

An outline of the nematode and trematode parasites noted in the dog and cat is provided in Table 16-3, although some authors vary on the sizing of the larvae. If specific identification is required, it is recommended to seek expert opinion.

Although eosinophilic inflammation may be expected with these organisms, many patients will present with neutrophilic inflammation only.[67,68]

Oslerus osleri (Filaroides osleri) and *Filaroides hirthi* ova and larvae noted in respiratory washings are very similar in appearance (see Figure 16-14). Differentiation may be undertaken by identification of nodules formed by *O. osleri*, particularly at or in the area surrounding the bifurcation of the trachea,[67] whereas *F. hirthi* are more likely to form subpleural nodules.[69] The airway nodules may be noted on bronchoscopy, and either may be noted on radiography. In some instances the nodules may be difficult to distinguish radiographically from neoplastic foci.

Angiostrongylus vasorum is reported in many areas worldwide; considered endemic in France, Ireland, and Denmark, it has been noted with increasing frequency in the United Kingdom in the last few years.[68] Associated clinical signs may include hypercalcemia and bleeding diatheses due to prolongation of prothrombin time and/or activated partial thromboplastin time, which resolve on successful treatment of the worm burden.

Toxoplasma gondii infection in cats may frequently involve the lung. Identification of tachyzoites both extracellularly and within macrophages, which may be numerous, have been reported in the BAL samples of cats with both experimentally induced[70] and spontaneous[71,72] clinical disease. *T. gondii* tachyzoites appear as small crescent-shaped bodies with a light blue cytoplasm and a dark-staining pericentral nucleus (see Figure 16-25).

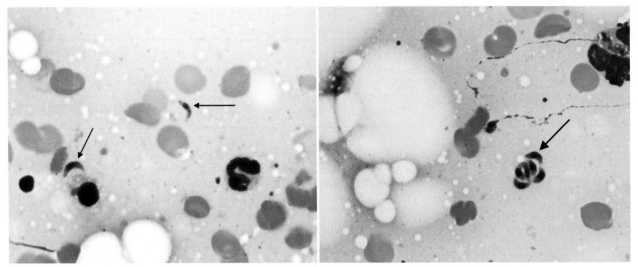

Figure 16-25 TW/BAL from a cat with toxoplasmosis. *Toxoplasma gondii* tachyzoites *(arrows)* appear as small crescent-shaped bodies with a light blue cytoplasm and a dark-staining pericentral nucleus. *(Courtesy Dr. R.L. Cowell, IDEXX Laboratories.)*

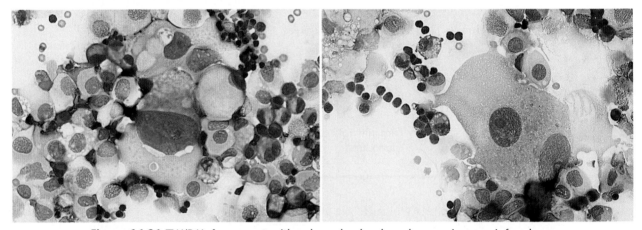

Figure 16-26 TW/BAL from a cat with a bronchoalveolar adenocarcinoma. A few large epithelial cells showing macronuclei and large prominent nucleoli are amongst inflammatory cells. (Wright's stain, original magnification 160×.)

Viral Diseases

Many viral respiratory diseases can cause lung damage and allow for secondary bacterial infection. Cytologically, increased numbers of neutrophils indicate inflammation. Lymphocytes may be increased, but the numbers are often low and nonspecific. If a secondary bacterial infection has occurred, bacterial organisms may be seen intracellularly and extracellularly on the slides.

Neoplasia

Neoplasia may exist as a single, solitary nodule or a diffuse infiltration. Solitary lesions are rare in metastatic lung tumors but common in primary lung tumors. Most solid tissue pulmonary neoplasms (i.e., not lymphoid) are metastatic nodules from malignant tumors at sites other than the lungs. Because metastatic lung tumors are generally interstitial, neoplastic cells are not collected by a TW/BAL unless the tumor has invaded the bronchial tree and that portion of the bronchial tree is not clogged by secretions or is so peripherally located that its cells cannot be collected by a TW/BAL. Primary lung tumors that involve the bronchial tree are more likely to exfoliate cells that are collected by routine washings (Figure 16-26).

Carcinomas compose 80% or more of all primary lung tumors in dogs and cats.[73,74] Lung carcinomas tend to appear in the following three areas[74]:
- Hilus of the lungs
- Multifocal and often peripheral sites (most commonly)
- In an entire lobe or lobes

Carcinomas are epithelial cell tumors; when cytologic evidence of acini formation or secretory product production is seen, they are classified as adenocarcinomas.

Lymphoma is a common neoplasm in both dogs and cats. It is typically multicentric and may involve the pulmonary parenchyma in dogs. Large numbers of lymphoblasts may be diagnostic of lymphoma. Scattered large lymphoid cells, when part of a generalized inflammatory

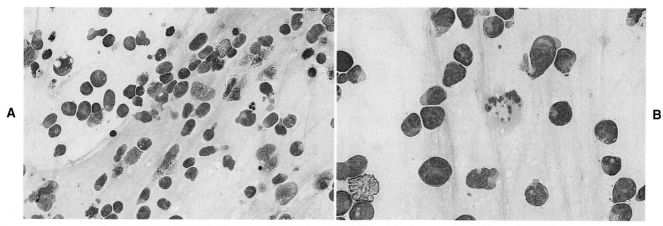

Figure 16-27 TW/BAL from a dog with multicentric lymphoma. **A,** Highly cellular slide containing many lymphoid cells in strands of mucus. (Wright's stain, original magnification 160×.) **B,** Higher magnification of the slide in **A.** The lymphoid cells are a population of pleomorphic lymphoblasts. A cluster of goblet cell granules is also present in the center of the field. (Wright's stain, original magnification 250×.)

reaction, are not sufficient for a diagnosis. TW/BAL specimens can be useful in diagnosing pulmonary involvement of lymphoma (Figure 16-27). In one study, 31 of 47 dogs with multicentric lymphoma (66%) had pulmonary involvement based on examination of BAL fluid collected with a bronchoscope.[75] In the same group of dogs, examination of TW fluid (collected by passing a urinary catheter through a sterile endotracheal tube) was much less sensitive, documenting pulmonary involvement in only 4 of the 46 dogs tested.

References

1. Moise NS, et al: Clinical, radiographic, and bronchial cytologic features of cats with bronchial disease: 65 cases (1980-1986). *J Am Vet Med Assoc* 194:1467-73, 1989.
2. Padrid P, et al: Canine chronic bronchitis. *J Vet Intern Med* 4:172-180, 1990.
3. Hawkins EC, et al: Demographic, clinical, and radiographic features of bronchiectasis in dogs: 316 cases (1988-2000). *J Am Vet Med Assoc* 223:1628-35, 2003.
4. Johnston W: Cytologic diagnosis of lung cancer: Principles and problems. *Path Res Pract* 181:1-36, 1986.
5. Creighton S, Wilkins R: Transtracheal aspiration biopsy: Technique and cytologic evaluation. *J Am Anim Hosp Assoc* 10:219-226, 1974.
6. Turnwald: in Proc 53rd Ann Mtg AAHA 52-55 (1986).
7. Cooper ES, Schober KE, Drost WT: Severe bronchoconstriction after bronchoalveolar lavage in a dog with eosinophilic airway disease. *J Am Vet Med Assoc* 227:1257-62, 2005.
8. Saunders HM, Keith D. In King LG (ed): *Textbook of Respiratory Disease in Dogs and Cats.* St. Louis, Saunders, 2004.
9. Hamilton TA, Hawkins EC, DeNicola DB: Bronchoalveolar lavage and tracheal wash to determine lung involvement in a cat with cryptococcosis. *J Am Vet Med Assoc* 198:655-6, 1991.
10. Hawkins EC, DeNicola D: Cytologic analysis of tracheal wash specimens and bronchoalveolar lavage fluid in the diagnosis of mycotic infections in dogs. *J Am Vet Med Assoc* 197:79-83, 1990.
11. McCullough S, Brinson J: Collection and interpretation of respiratory cytology. *Clin Tech Small Anim Pract* 14:220-226, 1999.
12. Hawkins EC: In King LG (ed): *Textbook of Respiratory Disease in Dogs and Cats.* St Louis, Saunders, 2004, pp 118-128.
13. Roudebush P: Tracheobronchoscopy. *Vet Clin North Am Small Anim Pract* 20:1297-314, 1990.
14. Hawkins EC, DeNicola DB, Kuehn NF: Bronchoalveolar lavage in the evaluation of pulmonary disease in the dog and cat: State of the art. *J Vet Intern Med* 4:267-274, 1990.
15. Boon D. In AAHA 52nd Annual Meeting 388-394 (1985).
16. O'Brien: Transtracheal aspiration in dogs and cats. *Mod Vet Pract* 64:412-413, 1983.
17. Hawkins EC, Berry CR: Use of a modified stomach tube for bronchoalveolar lavage in dogs. *J Am Vet Med Assoc* 215:1635-1639, 1999.
18. Hawkins EC, DeNicola DB: Collection of bronchoalveolar lavage fluid in cats, using an endotracheal tube. *Am J Vet Res* 50:855-889, 1989.
19. Vail DM, Mahler PA, Soergel BS: Differential cell analysis and phenotypic subtyping of lymphocytes in bronchoalveolar lavage fluid from clinically normal dogs. *Am J Vet Res* 56:282-285, 1995.
20. Amis TC, McKiernan BC: Systematic identification of endobronchial anatomy during bronchoscopy in the dog. *Am J Vet Res* 47:2649-2657, 1986.
21. Padrid P: Bronchoalveolar lavage in the evaluation of pulmonary disease in the dog and cat. *J Vet Intern Med* 5:52-55, 1991.
22. Hawkins EC, et al: Cytologic characterization of bronchoalveolar lavage fluid collected through an endotracheal tube in cats. *Am J Vet Res* 55:795-802, 1994.
23. Pinsker K, et al: Cell content in repetitive canine bronchoalveolar lavage. *Acta Cytologica* 24:558-563, 1980.
24. McCauley M, et al: Unguided bronchoalveolar lavage techniques and residual effects in dogs. *Aust Vet J* 76:161-165, 1998.
25. Moise B: Bronchial washings in the cat: Procedure and cytologic evaluation. *Comp Cont Ed* 5:621-7, 1983.
26. Hawkins EC, et al: Cellular composition of bronchial brushings obtained from healthy dogs and dogs with chronic cough and cytologic composition of bronchoalveolar lavage fluid obtained from dogs with chronic cough. *Am J Vet Res* 67:160-167, 2006.
27. Lotti U, Neibauer GW: Tracheobronchial foreign bodies of plant origin in 153 hunting dogs. *Compend Cont Vet Ed* 14:900-905, 1992.
28. Silverstein D, et al: Pulmonary alveolar proteinosis in a dog. *J Vet Int Med* 14:546-551, 2000.

29. Rebar A, DeNicola D, Muggenburg B: Bronchopulmonary lavage cytology in the dog: Normal findings. *Vet Path* 17: 294-304, 1980.

30. Thompson A, et al: Preparation of bronchoalveolar lavage fluid with microscope slide smears. *Eur Respir J* 9:603-608, 1996.

31. Henderson RF: Use of bronchoalvelolar lavage to detect lung damage. *Env Health Perspec* 56:115-129, 1984.

32. Carre P, et al: Technical variations of bronchoalveolar lavage (BAL): Influence of atelectasis and the lung region lavaged. *Lung* 163:117-125, 1985.

33. Damiano V, et al: A morphologic study of the influx of neutrophils into dog lung alveoli after lavage with sterile saline. *Am J Pathol* 100:349-364, 1980.

34. Mills PC, Litster AL: Using urea dilution to standardise components of pleural and bronchoalveolar lavage fluids in the dog. *N Z Vet J* 53:423-428, 2005.

35. Thornton DJ, Sheehan JK: From mucins to mucus: Towards a more coherent understanding of this essential barrier. *Proc Am Thorac Soc* 1:54-61, 2004.

36. Young KM: Eosinophils. In Feldman BF, Zinkl JG, Jain NC (eds): *Schalm's Veterinary Hematology*, ed 5. Philadelphia, Lippincott Williams & Wilkins, 2000.

37. Baldwin F, Becker A: Brochoalveolar eosinophilic cells in a canine model of asthma: Two distinctive populations. *Vet Pathol* 30:97-103, 1993.

38. Hirshman C, et al: Increased metachromatic cells and lymphocytes in bronchoalveolar lavage fluid of dogs with airway hyperreactivity. *Am Rev Resp Dis* 133:482-487, 1986.

39. Slauson D, Cooper B: *Mechanisms of Disease: A Textbook of Comparative General Pathology*. St Louis, Mosby, 2002.

40. Nunez-Ochoa L, Desnoyers M, Lecuyer M: What is your diagnosis? Iatrogenic aspiration of barium sulphate preparation. *Vet Clin Path* 22:122, 1993.

41. Nyby M, et al: Incidence of *Simonsiella* in the oral cavity of dogs. *J Clin Microbiol* 6:87-88, 1977.

42. Lecuyer M, et al: Bronchoalveolar lavage in normal cats. *Can Vet J* 36:771-773, 1995.

43. Padrid PA, et al: Cytologic, microbiologic, and biochemical analysis of bronchoalveolar lavage fluid obtained from 24 healthy cats. *Am J Vet Res* 52:1300-1307, 1991.

44. Mayer P, Laber G, Walzl H: Bronchoalveolar lavage in dogs: Analysis of proteins and respiratory cells. *J Vet Med Assoc* 1990: 392-399, 1990.

45. Brown N, Noone K, Kurzman I: Alveolar lavage in dogs. *Am J Vet Res* 44:335-337, 1983.

46. Baudendistel L, et al: Bronchoalveolar eosinophilia in random-source versus purpose-bred dogs. *Lab Anim Sci* 42:491-496, 1992.

47. Clercx C, et al: An immunologic investigation of canine eosinophilic bronchopneumopathy. *J Vet Intern Med* 16: 229-237, 2002.

48. Boothe HW, et al: Evaluation of the concentration of marbofloxacin in alveolar macrophages and pulmonary epithelial lining fluid after administration in dogs. *Am J Vet Res* 66:1770-1774, 2005.

49. deHeer H, McManus P: Frequency and severity of tracheal wash haemosiderosis and association with underlying disease in 96 cats: 2002-2003. *Vet Clin Path* 34:17-22, 2005.

50. McKiernan BC, Smith AR, Kissil M: Bacterial isolates from the lower trachea of clinically healthy dogs. *J Am Anim Hosp Assoc* 20:139-142, 1984.

51. Randolph J, et al: Prevalance of mycoplasmal and ureaplasmal recovery from tracheobronchial lavages and prevalance of mycoplasmal recovery from pharyngeal swab specimens in dogs with or without pulmonary disease. *Am J Vet Res* 54:387-391, 1993.

52. Creighton S, Wilkins R: Bacteriologic and cytologic evaluation of animals with lower respiratory tract disease using transtracheal aspiration biopsy. *J Am Anim Hosp Assoc* 10:227-232, 1974.

53. Peeters DE, et al: Quantitative bacterial cultures and cytological examination of bronchoalveolar lavage specimens in dogs. *J Vet Int Med* 14:534-541, 2000.

54. Clercx C, et al: Eosinophilic bronchopneumopathy in dogs. *J Vet Intern Med* 14:282-291, 2000.

55. Bart M, et al: Feline infectious pneumonia: A short literature review and a retrospective immunohistological study on the involvement of *Chlamydia* spp. and distemper virus. *Vet J* 159:220-230, 2000.

56. Bauer N, et al: Calcospherite-like bodies and caseous necrosis in tracheal mucus from a dog with tuberculosis. *Vet Clin Path* 33:168-172, 2004.

57. Carter GR, Wise DJ: *Essentials of Veterinary Bacteriology and Mycology*. Ames, Iowa, Blackwell, 2004.

58. Williams M, Olver C, Thrall MA: Transtracheal wash from a puppy with respiratory disease. *Vet Clin Pathol* 35:471-473, 2006.

59. Foster SF, et al: Pneumonia associated with *Mycoplasma* spp. in three cats. *Aust Vet J* 76:460-444, 1998.

60. Muntz F: Oxalate-producing pulmonary aspergillosis in an alpaca. *Vet Pathol* 36:631-632, 1999.

61. Legrende A, Walker M: Canine blastomycosis: A review of 47 clinical cases. *J Am Vet Med Assoc* 178:1163-1168, 1981.

62. Armstrong P, DiBartola S: Canine cocciodiomycosis: A literature review and report of eight cases. *J Am Anim Hosp Assoc* 19:937-945, 1983.

63. Ford R: Canine histoplasmosis. *Comp Cont Ed* 11:637-642, 1980.

64. McCully R, et al: Canine *Pneumocystis* pneumonia. *J South Afr Vet Assoc* 50:207-213, 1979.

65. Lobetti R: Common variable immunodeficiency in miniature dachshunds affected with *Pneumonocystis carinii* pneumonia. *J Vet Diagn Invest* 12:39-45, 2000.

66. Watson PJ, et al: Immunoglobulin deficiency in Cavalier King Charles Spaniels with *Pneumocystis* pneumonia. *J Vet Intern Med* 20:523-527, 2006.

67. Outerbridge CA, Taylor S: *Oslerus osleri* tracehobronchitis: Treatment with ivermection in 4 dogs. *Can Vet J* 39: 238-240, 1998.

68. Chapman PS, et al: *Angiostrongylus vasorum* infection in 23 dogs (1999-2002). *J Small Anim Pract* 45:435-440, 2004.

69. Carrasco L, et al: Massive *Filaroides hirthi* infestation associated with canine distemper in a puppy. *Vet Rec* 140: 72-73, 1997.

70. Hawkins EC, et al: Cytologic identification of *Toxoplasma gondii* in bronchoalveolar lavage fluid of experimentally infected cats. *J Am Vet Med Assoc* 210:648-650, 1997.

71. Brownlee L, Sellon RK: Diagnosis of naturally occurring toxoplasmosis by bronchoalveolar lavage in a cat. *J Am Anim Hosp Assoc* 37:251-255, 2001.

72. Barrs VR, Martin P, Beatty JA: Antemortem diagnosis and treatment of toxoplasmosis in two cats on cyclosporin therapy. *Aust Vet J* 84:30-35, 2006.

73. Hahn F, Muggenburg B, Griffith W: Primary lung neoplasia in a Beagle colony. *Vet Pathol* 33:633-638, 1996.

74. Moulton J, von Tscharner C, Schnieder R: Classification of lung carcinomas in the dog and cat. *Vet Pathol* 18:513-528, 1981.

75. Hawkins EC, et al: Cytologic analysis of bronchoalveolar lavage fluid from 47 dogs with multicentric malignant lymphoma. *J Am Vet Med Assoc* 203:1418-1425, 1993.

76. Bacha WJ Jr, Bacha LM: *Color Atlas of Veterinary Histology*. New York, Lippincott Williams and Wilkins, 2000.

77. Anderson RC: *Nematode Parasites of Vertebrates: Their Development and Transmission.* Wallingford, UK, CABI, 2000.

78. Andreasen CB: Bronchoalveolar lavage. *Vet Clin North Am Small Anim Pract* 33:69-88, 2003.

79. Cobb MA, Fisher MA: *Crenesoma vulpis* infection in a dog. *Vet Rec* 130:452, 1992.

80. Rakich PM, Latimer KS: Cytology of the respiratory tract. *Vet Clin North Am Small Anim Pract* 19:823-850, 1989.

81. Thienpont D, Rochette F, Vanparijs OFJ: *Diagnosing Helminthiasis by Coprological Examination.* Titusville, NJ, Janssen Research Foundation, 1986.

82. Pechman R: Pulmonary paragonimiasis in dogs and cats: A review. *J Small Anim Pract* 21:87-95, 1980.

83. Bolt G, et al: Canine angiostrongylus: A review. *Vet Rec* 135:447-452, 1994.

84. Andreasen CB, Carmichael P: What is your diagnosis? *Filaroides hirthi. Vet Clin Pathol* 21:77-78, 1992.

The Lung and Intrathoracic Structures

R.L. Cowell, R.D. Tyler, J.H. Meinkoth, and D. DeNicola

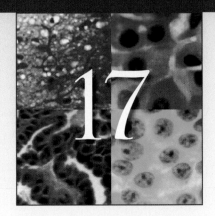

CHAPTER

Percutaneous transthoracic fine-needle aspirates (FNAs) or fine-needle biopsy (FNB) of the lung and mediastinal masses may be extremely useful in patients with diffuse pulmonary lesions or lung and intrathoracic masses that can be localized radiographically or by ultrasound.[1,2] It is a rapid, relatively safe procedure that can be used to collect material for cytologic evaluation and to obtain material for culture (Box 17-1). Neoplasms, hypersensitivity conditions, inflammatory lesions, and specific infectious agents (mycotic, protozoal, bacterial) may often be detected.[1-3] In human patients, FNB of the lung is 96% successful in diagnosing malignant neoplasms and 77% successful in obtaining material that yielded an infectious agent from immunosuppressed patients with a focal, pneumonic infiltrate.[3]

Although FNAs can generally be obtained with little risk, less invasive procedures, such as transtracheal/bronchoalveolar wash, thoracic radiography, and hematologic examination, should be performed first.[2,4] Transthoracic pulmonary fine-needle aspiration is contraindicated in animals with bleeding disorders, cystic or bullous lung diseases, pulmonary hypertension, and diseases producing forceful breathing and coughing that cannot be temporarily controlled (Table 17-1).[2-4] The procedure is also contraindicated in intractable patients. Hemorrhage, pneumothorax, and/or lung laceration are the primary complications.[2-4] In people, tumor seeding along the needle tract after FNB of a pulmonary mass has occurred in a few instances.[5]

Ultrasonography has become a common tool for assisting collection of cytology and biopsy specimens from lung and mediastinal lesions. It allows sampling of localized lesions and better visualization of lesions that may be difficult to visualize radiographically due to fluid accumulation in the chest.[1]

If ultrasound guidance is not available, the dorsal portion of the right caudal lobe is the preferred site for aspiration in patients with diffuse lung lesions.[3] Because the lung parenchyma is thickest in the caudal lobe, parenchymal aspirates are obtained more easily from this area and the likelihood of penetrating another vital structure is minimized.[3]

Although several positions can be used, standing and sternal positions have the following advantages with or without the assistance of ultrasound guidance:

- The dorsal lung is in a nondependent (high) area, which results in greater negative pressure and greater distension of alveoli; therefore fewer alveoli rupture and the biopsy site seals more rapidly.
- If ventilation occurs during aspiration, caudal lung motion is less; therefore the likelihood and severity of lung laceration are reduced.
- The chance of hemorrhage is decreased because blood perfusion and pressure are less in nondependent lung regions.[6]

With localized lung disease, the lesion is located on radiographs, and proper needle placement is determined by counting the ribs and measuring from the vertebrae, sternum, or costochondral junction.

Utilization of ultrasound to visualize lesions and guide in the collection of cytologic and histologic specimens is common. This technique may be especially useful if there is fluid around a visible lesion or if the lesion has contact with the chest wall.[7] It is preferred over blind fine-needle aspiration when masses are located near vital structures (e.g., large vessels). In general, sedation is indicated to adequately restrain patients during the procedure. Patient preparation, postaspiration management (e.g., observation), and complications are similar to those described for fine-needle aspiration.[7]

TECHNIQUE

The technique described later is for non-ultrasound–guided fine-needle aspiration of the lung. The technique for ultrasound guided biopsies is not described in this chapter but can be found in numerous textbooks.[1]

Pulmonary aspirates can be obtained quickly with minimal equipment. If the lesion is localized and proper needle placement can be determined radiographically, the likelihood of obtaining a useful or diagnostic sample is high. In generalized lung disease, however, the needle may be placed in an uninvolved area and yield only normal or nondiagnostic cells on aspiration; therefore multiple attempts are more likely to be needed.

Indications for Performing a Fine-Needle Aspiration Biopsy of Lung Parenchyma

- Investigate the etiology of a large, solitary pulmonary mass or consolidated area
- Investigate the etiology of diffuse or generalized parenchymal disease
- Detect inflammatory lesions and obtain material for culture
- Detect a hypersensitivity reaction
- Confirm neoplasia
- Avoid the need for more invasive procedures (e.g., thoracotomy or biopsy)

TABLE **17-1**

Contraindications for Fine Needle Aspiration of Lung Parenchyma and Associated Complications

Contraindication	Complication
Uncooperative patient	Lung laceration
Uncontrollable coughing or forceful breathing	Lung laceration
Any bleeding disorder	Severe intrapulmonary or pleural hemorrhage
Pulmonary hypertension	Severe intrapulmonary or pleural hemorrhage
Cysts or bullous emphysema	Pneumothorax

The area to be aspirated depends on whether the lesion is localized or generalized. If generalized, the needle is inserted on the right side of the chest between the seventh and ninth ribs, two thirds of the way dorsal between the costochondral junction and the vertebral bodies.[3] For localized lesions, the area of needle insertion depends on the location of the lesion, which is identified by lateral, dorsoventral, and ventrodorsal radiographs.[3]

The hair is clipped, the area is scrubbed and draped, and an antiseptic is applied. Local anesthetic may be used if desired but is frequently not needed. Heavy sedation may be required in uncooperative patients; however, sedation should be avoided if possible because sedated patients cannot clear respiratory secretions or endobronchial hemorrhage that may result from the FNB procedure.[3]

The patient is restrained in the standing, sitting, sternal, or lateral recumbent position. Depending on the animal's size, a 23- to 25-gauge, ⅝- to 1½-inch needle, with a 10- to 20-ml syringe attached, is inserted aseptically through the chest wall at the cranial aspect of the rib, avoiding the intercostal vessels on the adjacent rib's caudal border. The nose and mouth are temporarily held closed to stop lung movement while the needle is advanced into the lung parenchyma (about 1 to 3 cm), and negative pressure is applied while the needle is moved back and forth (about 1 cm). Negative pressure is released and the needle is withdrawn. Some authors advocate maintaining negative pressure while the needle is withdrawn to help avoid leaving tissue along the needle tract.[2,3]

The needle is removed from the syringe and the syringe is filled with air. The needle is reconnected to the syringe and the material in the hub of the needle is forced onto a glass slide, smeared, and stained for cytologic evaluation. Chapter 1 describes general techniques for FNB (aspiration and nonaspiration techniques), slide preparation, and staining. An adequate sample for cytologic evaluation can generally be collected with one or two attempts.

The patient should be closely monitored for postaspiration complications. Thoracic radiographs, immediately and 24 hours postaspiration, have been suggested.[3] Pneumothorax is the most common complication, reported to occur in 20% of patients.[8] However, most involve mild asymptomatic pneumothorax, which resolves spontaneously.[3] Favorable patient positioning may inhibit pneumothorax progression.[6] Rotating the animal so that the lung puncture site is down (dependent position) for 3 minutes markedly decreases pneumothorax formation.[6] The clinician should be prepared to insert a chest tube if severe pneumothorax develops.[3]

Scrapings and impressions of lung parenchyma taken during surgical biopsy, lobectomy, or necropsy can be useful in determining disease processes or etiology. Scrapings and impression smears are evaluated for the same changes as described for FNAs.

CYTOLOGIC EVALUATION

Cell Types of the Lung

Cells seen in FNAs or impression smears of pulmonary parenchyma include leukocytes and red blood cells (RBCs), as well as specialized cells of the lung, such as ciliated and nonciliated columnar cells, ciliated and nonciliated cuboidal cells, goblet cells, alveolar macrophages, and alveolar epithelial cells. Ciliated and nonciliated columnar and cuboidal cells and alveolar macrophages are generally seen unless lesions obliterated normal lung parenchyma. Goblet cells are seen only occasionally in pulmonary aspirates, scrapings, and impression smears.

Columnar and Cuboidal Cells: Ciliated columnar cells (Figure 17-1) have an elongated or cone shape, with cilia on the flattened end and the other (basal) end containing the nucleus and often terminating in a tail. The nucleus is generally round to oval, with a finely granular chromatin pattern.[9] Ciliated cuboidal cells appear similar to ciliated columnar cells, except cuboidal cells are as wide as they are tall. Nonciliated columnar and cuboidal cells appear identical to their ciliated counterparts, except the cilia are absent.

Goblet Cells: Goblet cells are mucus-producing bronchial cells. Goblet cells are infrequently seen in specimens prepared from FNAs of the lung, but are commonly seen in scraping or impression smears of lung tissue. They are columnar cells that often have an elongated contour in cytologic preparations. The cells have a basally placed nucleus and round granules of mucin that frequently distend the apical cytoplasm. Occasionally, the cytoplasm

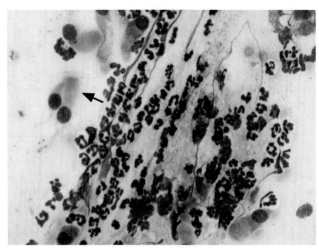

Figure 17-1 Impression smear of inflamed lung tissue. There are ciliated epithelial cells *(arrow)* and alveolar epithelial cells that lack cilia. There are many neutrophils in this inflammatory lesion.

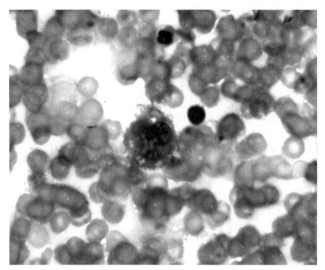

Figure 17-2 FNA of lung. A single alveolar macrophage containing phagocytosed red blood cells is surrounded by red blood cells in this hemorrhagic aspirate.

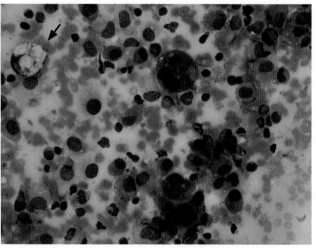

Figure 17-3 FNA from a lung mass. Most cells are neoplastic cells of histiocytic origin. The cells vary in size and have blue-stained, homogeneous to vacuolated cytoplasm. Nuclear size is variable and nuclei are occasionally lobulated or multiple. A single, nonneoplastic alveolar macrophage with vacuolated cytoplasm is present *(arrow)*.

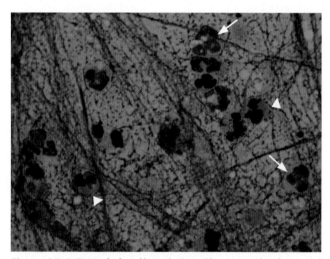

Figure 17-4 FNA of a focal lung lesion. The stringy background material is consistent with mucus. Both neutrophils *(arrow)* and eosinophils *(arrowhead)* are present. This suggests that allergy, hypersensitivity, or parasitism should be considered as a cause for this inflammatory lung lesion.

is so greatly distended that the cell appears round. The granules generally stain red or blue with Romanowsky-type stains. Mucin granules released from ruptured goblet cells may be free in the background. It is important to recognize these normal structures and differentiate them from mast cell granules, eosinophil granules, and infectious agents.

Alveolar Epithelial Cells: Alveolar epithelial cells (see Figure 17-1) are cuboidal to round cells that line alveoli. They have centrally to basally located round to oval nuclei. The nuclear chromatin is slightly coarse. Cytoplasm is light blue. Occasionally the cells appear elongated, especially in FNA, due to mechanical distortion during slide preparation. Some alveolar epithelial cells are present in most pulmonary cytology specimens.

Alveolar Macrophages: Alveolar macrophages (Figures 17-2 and 17-3) are readily found in pulmonary aspirates and impression smears from clinically normal animals. They are typically the predominant cell type. The nucleus is round to indented and eccentric. Occasional binucleate alveolar macrophages are seen in smears from clinically normal animals. Alveolar macrophages have abundant blue-gray, granular cytoplasm. Activated macrophages appear to have more abundant, vacuolated (foamy) cytoplasm and may contain phagocytized material.

Neutrophils: Neutrophils (Figure 17-4; see Figure 17-1) in pulmonary aspirates or impression smears look like peripheral blood neutrophils, although degenerative

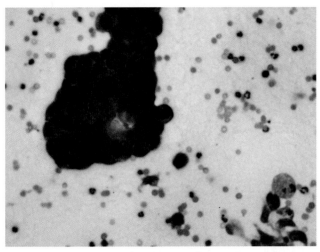

Figure 17-5 This aspirate from a dog with a pulmonary adenocarcinoma shows a group of large epithelial cells with variation in cell and nuclear size, coarse nuclear chromatin, large nucleoli, basophilic cytoplasm, and cytoplasmic vacuolation. Note how much larger the neoplastic cells are compared with the red blood cells, neutrophils, and alveolar macrophages that are in the background.

changes may be present. Some of the neutrophils are present because of blood contamination during aspiration or making of impression smears. The number of neutrophils present secondary to blood contamination depends on the degree of contamination and the number of neutrophils present in the peripheral blood. Generally, there is 1 white blood cell (WBC)/500 to 1000 RBCs. A relative increase in neutrophils for the amount of blood suggests inflammation, but this observation should always be compared with the peripheral leukogram to help distinguish between peripheral blood contamination and a true inflammatory cell infiltrate within the lung.

Eosinophils: Eosinophils are bone marrow–derived granulocytes containing intracytoplasmic lysosome granules. These granules have an affinity for the acid dye eosin, which stains them red or eosinophilic (see Figure 17-4). Typically eosinophils are present in very low numbers in lung specimens from clinically normal dogs and cats. Increased numbers of eosinophils indicate an allergic or hypersensitivity reaction.

Lymphocytes/Plasma Cells: Lymphocytes may be present in small numbers in pulmonary aspirates, scrapings, and impression smears from normal dogs and cats. With immune stimulation, lymphocytes become activated. Their cytoplasm becomes more abundant and stains deep blue because of increased protein synthesis. Also, some lymphocytes develop into plasma cells. Slight lymphocytosis or few reactive lymphocytes generally denote immune stimulation or chronic inflammation and are of limited diagnostic value because of the lack of etiologic specificity. Cellular aspirates primarily consisting of small lymphocytes may occur when a reactive pulmonary or mediastinal lymph node or thymoma is aspirated rather

than lung tissue. Lymphoma (although rare in the lung) should be suspected if >50% of cells are lymphoblasts.

Mast Cells: Mast cells are occasionally observed in pulmonary aspirates, scrapings, and impression smears from dogs and cats with many different inflammatory lung disorders. They are readily identified by their red-purple intracytoplasmic granules, which are frequently present in large numbers and may obscure the nucleus. Scattered granules from ruptured mast cells may be present free on the slide and should not be misinterpreted as bacteria. In low numbers, they are of little diagnostic significance. A high number of mast cells indicates pulmonary mast cell neoplasia, but this is an extremely uncommon finding.

Erythrocytes: Erythrocytes are always present in pulmonary aspirates, scrapings, and impression smears. Blood contamination during collection must be differentiated from true intrapulmonary hemorrhage. The presence of pulmonary macrophages with phagocytized RBCs or RBC-breakdown products, such as hematoidin, biliverdin, or hemosiderin (see Figure 17-2) helps differentiate blood contamination from intrapulmonary hemorrhage.

Neoplasia: Pulmonary neoplasia may be primary or metastatic. Carcinomas and adenocarcinomas (Figure 17-5) are the most common form of primary and metastatic pulmonary neoplasia.[10] Sarcomas, including histiocytic sarcoma and osteosarcoma, are more likely to be metastatic. Disseminated histiocytic neoplasms (see Figure 17-3) and malignant melanoma may also involve the lung and be detected in cytologic preparations. Cells retrieved on pulmonary aspirates, scrapings, or impression smears are evaluated for the criteria of malignancy such as variation in cell size (with a high proportion of large cells) and shape, large nuclei with prominent nucleoli and a coarse chromatin pattern, nuclear molding, and mitotic figures. Evaluating cells for neoplastic criteria is easier if inflammation is absent because inflammation readily induces metaplastic and dysplastic changes, which must be differentiated from neoplastic changes. Also, one must be careful not to confuse cells obtained by accidental aspiration of nonpulmonary tissue, such as accidental aspiration of the liver (especially when the caudal lung lobes are the attempted site of aspiration), with neoplastic cells.

Mesothelial Cells: In attempting to aspirate the lung parenchyma, cells from the lung or pleural surface may be aspirated (Figure 17-6). These cells are often in sheets, but may be individual. They may have polyhedral or angular contour and, in some cases, a pink-stained periphery, characteristic of mesothelial cells may be detected.

Miscellaneous Findings: Cornstarch (glove powder) is frequently seen on slides from pulmonary aspirates, scrapings, and impression smears. These are typically clear-staining, large, round to hexagonal particles with central fissures. Cornstarch is an incidental finding and should not be confused with an organism or cell.

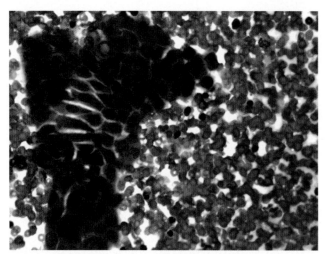

Figure 17-6 FNA from an attempted aspirate of the lung. A sheet of mesothelial cells from the pleural surface of the chest or the lung was aspirated. The polyhedral cells do not vary much in size, and a pink-stained, slightly fringed border can be seen along one edge of the aggregate of cells. These cells do not have cytologic features of malignancy and should not be mistaken for neoplastic epithelial cells.

Cell Types of Mediastinal Aspirates

Structures of the cranial mediastinum (the mediastinum that is cranial to the heart) include segments of the trachea, esophagus, and major large vessels and nerve trunks dorsally and lymph nodes and thymic tissue in the ventral portion. It is the structures of the ventral mediastinum that are usually evaluated cytologically. Cells of normal thymic tissue include a mixture of lymphoid cells, epithelial cells of Hassall's corpuscles with varying degrees of squamous differentiation, and a low number of mast cells.

Thymic Epithelial Cells: The epithelial cells of the thymus are located in the medullary portion of thymic lobules in structures called Hassall's corpuscles (Figure 17-7). They are angular to round and have variable amounts of blue-stained cytoplasm with a homogeneous (hyalinized) appearance. Rarely, they may be mineralized. Aspirates or scrapings of normal thymic tissue are rarely submitted for cytologic evaluation, but the presence of these epithelial cells in specimens from mediastinal masses is considered an important feature for identification of the site of origin.

Thymic Lymphoid Cells: Thymic lymphocytes are found in both the cortex and medulla of the thymus. The cortical lymphocytes are more densely arranged than those of the medulla. Cortical lymphocytes generally include both small and large lymphocytes. The lymphocytes of the medulla are typically small. Thymic lymphoma is usually characterized by proliferation of large lymphoid cells, although small cell lymphoma may occur at this site.

Mast Cells: Mast cells are seen in very low numbers in normal thymic tissue. They are common in aspirates of thymoma and are often used to support this diagnosis.

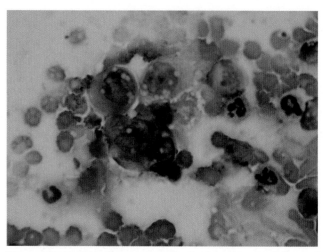

Figure 17-7 FNA from a mediastinal lesion. A cluster of epithelial cells with smudged cytoplasm having small, discrete vacuoles is consistent with the epithelial cells of Hassall's corpuscles.

Erythrocytes: As in specimens from other sites, RBCs are common in thymic specimens. In most specimens their presence is a result of peripheral blood contamination. Intrathymic hemorrhage may occur during thymic involution and may occur with rodenticide poisoning, but the presence of blood in thymic cytologic specimens is not diagnostic of these conditions.

Neoplasia: Primary mediastinal neoplasms include lymphoma (involving mediastinal lymph nodes and/or the thymus) and thymoma. Metastatic neoplasms, most commonly carcinoma or melanoma, may involve mediastinal lymph nodes.

Miscellaneous: Artifacts of specimen collection, including the presence of glove powder and ultrasound gel, may be present. Ultrasound gel, is purple, acellular, crystalline to granular, and in fragments of variable size.

CYTOLOGIC INTERPRETATION

Lung

Pulmonary aspirates, scrapings, and impression smears are interpreted according to the type, quantity, and proportion of cells recovered. They can generally be classified into the following categories:

- *Insufficient sample:* No cells are seen other than those from blood contamination.
- *Only normal cell types:* Blood and alveolar cells, macrophages with little evidence of phagocytic activity, and ciliated columnar epithelial cells are the only cells present.
- *Eosinophilic infiltrate:* The proportion of eosinophils in the aspirate is greater than the number of eosinophils expected from blood contamination.
- *Neutrophilic infiltrate:* The number of neutrophils in the aspirate is significantly greater than would occur from blood contamination.

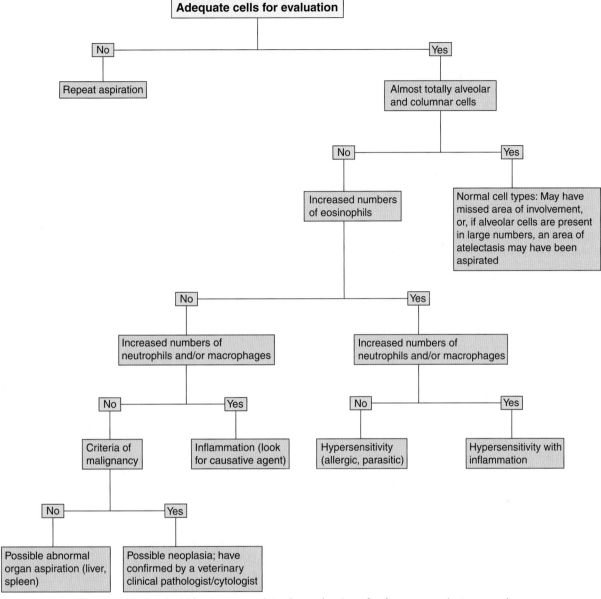

Figure 17-8 An algorithmic approach to the evaluation of pulmonary aspirates, scrapings, or impression smears.

- *Granulomatous inflammation:* Multinucleated inflammatory cells (giant cells) and/or epithelioid macrophages are present.
- *Histiocytic (macrophage) infiltrate:* The sample is very cellular and consists primarily of macrophages.
- *Hyperplasia/dysplasia (benign):* Atypical cells are seen, but insufficient criteria of malignancy are present for establishing a diagnosis of malignant neoplasia.
- *Malignant neoplasia:* Cells with sufficient criteria of malignancy to diagnose malignant neoplasia are present.
- *Ectopic aspirate:* Cells typical of an organ other than the lung are present.

These categories may overlap. Classification of pulmonary aspirates and impressions into one or more of these categories allows disease process(es) to be identified. Figure 17-8 presents an algorithm to aid evaluation

of pulmonary aspirates, scrapings, or impression smears. Integration of the patient history, physical examination findings, and clinical laboratory test results may allow further refinement of the diagnosis.

Mediastinal Lymph Nodes and Thymus

Aspirates, impression smears, or scrapings of mediastinal lymph nodes and the thymus are typically assessed only when there is clinically detectable organomegaly. Because both mediastinal lymph nodes and the thymus are lymphoid organs, differentiating between these two sites may be problematic. Specimens from these sites may be classified as follows:

- *Insufficient sample:* No cells are seen other than those from blood contamination.

- *Only normal cell types:* Normal cell types of the thymus include a mixture of lymphoid cells (mostly small) with occasional epithelioid cells of Hassall's corpuscles. Rare mast cells may be seen. Because normal thymic tissue is rarely sampled, seeing these cell types in a mass lesion of the cranial mediastinum is most consistent with thymoma. Mediastinal lymph nodes, as other lymph nodes, have a resident population of predominately small lymphocytes, with fewer large lymphocytes, lymphoblasts, and occasional plasma cells.
- *Inflammatory cell infiltrates:* Neutrophilic, eosinophilic, and histiocytic infiltrates may be seen in aspirates of mediastinal lymph nodes, but are unlikely to be seen in primary thymic lesions. Inflammatory cells are seen in mediastinal lymph node specimens, which usually reflects primary lung lesions or systemic disease involving multiple lymph nodes.
- *Neoplasia:* Cells with criteria for malignant neoplasia or the appropriate population of cells seen in thymoma are present.

LUNG SPECIMENS

Only Normal Cell Types Present

If the area of involvement is missed, only blood and normal cell types (i.e., alveolar cells, macrophages, and cuboidal and columnar cells) may be seen. Reaspiration should be attempted. If an area of involvement cannot be aspirated, a lung biopsy is indicated.

Large numbers of pulmonary macrophages and alveolar cells are frequently present when an area of atelectasis is aspirated. Because of the high cellularity of the aspirate and lack of an inflammatory response, neoplasia may be suspected; however, on careful evaluation of cell morphology, sufficient criteria of malignancy are not present to warrant such an interpretation.

Hypersensitivity

Eosinophils are important in defending against helminth infections and in modulating hypersensitivity reactions.[11] Eosinophils generally compose <5% of cells in pulmonary aspirates and impression smears from clinically normal dogs. The number of eosinophils present in pulmonary aspirates from clinically normal cats has not been published. However, bronchoalveolar lavage specimens from clinically normal cats have a much higher percentage of eosinophils than similar specimens from dogs, suggesting that higher numbers of eosinophils are in the lung parenchyma of cats. The expected proportion of eosinophils in feline lung specimens is, therefore, higher than it is in dog specimens. High proportions of eosinophils (i.e., >10% in dogs and 20% in cats) in pulmonary aspirates, scrapings, or impression smears indicate allergy or hypersensitivity. Parasitic antigens are the most common initiators of this type of reaction, but other causes of hypersensitivity, including inhaled antigens such as pollen or dust, may cause eosinophilic infiltration of the lung. Rarely, eosinophilic infiltrates may be associated with tumors or some fungal infections. These diseases can be diagnosed by identifying the neoplastic cells or fungal hyphae in the specimens.

Other inflammatory cells (neutrophils, macrophages) may be seen in association with infiltrates of eosinophils if tissue irritation is sufficient to induce an inflammatory response. Circulating and, likely, tissue eosinophil numbers are decreased by glucocorticoid administration. Therefore glucocorticoid therapy can mask the typical eosinophilic response seen cytologically with reaginic (immunoglobulin E) hypersensitivity.

Inflammation

A relative increase in the number of leukocytes (neutrophils, eosinophils, or lymphocytes) for the amount of blood is consistent with inflammation. Typically, 1 WBC/500 to 1000 RBCs is the expected WBC concentration from blood contamination. However, this WBC number may increase with peripheral leukocytosis, and the observation of a relative increase in neutrophils should be compared with the peripheral leukogram. Eosinophilic inflammation is described in the discussion of hypersensitivity earlier in this chapter. Although alveolar macrophages are normal inhabitants of the lung, even in the absence of an inflammatory response, a relative increase in macrophages suggests inflammation. A high proportion of neutrophils indicates inflammation (see Figure 17-1). Neutrophils may show degenerative changes because of bacterial toxins or may be smudged (ruptured) secondary to trauma from collection and preparation. Inflammation may be present because of infectious or noninfectious processes. Infectious causes of neutrophilic inflammation include bacterial, mycotic, viral, and protozoal diseases. Examples of noninfectious lesions associated with neutrophilic infiltrates include tissue necrosis secondary to inhalation of an irritating substance and ischemic necrosis, which occurs when a neoplasm that has outgrown its blood supply or blood flow to tissue is impaired due to thrombosis. Identification of neoplastic cells or the infectious agent provides an etiologic diagnosis.

Pulmonary aspirates characterized by many neutrophils and fewer macrophages suggest acute or chronic active inflammation. A specific diagnosis can be made if a causative agent is seen. Otherwise, the cytologic changes are interpreted as neutrophilic (purulent or suppurative) inflammation. There are many causes of neutrophilic inflammation. Causes include bacterial pneumonia, abscesses secondary to bacterial infections or foreign-body (i.e., plant or food) inhalation, necrotic tumors, and inhalation of toxic substances causing inflammation of the lung parenchyma without discrete abscess formation. Mycotic and protozoal agents frequently result in granuloma formation but may be associated with a neutrophilic response.

Very cellular samples consisting almost totally of pulmonary macrophages and alveolar cells are common when areas of atelectasis are aspirated or imprinted. Diseases such as lipid pneumonia and granulomatous pneumonia can result in cellular aspirates or imprints primarily consisting of macrophages. Large discrete vacuoles containing nonstaining material (lipid) may be present

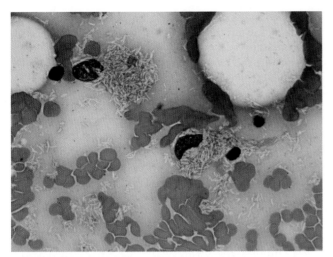

Figure 17-9 FNA from a lung lesion from a cat. Many macrophages with discrete, negative rod-shaped images are typical of mycobacterial lesions.

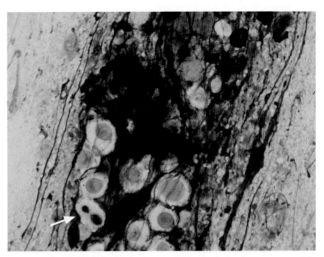

Figure 17-10 Scraping from the lung of a cat with cryptococcosis. There is mucinous material in the background and many organisms are present. The characteristic capsules are nonstaining in this preparation. One narrow-based budding yeast form is seen *(arrow)*.

within macrophages in lipid pneumonia. RBCs and/or RBC-breakdown products phagocytosed by macrophages may be seen with intrapulmonary hemorrhage or passive congestion of the lung (see Figure 17-2). Nonphagocytized RBCs are always present because of peripheral blood contamination. Macrophages are important in defending against microorganisms; phagocytized microorganisms, especially mycotic or protozoal organisms, may be seen.

Granulomatous reactions are characterized by a predominance of macrophages with fewer neutrophils and, occasionally, binucleate and multinucleate inflammatory giant cells. Although many disorders can cause granulomatous inflammation, foreign bodies and mycotic and protozoal agents are most common causes of this type of inflammation in dogs and cats.

Bacterial Diseases: Many different bacteria can cause pulmonary lesions. Bacterial pneumonia is generally caused by infection with a gram-negative rod.[12] Phagocytized and nonphagocytized bacteria may be found in aspirates, scrapings, and impression smears of lung parenchyma from animals with bacterial pneumonia or a lung abscess. Identifying the bacteria as rods or cocci helps in choosing initial antibacterial therapy while awaiting culture and sensitivity results. With hematologic stains, bacteria (both gram positive and gram negative) stain blue-black. If gram stains are applied to cytologic preparations, gram-positive bacteria will stain dark blue to black and gram-negative bacteria stain red or orange.

Most pneumonias caused by rod-shaped bacteria are due to infection with gram-negative rods. If rod-shaped bacteria, especially bipolar rods, are seen in cytologic preparations, a drug effective against gram-negative bacteria should be used while awaiting culture and sensitivity results. Filamentous rods suggestive of either *Actinomyces* spp., *Nocardia* spp., or, rarely *Fusobacterium* spp. are occasionally seen. *Mycobacterium* spp. may infect dogs or cats and are more difficult to identify cytologically because they do not stain with routine hematologic stains. On careful examination, however, the negative images of *Mycobacterium* spp.

can be seen (Figure 17-9). *Staphylococcus* and *Streptococcus* spp. are the cocci most often associated with pneumonia. Therefore, when bacterial cocci are seen cytologically, a drug effective against gram-positive bacteria should be used while awaiting culture and sensitivity results.

Mycotic and Protozoal Diseases: Many different mycotic and protozoal organisms can colonize the lungs.[13] A lung aspirate or biopsy and scraping or impression smear is indicated when generalized lung disease or a localized mass cannot be confirmed by less invasive techniques. Some of the common mycotic and protozoal organisms associated with lung lesions are *Blastomyces dermatitidis*, *Cryptococcus neoformans* (Figure 17-10), *Coccidioides immitis*, *Histoplasma capsulatum* (Figure 17-11), *Sporothrix* spp., *Aspergillus* spp. or other opportunistic fungi (Figure 17-12), *Toxoplasma gondii*, *Cytauxzoon felis*, and *Pneumocystis carinii*.

Viral Diseases: Many viral diseases can cause lung damage. Viral pneumonias may be associated with concurrent bacterial infection. It is difficult to make specific cytologic diagnoses of pure viral pneumonia. The inclusion bodies that are characteristic of viral infections such as canine distemper or canine adenovirus are rarely seen in lung aspirates. Failure to find viral inclusions does not rule out infection with these viruses. Other viral diseases such as feline infectious peritonitis, a corona virus that causes multifocal vasculitis, necrosis, and inflammation do not have intralesional inclusion bodies. With secondary bacterial infection, large numbers of neutrophils and bacterial organisms are present.

Atypical Cell Types

Atypical cells may be seen with pulmonary metaplasia, dysplasia, or neoplasia (primary or metastatic). If abdominal organs or nonpulmonary thoracic organs are

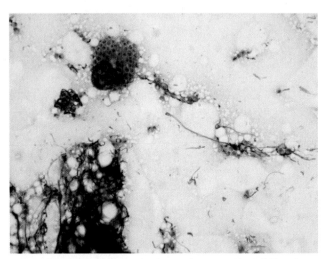

Figure 17-11 FNA from the lung of a cat with a diffuse lung lesion. Macrophages are filled with yeast consistent with *Histoplasma capsulatum*. Organisms, perhaps released from ruptured cells, are free in the lightly stained background material. Characteristically, these round to oval organisms are 1 to 4 μm in diameter with dark blue to purple stained nuclei surrounded by a thin, usually nonstaining capsule.

accidentally aspirated, cells in aspirates may be initially considered "atypical." Any atypical cells should be evaluated for malignant criteria.

Metaplasia: Metaplasia is an adaptive response of epithelial cells to chronic irritation.[11] Replacement of normal respiratory epithelial cells of the trachea, bronchi, and bronchioles with stratified squamous epithelium (squamous metaplasia) is an example of pulmonary metaplasia.[11] These metaplastic cells mimic maturing squamous epithelium and must not be confused with neoplasia.

Dysplasia: By definition, dysplasia is a nonneoplastic change that occurs because of an external influence altering cell proliferation, differentiation, and maturation. Conditions such as inflammation and tissue irritation can cause dysplasia; however, severely dysplastic changes are sometimes referred to as carcinoma in situ[11] or preneoplastic lesions. Dysplasia may indicate asynchrony in cell and tissue development. Dysplastic changes include variation in cell size and shape, increased nuclear-to-cytoplasmic ratio, altered (usually increased) staining intensity, and higher proportions of immature cells.[11] These changes can be difficult to differentiate from neoplasia and may progress to neoplasia.

Neoplasia: Neoplasms involving the lung may be solitary (focal) or multifocal (multinodular) or have a more diffuse, infiltrative distribution. Most primary lung tumors are solitary (focal) lesions. However, intrapulmonary metastasis, resulting in multiple nodules, may occur. The majority of tumors involving the lung are characterized by the presence of multifocal, nodular lesions and are metastatic. It is uncommon for a metastatic tumor from a site other than the lung to result in a solitary metastatic lesion. When evaluating cells for criteria of malignancy, care must be taken not to confuse inflammation-induced dysplasia or abnormal organ aspiration with neoplasia.

Primary lung tumors may be located at the hilus (suspected bronchial origin) or at the periphery of the lung (suspected bronchoalveolar origin) or may be diffuse.[13] Adenocarcinomas are by far the most common primary lung tumor.[10,14] Carcinomas and adenocarcinomas, whether primary to the lung or metastatic to the lung, are composed of large cell polyhedral to rounded (epithelial) cells that show the criteria of malignancy (see Chapter 2), such as a high nuclear-to-cytoplasmic ratio, marked variation in cell size with large cells present, and nuclear molding. When acinus or gland formation or production of secretory products is seen, the more specific classification of adenocarcinoma is used.

Carcinomas and adenocarcinoma are considered the most common type of tumor to metastasize to the lung, but other tumors, such as histiocytic sarcoma, osteosarcoma, hemangiosarcoma, and hematopoietic tumors may also involve the lung.

Anticancer Therapy: Irradiation and chemotherapy may result in such severe atypia of cells of the tracheobronchial epithelium, terminal bronchial epithelium, and alveolar epithelium that differentiation from neoplasia cannot be reliably made.[9] Pulmonary aspirates obtained after cancer therapy should be interpreted with caution.

MEDIASTINAL SPECIMENS

Specimens from the mediastinum are usually evaluated only if a mass lesion is present, and most of the time a neoplastic process is present. Inflammatory lesions are uncommon.

Lymph Nodes: Enlarged pulmonary and mediastinal lymph nodes may be identified as intrathoracic masses by radiographs or ultrasound. Cytologic interpretation of aspirates of pulmonary lymph nodes is the same as interpretation of peripheral lymph nodes.

Thymus: A thymoma is a neoplastic mass lesion of the cranial mediastinum. The cytologic challenge is to distinguish between thymoma and thymic lymphoma. Although lymphoma may occur in patients of any age, thymomas are more common in older dogs and cats.[15] When viewed radiographically or by ultrasound, lymphoma is more likely to be a solid lesion, whereas cystic lesions are more likely to be thymomas. Cytologic specimens of thymomas may be quite variable. They classically have a predominance of small lymphoid cells with fewer intermediate-sized lymphoid cells, epithelial cells (Hassall's corpuscles), macrophages, and mast cells (Figure 17-13). Malignant thymomas are invasive, but this is not a characteristic that can be evaluated in cytologic preparations. Radiographic or ultrasound evaluation is needed.

Thymic lymphoma is characterized by a homogeneous population of lymphoid cells, most often large cell type. Small cell and intermediate lymphomas of the thymus occur as well. The lack of a significant number of other

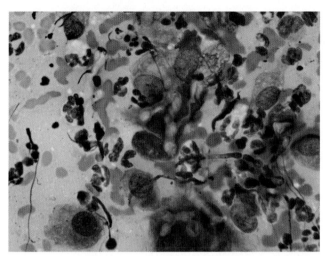

Figure 17-12 Impression smear from a nodular lung lesion. There is a mixture of inflammatory cells (neutrophils and macrophages) and many septate branching hyphae that are consistent with *Aspergillus* spp. Culture is needed for definitive identification of the fungal organism.

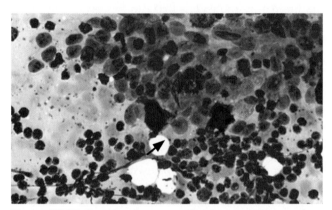

Figure 17-13 Scraping from a mediastinal mass from a dog. The mass consists of a mixture of small lymphocytes with epithelial cells *(arrow)* and few mast cells. This is characteristic of thymoma.

cell types is helpful in distinguishing thymic lymphoma from thymoma.

Fat: Mediastinal lipomas may radiographically appear as intrathoracic masses. Aspirated intrathoracic fat (lipoma or otherwise) grossly appears as a greasy, nondrying material. Cytologically, it appears identical to subcutaneous lipomas with fat spaces and some lipocytes constituting the majority of the smear.

Abdominal Organ Aspiration: Although the distal dorsal portion of the lung is the thickest, the needle can be forced deeply and through the lung, resulting

in aspiration of abdominal organs, usually the liver. Fragments of skeletal muscle (from the diaphragm) are seen less often. Consider that the caudal lung lobes extend caudal to the heart and the contour of the (diaphragmatic) caudal surface mirrors the contour of the cranial liver, only separated by the muscle of the diaphragm. Hepatocytes are large epithelial cells with a single, round nucleus and one or more small, round nucleoli. The cytoplasm is blue-gray and often granular. Bile or lipofucsin granules may be present. Care must be taken not to confuse accidentally aspirated hepatocytes with neoplastic cells.

References

1. Bahr R: Thorax. In Green RW (ed): *Small Animal Ultrasound.* Philadelphia, Lippincott-Raven, 1996, pp 89-104.
2. Silverstein D, Drobatz KJ: Clinical Evaluation of the Respiratory Tract. In Ettinger SJ, Feldman EC (eds): *Textbook of Veterinary Internal Medicine* St. Louis, Saunders, 2005, pp 1213-1215.
3. Roudebush P, et al: Percutaneous fine-needle aspiration biopsy of the lung in disseminated pulmonary disease. *J Am Anim Hosp Assoc* 17:109-116, 1981.
4. Shaw D, Ihle S: Pulmonary parenchymal diseases, pleural space and mediastinal disorders. In Shaw D, Ihle S (eds): *Small Animal Internal Medicine.* Baltimore, Williams & Wilkins, 1997, pp 222-237.
5. Anderson RW, Arentzen CE: Carcinoma of the lung. *Surg Clin North Am* 60:794-813, 1980.
6. Zidulka A, et al: Position may stop pneumothorax progression in dogs. *Am Rev Resp Dis* 126:51-53, 1982.
7. Nyland TG, Mattoon JS: *Veterinary Diagnostic Ultrasound.* Philadelphia, Saunders, 1995, pp 30-42.
8. Shure D, et al: Transbronchial needle aspiration in the diagnosis of pneumonia in a canine model. *Am Rev Resp Dis* 13:290-291, 1985.
9. Johnston WW: Cytologic diagnosis of lung cancer: Principles and problems. *Path Res Pract* 181:1-36, 1986.
10. Wilson DW, Dungworth DL: Tumors of the respiratory tract. In Meuten DJ (ed): *Tumors of Domestic Animals.* Ames, Iowa, Iowa State Press, 2002, pp 380-390.
11. Slauson DO, Cooper BJ: *Mechanisms of Disease*, ed 2. Baltimore, Williams & Wilkins, 1990, pp 204, 307.
12. Ford R: Bacterial pneumonia. In Bonagura J (ed): *Kirk's Current Veterinary Therapy XIII.* Philadelphia, Saunders, 1999, pp 812-815.
13. Legendre A, Toal R: Diagnosis and treatment of fungal diseases of the respiratory system. In Bonagura J (ed): *Kirk's Current Veterinary Therapy XIII.* Philadelphia, Saunders, 1999, pp 815-819.
14. Jacobs RM, Messick JB, Valli VE: Tumors of the hemolymphatic system. In Meuten J (ed): *Tumors of Domestic Animals.* Ames, Iowa, Iowa State Press, 2002, pp 165-166.
15. Moore LE, Biller DS: Mediastinal disease. In Ettinger SJ, Feldman EC (eds): *Textbook of Veterinary Internal Medicine.* St. Louis, Saunders, 2005, pp 1270-1271.

The Gastrointestinal Tract

J.L. Webb, P.M. Rakich, and K.S. Latimer

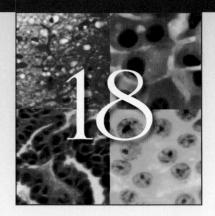

18

CHAPTER

Until recently, gastrointestinal (GI) cytology has largely been limited to rectal scrapings. With the increased popularity of endoscopy and ultrasound, however, GI cytology is becoming more commonplace. These diagnostic techniques allow more accurate determination of lesion location and also provide less invasive methods of obtaining cytologic samples than traditional laparotomy.

Dogs and cats with GI disease can present with a variety of clinical signs, including anorexia, weight loss, regurgitation, vomiting, diarrhea, constipation, tenesmus, hematemesis, melena, and hematochezia. Many of these clinical signs are nonspecific, and further ancillary testing (e.g., radiography with or without contrast media, ultrasound, occult blood testing) is needed to localize the disease to the GI tract.

TECHNIQUES TO OBTAIN CYTOLOGIC SPECIMENS FROM THE ALIMENTARY TRACT

Fine-needle aspirates (FNAs), endoscopic brushings, and biopsy imprints are used to obtain samples for most of the GI tract. All techniques have their advantages and disadvantages and these are summarized in Table 18-1. Descriptions of aspiration techniques, smear and imprint preparation, and staining are detailed in Chapter 1.

Fine-Needle Aspiration

Aspiration of the GI tract generally requires ultrasound guidance. FNAs are often used to sample masses, especially those that involve the submucosa and muscular wall that more superficial sampling techniques cannot reach. When obtaining FNAs, care should be taken to prevent or minimize contamination of the cytologic specimens with ultrasound gel because the gel stains intensely and can obscure cytologic details (Figure 18-1).

Endoscopic Brushings

Mucosal brushings can be obtained during endoscopy procedures. The technique involves passing a cytology brush through the endoscope and rubbing it on the desired area until slight bleeding is observed. The brush with its sample is then withdrawn from the endoscope and rolled onto a glass slide. Endoscopic brushings are an excellent technique to collect mucosal samples but they are limited by the length that can be reached and they can sample only the epithelial surface.[1]

Endoscopic and Surgical Biopsies

Making imprints from biopsy specimens is a common way to obtain cytologic samples for microscopic examination. Specimens can be prepared by touching or rolling the tissue along a glass microscope slide before the tissue is placed in formalin and processed for histologic examination. Either endoscopic or surgical full-thickness biopsy specimens can be used. Endoscopic biopsies have the advantage of being less invasive to collect but they usually sample only the mucosa and superficial submucosa. Full-thickness biopsies allow for examination of deeper layers but they are more invasive to collect and require open abdominal surgery.

Rectal Scrapings

Although most of the GI tract is difficult to reach for cytologic examination, the rectum is easily accessible for sampling. Mucosal scrapings are an easy, noninvasive method to obtain cytologic samples when large intestinal disease is suspected (Box 18-1). The object of a rectal mucosal scraping is to remove the overlying epithelium and obtain a sample from the lamina propria. Microscopic examination of this sample may reveal inflammation, infectious agents, or an infiltrating neoplasm. A rectal mucosal scraping is performed with a rigid instrument, such as a chemistry spatula, conjunctival scraper, or ear curette (Figure 18-2). Cotton swabs usually do not produce diagnostic samples because they are not abrasive enough to get a subepithelial sample. The rectum is first cleaned of feces so that a sample of mucosa, rather than adherent feces, is obtained. The instrument is guided into the rectum with a gloved finger as for performing a digital rectal examination. Lubricant is avoided or used sparingly because it stains intensely with Romanowsky stains and can obscure cytologic structures.

TABLE 18-1

Advantages and Disadvantages Associated with Techniques for Obtaining Cytologic Specimens from the Alimentary Tract

Technique	Advantages	Disadvantages
Fine-needle aspirates	Quick and easy Economical Noninvasive Minimal equipment (no anesthesia, +/- ultrasound guidance)	Largely restricted to mass lesions
Endoscopic brushings	Direct visualization of mucosal lesions Good sampling of epithelium	Samples only epithelium Samples only where endoscope can reach Requires sedation or anesthesia Moderately expensive
Impression smears – endoscopic biopsy	Direct visualization of mucosal lesions Less invasive than full-thickness biopsies	Samples only mucosa +/- superficial submucosa Samples only where the endoscope can reach Limited sampling of lesion Requires sedation or anesthesia Moderately expensive
Impression Smears – full-thickness surgical biopsy	All layers of intestinal wall can be examined Generally better sample quality than endoscopic biopsies	Most invasive method Requires general anesthesia Expensive

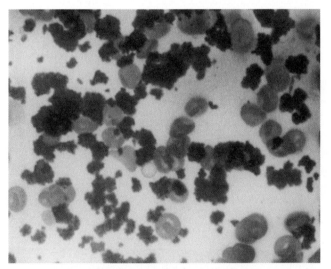

Figure 18-1 Ultrasound gel stains intensely magenta with Romanowsky stains and can obscure cellular detail. (Wright's stain.)

The instrument must be inserted far enough craniad to avoid the anus and reach the rectum. The instrument is drawn along the mucosa several times in a firm stroking motion. Scraping must be firm enough to remove the epithelium and collect material in the lamina propria but not so vigorous as to perforate the rectum. Perforation is especially a consideration in animals with chronic ulcerative colitis, in which the colon may be very friable. The scraper is removed from the rectum with the finger protecting the

BOX 18-1

Important Steps to Follow when Performing a Rectal Scraping

1. Clean rectum of feces before sampling
2. Avoid or use surgical lubricant sparingly
3. Use a rigid instrument for the scraping procedure (see Figure 18-2)
4. Sample far enough craniad to reach rectum and avoid anus
5. Scrape firmly enough to sample lamina propria but not so firmly as to cause perforation
6. Protect sample with gloved finger when removing from rectum

surface of the instrument so that the sample is not lost. The material is then placed on a glass slide and smeared with the scraping instrument or gently pressed with a second slide to make a smear consisting of a single layer of cells.

CYTOLOGIC EVALUATION OF THE ALIMENTARY TRACT

Esophagus

Normal Cytology: Esophageal disorders are uncommon in small animals and cytologic sampling of such disorders is rare. Normal cytologic findings from this region include nucleated squamous epithelial cells, occasionally

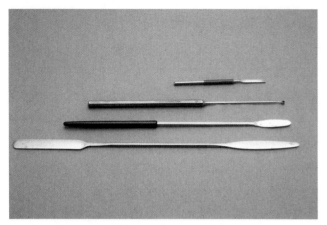

Figure 18-2 Various instruments used to perform rectal mucosal scrapings include *(top to bottom)* a conjunctival scraper, an ear curette, and two blunt chemistry spatulas.

with adherent bacterial flora. An occasional spindle cell from the muscular layer may be observed with a FNA or imprint of a biopsy specimen.

Neoplasia: Esophageal neoplasia accounts for less than 5% of all alimentary neoplasia. Squamous cell carcinoma, undifferentiated carcinoma, fibrosarcoma, osteosarcoma, and leiomyosarcoma have been reported in dogs and cats. There is a causal association between infection with the parasite *Spirocerca lupi* and development of esophageal sarcomas in dogs.[2,3]

Stomach

Normal Cytology: A normal gastric cytology specimen predominantly contains superficial mucus-secreting columnar epithelial cells. These cells will often be found in monomorphic honeycomb sheets or small strips of columnar cells (Figure 18-3). Individual cells contain a single, basally situated nucleus and finely granular cytoplasm. Chief and parietal cells will occasionally be seen. Chief cells can be recognized by their polygonal shape and numerous basophilic zymogen granules (Figure 18-4). Parietal cells are pyramidal and contain granular, eosinophilic cytoplasm.[4] FNAs or impression smears of deeper layers may also contain a few spindle-shaped smooth muscle cells or fibroblasts. These cells have an elongated nucleus with a dense chromatin pattern and attenuated, light blue cytoplasm. Various pieces of digesta and oral contaminants (mixed bacteria, including *Simonsiella* spp. and squamous cells) can sometimes be found along with an occasional neutrophil. Increased numbers of neutrophils may be associated with areas of ulceration.

Inflammation and Infection: Inflammatory conditions affecting the stomach may be the result of reactions to food antigens, microbial organisms, or self-antigens (Table 18-2).

Lymphocytic-Plasmacytic Gastritis: This is the most common form of gastric inflammation and is characterized cytologically by a moderate number of mature lymphocytes and plasma cells scattered amongst well-differentiated gastric epithelium.[5] Chronic hyperplastic

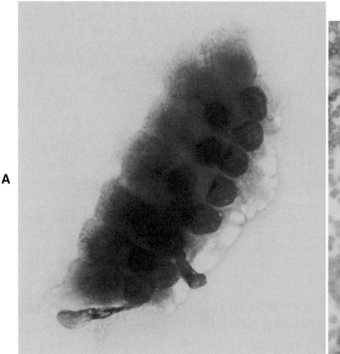

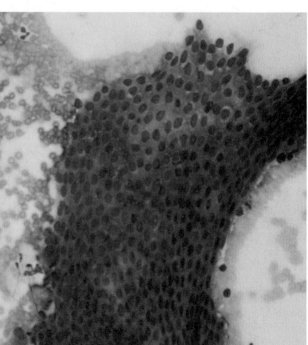

Figure 18-3 Normal gastric epithelium. **A,** When viewed from the side, epithelial cells appear as a strip of columnar cells with basal nuclei. **B,** When viewed from the top, these same cells appear as a monomorphic sheet of cells with densely packed nuclei and a thin border of cytoplasm. (Modified Wright's stain.)

gastritis, chronic superficial gastritis, atrophic gastritis, and *Helicobacter* infection are commonly associated with lymphocytic-plasmacytic inflammation.[5]

Eosinophilic Gastritis: Eosinophilic gastritis is less common and can be diagnosed by observing a mixed inflammatory population that is predominantly eosinophilic. Focal eosinophilic inflammation is found in association with migrating *Toxocara canis* larvae in dogs. Diffuse eosinophilic gastritis is thought to be allergic in nature but often the underlying cause is never found. It may be limited to the stomach or it may be part of a larger eosinophilic gastroenterocolitis complex. In cats, eosinophilic gastritis may also be part of the hypereosinophilic syndrome.[5] T-cell lymphoma, mast cell tumor, and pythiosis also may be associated with eosinophilic infiltration. Tumor cells will predominate over the eosinophils in cases of lymphoma and mast cell tumor, whereas pythiosis-related inflammation will also contain macrophages and other inflammatory cells.

Granulomatous Gastritis: Granulomatous gastritis is characterized by the presence of epithelioid macrophages and multinucleated giant cells and is rare in dogs and cats. This uncommon inflammatory infiltrate has been associated with mycobacteriosis and histoplasmosis.[5] *Mycobacterium* spp. are small, refractile, bacilli that do not stain with Romanowsky stains but may be visible as negative images against other material that does stain. Acid-fast stain can be applied to demonstrate the *Mycobacterium* spp. *Histoplasma capsulatum* organisms are described under "Rectal Scrapings."

Helicobacter: *Helicobacter* organisms are sometimes observed and their association, if any, with gastric disease is still debatable.[6] Cytologically, these bacteria have a typical corkscrew appearance (Figure 18-5). Organisms are more commonly seen, and in larger numbers, with cytologic as opposed to histologic specimens. The reason for this discrepancy is that *Helicobacter* spp. are associated with the luminal mucous layer. This layer is readily sampled with cytologic techniques but will often be lost by fluid agitation during formalin fixation and routine tissue processing for histologic examination.[7] *Helicobacter* bacteria are spiral-shaped, gram-negative rods that measure approximately 3.0 × 0.5 µm. Spiral-shaped bacteria can be present in cytologic specimens from healthy animals, but many more organisms usually are associated with gastritis. In addition, inflammation is present with gastritis.[8,9]

Pythiosis: Gastric pythiosis is infrequently diagnosed in dogs. The gastric wall is usually thickened by a proliferative inflammatory response that resembles a tumor-like mass. Aspiration of these lesions will obtain many eosinophils admixed with fewer neutrophils and macrophages. Hyphae of *Pythium insidiosum* stain poorly, if at all, with Romanowsky stains, but may appear as clear elongate structures surrounded by inflammatory cells (Figure 18-6, *A*). If necessary, Gomori's methenamine

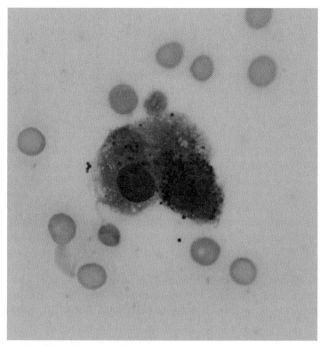

Figure 18-4 A gastric chief cell. This cell contains numerous basophilic zymogen granules. (Modified Wright's stain.)

TABLE 18-2

Inflammatory Conditions Affecting the Stomach of Dogs and Cats

	Incidence	Cytology	Associated Conditions
Lymphocytic-plasmacytic	Most common	Small lymphocytes and plasma cells	Chronic hyperplastic gastritis Chronic superficial gastritis Atrophic gastritis *Helicobacter* spp. infection
Eosinophilic	Less common	Mixed inflammation with eosinophils predominating	Allergy Parasites (migrating *Toxocara* spp. larvae) Fungal infection Pythiosis
Granulomatous	Rare	Epithelioid macrophages and/or multinucleated giant cells present	Mycobacteriosis Histoplasmosis

silver (GMS) stain may be applied to demonstrate the hyphae, which stain black (Figure 18-6, *B*).

Neoplasia: Gastric neoplasia accounts for <1% of all neoplasia in the dog and cat.[3,10] Malignant neoplasms predominate in dogs, with adenocarcinoma being most common followed by lymphosarcoma and leiomyosarcoma. Benign neoplasms are rare and include adenomas and leiomyomas.[11] Adenomas, often found in the pyloric region, cannot be differentiated from epithelial hyperplasia based

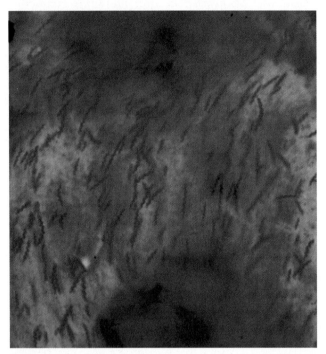

Figure 18-5 *Helicobacter* infection in a cat. Numerous *Helicobacter* spp. organisms are entrapped in mucus in a gastric biopsy imprint from a cat with ulcerative gastritis. (Wright's stain.)

on cytology alone because both lesions will exfoliate moderate numbers of normal-appearing epithelial cells. Lymphosarcoma is the most common gastric tumor in the cat; adenocarcinoma is rare.[11]

Gastric Adenocarcinoma: Adenocarcinomas typically occur in older dogs and cats and can present as a sessile polyp, ulcerated plaque, or diffuse thickening of the gastric wall.[10] These tumors may develop on the mucosal surface of the stomach or they may grow into the deeper layers. Consequently, brushings or impression smears of the mucosal surface may not always obtain a diagnostic sample. Neoplastic cells often have a lymphoid appearance (Figure 18-7). Individual cells are large and round and have a round nucleus, fine chromatin pattern, and one or two prominent nucleoli. A thin rim of dark blue and granular cytoplasm is present. In some tumors that elicit a connective tissue response (desmoplasia), scattered fibroblasts also may be present.

Lymphosarcoma: Gastric lymphosarcoma can present as multiple discrete masses or as a diffuse thickening of the mucosa with or without ulceration.[11] Cytologic diagnosis is based on the presence of a monomorphic population of lymphoblasts with a round to slightly indented nucleus, fine chromatin pattern, one or several prominent nucleoli, and a thin rim of dark blue cytoplasm (Figure 18-8). Small cell lymphomas also occur but are extremely difficult to differentiate cytologically from lymphocytic gastritis. Histopathology is often required in such cases to evaluate alterations in tissue architecture.

Smooth Muscle Neoplasms: Leiomyomas and leiomyosarcomas usually occur in dogs over 8 years of age, and the frequency of these tumors increases with age. Like most mesenchymal tumors, they often exfoliate poorly and may provide only a few cells to suggest a cytologic diagnosis. Leiomyomas are typically small tumors that produce few to no clinical signs. The cells are spindle-shaped and contain a thin, elongated nucleus with rounded ends (cigar-shaped). Leiomyosarcomas are large, slow-growing, solitary tumors. Cells vary from spindle-shaped to round

A
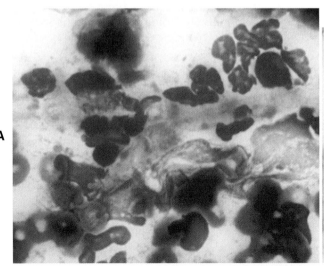
B
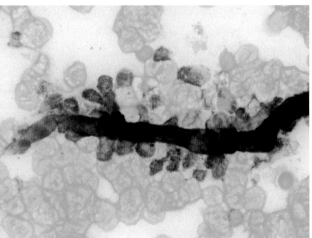

Figure 18-6 Gastric pythiosis in a dog. **A,** *Pythium insidiosum* appears as unstained, elongated structures surrounded by inflammatory cells in the Romanowsky-stained aspirate. (Wright's stain.) **B,** GMS staining reveals bulbous, poorly septate, branching hyphae that stain black.

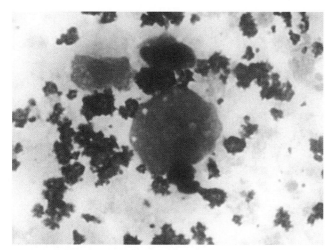

Figure 18-7 Gastric carcinoma in a cat. Notice that the neoplastic cell (center) is large and round, resembling a lymphoblast. (Wright-Leishman stain.)

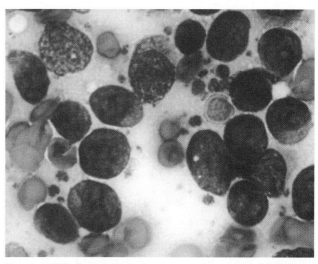

Figure 18-8 Gastric lymphosarcoma in a dog. Numerous large lymphoblasts have round nuclei, a fine chromatin pattern, and prominent nucleolar rings. (Wright's stain.)

and are pleomorphic with a high nuclear-to-cytoplasmic ratio. The nuclei vary in size but usually appear plump and have less aggregated chromatin. Mitotic figures may be observed.[3] Cytologic differentiation of leiomyoma, leiomyosarcoma, fibroma, fibrosarcoma, and other spindle cell sarcomas may be difficult (Figure 18-9). In such cases, immunocytochemistry or histologic evaluation with immunohistochemical staining may be necessary for a definitive diagnosis.

Intestine

Normal Cytology: Normal intestinal cytology consists of sheets of columnar epithelium and goblet cells. Columnar epithelial cells observed from the side appear rectangular with a round, basal nucleus that has a condensed chromatin pattern. The cytoplasm is light blue and more extensive toward the luminal surface. When aggregates of these cells are viewed from the top or bottom, the round nucleus is surrounded by a thin rim of cytoplasm, giving them a more cuboidal appearance. Goblet cells are elongated and have an apical accumulation of gray basophilic mucin granules and a basal nucleus. The proportion of goblet cells increases with progression from the small intestine to the large intestine.[4] FNAs and imprints of deeper layers may contain a few lymphocytes, plasma cells, occasional eosinophils, spindle-shaped fibroblasts (from the lamina propria and submucosa), and smooth muscle cells. A mixed bacterial population may be found in some samples, especially those from the large intestine. Intestinal conditions that can be diagnosed cytologically are classified as inflammatory, infectious, and neoplastic diseases.

Inflammation and Infection: Similar to the stomach, inflammatory infiltrates in the small and large intestine reflect an immune response to dietary, microbial, or self-antigens. Inflammatory cells infiltrate the lamina propria but frequently do not accumulate in the lumen. Therefore, a subepithelial specimen must be obtained to detect various cell populations and pathogens.

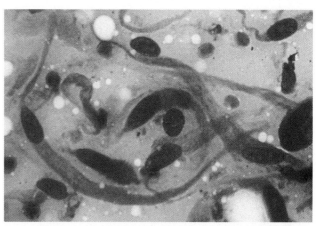

Figure 18-9 Gastric leiomyosarcoma in a dog. Plump spindle cells display moderate anisocytosis and anisokaryosis. A cytologic diagnosis of sarcoma was made, but the definitive diagnosis of leiomyosarcoma required histologic examination. (Wright's stain.)

Lymphocytic-Plasmacytic Enterocolitis: Lymphocytic-plasmacytic enteritis/colitis is the most common form of intestinal inflammation and is characterized by a mucosal infiltrate of mature lymphocytes and plasma cells.[5] A few eosinophils also may be present. Lymphocytic-plasmacytic inflammation has a more heterogeneous cell population but occasionally must be differentiated from early lymphosarcoma (see section on intestinal lymphosarcoma).

Eosinophilic Enterocolitis: Eosinophilic enteritis/colitis is the second-most common form of chronic inflammation and is characterized by a mixed inflammatory infiltrate in which eosinophils predominate (Figure 18-10).[5] In cats, eosinophilic inflammation may be part of the hypereosinophilic syndrome. Other conditions associated with eosinophilic intestinal infiltrates include parasitism, food allergy, pythiosis, T-cell lymphosarcoma, and mast cell tumor. In neoplasia, tumor cells usually predominate, however.

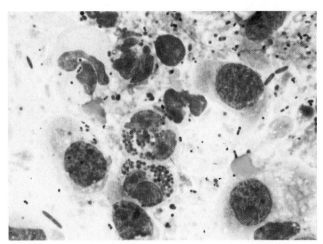

Figure 18-10 Eosinophilic enterocolitis in a dog. Scattered eosinophils in an intestinal imprint have red-brown granules as opposed to the bright red-orange granule color observed in blood smears. (Wright's stain.)

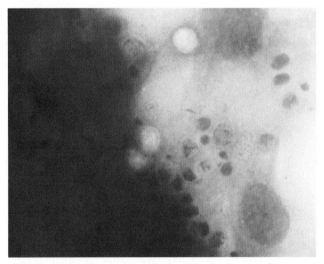

Figure 18-11 Cryptosporidiosis. Developing and mature sporocysts of *Cryptosporidium* spp. are present. The developing sporocysts are present in the apical ends of the columnar epithelial cells and appear basophilic, whereas mature sporocysts have a speckled eosinophilic appearance. (Wright's stain.)

Cryptosporidiosis: Intestinal cryptosporidiosis has been reported in dogs and cats, but is rarely diagnosed cytologically. Intestinal imprints may contain developing sporocysts of *Cryptosporidium parvum* contained within parasitophorous vacuoles in the apical end of enterocytes. Developing sporocysts will appear basophilic, whereas mature sporocysts will have a speckled, eosinophilic appearance with a clear cell wall. These organisms measure approximately 5 to 7 μm in diameter (Figure 18-11).

Coccidiosis: *Cystoisospora* spp. are members of the Apicomplexa family. Although coccidiosis usually is diagnosed by demonstration of sporocysts in fecal flotation specimens, sporozoites rarely may be observed in intestinal imprints taken during acute disease when hemorrhagic enteritis is present. During the early stages

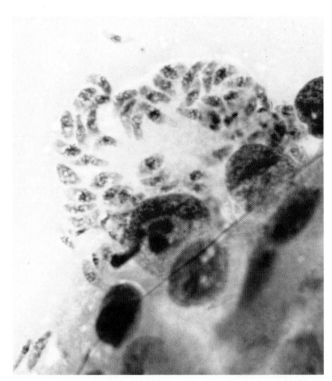

Figure 18-12 Sarcocystosis and esophageal carcinoma in a dog. Sporozoites from the family Apicomplexa are crescent-shaped and contain a small, central nucleus. (Wright's stain.)

of disease, the sporozoites multiply by binary fission and infect and destroy epithelial cells. These sporozoites are small, elongate to crescent-shaped, and have gently pointed ends. A small purple nucleus may be observed within a light blue cytoplasm (Figure 18-12).

Neoplasia: Intestinal neoplasia is uncommon in the dog and cat, but a variety of tumors can occur. Lymphosarcoma, intestinal adenocarcinoma, and mast cell tumors are the most common intestinal neoplasms in cats, both in the large and small intestines.[3] In dogs, intestinal adenocarcinoma is the most common small intestinal neoplasm. In contrast, adenoma, adenocarcinoma, and lymphosarcoma are the most common neoplasms of the large intestine.[2,3] In both dogs and cats, fibrosarcoma, leiomyosarcoma, leiomyomas, carcinoids, and plasma cell tumors rarely have been reported.[2] Most intestinal neoplasms are discrete but lymphosarcoma may infiltrate the bowel diffusely. The gross and cytologic features of some common intestinal tumors are summarized in Table 18-3.

Lymphosarcoma: Most cases of intestinal lymphosarcoma are diffuse but focal nodular forms do occur. In either case, a cytologic diagnosis can be made by demonstrating a monomorphic population of large lymphocytes. These lymphocytes are characterized by a fine chromatin pattern, one or several prominent nucleoli, and a thin rim of dark blue cytoplasm (Figure 18-13). In some instances, the neoplastic lymphocytes may contain fine to coarse azurophilic granules near the nuclear indentation (Figure 18-14). Such neoplasms are designated large granular lymphoma and may be associated with shorter

TABLE 18-3

Gross and Cytologic Features of Common Intestinal Tumors

Tumor	Gross Morphology	Cytology
Lymphosarcoma	Usually diffuse thickening of intestinal wall (occasionally nodular)	Monomorphic population of large lymphocytes with fine chromatin +/- nucleoli Figures 18-13 and 18-14
Adenocarcinoma	Mass or annular, constricting lesion	Clusters of round, oval, or columnar cells Anisocytosis, anisokaryosis Fine chromatin Prominent nucleoli Figure 18-15
Mesenchymal tumors	Nodular masses	Spindle-shaped cells Variable pleomorphism based on malignancy Figure 18-9

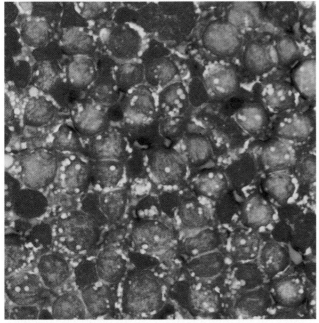

Figure 18-13 Intestinal lymphosarcoma in a dog. A monomorphic population of large lymphocytes have a fine chromatin pattern and cytoplasmic vacuoles. These cells are admixed with scattered small, well-differentiated lymphocytes. (Modified Wright's stain.)

patient survival time in cats. Unfortunately, many cases of intestinal lymphoma are accompanied by ulceration, and inflammation surrounds the neoplastic foci. Superficial cytology or biopsy specimens may sample only the inflammation and lead to an erroneous diagnosis of enteritis. If the neoplasm is sampled, it may be difficult to distinguish the neoplastic lymphocytes from routine inflammatory cells. Detecting lymphoma is particularly difficult, if not impossible, when the accompanying inflammation is lymphocytic. Histopathology and examination of tissue architecture is often needed in these cases to make a definitive diagnosis. The distinction between inflammation and neoplasia has become even less clear with the discovery that lymphocytic inflammation may predispose animals to developing lymphosarcoma.[12]

Intestinal Adenocarcinoma: Intestinal adenocarcinoma is most common in older animals and is usually found in the large intestine of dogs and the jejunum and ileum of cats. It may present as a mass or an annular, constricting lesion. Cytologically, neoplastic cells may appear round, oval, or slightly columnar. Anisocytosis and anisokaryosis are often present. Individual neoplastic cells have a round nucleus, fine chromatin pattern, one to two nucleoli, and light blue cytoplasm (Figure 18-15). Extensive desmoplasia is often present and fibroblasts can be observed cytologically. In such instances, spindle cells may be numerous and may confuse the cytologic diagnosis. Alternatively, if collagen deposition is abundant, the mass may not readily exfoliate neoplastic cells. Because of desmoplasia, transmural extension of the neoplasm may produce a large, ill-defined mass that incorporates adjacent organs and tissues.

Mesenchymal Tumors: Mesenchymal tumors include leiomyoma, leiomyosarcoma, fibroma, fibrosarcoma, schwannoma, gastrointestinal stromal tumors, and other ill-defined mesenchymal neoplasms. These neoplasms have a slow to moderate growth rate, are nodular tumors, and consist of spindle-shaped cells. Cytologically, it is difficult to distinguish between tumor types and determine their benign or malignant potential. Histopathology and immunohistochemical staining may be helpful in the diagnosis, but some neoplasms may defy classification.

Rectal Scrapings

Normal Cytology: A normal rectal scraping consists of clusters of columnar epithelial cells (Figure 18-16), a mixed bacterial population of rods and cocci of varying size, a small amount of mucus, and amorphous debris (Box 18-2). The amount of debris is minimal when feces are removed before scraping. Squamous epithelial cells indicate that the anus rather than the rectum was scraped, and the procedure may have to be repeated

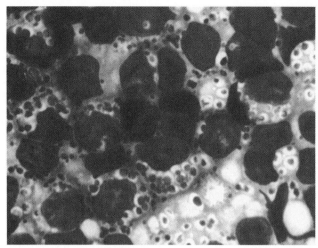

Figure 18-14 Large granular lymphoma in a cat. Aspirates of the intestinal mural mass contain a homogeneous population of lymphocytes with chunky purple cytoplasmic granules. (Wright's stain.)

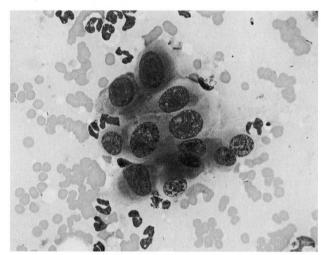

Figure 18-15 Intestinal carcinoma in a cat. Pleomorphic epithelial cells are characterized by anisocytosis, anisokaryosis, a high nuclear-to-cytoplasmic ratio and multiple, prominent nucleoli. Purulent inflammation is also present. (Wright's stain.) *(Courtesy Dr. F.S. Almy, University of Georgia, Athens, Ga.)*

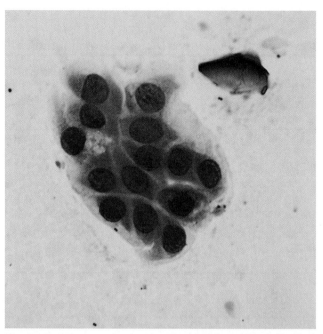

Figure 18-16 Normal rectal epithelium. Viewed from the top, the epithelial cells appear almost cuboidal. If viewed from the side, the same cells are columnar. (Modified Wright's stain.)

BOX 18-2

Findings in Normal Rectal Scrapings

Clusters of columnar epithelium
Mixed bacterial population (rods and cocci of varying sizes)
Small amount of mucus
Amorphous debris
Rare inflammatory cell
Blood ± (some bleeding may be induced by the scraping procedure)

(Figure 18-17). Inflammatory cells are rare in healthy animals and consist of lymphocytes, plasma cells, and mast cells. Neutrophils and red blood cells (RBCs) may be derived from the small amount of bleeding induced by the procedure, in which case they occur in an approximate WBC-to-RBC ratio of 1:500 to 1000. When lubricant jelly is used, the smear often contains varying amounts of bright pink to magenta amorphous, granular or fibrillar material (Figure 18-18). If a large amount of this material is present on a smear, it can obscure diagnostic structures. Occasionally, a section of mucosa containing a normal lymphoid follicle is scraped. This can be differentiated from lymphosarcoma by the presence of a heterogeneous population of lymphocytes consisting primarily of small lymphocytes, with fewer medium- and large-sized lymphocytes, and plasma cells.

Inflammation and Infection: Inflammation is commonly observed in diagnostic rectal scrapings. Occasionally pathogens may be seen following diligent microscopic examination of these specimens.

Eosinophilic Colitis: Eosinophilic colitis may occur as a primary disease of the colon or rectum or may be part of a more extensive syndrome designated eosinophilic gastroenterocolitis.[13] Rectal scrapings yield moderate to large numbers of eosinophils. Because ulceration occurs in this disease, many RBCs and neutrophils also may be seen.

Purulent Colitis: A predominance of neutrophils on a smear from a rectal scraping is a nonspecific finding because colitis due to any cause produces a layer of fibrin and neutrophils covering denuded foci (Figure 18-19). In some types of deep lesions that may cause extensive tissue necrosis (e.g., various malignant tumors), the mucosa is frequently ulcerated and infiltrated with neutrophils. For this reason, a scraping performed in any animal with ulcerative colitis is likely to yield many neutrophils and much fibrin. Fibrin is not stained with

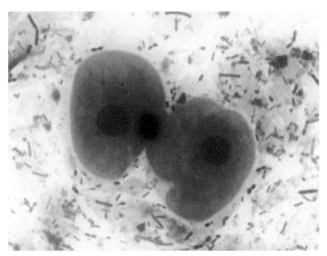

Figure 18-17 Normal anal epithelial cells. Squamous epithelial cells from a rectal scraping indicate that the anus, rather than the rectum, was scraped. (Wright's stain.)

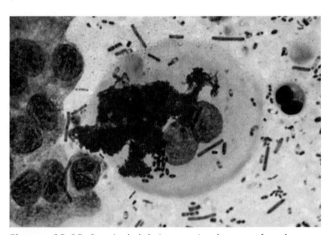

Figure 18-18 Surgical lubricant. A cluster of columnar epithelial cells and two squamous epithelial cells. The morphologic characterisics of the squamous epithelial cells are partially obscured by bright pink-staining surgical lubricant. (Wright-Leishman stain.)

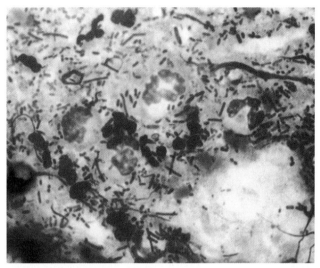

Figure 18-19 Purulent inflammation. Several degenerate neutrophils and a large, mixed population of bacteria are present. (Wright's stain.)

Romanowsky-type stains but may appear as pale granular or fibrillar material on new methylene blue–stained smears.

Clostridial Enterocolitis: Clostridial enterocolitis may be difficult to diagnose cytologically. A few clostridial bacilli may be observed in any rectal scraping. These organisms are large, blue-staining bacilli that may have a small, round, clear area that denotes spore formation. Organisms are abundant and associated with bloody diarrhea in clostridial enteritis.

Histoplasmosis: Disseminated histoplasmosis in dogs frequently causes chronic large intestinal diarrhea as well as signs referable to other affected organ systems.[13] A definitive diagnosis may be made by rectal scraping. *Histoplasma capsulatum* organisms are round to oval yeasts measuring 2 to 4 μm in diameter and consist of a basophilic center surrounded by a thin clear halo (Figure 18-20). There are usually multiple yeast organisms within macrophages and a few may be scattered

extracellularly. Macrophages without organisms, neutrophils, and a few lymphocytes and plasma cells are also usually present.

Cryptococcosis: *Cryptococcus neoformans* infects many tissues, but intestinal infection is uncommon. Large bowel involvement rarely occurs in dogs with disseminated cryptococcosis. The organisms are seen on smears as extracellular round to oval basophilic yeasts measuring 3.5 to 7.0 μm in diameter, with a clear capsule of variable thickness (1 to 30 μm). *Cryptococcus* spp. are rarely seen within macrophages.

Protothecosis: *Prototheca* is a colorless alga that is ubiquitous in the environment and rarely causes disease. In dogs, a disproportionate number of cases have been reported in Collies, but in cats, only the cutaneous form of the disease has been reported.[14] Protothecosis frequently causes intermittent and protracted bloody diarrhea in dogs, although the organism is usually widely disseminated throughout the body. Definitive diagnosis of protothecosis often can be made by rectal scraping. The organisms are round to oval, 1.3 to 13.4 μm wide, and 1.3 to 16.1 μm long. They have granular basophilic cytoplasm and a clear cell wall approximately 0.5 μm thick (Figure 18-21). A small nucleus is present in all but the small, immature forms. A single organism frequently consists of two, four, or more endospores. The organisms are predominantly extracellular, but small forms may be seen in macrophages and/ or neutrophils. Numerous organisms are usually present with a mixed population of inflammatory cells and blood.

Saccharomycopsis: *Saccharomycopsis* spp. are yeastlike ascomycetous fungi. Although these organisms are encountered more frequently in GI cytologic specimens from rabbits, they also may be observed in fecal smears of dogs with diarrhea. These yeasts are elongated structures that are often joined to form stick figures or are arranged in Y configurations (Figure 18-22). They possess a thin cell wall and a basophilic to azurophilic internal structure that may be slightly granular.

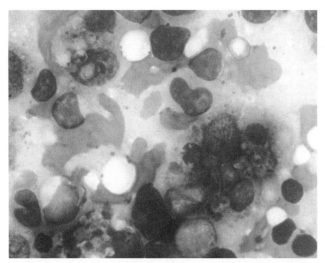

Figure 18-20 Histoplasmosis in a cat. Macrophages contain multiple *Histoplasma capsulatum* organisms characterized by a round, basophilic center and a thin, clear capsule. (Wright's stain.)

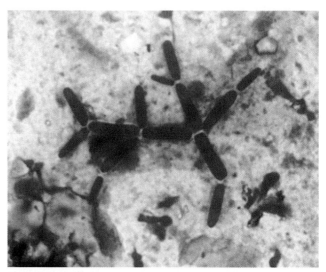

Figure 18-22 *Saccharomycopsis* in a dog with diarrhea. These elongate, basophilic yeasts often are arranged in stick figures. (Wright's stain.)

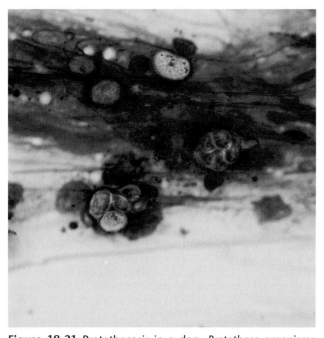

Figure 18-21 Protothecosis in a dog. *Prototheca* organisms vary in size and have granular, basophilic cytoplasm with a thin, clear cell wall. The organism on the right is compartmentalized and contains five endospores. (Wright's stain.)

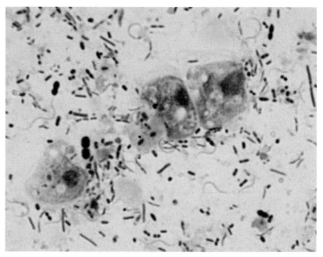

Figure 18-23 *Pentatrichomonas hominis* infection in a dog with large bowel diarrhea. The protozoa in this rectal scraping contain a nucleus and multiple cytoplasmic vacuoles. (Wright-Leishman stain.)

Protozoa: Protozoa are occasionally found in rectal scrapings. Not all protozoa in the intestinal tract are considered pathogenic, however. The tendency to produce disease depends on the virulence of the organism and host factors.

Pentatrichomonas hominis is a pyriform flagellate that inhabits the large intestines of people, dogs, cats, monkeys, and some rodents. *Tritrichomonas* spp. also has been reported in cats. The pathogenicity of these organisms is uncertain; they may be opportunist pathogens. Trichomoniasis is reported infrequently in dogs and cats.[15] The trophozoites measure 6 to14 μm by 4 to 6.5 μm and usually have five anterior flagella. Trichomonads have an undulating membrane that appears as an unstained curvilinear structure coursing the long axis of the organism on cytologic smears (Figure 18-23). The organisms have a dark nucleus and basophilic cytoplasm that may have small, clear vacuoles.

Giardia lamblia is usually diagnosed by examination of fecal wet mounts, where the characteristic rolling motion of the parasite is easily observed. Identification of this organism is difficult in Romanowsky-stained preparations because the small, pyriform organisms are often obscured by fecal debris.

Balantidium coli is the largest protozoan capable of infecting dogs. This ciliated protozoan can colonize the human and canine colon. Balantidiasis has not been

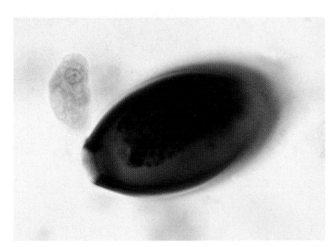

Figure 18-24 Entamoebiasis in a dog. An *Entamoeba histolytica* trophozoite (upper left) is irregular with a round nucleus and nucleolus and is adjacent to a much larger whipworm egg. (Trichrome stain.)

reported in cats.[16] The pig is the definitive host, and dogs become infected by eating pig feces. Canine balantidiasis may be complicated by concurrent trichuriasis. Damage to the colonic mucosa caused by whipworms may predispose to infection with *B. coli*. Balantidiasis can be diagnosed by fecal flotation, direct fecal smear, or rectal scraping. The organism may be seen in smears in two forms. Trophozoites are oval and usually measure 40 to 80 μm by 25 to 45 μm, but may be as large as 30 to 300 μm by 30 to 100 μm. They have spirally arranged, longitudinal rows of cilia and a large, oval nucleus. Round to oval cysts that measure up to 40 to 60 μm in diameter may also be seen. In each stage of the organism, diagnosis of balantidiasis is facilitated by the large size and prominent oval nucleus of the ciliate.

Entamoeba histolytica is an ameba that can occur as a commensal organism in the lumen of the colon or as a pathogen that invades the intestinal wall. It is primarily a parasite of people but can also invade the large intestine of dogs and cats. Infection with this organism is uncommon.[16] Trophozoites invade the mucosa through lytic action and produce colonic ulceration and inflammation with bloody mucoid diarrhea. Trophozoites measure 12 to 50 μm in diameter and cysts measure 10 to 20 μm in diameter. Trophozoites have a dark nucleus and basophilic cytoplasm that may contain clear vacuoles (Figure 18-24). The presence of ingested RBCs distinguishes *E. histolytica* from nonpathogenic amebae. Because of the cytoplasmic vacuoles and ingested RBCs, *E. histolytica* trophozoites may be mistaken for macrophages and overlooked if only a cursory examination of the smear is done.

Neoplasia: Lymphosarcoma in dogs is the neoplasm most commonly diagnosed by rectal scraping. In contrast, intestinal lymphosarcoma in cats usually involves the small intestine only, and rectal scraping is not diagnostic. Despite extensive colonic involvement in dogs, lymphosarcoma usually does not cause ulceration, and thus no hematochezia occurs. As with lymphosarcoma involving other tissues, the lymphoid population is monomorphic. The lymphocytes can vary from 8 to 15 μm in diameter in small cell neoplasms to 10 to 24 μm in diameter in large-cell neoplasms, but most lymphocytes are very similar in size in any single neoplasm. Nuclei can be round, indented, or cleaved. Chromatin clumping is variable, but nucleoli are usually prominent. Mitotic figures may be very few to frequent, and cytoplasm is scant to moderate in amount and stains intensely blue. Small clear vacuoles are occasionally present in the cytoplasm. Cytoplasmic projections and fragments and lysed or smudged cells may be numerous in some smears.

Although other tumors, such as leiomyomas, leiomyosarcomas, and adenocarcinomas, occur in the large intestine, rectal scrapings are usually not diagnostic. Generally, these tumors either originate within or penetrate the muscularis mucosa and involve the lamina propria only minimally. Likewise, scrapings of discrete masses that protrude into the intestinal lumen (e.g., polyps and adenomas) may also be nondiagnostic because material obtained by scraping the surface of such tumors is not necessarily representative of the entire mass. In such instances, a biopsy of the lesion is a more appropriate diagnostic technique.

References

1. Schiller KFR, et al. In Schiller KFR, et al: *Atlas of Gastrointestinal Endoscopy and Related Pathology*. Ames, Blackwell, 2002, p 38.
2. Crow SE: Tumors of the alimentary tract. *Vet Clin North Am Small Anim Pract* 15:577-587, 1985.
3. Head, Else and Dubielzig. In Meuten J: *Tumors of Domestic Animals*. Ames, Iowa, Blackwell, 2002, pp 401-482.
4. Jhala and Jhala. In Atkinson BF: *Atlas of Diagnostic Cytopathology*. Philadelphia, Saunders, 2003, pp 199-203.
5. Gelberg. In McGavin MD, Carlton WW, Zachary JF: *Thomson's Special Veterinary Pathology*. St. Louis, Mosby, 2001, pp 1-79.
6. Neiger R, Simpson KW: *Helicobacter* infection in dogs and cats: Facts and fiction. *J Vet Intern Med* 14:125-133, 2000.
7. Jergens AE, et al: Cytologic examination of exfoliative specimens obtained during endoscopy for diagnosis of gastrointestinal tract disease in dogs and cats. *J Am Vet Med Assoc* 213:1755-1759, 1998.
8. Happonen I, et al: Detection and effects of helicobacters in healthy dogs and dogs with signs of gastritis. *J Am Vet Med Assoc* 213:1767-1774, 1998.
9. Papasouliotis K, et al: Occurrence of gastric *Helicobacter*-like organisms in cats. *Vet Rec* 140:369-370, 1997.
10. Swann HM, Holt DE: Canine gastric adenocarcinoma and leiomyosarcoma: A retrospective study of 21 cases and literature review. *J Am Anim Hosp Assoc* 38:157-164, 2002.
11. Gualtieri M, Monzeglio MG, Scanziani E: Gastric neoplasia. *Vet Clin North Am Small Anim Pract* 29:415-425, 1999.
12. French RA, Seitz SE, Valli VE: Primary epitheliotrophic alimentary T-cell lymphoma with hepatic involvement in a dog. *Vet Pathol* 33:349-352, 1996.
13. Washabau and Holt. In Ettinger SJ, Feldman EC: *Textbook of Veterinary Internal Medicine*. St. Louis, Saunders, 2005, pp 1388-1389.
14. Greene RW, Rakich and Latimer. In Greene RW: *Infectious Diseases of the Dog and Cat*. St. Louis, Saunders, 2006, pp 659-665.
15. Gokin. In Greene RW: *Infectious Diseases of the Dog and Cat*. St. Louis, Saunders, 2006, pp 745-748.
16. Barr. In Greene RW: *Infectious Diseases of the Dog and Cat*. St. Louis, Saunders, 2006, pp 742-745.

The Pancreas

D. Borjesson

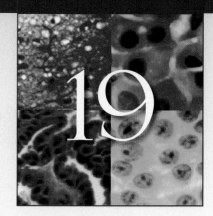

CHAPTER

19

Cytologic evaluation of the pancreas is becoming increasingly common as a tool to help clinicians distinguish between pancreatic disorders. This increase in pancreatic aspiration for cytologic evaluation may be due to an increase in clinician comfort with pancreatic manipulation and the ongoing utility of pancreatic aspiration with minimal complications in human medicine. Previous perceptions that pancreatic manipulation may result in secondary pancreatitis have largely been unsubstantiated.

Currently, no single test provides conclusive discrimination between inflammatory, cystic, neoplastic, and infectious diseases involving the pancreas. Patients with pancreatic disorders, with the exception of pancreatic insufficiency, often have similar histories and clinical signs. Clinicopathologic testing can frequently identify the presence of pancreatic disease in the dog; however, in the cat, serum chemistry tests are often less useful.[1-3] In both dogs and cats, abdominal ultrasound is a useful diagnostic tool to visualize and assess an abnormal pancreas. As with biochemical tests, however, the use of abdominal ultrasound to definitively distinguish between pancreatic diseases has variable sensitivity and specificity.[2,4] Once visualized, ultrasound-guided fine-needle biopsy (FNB) of the pancreas is a safe and effective adjunct to imaging in the diagnosis of pancreatic disorders. The pancreas exfoliates well, and cytologic examination of the pancreas in small animals has proved useful in the diagnosis of both neoplastic and nonneoplastic lesions, including abscesses, cysts, and pancreatitis.

NORMAL PANCREAS STRUCTURE

Anatomy and Histology

The pancreas consists of a right (duodenal) and left (transverse or splenic) limb joined at the head. The number and position of the pancreatic duct(s) opening into the duodenum and the location of the duct(s) to the common bile duct varies among species and among individuals in each species.[5] The pancreas consists of endocrine and exocrine components. Numerous tubuloacinar secretory units form the exocrine component of the organ. These secretory units drain into long, narrow intercalated ducts

lined by elongated, cuboidal cells. Intercalated ducts communicate directly with interlobular ducts.[6] Functionally, the tubuloacinar secretory units (exocrine pancreas) secrete digestive enzymes in an inactive proenzyme form. Pancreatic enzymes are activated by trypsin secreted by the duodenum.

The endocrine islets of Langerhans are clusters of epithelial cells scattered among the secretory units. Normal pancreatic islets contain four cell types, each secreting different pancreatic polypeptides: Alpha cells secrete glucagon, beta cells secrete insulin, D cells secrete somatostatin, and F cells secrete pancreatic polypeptide. Beta cells are the most numerous islet cells (composing 60% to 70% of the islet cells) and they are generally concentrated in the central part of the islet. The alpha cells compose about 20% of the islet cells and are generally located peripherally.[5]

SAMPLING TECHNIQUE

Methods

In veterinary medicine, percutaneous, ultrasound-guided fine-needle aspiration (FNA) of the pancreas is the most common method of tissue sampling although intraoperative sampling can also be performed.[7] FNB of the pancreas permits extensive sampling and, in people, is associated with a low risk of morbidity and mortality. It is especially useful in discriminating between pancreatic neoplasia and inflammation, with minimal complications. In human medicine, FNA is the diagnostic method of choice for patients with a pancreatic mass. The most common methods of sample procurement are computed tomographically guided or endoscopic ultrasound-guided aspiration. The vast majority of human pancreatic masses are neoplastic; as such, FNB is used to establish a rapid tissue diagnosis before chemotherapy and/or surgery.

Methods to obtain a FNB of the pancreas are outlined in Box 19-1. The described methods for sample procurement are closely based on methods originally published by Bjorneby and Kari.[7] In brief, the pancreas and surrounding abdominal structures should be thoroughly evaluated with ultrasound to visualize the area to be aspirated. If a mass is present, multiple areas within the mass and surrounding tissue should be aspirated. In dogs, inflammation (purulent

BOX 19-1

Outline of Fine-Needle Biopsy Technique*

- Use ultrasound to visualize the area to be aspirated
- Set out and label 6 to 10 clean glass slides
- Draw 1 mL of air into a 3-mL syringe
- Attach a 1½- to 3-inch 22-gauge needle to the syringe
- Guide the needle attached to the syringe into the pancreas
  - AVOID redirecting the needle; negative pressure is *not* needed
- Quickly expel the sample onto a slide
- Prepare multiple smears using a variety of gentle techniques
  - Include squash preparations and blood smear techniques
- Sample multiple sites within the lesion
- Rapidly air-dry the smears
- Submit air-dried, labeled slides to a veterinary clinical pathologist

*The technique described is adapted from Bjorneby JM, Kari S: Cytology of the pancreas. In Cowell RL, ed: *Vet Clin North Am Small Anim Pract* 32(6):1293-1312, 2002.

or lymphocytic) has been shown to occur in discrete areas throughout the pancreas (right and left limb).[7] Therefore, there is no preferential site to sample the pancreas (and confirm pancreatitis) in the absence of a visible lesion. Label clean glass slides, preferably with frosted edges, with patient identification and site of aspiration. Draw 1 ml of air into a 3-ml syringe. Attach a 1½- to 3-inch 22-gauge needle to the syringe. This needle/syringe combination may permit more accurate needle placement and angle control.[7] Using a guide or freehand, move the needle back and forth within the pancreas. Be careful to maintain the needle in the same tract. For sample procurement, no additional negative pressure is required. Do not attempt to redirect the needle because the tip of the needle may lacerate the tissue and cause excessive hemorrhage and leakage of pancreatic enzymes.[7] To minimize cell disruption, sample expulsion and smear preparation should be as gentle as possible. To ensure full evaluation of the cells present, expel the sample onto the middle of the slide where cells are most readily stained and visualized. Sample three to four different sites within the lesion if possible. To ensure the best quality sample (and thus the likelihood of a cytologic diagnosis), make multiple smears using a variety of smear techniques that result in both thin and thick preparations. Slide preparation techniques include the squash smear (slide-over-slide) or blood smear technique. The smears should be air-dried and submitted to a veterinary clinical pathologist.[7]

Troubleshooting

In general, pancreatic tissue exfoliates well for FNB. If you have any concerns regarding sample quality, talk with your cytopathologist regarding sample attainment and preparation. Ruptured cells can be the result of negative pressure in the syringe while aspirating or too much pressure on slides while making preparations.[7] Rapid drying of slides reduces refractile artifact on the slides. Hemodilution is common and generally will not confound diagnosis. However, if hemodilution is obscuring the diagnosis (especially distinguishing between blood contamination and inflammation), decrease the number of times the needle is moved within the pancreas. However, the trade off may be poor cytologic yield, which can occur if the needle biopsy technique is not aggressive enough. If clots tend to form, the needle and syringe can be flushed with an anticoagulant (i.e., ethylene-tetra-acetic acid [EDTA]) prior to organ aspiration. Nondiagnostic samples due to poor cellularity can occur when lesions are fibrous or if the lesion was missed during aspiration. Nondiagnostic samples should be interpreted in light of imaging findings. Reaspiration can always be attempted if the pancreas appears active and enlarged. However, if fibrosis appears possible, intraoperative biopsy will likely be superior for obtaining a diagnosis. Always interpret cytologic findings in light of imaging, physical examination, and biochemical findings. For example, if poorly cellular, proteinaceous fluid is obtained and the lesion on imaging is compatible with a cyst, then further diagnostics may not be warranted (Figure 19-1). However, if poorly cellular, proteinaceous fluid is obtained and the lesion is primarily solid or infiltrative with cystic or necrotic areas, then reaspiration may be indicated because the primary lesion may not be represented.

Complications

Significant adverse effects secondary to percutaneous FNB of the pancreas in dogs or cats have not been reported. Rarely, FNB of the pancreas, in human beings, has been reported to cause complications, such as needle tract seeding of tumors, fistula formation, and ascites.[7] In one human study, complications arising from FNB of both solid and cystic lesions of the pancreas were noted in only 4 of 248 (1.2%) patients. These complications included acute pancreatitis and aspiration pneumonia and were noted only after aspiration of cystic lesions.[8] Recommendations from this study included avoiding needle passage through the main pancreatic duct or branch ducts dilated proximal to an obstruction. In addition, aspiration was terminated if blood became visible in the syringe or if there was obvious hemorrhage within the target lesion.[8]

CYTOLOGIC EVALUATION

Normal

A decision tree to help guide initial cytologic evaluation of the pancreas is depicted in Figure 19-1. Exocrine epithelial cells are the most common cell type found on cytologic specimens from the pancreas. The background of the slide may contain blood from iatrogenic contamination, or it may be light pink indicating a small amount of protein. Normal exocrine epithelial cells are found in small clusters to large sheets that may form tubular and acinar structures (Figure 19-2). On low magnification, the cytoplasm appears

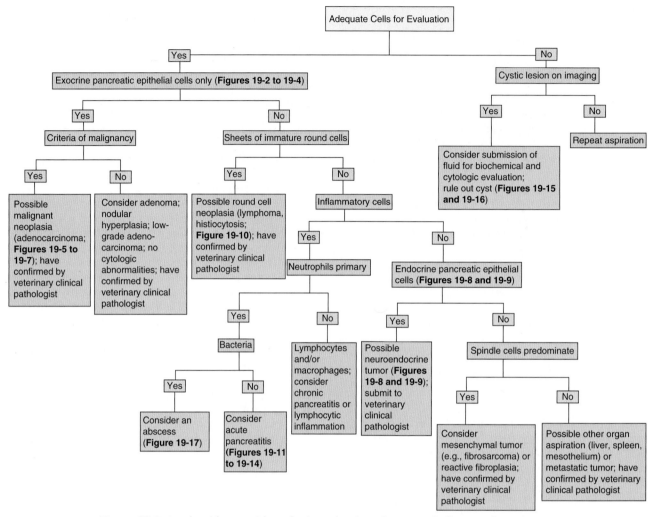

Figure 19-1 An algorithm to aid cytologic evaluation of pancreatic fine-needle aspirates.

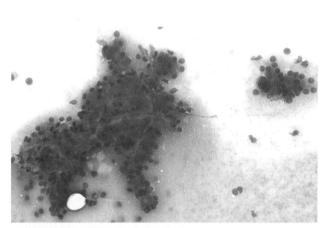

Figure 19-2 FNB of normal canine pancreas. Exocrine epithelial cells predominate and often exfoliate in small sheets and large clusters with acinar and tubular formations. Cells are polyhedral, cytoplasm is abundant, nuclear:cytoplasmic ratios are low, and nuclei are uniform. (Wright-Giemsa stain, original magnification 200×.)

grainy with a pink hue due to the presence of small, pink granules. Unlike intestinal epithelial cells, cell-to-cell junctions are not prominent, giving cells a more indistinct, fluffy appearance (Figure 19-3). The cells are polyhedral with abundant cytoplasm and a low nuclear-to-cytoplasmic ratio (Figures 19-2 to 19-4). Nuclei are basilar in location, uniform, and round to oval. Chromatin is stippled to reticulate and a single, small, occasionally prominent nucleolus can be noted (see Figures 19-3 and 19-4). On high magnification, abundant pink, cytoplasmic granules, most consistent with membrane-bound zymogen granules, are noted. In preparations with abundant cell rupture, these granules can fill the background of the slide, giving a mottled blue and pink appearance (see Figure 19-4). In a FNB of normal pancreas, no other cell populations will be present in high numbers. Occasionally, hematopoietic precursors, indicative of extramedullary hematopoiesis, small ductal cells, or uniform endocrine epithelial cells, will be seen. The number of leukocytes present in the aspirate should be interpreted in light of peripheral blood cell counts to avoid interpreting peripheral neutrophilia or lymphocytosis as pancreatic inflammation.

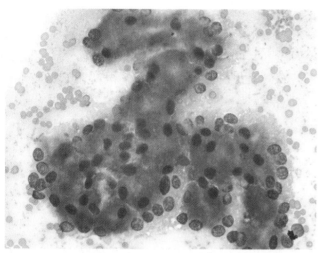

Figure 19-3 FNB of normal feline pancreas. The nuclei of exocrine epithelial cells often show a basilar distribution. Clear cell-to-cell junctions are not apparent. Nuclei are round to oval, chromatin is stippled, and single, small, uniform nucleoli can be present. (Wright-Giemsa stain, original magnification 500×.)

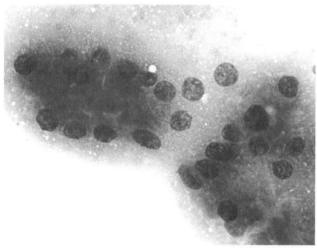

Figure 19-4 FNB of normal canine pancreas. Exocrine epithelial cells are characterized by apical, abundant, small, pink cytoplasmic granules, most consistent with membrane-bound zymogen granules. These granules give densely packed pancreatic exocrine epithelial cells a pink hue at lower magnification. (Wright-Giemsa stain, original magnification 1000×.)

Pancreatic Lesions

A summary of the World Health Organization scheme for histologic classification of pancreatic lesions of domestic animals is summarized in Box 19-2.[9]

Neoplasia

Adenoma: Benign exocrine epithelial tumors (i.e., exocrine adenomas, ductal [tubular] adenomas, or acinar adenomas) are rare in small animals and far less common than their malignant counterparts. They are generally small, solitary lesions found incidentally on imaging or

---

BOX 19-2

Summary of World Health Organization Classification of Pancreatic Lesions in Small Animals

Neoplastic lesions

Exocrine epithelial tumors
    Benign (e.g., adenoma)
    Malignant (e.g., adenocarcinoma)
Endocrine tumors (e.g., insulinoma, gastrinoma)
Non-epithelial tumors (e.g., fibrosarcoma, metastatic lymphoma, hemangiosarcoma)

Nonneoplastic lesions

Nodular hyperplasia of acinar cells
Acute pancreatitis
Chronic pancreatitis
Cyst (e.g., pseudocyst, congenital)
Abscess

---

necropsy examination. Histologically, they are partially or totally encapsulated, distinguishing them from the more common lesion of nodular hyperplasia.[5,9,10] Cytologically, adenomas cannot be distinguished from normal or hyperplastic pancreatic tissue (see Figure 19-1). If abundant, uniform pancreatic exocrine epithelial cells are noted in concert with imaging findings suggestive of a solitary, solid lesion, differential diagnoses should include an adenoma, well-differentiated carcinoma, or a hyperplastic nodule (see Figure 19-1).

Adenocarcinoma: Malignant tumors of the exocrine pancreas (i.e., adenocarcinomas, ductal [tubular] adenocarcinomas, or exocrine carcinomas) are rare in the dog and cat with incidences of 17.8 in 100,000 patient years at risk in the dog and 12.6 in 100,000 patient years at risk in the cat.[10,11] This is in contrast to human medicine in which pancreatic malignant tumors are the fifth leading cause of cancer-related death in the United States, with ductal adenocarcinomas accounting for >90% of these malignancies.[11] The histogenesis of adenocarcinomas in small animals remains uncertain. One author suggests that a ductular origin is suggested based on tubular architecture, but ultrastructural analysis indicates that acinar cells may be the originator cell type,[10] whereas other authors suggest that they can arise from either ductular or acinar epithelium, and often have features of both.[5]

In dogs, there is an increased incidence of pancreatic adenocarcinoma with aging, and Airedale terriers, boxers, Labrador Retrievers, and Cocker Spaniels may be at increased risk.[11] In one study of 13 dogs and cats, the average age at diagnosis was 9 and 10 years of age for dogs and cats, respectively.[12] Distant metastases are common at the time of diagnosis. In one study, 85% of the dogs and cats with pancreatic adenocarcinoma had distant metastases at the time of diagnosis, and 88% of the patients had metastatic disease at the time of necropsy.[12] Common metastatic sites include abdominal or thoracic lymph nodes, mesentery, adjacent gastrointestinal (GI) organs (including liver, duodenum, and jejunum), lungs, and less frequently, spleen, kidney, and diaphragm.[12] Local, destructive infiltration may destroy the common bile duct.

Clinical signs at the time of presentation are nonspecific but weight loss, vomiting, abdominal pain, and anorexia are common. Jaundice and cholestasis can result from obstruction of the bile duct by tumor and/or secondary liver disease. Clinicopathologic tests can show increases in pancreatic enzyme activity but evidence of extrahepatic biliary obstruction is more frequently seen, including elevations in alkaline phosphatase (ALP) and alanine aminotransferase (ALT) activities. Neutrophilia is often noted.[12] Described paraneoplastic syndromes include alopecia,[13] exocrine pancreatic insufficiency,[14] and cutaneous and visceral necrotizing panniculitis and steatitis.[15]

In dogs, pancreatic tumors frequently produce a mass, often in the midportion of the pancreas. In cats, tumors can be more diffuse and resemble nodular hyperplasia or chronic pancreatitis. Leakage of proteolytic enzymes from adenocarcinomas can be corrosive and may result in cystic change in the primary tumor and necrotizing steatitis in the omental and peritoneal fat.[10] Histopathologically, pancreatic adenocarcinomas show a tremendous range of differentiation. Some are well-differentiated tubular adenocarcinomas that form acinar structures, whereas others may form more solid sheets of poorly differentiated cells that no longer resemble pancreatic acini. They may be associated with a dense supporting stroma with a resultant scirrhous reaction. Focal hemorrhage and necrosis can occur along with focal accumulations of inflammatory cells, including T-lymphocytes.[10]

Although pancreatic adenocarcinoma is far less common in dogs and cats than it is in people, similar to people, the majority of pancreatic neoplasms are malignant. Several studies of human pancreatic carcinoma have established objective cytologic criteria for the diagnosis of pancreatic carcinoma. The implementation of these criteria have resulted in a relatively high diagnostic sensitivity and specificity for the diagnosis of pancreatic adenocarcinoma ranging from 80% to 98% and of 93% to 100%, respectively.[16] Similar standard criteria have not been developed in veterinary medicine. Given the increasing popularity of pancreatic FNB, objective cytologic criteria to diagnose pancreatic malignancy could be established for dogs and cats. Until that time, the criteria stated in human-based studies are compatible with important criteria of malignancy noted by the author.

Criteria of malignancy defining pancreatic adenocarcinoma are listed in Box 19-3. In the initial study, major criteria of malignancy included nuclear crowding and overlap (nuclei became oval, angular, and polygonal rather than round), nuclear membrane contour irregularities (grooving, notching), and irregular chromatin distribution (more applicable with alcohol-fixed specimens). Minor criteria included nuclear enlargement (or anisokaryosis, defined as a nucleus > 2.5 times the size of a red blood cell), single epithelial cells, necrosis, and mitosis.[17] Later studies confirmed the utility of these initial criteria and suggested additional criteria including increased cellularity, anisocytosis, prominent or macronucleoli

BOX **19-3**
Cytologic Criteria of Malignancy
Nuclear crowding and overlap (oval, polygonal, angular nuclei)
Anisokaryosis
Nuclear membrane contour irregularities
Prominent nucleoli (large and irregular)
Single cells/loss of cellular cohesion
Mitotic figures, especially aberrant mitoses
Increased nuclear:cytoplasmic ratio

(large and irregular), cytoplasmic vacuolation, and coarsely clumped chromatin patterns. Mitoses, especially abnormal mitoses, favored malignancy.[18,19] Combined, the strongest indicators of malignancy that define human pancreatic adenocarcinomas include anisokaryosis, loss of cellular cohesion (single cells are common), irregular nuclear contours, nuclear crowding, prominent nucleoli, and aberrant mitoses[16-19] (see Box 19-3).

Aspirates of pancreatic carcinoma in small animals are characterized by high cellularity (see Figure 19-1; Figures 19-5 and 19-6). Individual cells have an increased nuclear-to-cytoplasmic ratio and anisokaryosis is frequently marked (Figures 19-4 to 19-7). Irregular nuclear contours and nuclear molding can be noted along with polygonal and angular nuclei (see Figures 19-5 through 19-7). Although cytoplasmic vacuolization is frequently noted (see Figures 19-5 through 19-7), it also occurs with epithelial reactivity secondary to pancreatitis. Chromatin varies from reticulated to coarsely clumped and prominent, irregular and occasionally multiple nucleoli can be present (see Figures 19-6 and 19-7). The background can be necrotic, hemodiluted, inflamed (macrophages and small, lymphocytes; see Figure 19-6), or pink and cystic-appearing (see Figure 19-7). Well-differentiated adenocarcinomas of the pancreas can result in false-negative cytologic interpretations. In one study, well-differentiated adenocarcinomas were differentiated from high-grade adenocarcinomas by the absence of necrosis, mitoses, and macronuclei.[16] Differential diagnoses for large sheets or clusters of fairly well-differentiated pancreatic epithelial cells should include normal pancreas, adenoma, nodular hyperplasia, or well-differentiated carcinoma (see Figure 19-1).

Endocrine (Neuroendocrine) Tumors of the Pancreas: Neuroendocrine tumors of the pancreas (NETP) (i.e., tumors of pancreatic islet cells, islet cell adenomas, and islet cell adenocarcinomas) include insulinomas (beta cell neoplasms), gastrinomas, somatostatinomas, glucagonomas, and carcinoid tumors. In small animal patients, insulinomas are the most common NETP followed in frequency by gastrinoma. Somatostatinoma, glucagonoma, and carcinoid tumor are rarely or not yet reported in small animals. Most NETPs are multihormonal; as such, they may secrete/express one or more neuroendocrine markers including pancreatic hormones (e.g., insulin, glucagon,

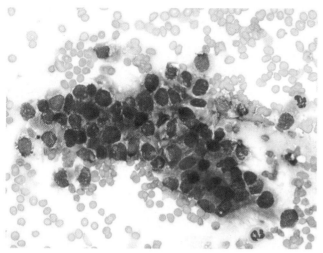

Figure 19-5 FNB of pancreatic adenocarcinoma in a cat. These cells show a markedly increased nuclear-to-cytoplasmic ratio and anisokaryosis. Additional criteria of malignancy include polygonal nuclei, nuclear overlap, irregular nuclear membranes, cytoplasmic vacuolization, and rare nucleoli. (Wright-Giemsa stain, original magnification 500×.)

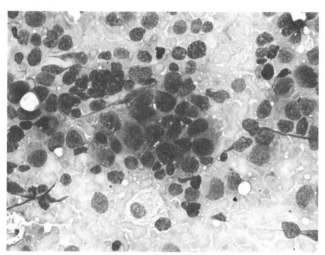

Figure 19-6 FNB of pancreatic adenocarcinoma in a dog. Cells from this sample exfoliated in loosely cohesive sheets with many single cells present. Additional criteria of malignancy included marked anisokaryosis, increased nuclear:cytoplasmic ratios, nuclear crowding and molding, polygonal nuclei, punctate cytoplasmic vacuoles, and occasional nucleoli. (Wright-Giemsa stain, original magnification 500×.)

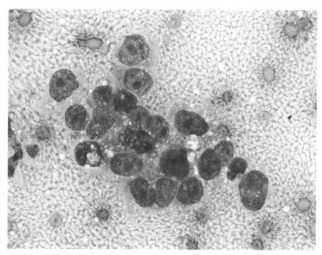

Figure 19-7 FNB of pancreatic adenocarcinoma in a cat. This cluster of cells show marked nuclear and nucleolar criteria of malignancy. Note the markedly elevated nuclear-to-cytoplasmic ratio, marked nuclear enlargement, irregular nuclear membrane contours, and prominent, deeply basophilic, single to multiple, occasionally irregular nucleoli. The dense, pink, stippled background of the slide may represent a cystic component to this neoplasm. (Wright-Giemsa stain, original magnification 1000×.)

pancreatic polypeptide, and somatostatin) and hormones not normally expressed in mammalian pancreas (e.g., gastrin, adrenocorticotropic hormone, and calcitonin). The majority of NETPs are immunohistochemically positive for insulin (89%) with around 30% positive for somatostatin, glucagon, and pancreatic polypeptide.[20] Amyloid deposits may be found in 17% to 32% of NETPs.[20]

Cytopathologists examining tissue from a pancreatic mass can generally readily discriminate between tumors of the exocrine and endocrine (NETPs) pancreas (see Figure 19-1). However, the biologic behavior of

NETPs can be difficult to predict. The degree of multi-hormonality and growth pattern show no correlation with biologic behavior.[20] In addition, cytologic features of the neoplastic cells are generally not helpful in differentiating between benign NETPs (islet cell adenomas) and their malignant counterparts (islet cell carcinomas) unless there are profound criteria of malignancy. The absence of anaplastic features cannot be used to rule out malignancy. Histologic evidence of invasion by the tumors cells through the capsule and into adjacent pancreatic parenchyma or lymphatics, or metastatic disease, are the most important criteria of malignancy for NETPs.[21,22] When the cytologic specimen is characterized by minimally pleomorphic neuroendocrine cells, in the absence of history or clinical findings, the cytologic diagnosis of neuroendocrine tumor or islet cell tumor is most appropriate.

Insulinomas are seen most frequently in dogs from 5 to 12 years of age. Grossly, they appear as single, small nodules visible from the serosal surface of the pancreas; however, malignant tumors may be larger and multilobular and show extensive invasion into the adjacent parenchyma. Malignant insulinomas are more common than benign insulinomas in dogs.[21] In one study, 45% to 55% of insulin-producing NETPs were malignant in dogs (in contrast to 10% to 15% in human beings).[20] Metastasis to regional lymph nodes, liver, mesentery, and omentum is noted in about 50% of cases.[23] Many different breeds are affected; however, Boxers, Fox Terriers, standard poodles and German shepherds appear to be overrepresented. Both sexes appear to be affected equally.[21] Because most insulinomas are secretory, a tentative diagnosis can be made by demonstrating profound hypoglycemia and an abnormal insulin:glucose ratio. Surgical removal (partial

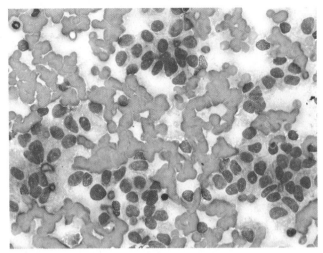

Figure 19-8 FNB of a malignant insulinoma in a dog. The sample is highly cellular, with cells found in loosely cohesive groups. Cell-to-cell borders are indistinct, and free nuclei appear scattered in a mass of shared cytoplasm. Compared with adenocarcinomas, anisokaryosis is relatively mild, although rare large nuclei are noted. Overall, the cells have a monomorphic appearance. As with other neuroendocrine tumors, individual cells are generally nondescript. Definitive tumor classification can be made only in light of imaging findings, physical examination findings, and clinicopathologic data. This patient had a persistently low glucose of 23 mg/dl (reference interval: 70-120 mg/dl) and a fasting insulin concentration of 138 IU/ml (reference interval: 5-15 IU/ml). Necropsy confirmed metastases to mesenteric lymph nodes and liver. (Wright-Giemsa stain, original magnification 500×.)

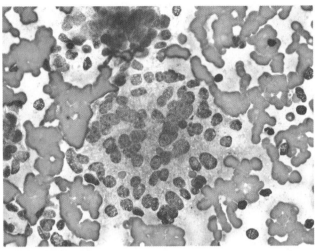

Figure 19-9 FNB of a malignant insulinoma in a dog. A large cluster of cells is noted with free nuclei in a hemodiluted background. Individual cells have indistinct cytoplasmic borders, giving the appearance of naked nuclei in a sea of cytoplasm. In this case, anisokaryosis is moderate, nuclear crowding is evident and single to multiple, small, deeply basophilic nucleoli are noted. Necropsy confirmed multiple metastatic lesions and positive immunohistochemical staining for insulin. (Wright-Giemsa stain, original magnification 500×.)

pancreatectomy) may significantly increase median survival time.[23] In one study of dogs with insulinomas, it was reported that (1) dogs with higher preoperative serum insulin levels had shorter survival times, (2) dogs with tumors confined to the pancreas had longer disease-free intervals, and (3) younger dogs had significantly shorter survival time than did older dogs.[24] Gastrinomas, although a rare tumor in veterinary medicine, frequently metastasize to regional lymph nodes and liver. Prognosis is considered grave.[22]

The cytologic appearance of NETPs is typical of other neuroendocrine tumors. They are generally highly cellular with prominent cellular dissociation, consisting of many single cells and/or small, poorly cohesive groups (Figures 19-8 and 19-9). Aspirates frequently contain free (naked) nuclei embedded in a background of lightly basophilic cytoplasm (see Figures 19-8 and 19-9). Intact cells are of medium to large size with poorly defined cytoplasmic borders (see Figure 19-8). The cytoplasm of intact cells is generally pale blue and may contain numerous small, punctate vacuoles (see Figure 19-9). Anisokaryosis is usually mild to moderate, giving a monomorphic appearance to the cells (see Figures 19-8 and 19-9). Additional nuclear features may include nuclear molding, eccentrically placed nuclei (giving a plasmacytoid appearance), and binucleation. Chromatin is generally fine and granular with a single prominent nucleolus (see Figures 19-8 and 19-9).[5,23,25,26]

Nonepithelial Tumors: Nonepithelial pancreatic tumors in small animals are rare (see Figure 19-1). Fibrosarcoma and multicentric system disease, including malignant histiocytosis,[27] lymphoma (Figure 19-10), hemangiosarcoma, liposarcoma, malignant nerve sheath tumor, and malignant melanoma, have been described.[5,10] Blood-borne metastasis from thyroid and mammary gland carcinoma, and direct extension from contiguous organs in alimentary lymphoma and from carcinoma of gastric adenocarcinoma,[28] duodenum, or common bile duct, have been noted.[9]

Nonneoplastic Lesions

Nodular Hyperplasia of Acinar Cells: Nodular hyperplasia of acinar cells (i.e., pancreatic exocrine nodular hyperplasia) is a common, often incidental, lesion in older dogs and cats (up to 80% of dogs may have nodular hyperplasia at necropsy).[29] In one study, the mean age of dogs with nodular hyperplasia was 9.5 years, whereas the mean age of dogs without nodular hyperplasia was 3.4 years.[29] Grossly, the lesion may be a solitary nodule or, more commonly, may appear as multiple, small, white to tan, well-circumscribed nodules. Histologically, they are distinguished from adenomas by their multiplicity, small size, lack of a capsule, and close resemblance to normal exocrine pancreatic tissue.[10,21] These lesions are not preneoplastic and patients are generally asymptomatic. Cytologically, nodular hyperplasia consists of sheets of well-differentiated exocrine pancreatic epithelial cells and, as such, is not distinguishable from an adenoma or well-differentiated carcinoma (see Figure 19-1). In these cases, cytologic interpretation should be done in light of imaging findings.

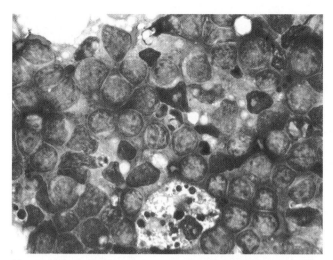

Figure 19-10 FNB of pancreatic lymphoma in a dog. The sample is highly cellular; however, only rare pancreatic epithelial cells were noted in the aspirate (none are depicted in the image) as the pancreas was infiltrated with neoplastic lymphocytes. Individual lymphocytes are large and round with a small rim of basophilic cytoplasm. Chromatin is smooth, and single to multiple pale nucleoli are noted. A large macrophage/histiocyte is noted along with occasional dark, condensed, apoptotic cells. This patient had multisystemic lymphoma involving the liver, spleen, and pancreas at the time of presentation. (Wright-Giemsa stain, original magnification 1000×.)

Pancreatitis

Acute Pancreatitis: In human beings, a uniform classification system has been developed for pancreatitis.[30] Acute pancreatitis is defined as an acute inflammatory process (usually neutrophilic) of the pancreas with variable involvement of other regional tissues or remote organ systems that does not lead to permanent changes. Chronic pancreatitis is defined as a chronic inflammatory process (usually lymphocytic) of the pancreas with variable involvement of other regional tissues or remote organ systems that leads to permanent changes, mainly fibrosis or atrophy and adhesions.[30] In addition, acute necrotizing pancreatitis is a severe form of acute pancreatitis characterized by extensive pancreatic and peripancreatic necrosis with severe forms progressing to dissolution of pancreatic parenchyma with accompanying hemorrhage, interstitial fluid accumulation, and deposition of fibrin and leukocytes.[31] This classification scheme can be loosely applied to both cats and dogs that manifest acute, uncomplicated pancreatitis; acute necrotizing pancreatitis; and chronic (fibrosing) pancreatitis.[5]

Pancreatitis is the most frequent disease process of the exocrine pancreas in the dog. For many canine patients, physical examination, biochemical testing, and imaging studies are satisfactory to support the diagnosis of acute pancreatitis in the absence of pancreatic cytologic evaluation. However, increasingly, FNB of the pancreas is recommended to confirm the diagnosis and/or rule out secondary disease processes, including underlying neoplasia.

Acute pancreatitis appears to be both less common and more difficult to diagnose in the cat.[1,2] Ultrasonography is of only moderate utility in the diagnosis of pancreatitis in cats. In one study, results of ultrasonography were consistent with a diagnosis of pancreatitis in only 7 of 20 cats with acute pancreatic necrosis.[2] In addition, in cats with clinical signs of pancreatitis, serum concentration of feline trypsin-like immunoreactivity was poorly associated with histopathologic diagnosis.[3] Together, findings suggest that feline acute necrotizing pancreatitis and chronic nonsuppurative pancreatitis cannot be reliably distinguished from each other or from other primary pancreatic diseases on the basis of history, physical examination findings, clinicopathologic testing, radiographic abnormalities, or ultrasonographic abnormalities.[1] As such, cytology may play a larger role in distinguishing between pancreatic inflammation and other pancreatic disorders (especially neoplasia) in feline patients. Pancreatitis, pancreatic necrosis, and/or pancreatic degeneration in the cat can also occur in association with other diseases including toxoplasmosis, hepatic lipidosis, feline infectious peritonitis, Easter lily toxicosis,[32] and virulent systemic feline calicivirus infection.[33] Therefore, concurrent cytologic evaluation of the pancreas and other organs, notably the liver and/or GI system, may prove useful for evaluating pancreatic manifestations of systemic disease. However, as with dogs, some degree of pancreatic inflammation, necrosis, and/or fibrosis is a very common histopathologic finding at necropsy, even with no clinical evidence of pancreatic disease. As such, the cytologic diagnosis of pancreatic inflammation should not be based solely on the number of inflammatory cells present but also on concurrent abnormalities including necrosis, hemorrhage, and/or epithelial reactivity.

Aspirates are generally highly cellular and characterized by abundant exocrine epithelial cells and a population of inflammatory cells (see Figures 19-1 and 19-11). Neutrophils predominate in acute or acute necrotizing pancreatitis. The neutrophils are classically nondegenerate; however, they can appear ragged and mild to moderately degenerate, likely secondary to concurrent necrosis (see Figures 19-11 and 19-12). Neutrophils are frequently noted in large aggregates, occasionally embedded in necrotic or cystic-appearing debris (see Figures 19-11 and 19-13). The background may contain amorphous blue to pink material consistent with necrosis (Figure 19-14) or aggregates of crystalline, clear material consistent with calcific debris (see Figure 19-13). Necrosis may be accompanied by hemorrhage as evidenced by activated, vacuolated, and hemosiderin-laden macrophages. Golden heme breakdown products can also be noted (see Figure 19-14). Epithelial cells often appear atypical and reactive. They may have deeply basophilic cytoplasm (with fewer distinct pink granules), cytoplasmic vacuolation, increased nuclear:cytoplasmic ratios, and even prominent or small multiple nucleoli (see Figure 19-12). Although generally mild, the epithelial atypia can be fairly marked and may result in a false-positive diagnosis of pancreatic carcinoma if inflammatory cells or other evidence of pancreatitis are lacking (e.g., necrosis, hemorrhage, or fibrosis). Thus, distinguishing between pancreatitis with marked epithelial reactivity and pancreatic carcinoma with secondary inflammation and necrosis may present a challenge and should be recognized as a potential pitfall in the cytologic diagnosis of pancreatic disease. Finally, pancreatitis can be

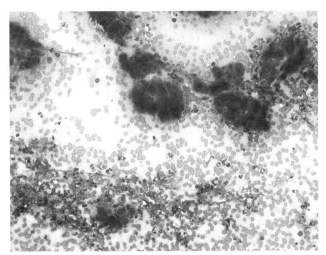

Figure 19-11 FNB of acute pancreatitis in a dog. The sample consists of multiple cell populations, including exocrine pancreatic epithelial cells and mixed, primarily neutrophilic, inflammatory cells. Epithelial cells are highly cohesive. They have abundant pink/blue cytoplasm and a low nuclear-to-cytoplasmic ratio. Inflammatory cells are present in large aggregates surrounding and adjacent to epithelial cells. (Wright-Giemsa stain, original magnification 200×.)

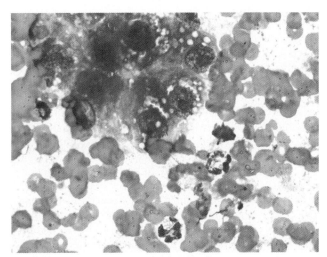

Figure 19-12 FNB of acute pancreatitis in a dog. The sample consists of multiple cell populations. Note that the neutrophils appear ragged and one neutrophil contains clear, punctate cytoplasmic vacuoles. Epithelial cells are atypical and reactive (deeply basophilic) with some criteria of malignancy, including prominent nucleoli. In the absence of inflammation, these cellular changes could be mistaken as indicative of malignancy. (Wright-Giemsa stain, original magnification 1000×.)

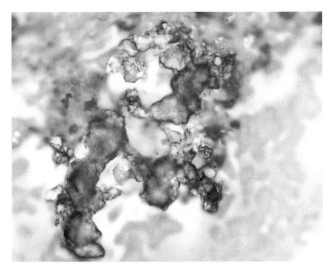

Figure 19-13 Calcific/mineralized debris obtained from FNB of canine pancreas. This debris is often multidimensional and refractile. It can be noted in large chunks, as depicted, or scattered throughout the background as crystalline material. It appears to be primarily associated with necrosis; however, it is not indicative of any specific pancreatic disorder. In this case, it was associated with necrotizing pancreatitis; however it can also be noted if the necrotic center of a pancreatic adenocarcinoma is aspirated. (Wright-Giemsa stain, original magnification 500×.)

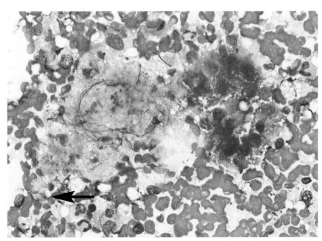

Figure 19-14 FNA of acute pancreatitis in a dog. This aspirate was characterized by reactive, deeply basophilic, and atypical epithelial cells admixed with mixed inflammatory cells in a background of amorphous pink and blue material consistent with necrotic and cystic debris. Golden heme breakdown products were also noted consistent with hemorrhage *(arrow)*. (Wright-Giemsa stain, original magnification 500×.)

accompanied by ascites. This effusion is generally a modified transudate or a nonseptic, purulent exudate with neutrophils that have punctate clear, cytoplasmic vacuoles. The effusion may have a proteinaceous background that is basophilic or "dirty" and may indicate saponified fat.

Chronic Pancreatitis/Lymphocytic Inflammation: Histopathologically, chronic pancreatitis is characterized by focal aggregation of ducts and endocrine cells set in fibrous tissue infiltrated by chronic inflammatory cells.[9] On imaging, the pancreas may appear fibrotic, nodular, or atrophied. As such, FNB of the lesions associated with chronic pancreatitis is rarely performed. Described morphologic features of chronic pancreatitis include low numbers of mixed acinar and ductal epithelial cells; mild epithelial reactivity or atypia (demonstrated by slight nuclear enlargement and slight nuclear contour irregularities); mixed inflammatory cells, especially small lymphocytes; calcified debris; and, possibly, wispy pink fibrous material (see Figure 19-1).[34] Unfortunately, underlying carcinoma can be associated with, or surrounded by, lesions compatible with acute and chronic pancreatitis leading to a potential sample bias.

Occasionally, lymphocytic inflammation of the pancreas can be noted that may not be associated with chronic pancreatitis. Considerations for increased numbers of small, well-differentiated lymphocytes in a pancreatic aspirate include lymphocytic inflammation of pancreatic islets associated with diabetes,[35] underlying viral disease, or small cell lymphoma (see Figure 19-1). With the diabetic cat, it was hypothesized that immune-mediated islet cell destruction could have contributed to beta cell depletion.[35] However, inflammatory destruction of insulin-producing cells has not been proven to be involved in development of diabetes in cats.

Pancreatic Cysts: Pancreatic cysts are subcategorized into congenital cysts, acquired retention cysts, and pseudocysts. Congenital cysts have been rarely described in small animals.[36] Similarly, acquired retention cysts are rare. Pseudocysts are also rare but are the most common pancreatic cystic lesion seen in small animals.[36,37] In human beings, pseudocysts are a common sequelum to acute and chronic pancreatitis. Pseudocysts are lined by granulation tissue and contain pancreatic enzymes and debris. They are suspected to result from the release of pancreatic secretions into the periductular connective tissue during an episode of acute pancreatitis. This may also hold true with dogs and cats; in one retrospective study, all six animals had a clinical diagnosis of pancreatitis.[37] Pseudocysts can be safely aspirated.[37,38] In addition, there may be preferential localization of pseudocysts to the left pancreatic limb.[37,38] Their fluid contents can be measured for amylase and lipase activities and cytology can be performed to rule out an abscess. In one retrospective study, six animals had high lipase activity in the pseudocyst fluid, and in two dogs and one cat the lipase activity in the fluid was greater than in serum.[37] Low pancreatic enzyme activity suggests a cystic neoplasm, whereas high levels of pancreatic enzyme activity suggest a pseudocyst. In human beings, many pseudocysts resolve spontaneously; however, they may also hemorrhage, rupture, or become secondarily infected.

Regardless of ontogeny, the cytologic appearance of cyst fluid derived from the pancreas is similar to that of cysts from any organ/structure. Aspirated samples are generally of low cellularity with a light pink to deep blue background that may contain abundant amorphous or crystalline debris (see Figure 19-1; Figures 19-15 and 19-16). Nucleated cells consist of rare nondegenerate neutrophils and occasional macrophages (see Figure 19-16). Macrophages may be cytophagic including erythrophagocytic or hemosiderin-laden if hemorrhage is present (see Figure 19-16). Pseudocyst fluid is aseptic and may have elevated total protein concentration. Cytologic evaluation of cystic fluid from the pancreas is most useful in ruling out other significant differential diagnoses for fluid-filled masses of the pancreas including abscesses and cystic neoplasms.

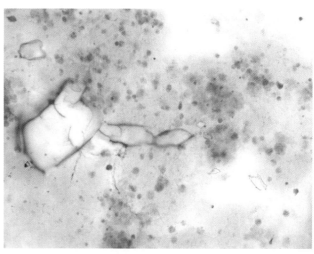

Figure 19-15 FNA of a pancreatic cyst in a dog. The sample is of low cellularity with amorphous cellular and crystalline debris in a dense pink background. Epithelial cells are generally absent. Differential diagnoses should include a primary cyst (the type of cyst cannot be determined on cytologic examination alone) or cystic neoplasm. (Wright-Giemsa stain, original magnification 500×.)

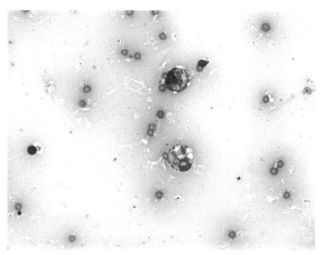

Figure 19-16 FNA of a pancreatic cyst with mild hemorrhage in a cat. Samples are characterized by low cellularity, primarily activated, erythrophagocytic macrophages. The background contains rare red blood cells and pink stippling consistent with increased protein. (Wright-Giemsa stain, original magnification 500×.)

Pancreatic Abscesses: Primary pancreatic abscesses in small animals are rare. Sources of infection for abscesses include the biliary tract, the transverse colon, or the bloodstream. Aspirates of abscesses are highly cellular and dominated by degenerate neutrophils (see Figures 19-1 and 19-17). Due to cell fragility, the slide background is frequently characterized by lysed nuclear and cellular debris. Neutrophil nuclei are swollen (degenerate) and intracellular bacteria may be seen (see Figure 19-1; Figure 19-17, *arrow*). The absence of bacteria does not rule out an abscess; as such, if an abscess is suspected based on clinical or imaging findings, culture and sensitivity

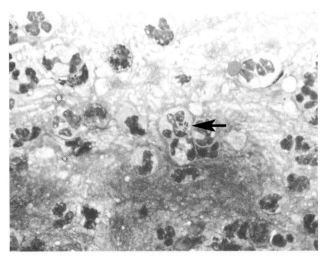

Figure 19-17 FNA of a pancreatic abscess in a dog. The sample is highly cellular and dominated by degenerate neutrophils with swollen nuclei. Intracellular coccoid bacteria are present *(arrow)*. As a result of cell fragility, the background contains abundant lysed nuclear and cellular material. This dog had a history of chronic pancreatic cyst. (Wright-Giemsa stain, original magnification 1000×.)

are warranted. The cytologic distinction between an abscess and acute pancreatitis is not always straightforward. Occasionally, an abscess may be characterized by nondegenerate neutrophils and scattered reactive epithelial cells in the absence of bacteria. This is most likely if the patient has been, or is currently being, treated with antibiotics. As such, differential diagnoses for purulent inflammation should include an abscess or acute pancreatitis in the absence of additional cytologic clues.

ACKNOWLEDGEMENTS

The author would like to thank Dr. Kari Anderson for helpful review of the sampling technique section and Dr. Jed Overmann for input and review of images.

References

1. Ferreri JA, et al: Clinical differentiation of acute necrotizing from chronic nonsuppurative pancreatitis in cats: 63 cases (1996-2001). *J Am Vet Med Assoc* 223:469, 2003.
2. Saunders HM, et al: Ultrasonographic findings in cats with clinical, gross pathologic, and histologic evidence of acute pancreatic necrosis: 20 cases (1994-2001). *J Am Vet Med Assoc* 221:1724, 2002.
3. Swift NC, et al: Evaluation of serum feline trypsin-like immunoreactivity for the diagnosis of pancreatitis in cats. *J Am Vet Med Assoc* 217:37, 2000.
4. Hess RS, et al: Clinical, clinicopathologic, radiographic, and ultrasonographic abnormalities in dogs with fatal acute pancreatitis: 70 cases (1986-1995). *J Am Vet Med Assoc* 213:665, 1998.
5. Jones T, Hunt R, King N: *Veterinary Pathology,* ed 6, Baltimore, Williams & Wilkins, 1997.
6. Bacha W, Bacha L: *Color Atlas of Veterinary Histology,* ed 2, Baltimore, Lippincott Williams & Wilkins, 2000.
7. Bjorneby JM, Kari S: Cytology of the pancreas. In Cowell RL, ed: *Vet Clin North Am Small Anim Pract* 32(6): 1293-1312, 2002.
8. O'Toole D, et al: Assessment of complications of EUS-guided fine-needle aspiration. *Gastrointest Endosc* 53:470, 2001.
9. Head K, et al: *WHO Histological Classification of Tumors of the Alimentary System of Domestic Animals,* Washington DC, Armed Forces Institute of Pathology, 2003.
10. Head K, Else R, Dubielzig R: Tumors of the alimentary tract. In Meuten D, ed: *Tumors in Domestic Animals,* Ames, Iowa, Iowa State Press, 2002.
11. Priester WA: Data from eleven United States and Canadian colleges of veterinary medicine on pancreatic carcinoma in domestic animals. *Cancer Res* 34:1372, 1974.
12. Bennett PF, et al: Ultrasonographic and cytopathological diagnosis of exocrine pancreatic carcinoma in the dog and cat. *J Am Anim Hosp Assoc* 37:466, 2001.
13. Tasker S, et al: Resolution of paraneoplastic alopecia following surgical removal of a pancreatic carcinoma in a cat. *J Small Anim Pract* 40:16, 1999.
14. Bright JM: Pancreatic adenocarcinoma in a dog with a maldigestion syndrome. *J Am Vet Med Assoc* 187:420, 1985.
15. Fabbrini F, et al: Feline cutaneous and visceral necrotizing panniculitis and steatitis associated with a pancreatic tumour. *Vet Dermatol* 16:413, 2005.
16. Lin F, Staerkel G: Cytologic criteria for well differentiated adenocarcinoma of the pancreas in fine-needle aspiration biopsy specimens. *Cancer* 99:44, 2003.
17. Robins DB, et al: Fine needle aspiration of the pancreas: In quest of accuracy. *Acta Cytol* 39:1, 1995.
18. Ylagan LR, et al: Endoscopic ultrasound guided fine-needle aspiration cytology of pancreatic carcinoma: A 3-year experience and review of the literature. *Cancer* 96:362, 2002.
19. Eloubeidi MA, et al: Yield of endoscopic ultrasound-guided fine-needle aspiration biopsy in patients with suspected pancreatic carcinoma. *Cancer* 99:285, 2003.
20. Minkus G, et al: Canine neuroendocrine tumors of the pancreas: A study using image analysis techniques for the discrimination of metastatic versus nonmetastatic tumors. *Vet Pathol* 34:138, 1997.
21. Capen C: Tumors of the endocrine glands. In Meuten D (ed): *Tumors in Domestic Animals,* Ames, Iowa, Iowa State Press, 2002.
22. Tobin RL, et al: Outcome of surgical versus medical treatment of dogs with beta cell neoplasia: 39 cases (1990-1997). *J Am Vet Med Assoc* 215:226, 1999.
23. Caywood D, et al: Pancreatic insulin-secreting neoplasms: Clinical, diagnostic, and prognostic features in 73 dogs. *J Am Anim Hosp Assoc* 24:577, 1988.
24. Green RA, Gartrell CL: Gastrinoma: A retrospective study of four cases (1985-1995). *J Am Anim Hosp Assoc* 33:524, 1997.
25. Ardengh JC, de Paulo GA, Ferrari AP: EUS-guided FNA in the diagnosis of pancreatic neuroendocrine tumors before surgery. *Gastrointest Endosc* 60:378, 2004.
26. Jimenez-Heffernan JA, et al: Fine needle aspiration cytology of endocrine neoplasms of the pancreas: Morphologic and immunocytochemical findings in 20 cases. *Acta Cytol* 48:295, 2004.
27. Hayden DW, et al: Disseminated malignant histiocytosis in a golden retriever: Clinicopathologic, ultrastructural, and immunohistochemical findings. *Vet Pathol* 30:256, 1993.
28. Swann HM, Holt DE: Canine gastric adenocarcinoma and leiomyosarcoma: A retrospective study of 21 cases (1986-1999) and literature review. *J Am Anim Hosp Assoc* 38:157, 2002.

29. Newman SJ, et al: Correlation of age and incidence of pancreatic exocrine nodular hyperplasia in the dog. *Vet Pathol* 42:510, 2005.

30. Bradley EL, 3rd: A clinically based classification system for acute pancreatitis: Summary of the International Symposium on Acute Pancreatitis, Atlanta, Ga, September 11 through 13, 1992, *Arch Surg* 128:586, 1993.

31. Newman S, et al: Localization of pancreatic inflammation and necrosis in dogs. *J Vet Intern Med* 18:488, 2004.

32. Rumbeiha WK, et al: A comprehensive study of Easter lily poisoning in cats. *J Vet Diagn Invest* 16:527, 2004.

33. Pesavento PA, et al: Pathologic, immunohistochemical, and electron microscopic findings in naturally occurring virulent systemic feline calicivirus infection in cats. *Vet Pathol* 41:257, 2004.

34. Afify AM, et al: Endoscopic ultrasound-guided fine needle aspiration of the pancreas: Diagnostic utility and accuracy. *Acta Cytol* 47:341, 2003.

35. Hall DG, et al: Lymphocytic inflammation of pancreatic islets in a diabetic cat. *J Vet Diagn Invest* 9:98, 1997.

36. Coleman MG, Robson MC, Harvey C: Pancreatic cyst in a cat. *N Z Vet J* 53:157, 2005.

37. VanEnkevort BA, O'Brien RT, Young KM: Pancreatic pseudocysts in 4 dogs and 2 cats: Ultrasonographic and clinicopathologic findings. *J Vet Intern Med* 13:309, 1999.

38. Hines BL, et al: Pancreatic pseudocyst associated with chronic-active necrotizing pancreatitis in a cat. *J Am Anim Hosp Assoc* 32:147, 1996.

The Liver

T.W. French, T. Stokol, and D. Meyer

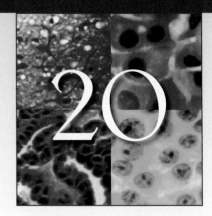

CHAPTER 20

Cytologic examination of samples from the hepatobiliary system complements other diagnostic procedures and, in some cases, provides the specific diagnosis. Specimens for cytologic examination can be collected by percutaneous fine-needle aspiration, percutaneous needle core biopsy, or surgical biopsy. Cytologic examination of material collected by fine-needle aspiration and needle biopsy, which are relatively inexpensive and safe procedures, can determine whether exploratory surgery is warranted. Collection and examination of cytologic samples are most commonly performed on patients with nodular lesions, abnormal echogenicity, or generalized or lobar liver enlargement. The increasing availability of imaging procedures, such as ultrasonography and computed tomography, to direct the collection of needle aspiration and biopsy has increased the accuracy of sampling nodular lesions, thereby extending the diagnostic usefulness of liver cytology.

Cytologic evaluation of hepatobiliary tissue should be preceded by assessment for abnormal liver size or function by physical examination, hematologic and clinical chemistry enzyme and function tests, and radiographic or ultrasound examinations. Cytologic examination is a logical next step in the differential diagnoses of suspected degenerative, inflammatory, or neoplastic liver disease.

TECHNIQUES (Box 20-1)

Various techniques for percutaneous sampling of the hepatobiliary system have been described.[1-4] Complications following these procedures are rare and include hemorrhage and potential seeding of needle tracts by neoplastic cells. Because compromised hemostasis is a life-threatening concern in animals with liver disease, the risk for excessive bleeding should be assessed particularly in cats with prolonged anorexia and in severely ill patients.[4,5] A thorough history should include questioning the owner about prior bleeding episodes and treatment with over-the-counter anticoagulant drugs, such as aspirin. This is followed by a complete physical examination and laboratory testing to evaluate platelet number (a platelet count or estimate from a blood smear), a buccal mucosal bleeding time (BMBT), and coagulation assays (prothrombin time, activated partial thromboplastin time, and possibly

protein-induced vitamin K absence). Abnormal test results do not reliably predict a bleeding tendency, and hemorrhage can occur in animals with normal profiles.[6] It is pragmatic to avoid aspirating the highly vascular liver if there are severe coagulation abnormalities and/or clinical signs of hemorrhage elsewhere in the body. If a liver aspirate is deemed an acceptable risk in a patient with mildly prolonged coagulation tests, it is prudent to perform it early in the day so that the hematocrit can be followed and interventional abdominal surgery performed if excess bleeding is detected.

Aspiration and needle biopsy are usually performed with the patient in dorsal or right lateral recumbency, but can be performed with the patient standing. Chemical restraint is unnecessary for many patients. With the patient in dorsal recumbency, a blind biopsy is performed by inserting (at a 30- to 45-degree angle to the skin in dogs, and almost vertically in cats) midway between the left costal arch and the end of the xiphoid process.[1] If the animal is standing or lying on the right side, the collection site is found by percussing the intercostal spaces to locate the liver beneath the rib cage. The next intercostal space caudal to the space where the sound of percussion changes from resonant to dull is usually a satisfactory site for aspiration. The collection site can be determined by palpation if an enlarged liver extends beyond the rib cage. Increasingly, sensitive imaging procedures such as ultrasound are used to facilitate accurate sampling of the liver, including sites with normal and abnormal echogenicity.[3,4]

Cells from the hepatobiliary system can be aspirated using a 21- to 22-gauge, 1 to 2½-inch hypodermic needle and a 6- or 12-ml syringe. Alternatively, a 22-gauge spinal needle with a stylet can be used. The stylet prevents obstruction of the needle as it penetrates the body wall. With the needle in the liver, samples are aspirated by rapidly withdrawing the plunger of the syringe to the 5- or 6-ml mark. The suction is gently released before the needle is withdrawn. The specimen will consist of small pieces of parenchymal tissue mixed with fresh blood.

Once the needle is withdrawn, the syringe should be detached and filled with 1 to 2 ml of air. After reattaching the syringe to the needle, a small drop of sample (6 to 8 mm diameter) is expelled onto each of several glass slides. Place the drops near the center of the slides; sample that is smeared close to the end may not be stained by automated stainers and is difficult to evaluate microscopically. The sample is best spread gently into a smear by the squash method (see Chapter 1).

The liver can also be sampled by a nonaspiration technique, using a 26-gauge needle only, as described in Chapter 1. This method may reduce the likelihood of contaminating the specimen with excessive amounts of blood.

Smears of biopsies are prepared by imprinting the tissue on clean glass slides or by gently rolling a core of tissue along a slide. The surface of the tissue to be imprinted should be lightly blotted with absorbent, lint-free tissue before the smears are made. Small fragments of tissue can be manipulated with fine forceps or skewered on a clean 25-gauge hypodermic needle, which provides a convenient handle for touching the cut surface of the tissue to the slides. Two to three impressions should be made on each of several slides.

Smears should be dried quickly and protected from exposure to formalin fumes or liquid for optimal staining. Typically, if several smears are available, one or two are stained with a routine Romanowsky-type (blood) stain and then examined. Retain additional unstained smears so that special stains can be performed if indicated. A well-made squash smear of a highly cellular aspirate is shown (Figure 20-1).

NORMAL FINDINGS

Aspirates and impressions from normal livers consist largely of hepatocytes and variable amounts of peripheral blood. Hepatocytes exfoliate readily and are distributed in the smear as single cells and in cords and clusters. Normal hepatocytes (Figures 20-2 and 20-3) are large, round or slightly oval to polyhedral cells that have round nuclei and abundant cytoplasm. Slight variation in cell size is normal. Their cytoplasm contains many ribosomes, which stain blue, and other organelles that are unstained or slightly pink. Therefore, the overall color of the cytoplasm in most normal hepatocytes is light blue or lavender, with light pink cytoplasmic granules. The intensity of the color is variable and depends on the degree to which the cell has been spread. Hepatocytes in large clusters, which resist flattening, have a deeper blue cytoplasm than single

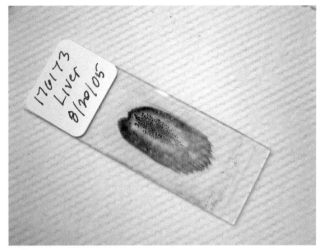

Figure 20-1 An optimal smear of a liver aspirate resembles a good bone marrow preparation and consists of gently spread tissue surrounded by fresh blood.

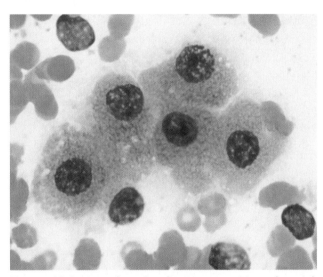

Figure 20-2 Normal canine hepatocytes. Note the pink granularity of the cytoplasm and the uniform round nuclei. These could have been collected from a normal liver or from an unaffected area of a diseased liver. (Wright's stain, 1000×.)

cells or cells in flattened sheets. In older animals, lipofuscin pigment granules may be seen in the cytoplasm of the hepatocytes (see Pigments).

Nuclei typically are centrally located, are quite uniform in size, and have coarsely reticular chromatin. A single nucleolus often is visible; in some intact cells this can be obscured by heterochromatin. The nucleoli are more easily seen in the nuclei of ruptured or understained cells. A low number of binucleate hepatocytes is normal. Rectangular crystalline intranuclear inclusions are seen occasionally; these are of no known pathologic significance (see Figure 20-3).

Biliary tract epithelial cells typically are few in aspirates of normal liver. These appear as cuboidal to columnar cells in small clusters or flat sheets (Figure 20-4). Rarely, distinct tubular arrangements may be seen (Figure 20-5). The cells have round, central nuclei and scant amounts

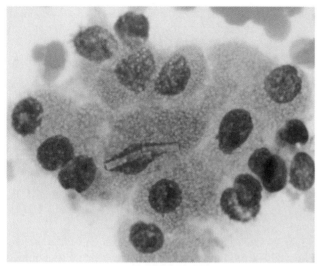

Figure 20-3 Normal canine hepatocytes. One hepatocyte in the field contains two crystalline intranuclear inclusions. This is an occasional finding of no known significance. (Wright's stain, 1000×.)

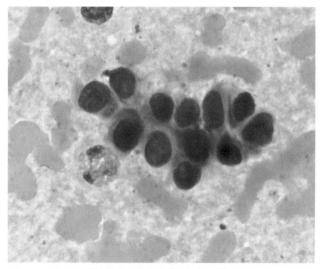

Figure 20-4 Epithelial cells of the biliary tract are cuboidal to low columnar cells and are usually seen as small flattened sheets. (Wright's stain, 1000×.)

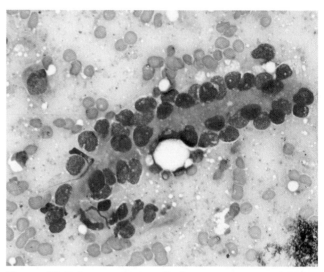

Figure 20-5 An uncommon finding, a segment of intact bile duct is present in this aspirate. Bile duct hyperplasia is not reliably detected by fine-needle aspiration cytology. (Wright's stain, 500×.)

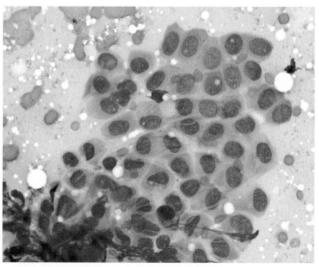

Figure 20-6 Sheets of freshly exfoliated mesothelial cells are seen occasionally in liver aspirates. These appear as a mosaic arrangement of angular, polygonal cells with pale blue cytoplasm and uniformly sized round to oval nuclei. (Wright's stain, 500×.)

of light blue cytoplasm, which distinguishes them from the larger, granular hepatocytes. Their chromatin is dense and smooth and nucleoli are not visible.

Mechanically exfoliated mesothelial cells may be seen in aspirates from some animals. These can be difficult to distinguish from biliary epithelial cells, but are generally larger, polygonal to spindloid, and found in flat sheets with a mosaic pattern (Figure 20-6). Occasional samples may include some amount of extrahepatic tissue such as adipocytes and/or lipid aspirated from mesenteric fat.

Resident hepatic macrophages, Kupffer cells, are few or absent in smears of normal liver. Rare lipid-laden Ito cells may be identified in some aspirates. In cats, low numbers of lymphocytes may also be seen and are of equivocal significance because a few lymphocytes can be found

in the portal triads in healthy animals.[7] Low numbers of resident mast cells are seen in many samples. These are small, often polygonal cells with a round blurry nucleus and lightly granulated cytoplasm (Figure 20-7). At lower magnifications, they will appear as small purple splotches nestled within the cords of hepatocytes.

PIGMENTS

Several different pigments can be seen within hepatocytes in cytologic preparations (Table 20-1). Their presence can be a normal finding or be associated with extrahepatic or hepatic disease. Differentiating among these based solely on routinely stained smears can be difficult. Special stains and microscopy methods can be employed for specific identification. Typically this is necessary only when excess copper is suspected because this may be of direct diagnostic significance.

Lipofuscin

Lipofuscin is a "wear and tear" pigment, consisting of indigestible residue accumulated within autophagolysosomes. Large amounts may be seen in hepatocytes from older cats and dogs. This is a normal feature of aging and does not represent a pathologic process. Granules of lipofuscin (Figure 20-8) are similar in size to bile pigment and hemosiderin

and range from brownish to blue-green in color. Based on one study, lipofuscin is the pigment most commonly observed within canine hepatocytes.[8] The same is true in cats. Presumptive identification of hepatocyte pigment as lipofuscin, and not bile, is justified if other evidence of cholestasis (i.e., bile casts, hyperbilirubinemia, bilirubinuria) is absent. More direct identification of lipofuscin is seldom needed but can be achieved by examining unstained smears for autofluorescence under ultraviolet light at various wavelengths (Figure 20-9).[8] Among the pigments discussed here, autofluorescence is specific for lipofuscin. Lipofuscin granules also specifically stain red with a modified Ziehl-Neelsen stain (Figure 20-9) or Luxol fast blue.

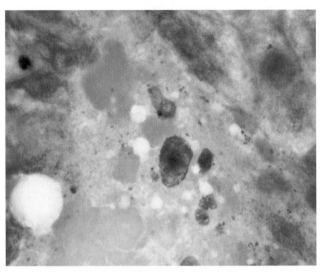

Figure 20-7 A single resident-type mast cell is at the center. These can be seen in varying numbers scattered through smears from normal and abnormal livers. They are small cells with fine purple cytoplasmic granules and condensed nuclei. (Wright's stain, 1000×.)

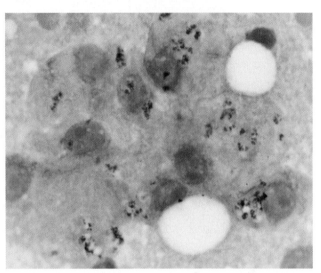

Figure 20-8 The dark pigment in these canine hepatocytes is lipofuscin. The cells were aspirated from a hyperplastic nodule in the liver of a 12-year-old dog. Images in Figure 20-9 are from the same aspirate. (Wright's stain, 1000×.)

TABLE 20-1

Hepatocellular Pigments

Pigment	Cytologic Appearance	Significance and Common Causes	Confirmatory Tests
Lipofuscin	Dark green to blue-green granules in hepatocytes and/or macrophages. Difficult to distinguish from bile.	No pathologic significance – increases with aging. Most common pigment in canine and feline hepatocytes.	Ultraviolet microscopy, modified Ziehl-Neelsen, Luxol fast blue
Bile pigments	Dark green granules in hepatocytes. Difficult to distinguish from lipofuscin.	Cholestasis – may be localized or widespread, intrahepatic or extrahepatic.	Concurrent bile casts, high serum/urine bilirubin and cholestatic enzymes, Hall's stain
Hemosiderin	Brownish-gold to black granules in hepatocytes and/or macrophages.	Anemias – immune-mediated hemolytic or nonregenerative, chronic disease, aplastic; localized hemorrhage.	Prussian blue stain
Copper	Light blue-green, refractile granules in hepatocytes. Focus up and down to facilitate visualization.	Small amounts can be secondary to chronic cholestasis. Large amounts suggest primary copper-induced hepatopathy.	Rubeanic acid stain, measure tissue copper levels

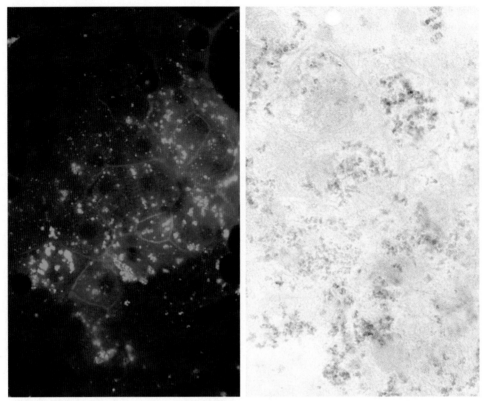

Figure 20-9 Lipofuscin. When an unstained, unfixed smear is viewed under ultraviolet light using a FITC filter, a bright green autofluorescence is observed *(left)*. (490 nm, 500×.) Stained with a modified Ziehl-Neelsen procedure, lipofuscin appears as red granular material *(right)*. (500×.)

Bile Pigment

Bile accumulation within hepatocytes is recognized as small, dark green to black granules (Figure 20-10) and can be found in various hepatobiliary disorders. Abundant intracytoplasmic bile pigment is suggestive of cholestasis, although the process may not be severe enough to cause hyperphosphatasemia, hyperbilirubinemia, or icterus. Because of the similarity to lipofuscin with routine stains, however, cholestasis is confirmed only when solid, dark green or black bile casts, also called bile plugs or thrombi, are observed between contiguous hepatocytes (Figure 20-11). These represent accumulated bile in biliary canaliculi. Cast fragments may litter the background of the smears. In some cases, the cause of cholestasis may be evidenced by an accompanying inflammatory or neoplastic infiltrate.

Hemosiderin

Hemosiderin is recognized as golden to golden-brown granules in hepatocytes (Figure 20-12). Hemosiderin can be distinguished from other pigments by applying a Prussian blue reaction to a methanol-fixed smear, which stains hemosiderin granules blue. In many cases, increased iron content in hepatocytes is associated with increased iron turnover caused by hemolytic anemia or ineffective erythropoiesis (e.g., immune-mediated nonregenerative

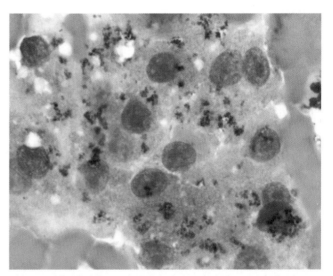

Figure 20-10 These hepatocytes contain a dark green to black granular pigment. Based solely on morphologic features, this could be either bile pigment (suggestive of cholestasis) or lipofuscin (no significance). In this instance, the concurrent findings of canalicular casts (see Figure 20-11) and serum biochemical evidence of cholestasis support the likelihood that it is bile. (Wright's stain, 1000×.)

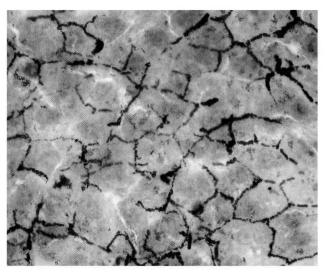

Figure 20-11 Bile casts fill the canaliculi between contiguous hepatocytes in this aspirate of dog liver. This is a clear indication of (minimally) localized cholestasis. Depending on its extent, this abnormality may or may not be reflected by changes in serum enzymes or bilirubin. (Wright's stain, 500×.)

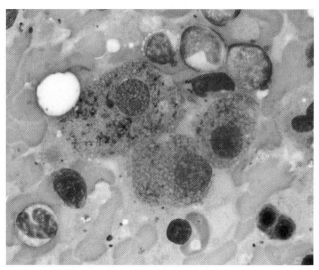

Figure 20-12 Hemosiderin appears as a brown-gold pigment in these hepatocytes from a beagle with chronic hemolytic anemia. The surrounding erythroid and myeloid precursors indicate hepatic extramedullary hematopoiesis, in this case related to the anemia. (Wright's stain, 1000×.)

anemia). Iron also can accumulate due to decreased iron utilization associated with severely decreased erythropoiesis (e.g., pure red cell aplasia, aplastic anemia). Repeated blood transfusions and administration of iron-containing compounds (especially by injection) also can increase hepatic iron content. In macrophages, hemosiderin can vary from gold to brown-black in color, depending on the amount within the cell. Macrophages containing phagocytized red cells or hemosiderin or both are concomitant findings in many patients with hemolytic disease.

Copper

When present in excessive amounts, copper can become visible in hepatocytes as refractile, pale blue-green cytoplasmic granules (Figure 20-13). Smears can be stained with rubeanic acid to confirm the presence of copper (Figure 20-14). This procedure can be used even if the slide was first stained with Romanowsky-type stains. Small amounts of copper can accumulate secondary to prolonged cholestatic liver disease. If large amounts of copper are observed, a primary copper-accumulation hepatopathy should be suspected. This has been reported as a familial condition in Bedlington terriers, West Highland white terriers,[9] Skye terriers,[10] and Dalmations.[11] In some breeds, such as the Doberman Pinscher, it remains unclear whether the increased copper represents a primary or secondary storage disorder.[12] Copper-associated hepatopathy in a young Siamese cat has also been reported.[13]

NONNEOPLASTIC CONDITIONS AND DISEASES

Hepatocellular Cytoplasmic Vacuolation

Morphologically, two types of cytoplasmic vacuolation are commonly seen: lipid and nonlipid (Table 20-2). Lipid vacuolation results from accumulation of triglycerides and is most often seen in aspirates of feline liver. Nonlipid vacuolation results from accumulation of glycogen and/or water, and is most often seen in aspirates of canine liver.

Lipid Vacuolation: The cytoplasm of affected hepatocytes contains round, empty-appearing, sharply delineated vacuoles of varying sizes (Figure 20-15). This appearance is termed fatty change or steatosis. The smear background may be punctuated with similar vacuoles. In severe cases, there are so many lipid vacuoles within the cells that little cytoplasm is visible. In some cells, a single very large vacuole may displace the nucleus to the periphery of the cell such that it resembles an adipocyte. The cells often are remarkably swollen by the lipid accumulation, which can contribute to cholestasis by compression of the canalicular spaces. Bile casts may be seen as a reflection of this effect. Lipid presence can be confirmed by staining an unfixed smear with Sudan III, Oil red O, or new methylene blue.

Fatty change of variable degree can be seen as a nonspecific indicator of liver injury in all species. In cats, hepatomegaly due to fatty change is most commonly seen as the central feature in the cholestatic syndrome of feline hepatic lipidosis (FHL). Development of this disorder almost always is triggered by the presence of an underlying disease process causing a catabolic state.[14] Affected cats are usually icteric and have livers that are enlarged by extensive, diffuse accumulation of lipid in hepatocytes. Most cats with hepatic lipidosis have markedly increased serum alkaline phosphatase activity and hyperbilirubinemia (mostly direct/conjugated) with no or only a slight increase in gamma glutamyltransferase activity. Hepatomegaly caused by lipid accumulation in hepatocytes is uncommon in dogs. Mild to moderate lipid vacuolation can develop secondary to various metabolic disorders in dogs and cats, especially diabetes mellitus. Severe hepatic lipidosis and hypoglycemia can occur subsequent to anorexia in puppies of toy dog breeds.[15] Dogs

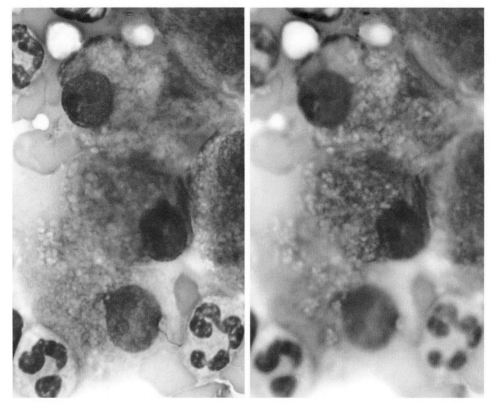

Figure 20-13 This is an imprint of a liver biopsy from a 3-year-old mixed breed dog with copper-associated hepatopathy. The pale green refractile granules in the hepatocytes contain copper. Note how the granules are best seen slightly above the plane of focus of the cells *(right).* Focusing up and down helps to visualize suspected granules. (Wright's stain, 1000×.)

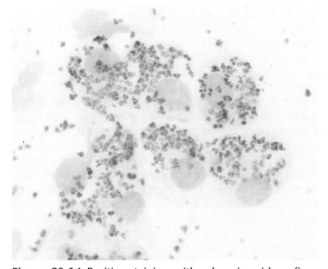

Figure 20-14 Positive staining with rubeanic acid confirms that the cytoplasmic granules seen in the preceding image are composed of copper. The presence of copper in such large amounts suggests it likely is the cause, rather than the effect, of liver disease. (Rubeanic acid stain, 1000×.)

with aflatoxicosis develop severe hepatic lipidosis; their liver aspirates resemble those of cats with FHL.

Nonlipid Vacuolation: The cytoplasm of affected hepatocytes has a lacey, wispy vacuolation or rarefaction often associated with mild to marked cell swelling (Figure

20-16). This appearance can be due to hepatocellular injury and has been attributed to increased cytoplasmic water. In dogs, a similar morphology can be due to glycogen accumulation, most notable and extensive in association with exogenous or endogenous glucocorticoid excess.

A variety of liver-related conditions, including ischemia, inflammation/infection, cholestasis, and toxins, can result in nonlipid vacuolar change. The vacuolar change may be nonuniform, affecting some hepatocyte clusters more than others. It may also vary in degree, within and between clusters. Associated cytologic findings may include evidence of necrosis, various inflammatory cells, infectious agents, and bile casts. It can also be a feature of aspirates from hyperplastic and regenerative nodules, possibly secondary to localized abnormalities of blood supply or bile flow.

In dogs, nonlipid vacuolar change can also be caused by high plasma concentrations of glucocorticoid hormones. The altered morphology is related to the increased volume of unstained glycogen that displaces the blue-staining, RNA-containing organelles. The periodic acid–Schiff stain for glycogen can be used to demonstrate this as the cause. In some patients, vacuolar hepatopathy of this type can be attributed to hyperadrenocorticism (HAC) or exogenous corticosteroid therapy, which has been called a *steroid hepatopathy*. These patients generally have characteristic accompanying clinical signs (e.g., polyuria, polydipsia, polyphagia) and very high serum alkaline phosphatase activity without

TABLE 20-2

Hepatocellular Vacuolation

Cytoplasmic Change	Appearance	Common Causes	Confirmatory Measures
Lipid vacuolation	Variably sized, sharply defined, empty appearing vacuoles. Marked cell swelling possible in severe cases.	Feline hepatic lipidosis, diabetes mellitus, hepatocellular injury of many causes.	New methylene blue, Oil red O, Sudan III
Nonlipid vacuolation	Lacy vacuoles or rarefaction of cytoplasm. Marked cell swelling possible in severe cases.	Hyperadrenocorticism, exogenous glucocorticoids, stress of chronic illness, hepatocellular injury of many causes.	PAS for glycogen: positive indicates glycogen accumulation, negative suggests hydropic change

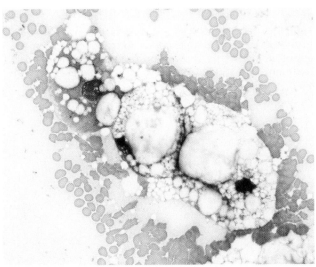

Figure 20-15 These greatly swollen hepatocytes are filled with many discrete vacuoles of varying sizes. The empty, sharply demarcated appearance of the vacuoles indicates that they contain lipid. Nearly all the hepatocytes aspirated were comparably affected. Collected from an icteric cat with hepatomegaly, the aspirate was diagnostic for feline hepatic lipidosis. (Wright's stain, 500×.)

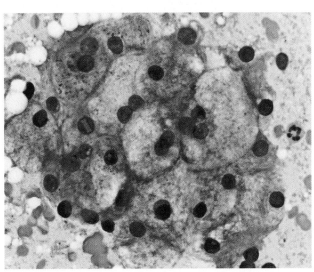

Figure 20-16 The canine hepatocytes in this field show marked swelling and nonlipid, vacuolar change that could be caused by glycogen accumulation associated with glucocorticoid excess or water accumulation (hydropic change) caused by cellular injury (e.g., ischemia, hepatotoxins.). The cells shown in this instance are from a dog with HAC and hypothyroidism. (Wright's stain, 500×.)

hyperbilirubinemia. Hepatomegaly commonly is present, and hepatocytes aspirated from such dogs often are several-fold larger than normal hepatocytes. Nonlipid vacuolar change and high alkaline phosphatase also are common findings in dogs secondary to chronic stress associated with a variety of diseases (e.g., neoplasia, congenital or acquired hepatobiliary disease).[16]

Amyloidosis

The liver is a major site of amyloid deposition in dogs with reactive, or secondary, amyloidosis. Amyloid accumulation in Disse's space in liver and other tissues, such as kidney, spleen, lymph node, and skin, can develop secondary to prolonged, intense systemic inflammation. In some animals, the primary disease is infectious (e.g., systemic mycosis or leishmaniasis). A familial inflammatory disorder culminating in severe amyloidosis is recognized in Chinese Shar Pei, some of which have severe liver

dysfunction.[17] Hepatic hemorrhage and rupture are major causes of morbidity and death in Oriental shorthair and Siamese cats with systemic amyloidosis.[18] In smears of affected liver or other tissue, amyloid appears as amorphous, pink, extracellular material found between hepatocytes and can resemble necrotic cellular debris (Figure 20-17).

Extramedullary Hematopoiesis

Hematopoietic foci in the livers of dogs and cats can develop concurrently with accelerated hematopoiesis in marrow, usually in response to anemia or systemic inflammatory diseases. Occasionally, evidence of hepatic hematopoiesis is found in nonanemic dogs with chronic hepatitis or nodular hyperplasia. It can also be a normal finding in some older animals. Extramedullary hematopoiesis is recognized by the presence of hematopoietic cells at all stages of maturation (see Figure 20-12). The

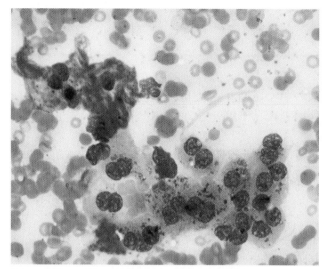

Figure 20-17 The pink, amorphous, extracellular material beside the hepatocytes in this field is amyloid. The sample was aspirated from a Shar-Pei with hepatomegaly. Amyloid deposition was confirmed by staining sections of the liver with Congo red. The pigment in the hepatocytes is probably lipofuscin. (Wright's stain, 500×.) *(Slide courtesy Dr. C. Mesher.)*

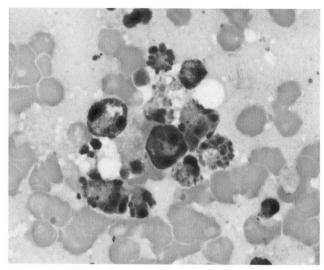

Figure 20-18 Cell death via apoptosis is seen in a liver aspirate from a dog with metastatic pancreatic carcinoma. Numerous apoptotic bodies are shown, most of which contain nuclear fragments in addition to cytoplasm and organelles. (Wright's stain, 1000×.)

erythroid line is usually the predominant cell line and, in most cases, is accompanied by immature neutrophils. The hematopoietic cells are normal in appearance, and intermediate to late stages of maturation should be more numerous than earlier stages. Myelolipomas, which are tumor-like nodular masses composed of lipid-containing stromal cells and hematopoietic cells, are rarely encountered. Material aspirated from myelolipomas is cytologically indistinguishable from normal marrow.

Hepatocellular Death and Regeneration

Irreversible injury leading to death of hepatocytes can occur secondary to a wide variety of toxins (e.g., aflatoxins, cycad toxicity), drugs (e.g., tetracycline and diazepam in cats, rimadyl and xylitol in dogs), immune-mediated disease, metabolic disturbances, ischemia, neoplasia, and infectious agents. Cell death can occur via two pathways, apoptosis and necrosis. The two are largely distinct in terms of their morphologic features. However, apoptosis and necrosis can be mediated through similar/shared biochemical pathways and both can occur simultaneously in response to some stimuli.[19,20]

Apoptosis (programmed cell death) is a physiologic process important both in development and in homeostasis of renewable cell populations such as leukocytes and intestinal crypt cells. However, it also can be triggered by a variety of injurious stimuli. Whether a cell dies through apoptosis or necrosis depends on a range of factors, including the nature, severity, and duration of the injury and the underlying physiology of the cell. In cytologic specimens, apoptotic cells have pyknotic or karyorrhectic nuclei but intact cell membranes and cytoplasmic features. With time, cytoplasmic blebbing results in the formation of membrane-delimited apoptotic bodies, which may or may not contain nuclear remnants (Figure 20-18). They

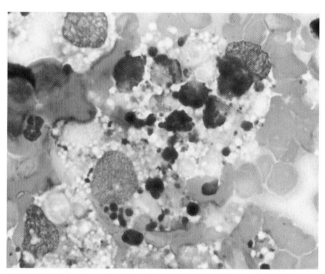

Figure 20-19 Intact apoptotic bodies are avidly phagocytized by macrophages. Because the release of cytoplasm from the dead cells into the interstitium is minimized, apoptosis incites less inflammation as compared with necrosis. (Wright's stain, 1000×.)

are subsequently phagocytized by resident Kupffer cells and/or macrophages (Figure 20-19). Apoptosis typically does not incite an inflammatory response, as the contents of the dead cell are not released.

Necrosis, on the other hand, is always a pathologic process—the end stage of irreversible cell injury. The cells may swell initially but eventually condense. Cytoplasm becomes more pink in color due to loss of RNA and denaturation of cytoplasmic proteins. Subsequently enzymatic digestion leads to the breakdown of cell membranes. Nuclei may be pyknotic or karyorrhectic and eventually disappear (karyolysis). Coagulative and liquefactive are the most commonly encountered types of necrosis.

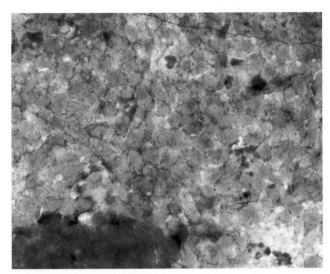

Figure 20-20 Coagulative necrosis is seen in the same smear from which Figures 20-18 and 20-19 were taken. Note that shrunken cell outlines still are visible, although the nuclei have faded (karyolysis) and the cytoplasm has a pink homogenous appearance. Soon the membranes will fail, releasing cytoplasm from the dead cells. (Wright's stain, 500×.)

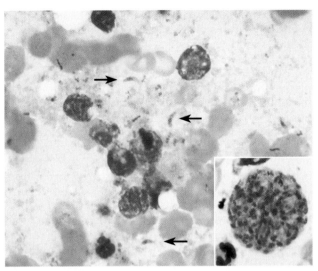

Figure 20-21 Necrosis in an aspirate of liver from an 11-year-old dog with fever and icterus. Bare hepatocyte nuclei with condensed chromatin are seen on a background of cell debris. Also present are banana-shaped tachyzoites typical of *Toxoplasma gondii (arrows)*, which was the inciting cause. The inset shows a tissue cyst, many of which were seen scattered through the smear. (Wright's stain, 1000×.)

Coagulative necrosis, which occurs when protein denaturation dominates, is recognized by the presence of hepatocytes with glassy pink cytoplasm, which retain distinct cellular outlines for a time (Figure 20-20). Liquefactive necrosis occurs when enzymatic digestion prevails. This results in earlier breakdown of cell membranes and complete disintegration of the cells, such that they are seen only as amorphous pink to light purple debris (Figure 20-21). In contrast to apoptosis, necrosis does incite an inflammatory response consisting of macrophages or Kupffer cells or a mixture of macrophages, lymphocytes, and neutrophils. Proliferative macrophages/Kupffer cells are often seen in small aggregates and contain phagocytized cellular debris and erythrocytes (if hemorrhage occurs secondary to necrosis). Lipofuscin pigment may also be prominent within these phagocytic cells.

Regenerating hepatocytes during the reparative process subsequent to injury are pleomorphic. They may display cytologic criteria of malignancy, including marked anisokaryosis, multinucleation, increased cytoplasmic basophilia, and prominent large nucleoli (Figure 20-22), and can be mistaken for hepatocellular neoplasia. Concurrent cytologic evidence of necrosis and/or inflammation and cholestasis, however, should raise a flag of caution. A presumptive cytologic diagnosis of hepatocellular regeneration secondary to necrosis should be made and follow-up by histologic examination considered.

Nodular Hyperplasia

Single or multiple spherical masses composed of hepatic parenchyma are commonly found in old dogs. In livers of otherwise normal size and contour, these masses are called hyperplastic nodules. In many dogs, these changes are incidental findings, often detected during

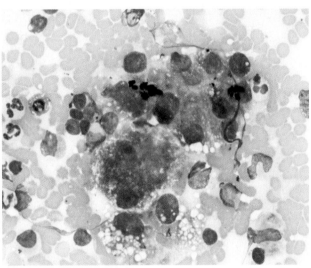

Figure 20-22 Aspirate of a hepatic necroinflammatory lesion in a dog. A cluster of atypical hepatocytes is seen surrounded by mixed inflammatory cells. Abnormal features include high nuclear-to-cytoplasmic ratios, excessive cytoplasmic basophilia and vacuolation, moderate to marked anisocytosis, and anisokaryosis with multiple large nucleoli. These changes can mimic the appearance of malignant cells but in this case are reflective of a regenerative response to necrosis and inflammation. (Wright's stain, 500×.)

abdominal ultrasonography. Concurrent mild to moderate increases in liver enzymes, especially alkaline phosphatase, may be seen. Nodular hyperplasia can also be a sequela to chronic inflammation and/or necrosis. In tissue smears collected from hyperplastic nodules or areas of regenerative hyperplasia, the hepatocytes may be indistinguishable from normal. In other cases, mild to moderate nonlipid vacuolar change may be seen. Other cytologic features characteristic of hyperplastic tissue include slightly increased cellular and nuclear size, increased nuclear-to-cytoplasmic ratios, mild anisocytosis and anisokaryosis, and increased basophilia of the cytoplasm. Binucleate hepatocytes are more numerous than in normal tissue (Figure 20-23). Focal accumulations of lipid- or lipofuscin-laden macrophages (lipogranulomas) may be seen. Hyperplastic masses can closely resemble primary or metastatic tumors radiographically and ultrasonographically. Furthermore, the cytologic features of such masses can be indistinguishable from those of hepatocellular adenoma and well-differentiated carcinoma (see the discussion of epithelial tumors later in this chapter). In some cases, hyperplastic nodules can be differentiated from hepatocellular tumors if cytologic findings are considered in light of clinical history and results of other diagnostic procedures. In

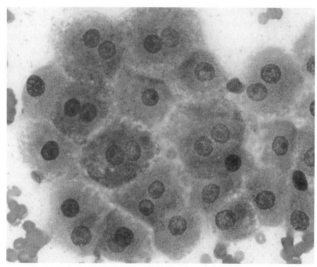

Figure 20-23 Aspirate from one of the multiple regenerative nodules in the liver of a dog with a history of chronic liver disease. Variation in cell size is greater than normal. The proportion of binucleated cells is increased (nearly 50% in this field), but the individual nuclei are of normal morphologic appearance. (Wright's stain, 500×.)

other cases, histologic examination of liver biopsies to determine the architecture of the mass is needed for definitive diagnoses.

Inflammatory Disorders

Reports vary with regard to the relative sensitivity of cytology compared with histologic evaluation in the diagnosis of various inflammatory diseases of the liver.[21,22,23] Owing to the typically smaller sample, however, it seems logical that cytology of fine-needle aspirates would be less sensitive for conditions with minimal cellular infiltrates (e.g., low-grade chronic hepatitis or mild focal to multifocal lesions). The same effect of sample size applies when comparing histologic evaluation of needle and wedge biopsy specimens.[24] Therefore, if inflammatory cells in a smear are not sufficient for determining inflammation by cytology, an inflammatory process in the liver cannot be excluded. Additionally, it is difficult to diagnose inflammation cytologically when evaluating blood-contaminated liver aspirates from animals, particularly in cases with a marked leukocytosis, because the neutrophils contributed by the blood may be mistaken as infiltrating cells. Comparing the leukocyte numbers in areas surrounding clusters of hepatocytes with those in areas consisting only of blood can help in deciding whether an interpretation of inflammation is warranted (Table 20-3). Additional evidence of inflammation is the presence of cells not found in blood (e.g., macrophages and plasma cells), observing neutrophils that are intercalated between hepatocytes in clusters, and the presence of neutrophils with pyknotic and fragmented nuclei or degenerative changes produced by exposure to bacterial toxins.

Suppurative Inflammation: Suppurative exudates are almost entirely composed of neutrophils. Macrophages and lymphocytes usually compose less than 10% of the cells in suppurative exudates. Suppurative exudates often represent bacterial infections, which may reach the liver by ascending the biliary tree, causing cholangiohepatitis, or (less commonly) spreading hematogenously and producing focal or multifocal hepatic abscesses. Aspirates

TABLE **20-3**

Inflammatory Infiltrates

Type of Inflammation	Cell Types Present*	Some Possible Causes
Suppurative inflammation	Neutrophils predominate (>90% of inflammatory cells). Hepatocytes may be absent with abscesses. Few lymphocytes and macrophages.	Suppurative cholangiohepatitis (± bacteria), hepatic abscess secondary to necrosis.
Mixed inflammation	Neutrophils, eosinophils, macrophages, lymphocytes, plasma cells, multinucleated giant macrophages in variable proportions.	Infectious diseases—viral (feline infectious peritonitis), mycotic, mycobacterial, protozoal; drug and toxic injury; and systemic immune-mediated disorders.
Nonsuppurative inflammation	Primarily small, mature-appearing lymphocytes and fewer plasma cells.	Lymphocytic, lymphoplasmacytic cholangiohepatitis. Rule out chronic lymphocytic leukemia and small cell lymphoma (see text).

*Minimal and/or multifocal infiltrates of any type are not reliably detectable by fine-needle aspiration cytology.

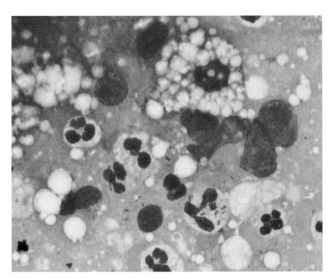

Figure 20-24 Numerous neutrophils are seen below a cluster of lipid-laden hepatocytes. Note the intracellular bacteria in one of the neutrophils. The cytologic diagnosis was suppurative inflammation associated with bacterial infection. This dog had pancreatitis, cholestasis, and ascending bacterial cholangiohepatitis. (Wright's stain, 1000×.)

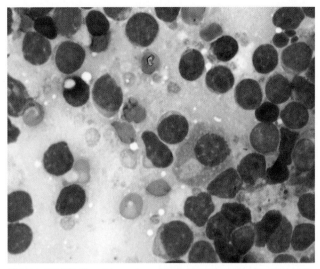

Figure 20-25 Small lymphocytes and a plasma cell are seen in this liver aspirate from an icteric cat. This finding could represent nonsuppurative inflammation or infiltration with neoplastic cells of well-differentiated lymphoma or chronic lymphocytic leukemia. The histologic diagnosis was lymphocytic plasmacytic cholangiohepatitis. (Wright's stain, 1000×.)

from livers with suppurative cholangiohepatitis typically include hepatocytes in addition to inflammatory cells (Figure 20-24). Abundant intracellular bile pigment and many bile casts are usually present because cholestasis is a common outcome of cholangiohepatitis. In most cases, aspiration of a suppurative exudate from a focal lesion indicates a hepatic abscess, and hepatocytes are few or absent in such aspirates. Phagocytized and extracellular bacteria are found in some aspirates.

Mixed Inflammation: Mixed inflammatory cell exudates are composed of neutrophils, eosinophils, macrophages, lymphocytes, plasma cells, and in some cases, multinucleated giant macrophages. The proportion of the exudate composed of each type of cell is variable and depends on the cause. Examples of diseases with mixed cell inflammation include feline infectious peritonitis, mycotic infection (i.e., coccidioidomycosis, histoplasmosis, aspergillosis), mycobacterial infection, protozoal infection (i.e., hepatozoonosis, leishmaniasis, cytauxzoonosis, and toxoplasmosis [see Figure 20-21]), drug and toxic injury, and systemic immune-mediated disorders. In some cases, the specific cause of mixed inflammation is still undetermined after liver biopsies have been examined histologically. The presence of many macrophages can be associated not only with inflammation, but also with hemolytic disease, necrosis, hemorrhage, or neoplasia.

Lymphocytic (Nonsuppurative) Inflammation: Hepatic infiltrates composed of numerous small lymphocytes and a few plasma cells are commonly recognized in cats (Figure 20-25), and in many cases, morphologic and biochemical evidence of cholestasis is present. These cytologic findings are typical of lymphocytic cholangiohepatitis in cats, but are also consistent with certain forms of lymphoid neoplasia (i.e., chronic lymphocytic leukemia [CLL] and small cell lymphoma). The lymphocytes in CLL and small cell lymphoma are morphologically indistinguishable from nonneoplastic lymphocytes; therefore other information must be considered to reach the correct diagnosis. CLL occurs in middle-aged to elderly cats and dogs and is characterized by persistent lymphocytosis and splenomegaly. Small cell lymphoma can usually be differentiated from lymphocytic cholangiohepatitis by examining a liver biopsy histologically and by immunophenotyping. If an infiltrate consists mostly of a single lymphoid lineage (e.g., CD3+ T-cells), lymphoma is likely, whereas a mixed lymphoid infiltrate (T- and B-cells) are more characteristic of inflammatory diseases. Lymphocytic cholangiohepatitis is more prevalent than either of the neoplastic lymphoproliferative disorders that can mimic its cytologic pattern. In most cases of hepatic lymphoma, the morphologic features of the infiltrating cells are sufficiently abnormal (i.e., they are typically large blasts) to distinguish them from inflammatory cells.

Eosinophilic Inflammation: A few conditions elicit a mixed-cell exudate rich with eosinophils. Liver fluke infestation, which is seen in cats in Florida and Hawaii, typically produces an exudate with a high percentage of eosinophils. Periportal infiltrates of eosinophils, lymphocytes, and plasma cells are found in some dogs and cats with eosinophilic enteritis.

NEOPLASTIC CONDITIONS (Table 20-4)

Differentiating primary and metastatic hepatobiliary tumors from the nonneoplastic diseases that resemble them poses a common diagnostic challenge. Other sources[25-29] provide the clinical and histologic characteristics of the

TABLE 20-4

Hepatic Neoplasms

Cell Type	Tumors
Discrete or round cell tumors (hemolymphatic)	Lymphoma, acute leukemias, mast cell tumor, histiocytic sarcoma, extramedullary plasmacytoma, multiple myeloma
Mesenchymal tumors	Primary hepatic: hemangiosarcoma, fibrosarcoma, leiomyosarcoma, osteosarcoma
	Metastatic: hemangiosarcoma, fibrosarcoma, melanosarcoma, osteosarcoma, leiomyosarcoma
Epithelial tumors	Primary hepatic: hepatoma, hepatocellular carcinoma, cholangioma, cholangiocarcinoma, cystadenoma, cystadenocarcinoma
	Metastatic: pancreatic, gastric, colon, renal, and mammary carcinomas
Endocrine/neuroendocrine tumors	Primary hepatic: carcinoid
	Metastatic: insulinoma, gastrinoma, phaechromocytoma, thyroid carcinoma, intestinal carcinoid

tumors and tumor-like masses, the cytologic features of which are described in this chapter.

Epithelial Tumors

Primary epithelial tumors of the hepatobiliary system in dogs and cats are hepatocellular adenomas and carcinomas and bile duct (cholangiocellular) adenomas and carcinomas. Hepatocellular and intrahepatic cholangiocellular carcinomas are classified based on gross appearance (i.e., massive, nodular, or diffuse).[30,31] Massive carcinomas produce one markedly enlarged liver lobe, which is the left lobe in many cases. Nodular carcinomas form multiple, discrete masses of different sizes that are distributed through several lobes and can resemble the multiple, regenerative nodules of cirrhotic livers. Diffuse carcinomas infiltrate large areas of the liver and are unencapsulated. Bile duct carcinomas also occur in extrahepatic bile ducts and gallbladder.

Most animals with diffuse and nodular carcinomas have extrahepatic metastases at the time of diagnosis. The lungs, peritoneum, and lymph nodes are common sites of metastases from these primary hepatobiliary carcinomas. The metastatic rate of the massive form is much lower than those of the nodular and diffuse forms and liver lobectomy greatly reduces tumor-related mortality.[32]

The liver itself receives metastases from carcinomas arising in other tissues. In many cases, cytologic examination of aspirates or imprints from hepatic masses can distinguish hepatocyte or biliary origin as opposed to metastatic.

Hepatocellular Neoplasia: Smears of aspirates and imprints of epithelial tumors typically are cellular and contain large multicellular clusters. Cells from hepatocellular adenomas and many carcinomas are sufficiently differentiated for their hepatocytic origin to be recognized. However, cells from adenomas and some well-differentiated hepatocellular carcinomas may be cytologically indistinguishable from normal hepatocytes or those from hyperplastic nodules. Features evident radiographically or ultrasonographically

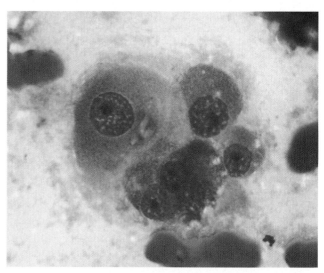

Figure 20-26 Hepatocellular carcinoma cells aspirated from one of several large nodules in the liver of a dog. The cells are recognizable as hepatocytes but display markedly atypical features indicative of malignancy. There is increased cytoplasmic basophilia and marked variation in cell size, nuclear size, and nuclear-to-cytoplasmic ratio. Nucleoli are very prominent. No inflammatory component is present. (Wright's stain, 1000×.)

may be similarly inconclusive. In these cases, histologic assessment of the architectural features of affected tissues offers the best chance for definitive diagnoses. The presence of hepatocytes with marked cytologic atypical (i.e., very large nuclei, high nuclear-to-cytoplasmic ratios, large nucleoli, deep blue cytoplasm, and marked variation in cellular and nuclear size within the population) provides a reasonable basis for a cytologic diagnosis of hepatocellular carcinoma (Figure 20-26). These tumors are not typically inflamed or necrotic, which helps distinguish them from hepatocellular regeneration in response to necrosis. If hepatocytes from a liver mass are not markedly atypical, the cytologic interpretation should acknowledge the possibility of nodular hyperplasia, hepatocellular adenoma, or well-differentiated carcinoma.

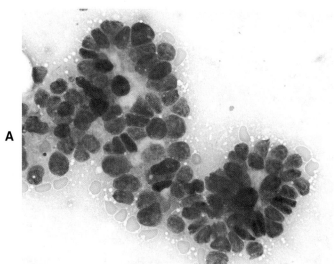

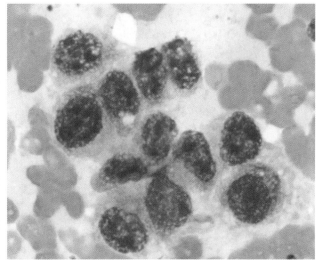

Figure 20-27 A, Aspirate from one of the many metastatic nodules in the liver of a dog with a pancreatic carcinoma. Note the acinar-like arrangement of the tumor cells. (Wright's stain, 500×.) **B,** Fine pink zymogen granules are present in the cytoplasm of these cells from a metastatic pancreatic carcinoma. Also note the high nuclear-to-cytoplasmic ratios and multiple prominent nucleoli. (Wright's stain, 1000×.)

Biliary Neoplasia: Cells exfoliated from well-differentiated cholangiocellular tumors (benign or malignant) are cuboidal to low columnar cells that are smaller than hepatocytes and arranged in sheets and clusters. Cells from these tumors can closely resemble normal biliary epithelia (see Figure 20-4). Tubular and acinar arrangements are evident in smears from some tumors. Nuclei are round to oval and have smooth, finely reticular chromatin. Nucleoli are inapparent in intact cells, and cellular and nuclear size are usually about that of normal biliary tract cells. Poorly differentiated biliary carcinomas cannot be clearly distinguished from other carcinomas by cytology alone (see subsequent discussion). Some benign and malignant cholangiocellular tumors contain cysts filled with acellular, yellow, watery or slightly mucinous fluid.

Aspirates from biliary cystadenomas and cystadenocarcinomas often consist primarily of fluid that may be mucinous, hemorrhagic, or clear. Similar fluid can be aspirated from nonneoplastic cysts and some cholangiocellular tumors; hence, aspirates of this type usually are inconclusive.

Metastatic Carcinomas: The cells of many carcinomas metastatic to liver are clearly identifiable as malignant but lack sufficient differentiation for a cytologic determination of specific tissue of origin (see subsequent discussion). In some cases of metastatic pancreatic carcinoma, acinar structures may be seen and tiny pink zymogen granules can be seen in the cytoplasm of highly basophilic epithelial cells (Figure 20-27) consistent with pancreatic tissue.

Undifferentiated Neoplasia: Aspirates and imprints from some hepatic masses consist of cells that are too poorly differentiated to be specifically identified as hepatocellular, cholangiocellular, or metastatic. Smears of anaplastic carcinomas usually contain large, dense clusters of adherent cells, indicating an epithelial origin (Figure

20-28). Individual cells are typically round and have high nuclear-to-cytoplasmic ratios, finely reticular chromatin, visible nucleoli in intact cells, and scant rims of blue cytoplasm. These features warrant a cytologic diagnosis of carcinoma of undetermined origin.

Neuroendocrine and Endocrine Tumors

Neuroendocrine tumors, or carcinoids, are derived from amine precursor uptake and decarboxylation (APUD) cells of the biliary system and occur in both dogs and cats.[33-35] In most cases, these tumors are found as multiple nodular masses dispersed throughout the liver, but they can also form masses in the extrahepatic bile ducts and gallbladder.[36] Metastatic tumors are present at diagnosis in nearly all animals with hepatobiliary carcinoids. Endocrine and neuroendocrine tumors that have metastasized from other sites also produce widely dispersed nodules. Pancreatic islet cell tumors are the most common type of metastatic endocrine tumor, but others include pheochromocytomas, gastrinomas, intestinal carcinoids, and thyroid carcinomas. Cells in smears generally can be identified as originating from neuroendocrine or endocrine tumors, but cytologic features alone are not specific enough to reliably differentiate among the several types. Cells are determined to originate from neuroendocrine tumors if they contain argyrophilic granules in sections stained with Grimelius' stain or argentaffin granules in sections stained with Fontana-Masson stain. The use of immunohistochemical procedures to demonstrate the presence of different hormones, such as gastrin, can also be helpful in identifying specific tumors.[34,35]

Smears of aspirates and imprints of neuroendocrine and endocrine tumors are usually very cellular, but the cells are quite fragile. Typically, a high percentage of the cells are partly or completely disrupted during smear preparation, and bare nuclei outnumber intact cells in some

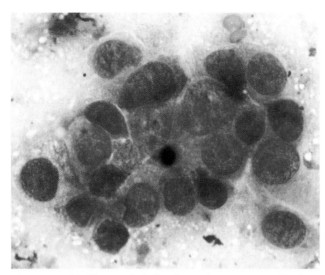

Figure 20-28 The epithelial cells in this aspirate of a liver mass from a dog are poorly differentiated and show cytologic features of malignancy. The cytologic diagnosis was carcinoma, further classified histologically as biliary carcinoma. (Wright's stain, 1000×.)

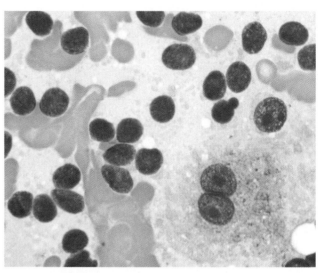

Figure 20-29 Aspirate from one of the numerous metastases in the liver of a dog with pancreatic gastrinoma. Note the numerous, bland, bare nuclei and the uniformity of nuclear size. Intact tumor cells had small amounts of pale blue cytoplasm. Two hepatocytes are at lower right. (Wright's stain, 1000×.)

smears (Figure 20-29). Cells in imprints tend to form a mosaic pattern. Aspirated cells occur individually, in small flat sheets or packets. Intact cells are round to polyhedral, with small to moderate amounts of pale blue or pink cytoplasm that may contain numerous vacuoles. Nuclei are round and centrally placed in many cells, and nuclear size variation often is minimal. Chromatin is lightly to coarsely stippled and nucleoli are not prominent.

Sarcomas

Malignant tumors of connective tissue origin can arise in the liver, but metastatic sarcomas are much more common. Hemangiosarcoma is the most common sarcoma involving the liver, where it can be either a primary or metastatic tumor. Smears of aspirates or imprints of hepatic sarcomas may contain few to many tumor cells, mostly depending on the density of cells in the sampled tissue and the amount of collagen surrounding the tumor cells. Frequently, aspirates from hemangiosarcomas consist largely of blood from cavernous sinuses within the tumor mass, with few to no identifiable tumor cells. Many erythrophagocytic macrophages may be present in such specimens. When present in smears, the tumor cells are spindle-shaped or stellate with tapering extensions of blue cytoplasm. Cell borders are indistinct, and nuclei are typically oval and placed near the center of the cell. Chromatin can be moderately condensed to finely reticular. Nucleoli can be inapparent or very prominent and large. Some sarcomas are quite uniform in cellular and nuclear size, whereas others display marked anisocytosis and anisokaryosis (Figure 20-30). Streaming bands of pink fibrillar extracellular matrix material (collagen) can be entwined between and around cells in many sarcomas, including hemangiosarcomas. Generally, the features of individual cells from the various sarcomas are not sufficiently distinctive for a specific diagnosis as to cell type of origin.

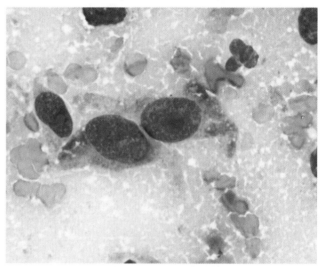

Figure 20-30 The aspiration of a liver mass from a cat collected numerous spindle cells as shown in this field. Marked anisocytosis and anisokaryosis with macronucleoli indicate a cytologic diagnosis of sarcoma; the histologic diagnosis was hemangiosarcoma. (Wright's stain, 1000×.)

Hemolymphatic Neoplasia

Lymphoma: Lymphoma is the most common neoplastic disease involving the liver in dogs and cats. In a small percentage of cases, the neoplastic lymphocytes are small, mature cells that are indistinguishable from normal lymphocytes. The differentiation of chronic lymphocytic leukemia from well-differentiated small cell lymphoma and lymphocytic cholangiohepatitis is discussed in the section on nonsuppurative inflammation. In most cases of hepatic lymphoma, the infiltrating lymphocytes have the cytologic features of blast cells, are larger than normal lymphocytes, and have finely or coarsely reticular chromatin and variable

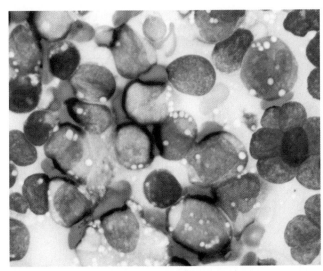

Figure 20-31 Aspirate from the liver of an 8-year-old dog. The neoplastic round cells have vacuolated cytoplasm and pleomorphic nuclei, but most resemble lymphoblasts. The cytologic diagnosis of lymphoma was confirmed on histologic examination. (Wright's stain, 1000×.)

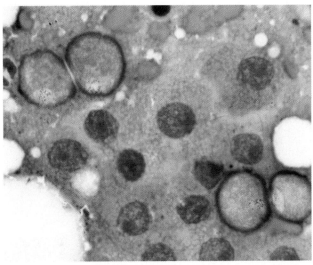

Figure 20-32 A cluster of hepatocytes is flanked by four large round cells in this aspirate from a 16-year-old Siamese cat with diffuse hepatomegaly. The cells have large nuclei with diffuse chromatin and visible nucleoli. Focal aggregates of fine red granules are clearly seen in three of these cells, which are diagnostic for a lymphoma of granular lymphocytes. (Wright's stain, 1000×.)

amounts of deep blue cytoplasm. Some hepatic lymphomas have nuclei with highly irregular contours that resemble monocyte nuclei (Figure 20-31). Cells from lymphoma of granular lymphocytes contain distinctive pink to red granules that vary in size, but are often found in a small area of cytoplasmic clearing adjacent to an indentation of the nucleus (Figure 20-32). Lymphoma of granular lymphocytes is a common neoplasm in cats and is less frequently seen in dogs. In cats, the tumor usually arises in the intestinal tract (jejunum, ileum, and duodenum) and metastasizes readily to the mesenteric lymph nodes, liver, and other sites. Most granular lymphomas in cats appear to be CD8+ cytotoxic T-cells, originating from an intraepithelial lymphocyte.[37] In some of these lymphomas, the granules can be quite large, red to magenta in color, and found within a distinct cytoplasmic vacuole. Lymphomas of granular lymphocytes can be misidentified as mast cells and, similar to poorly differentiated mast cells, rapid cytologic stains (e.g., Diff-Quik) will not stain the granules in some tumors. The presence of granular lymphocytes does not always indicate neoplasia; these cells can also be seen as part of an inflammatory response (e.g., secondary to hepatic necrosis).

Plasma Cell Tumors: These neoplasms of terminally differentiated B-cells can infiltrate the liver. Plasma cell tumors are of two types: extramedullary plasmacytomas (EMPs) and multiple myeloma.

EMPs are usually solitary dermal or mucocutaneous masses, often affecting the facial regions in dogs. The Cocker Spaniel appears to be predisposed. These tumors are considered benign and rarely metastasize. A visceral form of EMP has been reported in both dogs and cats. These typically arise in the gastrointestinal tract, including the rectum and stomach. Metastasis to the liver, local lymph nodes, and spleen can occur.

Multiple myeloma is a disseminated plasma cell neoplasm that predominantly involves the bone marrow.

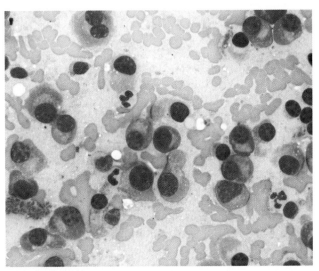

Figure 20-33 Neoplastic plasma cells aspirated from the liver of a 16-year-old cat with multiple myeloma. Although normal in size and echogenicity, both the liver and spleen had cytologically detectable infiltrates. The neoplastic cells are recognizable as plasma cells, but the cells and their nuclei are abnormally variable in size. (Wright's stain, 500×.)

Hepatic and splenic infiltrates are seen in some animals with multiple myeloma, particularly cats.[38] Plasma cells can be recognized by their characteristic morphologic features (i.e., eccentric round nuclei with coarsely clumped chromatin and a moderate amount of deep blue cytoplasm with a distinct perinuclear clear zone representing the Golgi apparatus) (Figure 20-33).

Aspirates of metastatic foci in the liver consist of numerous plasma cells, in the absence of significant numbers of lymphocytes. In some cases, the tumor cells show

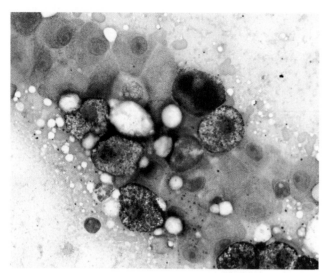

Figure 20-34 Numerous large, heavily granulated mast cells are seen interspersed among normal-appearing hepatocytes in this aspirate from the enlarged liver of a 17-year-old cat. Note the larger size and numbers of mast cells as compared with the normal resident type pictured in Figure 20-7. Splenomegaly and mastocytemia were concurrent findings. The diagnosis was systemic mastocytosis. (Wright's stain, 500×.)

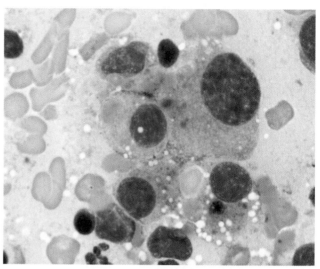

Figure 20-35 These cells were aspirated from one of the numerous nodular lesions in the liver of a 10-year-old Rottweiler with anemia and thrombocytopenia. Note the marked variation in nuclear size and the erythrophagocytic activity and hemosiderin in the cell at the lower right. The cytologic and histologic diagnosis was histiocytic sarcoma. The tumor also involved the spleen and bone marrow in this patient. (Wright's stain, 1000×.)

increased binucleation and anisokaryosis. The cells composing EMPs are often more variable than those in multiple myeloma; binucleated and multinucleated cells (with unequally sized nuclei) are common, as are pleomorphic nuclei. The tumor cells in both types of neoplasms can secrete excess quantities of a specific class of immunoglobulins, either IgA or IgG, resulting in a monoclonal gammopathy.

Acute Leukemias: The liver is a common site of infiltration in dogs and cats with acute leukemia (i.e., either acute myeloid leukemia [AML] or acute lymphoblastic leukemia [ALL]). In smears stained with routine blood stains, monoblasts and agranular myeloblasts can be indistinguishable from lymphoblasts; therefore additional information is needed to differentiate lymphoma from AML or ALL. Evaluating bone marrow and blood provides helpful information in many cases. Few to many blast cells circulate in the blood in all three diseases, but patients with acute leukemia are more likely than patients with lymphoma to have concurrent nonregenerative anemia, neutropenia, and/or thrombocytopenia. Cats with AML are likely to have macrocytosis. Bone marrow aspirates are definitive; marrows aspirated from most patients with AML or ALL are hypercellular with blast cells and almost completely lack cells of normal differentiation. Marrow from many patients with lymphoma contains a detectable, but highly variable, number of abnormal cells along with many normal hematopoietic cells. Cytochemical staining and immunophenotyping are other useful tools to identify the lineage of morphologically undifferentiated blast cells.

Mast Cell Tumors: Neoplastic mast cells can infiltrate the liver secondary to Grade II or III cutaneous mast cell

tumors or as part of the syndrome of visceral mastocytosis, which typically arises in the spleen and is unassociated with a primary skin tumor. Neoplastic mast cells must be differentiated from normal tissue residents. The latter are few in number in samples of normal liver, but can be quite numerous in certain inflammatory diseases or secondary to nonspecific hepatocellular injury. Resident mast cells typically are lightly granulated and have small round nuclei (see Figure 20-7 and discussion in Normal Findings section). Larger cells with more abundant cytoplasm are more likely to be neoplastic, particularly when seen in high numbers (Figure 20-34). Basophilic cytoplasm, binucleation, large/variably sized nuclei, and the presence of nucleoli are additional cytologic features that are indicative of malignancy. The number and size of the purple cytoplasmic granules are quite variable among individual cases and sometimes within the same tumor.

Histiocytic Neoplasia: Histiocytic sarcoma is a common tumor in Bernese Mountain dogs, Golden Retrievers, Labrador retrievers, and Rottweilers, arising from interstitial dendritic cells.[39] The tumor occurs in cats as well, but less frequently than in dogs.[40,41] Hepatic involvement has been reported with the disseminated form of this disease in both species. Cytologically, the tumor cells are generally large, round to oval cells with eccentric, oval to indented nuclei with lacey chromatin. The cytoplasm is abundant, light to medium blue, and often quite vacuolated. In some cases the tumor cells are highly hemophagocytic, resulting in a clinical presentation that must be distinguished from benign hemophagocytic and immune-mediated syndromes.[42,43] In many patients, the histiocytes have markedly abnormal features, such as giant, multiple nuclei; prominent nucleoli; and marked variation in cellular, nuclear, and nucleolar size (Figure 20-35). In other patients, the neoplastic cells do not appear remarkably different from inflammatory macrophages and the diagnosis can be more difficult. Demonstration of similar cells in other sites, such as the spleen (where they often are more abnormal in appearance) or bone marrow, helps support the diagnosis. In dogs, the immunophenotype CD18+, CD3-, and CD79a- is most useful in confirming a histiocytic origin in formalin-fixed histologic sections.[39] Cytochemical staining for nonspecific esterase activity is a useful adjunct for cytologic smears.

REFERENCES

1. Kristensen, et al: Liver cytology in cases of canine and feline hepatic disease. *Compend Cont Ed Pract Vet* 12:797-808, 1990.
2. Bunch SE, et al: A modified laparoscopic approach for liver biopsy in dogs. *J Am Vet Med Assoc* 187:1032-1035, 1985.
3. Nyland TG, Mattoon JS: *Small Animal Diagnostic Ultrasound*, ed 2. Philadelphia, Saunders, 2002, pp 30-48.
4. Hager DA, et al: Ultrasound-guided biopsy of the canine liver, kidney, and prostate. *Vet Radiol* 26:82-88, 1985.
5. Leveille R, et al: Complications after ultrasound-guided biopsy of abdominal structures in dogs and cats: 246 cases (1984-1991). *J Am Vet Med Assoc* 203:413-415, 1993.
6. Bigge LA, et al: Correlation between coagulation profile findings and bleeding complications after ultrasound-guided biopsies: 434 cases (1993-1996). *J Am Anim Hosp Assoc* 37:228-233, 2001.
7. Weiss DJ, et al: Characterization of portal lymphocytic infiltrates in feline liver. *Vet Clin Pathol* 24:91-95, 1995.
8. Scott M, Buriko K: Characterization of the pigmented cytoplasmic granules common in canine hepatocytes. *Vet Clin Pathol* 34(Suppl):281-282, 2005.
9. Rolfe DS, Twedt DC: Copper-associated hepatopathies in dogs. *Vet Clin North Am Small Anim Pract* 25:399-417, 1995.
10. Haywood S, et al: Hepatitis and copper accumulation in Skye terriers. *Vet Pathol* 25:408-414, 1988.
11. Webb CB, et al: Copper-associated liver disease in Dalmatians: A review of 10 dogs (1998-2001). *J Vet Intern Med* 16:665-668, 2002.
12. Mandigers PJ, et al: Association between liver copper concentration and subclinical hepatitis in Doberman pinschers. *J Vet Intern Med* 18:647-650, 2004.
13. Haynes JS: Wade PR: Hepatopathy associated with excessive hepatic copper in a Siamese cat. *Vet Pathol* 32:427-429, 1995.
14. Center SA: Feline hepatic lipidosis. *Vet Clin North Am Small Anim Pract* 35:225-269, 2005.
15. Van der Linde-Sipman et al: Fatty liver syndrome in puppies. *J Am Anim Hosp Assoc* 26:9-12, 1990.
16. Sepesy LM, et al: Vacuolar hepatopathy in dogs: 336 cases (1993-2005). *J Am Vet Med Assoc* 229:246-252, 2006.
17. Loeven KO: Hepatic amyloidosis in two Chinese Shar Pei dogs. *J Am Vet Med Assoc* 204:1212-1216, 1994.
18. Zuber: Systemic amyloidosis in Oriental and Siamese cats. *Aust Vet Pract* 23:66-70, 1993.
19. Kumar V, et al: *Robbins and Cotran Pathologic basis of disease*, ed 7. Philadelphia, Saunders, 2005, pp 3-46.
20. Zeiss CJ: The apoptosis-necrosis continuum: Insights from genetically altered mice. *Vet Pathol* 40:481-495, 2003.
21. Roth L: Comparison of liver cytology and biopsy diagnoses in dogs and cats: 56 cases. *Vet Clin Pathol* 30:35-38, 2001.
22. Wang KY: et al: Accuracy of ultrasound-guided fine-needle aspiration of the liver and cytologic findings in dogs and cats: 97 cases (1990-2000). *J Am Vet Med Assoc* 224:75-78, 2004.
23. Weiss DJ, et al: Cytologic evaluation of inflammation in canine liver aspirates. *Vet Clin Pathol* 30:193-196, 2001.
24. Cole TL, et al: Diagnostic comparison of needle and wedge biopsy specimens of the liver in dogs and cats. *J Am Vet Med Assoc* 220:1483-1490, 2002.
25. Hammer AS, Sikkema DA: Hepatic neoplasia in the dog and cat. *Vet Clin North Am Small Anim Pract* 25:419-435, 1995.
26. Thamm. In Withrow SJ, MacEwen D: *Small Animal Clinical Oncology*, ed 3. Philadelphia, Saunders, 2001, pp 327-334.
27. Strombeck and Guilford. In Guilford WG: et al: *Strombeck's Small Animal Gastroenterology*, ed 3. Philadelphia, Saunders, 1996, pp 847-859.
28. Patnaik AK: A morphologic and immunocytochemical study of hepatic neoplasms in cats. *Vet Pathol* 29:405-415, 1992.
29. Post G, Patnaik AK: Nonhematopoietic hepatic neoplasms in cats. *J Am Vet Med Assoc* 201:1080-1082, 1992.
30. Patnaik AK, et al: Canine hepatocellular carcinoma. *Vet Pathol* 18:427-438, 1981.
31. Patnaik AK, et al: Canine bile duct carcinoma. *Vet Pathol* 18:439-444, 1981.
32. Liptak JM, et al: Massive hepatocellular carcinoma in dogs: 48 cases. (1992-2002). *J Am Vet Med Assoc* 225:1225-1230, 2004.
33. Patnaik AK, et al: Canine hepatic carcinoids. *Vet Pathol* 18:445-453, 1981.
34. Patnaik AK, et al: Hepatobiliary neuroendocrine carcinoma in cats: A clinicopathologic, immunohistochemical, and ultrastructural study of 17 cats. *Vet Pathol* 42:331-337, 2005.
35. Patnaik AK, et al: Canine hepatic neuroendocrine carcinoma: An immunohistochemical and electron microscopic study. *Vet Pathol* 42:140-146, 2005.
36. Morrell CN, et al: A carcinoid tumor in the gallbladder of a dog. *Vet Pathol* 39:756-758, 2002.
37. Roccabianca P, et al: Feline large granular lymphocyte (LGL) lymphoma with secondary leukemia: Primary intestinal origin with predominance of a CD3/CD8αα phenotype. *Vet Pathol* 43:15-28, 2006.
38. Patel RT: et al: Multiple myeloma in 16 cats: A retrospective study. *Vet Clin Pathol* 34:341-352, 2005.
39. Affolter VK, Moore PF: Localized and disseminated histiocytic sarcoma of dendritic cell origin in dogs. *Vet Pathol* 39:74-83, 2002.
40. Affolter VK, Moore PF: Feline progressive histiocytosis. *Vet Pathol* 43:646-655, 2006.
41. Kraje AC, et al: Malignant histiocytosis in 3 cats. *J Vet Intern Med* 15:252-256, 2001.
42. Moore PF: et al: Canine hemophagocytic histiocytic sarcoma: A proliferative disorder of CD11d+ macrophages. *Vet Pathol* 43:632-645, 2006.
43. Weiss DJ: Flow cytometric evaluation of hemophagocytic disorders in canine bone marrow. *Vet Clin Pathol* 31:36-41, 2002.

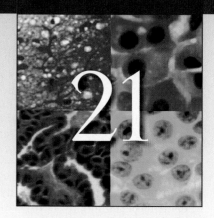

The Spleen

P.S. MacWilliams

CHAPTER 21

The spleen is part of the hemolymphatic system and consists of a cellular parenchyma of red and white pulp supported by a stroma of reticular fibers. It is surrounded by a connective tissue capsule containing variable amounts of smooth muscle. As a component of the hemolymphatic system, the spleen serves several purposes. In addition to an important role in the immune response, its functions include storage of platelets and mature red blood cells (RBCs); maturation of reticulocytes; phagocytosis and destruction of RBCs, platelets, white blood cells (WBCs), and foreign particles; and extramedullary hematopoiesis.[1] The nature of these functions causes the gross and microscopic appearance of the spleen to be affected by a variety of systemic inflammatory diseases and hematologic disorders. As with other organs, the spleen is subject to cell growth disturbances (e.g., hyperplasia, atrophy), circulatory abnormalities (e.g., hematoma, congestion, thrombosis, infarction), inflammation, and neoplasia (primary and metastatic).[2] Several of these processes, either alone or in combination, may result in splenic enlargement.

Splenomegaly is a common clinical abnormality in small animal practice and is usually detected by palpation or imaging techniques. Minor degrees of splenomegaly can be revealed radiographically or ultrasonographically. Depending on the cause, splenomegaly may be accompanied by hematologic abnormalities, such as hemolytic anemia, thrombocytopenia, leukopenia, leukemia, or hemolymphatic neoplasia.[3] A complete blood count and careful examination of RBCs, WBCs, and platelet morphology on a peripheral blood film are indicated. Causes of splenomegaly in dogs and cats are listed in Table 21-1.[2-4]

Once splenomegaly is detected, the specific cause should be determined, because splenic enlargement is usually a secondary manifestation of some other clinical problem. A complete physical examination and assessment of historic information are essential. Careful palpation and radiographic studies should reveal the severity of splenomegaly and whether the enlargement is diffuse and symmetric or localized to one area of the spleen (i.e., asymmetric). Ultrasonographic examination can be more sensitive and provides a more detailed assessment of architectural abnormalities in the spleen. By visualizing small nodules, target lesions, or changes in echogenicity in the spleen, ultrasound examination frequently reveals suspect areas of neoplasia, hyperplasia, inflammation, or extramedullary hematopoiesis that would not be visible radiographically. Indications for splenic aspiration are summarized in Box 21-1.[5]

Depending on presentation, a variety of diagnostic procedures may be useful. Immune-mediated causes of splenomegaly may be detected by tests for RBC antiglobulins (Coombs' test), antinuclear antibodies, or rheumatoid factor. Serologic tests may suggest fungal or protozoal infections. Blood films should be carefully searched for atypical WBC and RBC parasites, such as *Hemobartonella, Cytauxzoon,* or *Babesia* spp. Cytologic examination of bone marrow or lymph nodes is very useful in diagnosing hemolymphatic neoplasia and sometimes reveals infectious agents responsible for splenomegaly. Collection and cytologic evaluation of abdominal fluid are always indicated when splenomegaly is accompanied by peritoneal effusion. Serum chemistry assays and additional radiographic procedures may also contribute information to the diagnostic process.

COLLECTION OF SPLENIC SPECIMENS

Specimens for cytologic assessment of the spleen are derived from three sources: fine-needle aspirates, impression smears of surgical biopsies, and impression smears collected at necropsy.

Fine-Needle Aspiration

Aspiration of splenic samples through the abdominal walls of live animals should be carefully considered. An enlarged spleen can be turgid, friable, and engorged with blood. Profuse intraabdominal hemorrhage and tumor metastasis within the abdominal cavity are possible complications of this procedure; aspiration of the spleen should be considered carefully when hemangiosarcoma is suspected.[3,6] Recent studies in dogs and people concluded that thrombocytopenia, number of needle passes during collection, repeat aspirations, and core biopsies were not associated with an increase in the number or severity of complications.[7,8] In live dogs and cats, aspiration of

TABLE 21-1

Causes and Characteristics of Splenomegaly in Dogs and Cats[4]

Cause	Type of Enlargement	Severity of Enlargement
Hyperplasia	Symmetric	Mild to moderate
Infection		
Immunologic disease		
Extramedullary Hematopoiesis	Symmetric or nodular	Mild to moderate
Hemolymphatic Neoplasia	Symmetric	Moderate to severe
Lymphoproliferative neoplasms		
Myeloproliferative disorders		
Systemic mastocytosis		
Malignant histiocytosis		
Splenic Neoplasia	Asymmetric or nodular	Mild to severe
Hemangioma/hemangiosarcoma		
Fibrosarcoma		
Leiomyosarcoma		
Metastatic neoplasms		
Circulatory Disturbances		
Hematoma	Asymmetric	Mild to moderate
Portal hypertension	Symmetric	Mild to moderate
Torsion	Symmetric	Severe

BOX 21-1

Indications for Cytologic Examination of the Spleen[5]

Diffuse or symmetric enlargement
Splenic nodules or asymmetric enlargement
Radiographic evidence of abnormal splenic architecture
Abnormal ultrasonographic image of the spleen
   Hyperechoic or hypoechoic areas
   Abnormal variation in echogenicity
   Nodular or focal lesions
Detection of hemolymphatic neoplasia
Staging of hemolymphatic neoplasia

the spleen is indicated when the cause of splenomegaly cannot be determined by other means. The technique is especially useful in detecting splenic enlargement caused by hemolymphatic neoplasia and has some value in splenomegaly caused by infectious, immunologic, or hemolytic disease (see Table 21-1).

Aspiration of the spleen can usually be done without general anesthesia. The size and location of the spleen within the abdominal cavity determine the actual site for aspiration, and the surgical site is determined by where the spleen can be most easily apposed to the abdominal wall. The site is clipped and washed, and surgical disinfectant is applied. Infiltration of the abdominal wall with local anesthetic is usually unnecessary. Use of a 22- to 23-gauge needle with an attached 6- or 12-ml syringe is recommended. Needle length is determined by the size of the animal, but usually a 1- or 1½-inch needle is adequate.

The spleen is gently pressed against the abdominal wall at the prepared site. The needle with attached syringe is inserted through the skin and muscle layer into the spleen. Withdrawing the syringe plunger produces negative pressure while the needle is moved within the spleen along several axes. Maintaining suction while redirecting the needle in the parenchyma collects cells and tissue fragments from several areas. Negative pressure on the plunger should be released when a small amount of bloody fluid appears in the syringe tip. Excessive hemorrhage and dilution of the sample with blood should be avoided. It is very important to release the syringe plunger before the needle is withdrawn from the spleen. Immediately after withdrawing the needle from the animal, small drops of the aspirate are applied to glass slides. The consistency of the aspirated specimen determines the method of smear preparation.[9] Most splenic aspirates have the consistency of blood, and slides are prepared in the same manner as blood films. Specimens that are thick or contain tissue fragments are prepared by the squash technique, with the material gently compressed between two slides. The cells are spread by pulling the slides across each other. Chapter 1 contains a detailed description of slide preparation techniques.

Impression smears of splenic tissue from surgical biopsies or necropsy specimens have several uses. In some situations, an immediate diagnosis may be obtained. For example, a homogeneous population of large lymphoblasts (Figure 21-1) or a pure population of mast cells (Figure 21-2) confirms a diagnosis of lymphoma and mastocytoma, respectively. In other cases, cytologic findings may eliminate neoplasia from the differential diagnoses and allow other causes of splenomegaly to immediately be pursued.

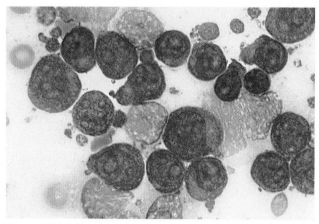

Figure 21-1 Fine-needle aspirate of spleen from a dog with lymphoma reveals a homogeneous population of lymphoblasts. Nucleoli are multiple and prominent. (Wright's stain, 1000×.)

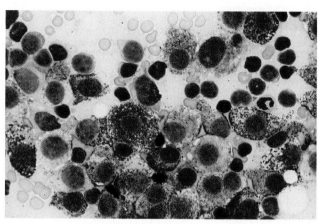

Figure 21-2 Fine-needle aspirate of spleen from a cat with marked symmetric splenomegaly caused by mast cell leukemia. The spleen is diffusely infiltrated with mast cells that have round nuclei and numerous intracytoplasmic purple granules. A group of small lymphocytes and a single neutrophil are noted in the upper right corner. (Wright's stain, 1000×.)

Impression Smears

Impression smears of splenic tissue reveal cellular details not visible in tissue sections and so are a valuable adjunct to histopathologic examination. Although tissue architecture is lost in collection, recognition of individual cell types, fungi, protozoa, RBC parasites, and neoplastic cell lines is sometimes easier on Wright's-stained slides and can complement histologic assessment. Impression smears and aspirates of spleen are especially valuable in differentiating various cell types (e.g., erythroid, granulocytic, lymphoid) of hemolymphatic neoplasms.

The most important aspect of making impression smears of splenic tissue is blotting the tissue on a paper towel to remove excess blood and tissue fluid before making tissue imprints on glass slides. A fresh-cut surface of the spleen is exposed by trimming the tissue with a scalpel blade. Cells are exfoliated by gently touching the blotted tissue surface to a glass slide.[9,10] Further details are described in Chapter 1.

Wright's stain or a similar Romanowsky stain (e.g., Diff-Quik) is the preferred stain for splenic cytology because it provides excellent definition of cytoplasmic features, and most veterinarians are familiar with its staining characteristics. Staining times with Wright's stain or Diff-Quik may need to be increased for slides that are more densely cellular than blood films. Chapter 1 contains specific information on staining techniques.

MICROSCOPIC EXAMINATION

Systematic examination of a well-stained slide that is representative of splenic parenchyma provides valuable information to identify the cause of splenomegaly or abnormalities in splenic imaging. Low-power objectives (4× and 10×) are used to assess cellularity and stain quality, locate cell clusters, and select slides and microscopic fields for further examination under higher magnification. The 40× and 100× objectives are used to assess general composition of the cell population and study nuclear and cytoplasmic details of individual cells. At these magnifications, it is helpful to find

a small lymphocyte or segmented neutrophil for size and color comparisons (Figures 21-3 to 21-5).

Interpretation of cytologic findings and differentiation of the various causes of splenomegaly require knowledge of the history, clinical signs, and laboratory results. Table 21-1 lists five general causes of splenic enlargement, but more than one mechanism may be operative in a given animal. For example, a dog with immune-mediated hemolytic anemia may have splenomegaly due to reactive hyperplasia and extramedullary hematopoiesis. Fine-needle aspirates of a symmetrically enlarged spleen are useful in identifying hyperplasia, extramedullary hematopoiesis, hemolymphatic neoplasia, and infectious agents such as *Histoplasma, Cytauxzoon,* and *Babesia* spp. For impression smears of biopsy or necropsy specimens, cytologic assessment is most useful for identifying protozoa and fungi and differentiating hyperplasia from extramedullary hematopoiesis, hemolymphatic neoplasia, and splenic neoplasia. Cytologic findings attributable to circulatory disturbances causing splenomegaly such as congestion, hematoma, torsion, or infarction are equivocal.

Figure 21-6 presents an algorithm for classification of splenic cytologic findings.

Normal Cytologic Features

Cytologic features of normal splenic aspirates and impression smears must be understood before abnormalities can be detected. Impression smears of normal splenic tissue have microscopic features similar to those of normal lymph nodes. Slides are usually very cellular because of a mixed population of small lymphocytes and lymphoblasts.[3,10] Variable shreds of connective tissue are often present consisting of fibrocytes and endothelial cells and adjacent lymphoid cells. Small lymphocytes predominate in most fields; however, because the spleen contains numerous lymphoid follicles with germinal centers, lymphoblasts may predominate in some microscopic fields

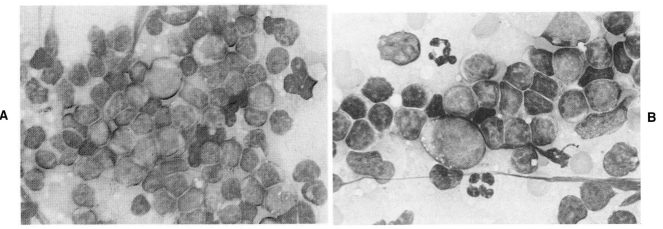

Figure 21-3 Impression smear of normal feline splenic tissue. **A,** The cell population is a mixture of small and large lymphocytes. The large cells in the center are lymphoblasts. The smaller cells with a small amount of light blue cytoplasm and smooth nuclear chromatin are small lymphocytes. (Wright's stain, 480×.) **B,** Higher magnification reveals several small lymphocytes, two neutrophils, and one lymphoblast (left). The lymphoblast is recognized by its large size, eccentric nucleus, and prominent nucleoli. (Wright's stain, 1000×.)

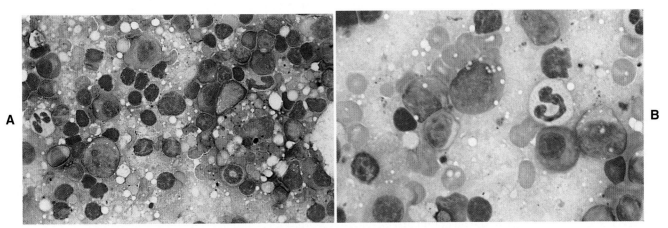

Figure 21-4 Fine-needle aspirate of hyperplastic splenic tissue from a dog with immune-mediated hemolytic disease. **A,** Small lymphocytes predominate, but increased numbers of lymphoblasts (lower left) and plasma cells (upper left) indicate hyperplasia. A large macrophage (lower right) contains many phagocytosed erythrocytes. (Wright's stain, 480×.) **B,** Higher magnification reveals two lymphoblasts (left) adjacent to a small lymphocyte. A neutrophil, plasma cell, and lymphoblast are located to the right of center. The plasma cell is recognized by its round, eccentric nucleus; smooth blue cytoplasm; and prominent Golgi zone. Compare the sizes of the neutrophil, plasma cell, lymphoblast, and lymphocyte. (Wright's stain, 1000×.)

using higher magnifications. Small lymphocytes are smaller than segmented neutrophils and have a round or slightly indented nucleus, dark condensed chromatin, and a thin rim of pale blue cytoplasm (see Figure 21-3). Lymphoblasts are identified by their large size, large irregular or indented nucleus, light-staining vesicular chromatin, multiple nucleoli, and basophilic cytoplasm. In addition to the lymphocyte population, a few macrophages and plasma cells may be observed, along with lesser numbers of neutrophils, mast cells, and platelet clumps. Some macrophages may contain cytoplasmic hemosiderin. The numbers of RBCs in

the background vary with the degree of splenic congestion and how well the cut tissue surfaces were blotted before making impression smears.

The microscopic appearance of fine-needle aspirates of splenic tissue is affected by the amount of hemodilution in the specimen. Experience with fine-needle aspirates of normal spleen is limited, and depending on the amount of blood contamination, the background contains varying numbers of RBCs, WBCs, and platelets. As in impression smears, the lymphoid population is mixed, with small lymphocytes predominating. Lesser numbers of

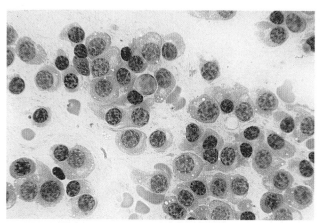

Figure 21-5 Impression smear of splenic tissue from a dog with multiple myeloma. The spleen is diffusely infiltrated by neoplastic plasma cells. With the exception of a small lymphocyte in the center, all of the cells are plasma cells. (Wright's stain, 480×.)

lymphoblasts are present, along with a few macrophages and plasma cells. Neutrophils, mast cells, endothelial cells, and fibrocytes are occasionally noted.[3,5]

Hyperplasia

Although considered a single category of splenomegaly, splenic hyperplasia results from a variety of inflammatory diseases, both septic and nonseptic. Mild to moderate degrees of splenomegaly are found in immune-mediated disorders and in systemic infectious diseases caused by bacteria, rickettsiae, protozoa, and fungi. Cytologic findings in hyperplastic splenomegaly depend on the causative agent, mechanism of disease, and host immune response. In general, splenic hyperplasia is characterized by increased numbers of macrophages, plasma cells, and lymphoblasts at the expense of small lymphocytes (see Figure 21-4).[3] Reduction in numbers of small lymphocytes is relative, however, and these cells remain the predominant cell type. A slight increase in neutrophil numbers is expected, and a marked increase in neutrophils indicates splenitis or abscessation. With chronic infections, the increase in macrophage and plasma cell numbers is often pronounced. When macrophages are prominent, it is important to examine their cytoplasm for cellular debris, pigment, phagocytized RBCs (see Figure 21-4), bacteria, and organisms such as *Histoplasma* (Figure 21-7, *A*) and *Leishmania* spp. (Figure 21-7, *B*). The RBCs in the background or within macrophages should be examined for *Mycoplasma (Haemobartonella)*, *Babesia* (Figure 21-8, *A*), and *Cytauxzoon* spp. (Figure 21-8, *B*) and Heinz bodies.[11] Leukocytes should be scrutinized for morulae of *Anaplasma phagocytophila (Ehrlichia)* (Figure 21-8, *C*) and *Hepatozoon* organisms (Figure 21-8, *D*).

Extramedullary Hematopoiesis

Extramedullary hematopoiesis is the development of sites of hematopoiesis outside of bone marrow and is frequently observed in dogs and cats with severe bone marrow disorders compromising production of blood cells or with chronic hemolytic anemias. The spleen is a frequent site of involvement, and splenomegaly and hypoechoic splenic foci are not unusual in animals with extramedullary hematopoiesis, either alone or in combination with reactive hyperplasia or neoplasia. In most situations, the predominant hematopoietic cell line is erythroid, with lesser numbers of megakaryocytes and granulocyte precursors.

Hematologic disorders frequently associated with extramedullary hematopoiesis include chronic hemolytic anemias, myeloproliferative disorders, lymphoproliferative neoplasia, and myelodysplastic syndromes.[12] Splenic hemangiosarcoma is usually accompanied by extramedullary hematopoiesis in dogs. In hemolytic anemias due to immunologic disease or infectious agents, the cytologic appearance is characterized by erythroid precursors (metarubricytes, rubricytes, prorubricytes, and a few rubriblasts) with a background of small and large lymphocytes (Figure 21-9). Macrophages containing hemosiderin and phagocytized RBCs are present. Metarubricytes are numerous and recognized easily, but the more immature erythroid cells can be confused with lymphoid cells. Features of immature RBCs differentiating them from lymphoid cells include a nearly round nucleus with irregularly clumped chromatin imparting a wheel-spoke or checkerboard appearance (see Figure 21-9). The cytoplasm is dark blue to blue-gray, depending on the stage of maturity, and may contain a juxtanuclear clear zone. When these cells are found in conjunction with myeloproliferative disease or lymphoid neoplasia in the spleen, erythroid precursors are mixed with the neoplastic cells. Asynchronous nuclear and cytoplasmic development is often present, especially in cats (see Figure 21-9).

Myelolipomas are benign nodular lesions that are observed incidentally in the spleen of dogs and occasionally in cats. Their cytologic appearance is characterized by marked extramedullary hematopoiesis with small groups of normal adipocytes. The key difference between myelolipomas and extramedullary hematopoiesis described previously is the presence of embedded fat tissue in the former.

Hemolymphatic Neoplasia

The normal spleen contains a mixed population of cells with a variety of sizes, shapes, and colors. When the spleen is enlarged because of lymphoproliferative neoplasia or a myeloproliferative disorder, the hallmark of the cytologic specimen is a very cellular slide containing a homogeneous population of neoplastic cells. Replacement of parenchyma with these cells is nearly complete, leaving only a few normal lymphoid cells and macrophages. The microscopic appearance of neoplastic cells depends on their cell type. Neoplasms identified frequently in the spleen include those derived from lymphocytes, erythroid precursors, granulocytes, histiocytes, and undifferentiated cells. Hematologic assessment, including blood and bone marrow and a battery of immunocytochemical stains, is sometimes necessary for definitive diagnosis.

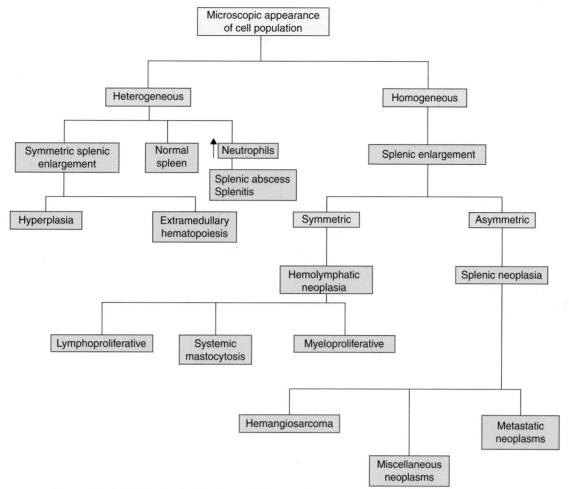

Figure 21-6 Cytologic classification of fine-needle aspirates and impression smears from the spleens of dogs and cats.

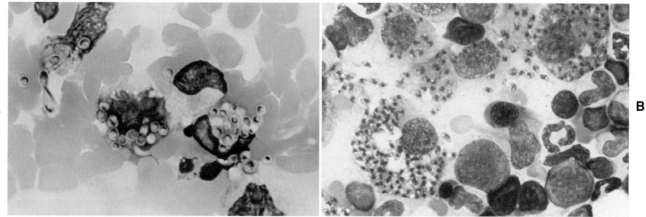

Figure 21-7 Recognition of infectious agents in spleen aspirates. **A,** Fine-needle aspirate of spleen from a dog with histoplasmosis. Macrophages contain phagocytosed *Histoplasma* organisms. One organism in the background (upper left) is budding. (Wright's stain, 1000×.) **B,** Impression smear of spleen from a dog with leishmaniasis. Numerous *Leishmania* amastigotes are present in macrophage cytoplasms and in the background. Plasma cells, neutrophils, and a few immature granulocytes are also noted. (Wright's stain, 1000×.)

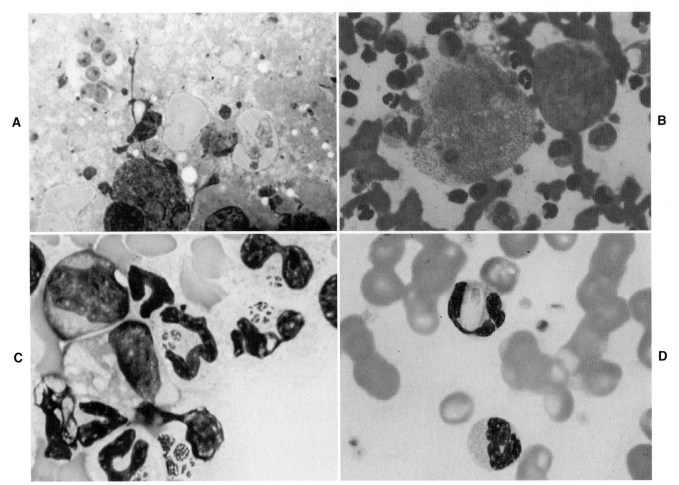

Figure 21-8 Hemotropic parasites that are observed occasionally in splenic aspirates or impression smears. Organisms that can be seen in the erythrocytes or leukocytes include *Babesia canis*, *Anaplasma phagocytophila*, and *Hepatozoan* spp. **A,** Impression smear of the spleen the from a dog with babesiosis. *B. canis* organisms are present in an erythrocyte and in the background. (Wright's stain, 1000×.) **B,** Two huge mononuclear cells with abundant cytoplasm, eccentric nuclei, and prominent nucleoli. These cells are macrophages containing many developing *Cytauxzoon* merozoites, which appear as either small, dark-staining bodies or larger irregularly defined clusters. (Wright's stain.) **C,** Morulae of *A. phagocytophila* are present on the cytoplasm of several neutrophils. (Wright's stain, 1000×.) **D,** A *Hepatozoon* organism is present in the cytoplasm of a neutrophil. Infected leukocytes can be seen in peripheral blood and may become entrapped in splenic sinusoids. Fine-needle aspirates of spleen are often diluted with peripheral blood. Red blood cells and platelets are present, indicating that some hemodilution has occurred. (Wright's stain, 1000×.)

In most dogs and cats with lymphoma and acute lymphocytic leukemia, normal cells are replaced by a homogeneous population of large, hyperchromatic lymphoblasts with abundant dark blue cytoplasm and large, round or indented nuclei containing multiple nucleoli (see Figure 21-1). Chronic lymphocytes, leukemia, and small cell lymphomas are more difficult to identify cytologically because these neoplasms have an abundance of small lymphocytes, which can be difficult to differentiate from the normal lymphoid population.

Splenic impression smears from cats with erythremic myelosis have numerous large round cells with round eccentric nuclei, fine granular chromatin, a single nucleolus, and dark blue cytoplasm containing a few fine red granules. In some cells, the cytoplasm contains a small localized clear zone (Figure 21-10). A few rubricytes and metarubricytes are present, with frequent examples of asynchronous maturation of the nucleus and cytoplasm.

Neoplastic cells can be derived from granulocytes, monocytes, plasma cells, mast cells, histiocytes, or primitive, undifferentiated cells. Splenic cytology is characterized by a monotonous population of the involved cell type displacing normal cells (see Figures 21-2, 21-5, 21-11, and 21-12).

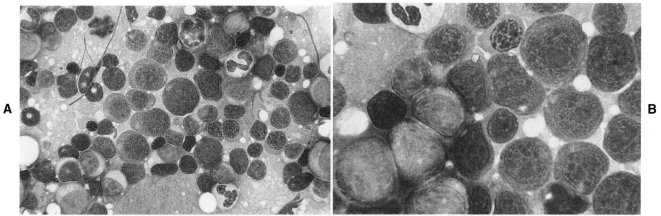

Figure 21-9 Feline splenic tissue with extramedullary hematopoiesis. **A,** Most of the cells are erythroid precursors at various stages of development, with a few neutrophils and several lymphocytes (lower right). The large round cells in the center are rubriblasts and prorubricytes. (Wright's stain, 480×.) **B,** Comparison between lymphoid cells (lower left) and erythroid precursors. An immature erythroid cell at the rubriblast and prorubricyte stage has a round nucleus, dark basophilic cytoplasm, coarse granular or loosely clumped chromatin, and when present, a single nucleolus. The metarubricyte at the top of the field has an immature nucleus in well-differentiated cytoplasm (nuclear-cytoplasmic asynchrony). (Wright's stain, 1200×.)

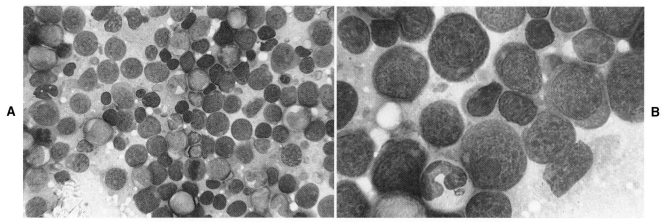

Figure 21-10 Impression smears of splenic tissue from a cat with erythremic myelosis. **A,** The normal cell population is displaced by many large hyperchromatic round cells. There is no differentiation toward more mature forms in the erythroid series. (Wright's stain, 480×.) **B,** The primitive cells in this myeloproliferative disorder are similar to rubriblasts. Morphologic features include a round nucleus with coarse granular chromatin, a large single nucleolus, and dark blue cytoplasm with a prominent clear zone. (Wright's stain, 1200×.)

Splenic Neoplasia

Primary neoplasms of the spleen include hemangiosarcomas, leiomyosarcomas, fibrosarcomas, undifferentiated sarcomas, and miscellaneous tumors.[12] Hemangiosarcomas can be recognized on impression smears. Specimens must be blotted well to remove excess blood, because these neoplasms have a rich blood supply. Slides made from scrapings of fresh-cut surfaces of tissue are frequently superior. The microscopic appearance of hemangiosarcomas is typical of mesenchymal neoplasms. Cells exfoliate individually or as aggregates associated with vascular structures. Tumor cells are very pleomorphic and hyperchromatic, with marked anisokaryosis. Some cells are fusiform, with indistinct borders, and others are irregularly shaped, with angular margins. Giant forms are not unusual. Nuclei are round to oval, with variable chromatin patterns and many large, pleomorphic nucleoli. Cytoplasm is light blue and clear (Figure 21-13). Erythroid precursors are often present, indicating extramedullary hematopoiesis.

Fibrosarcomas and leiomyosarcomas occur less frequently than hemangiosarcomas and have the cytologic appearance of spindle cell tumors. The diagnostic criteria discussed in Chapter 2 can be used to identify these tumors. Fibrosarcomas are further discussed in Chapter 5.

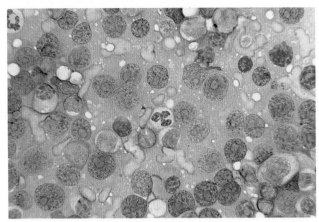

Figure 21-11 Impression smear of splenic tissue from a cat with an undifferentiated hemolymphatic neoplasm. A neutrophil and several small lymphocytes in the center are surrounded by primitive cells with indistinct cell margins, round nuclei, vesicular chromatin, and a single prominent nucleolus. (Wright's stain, 480×.)

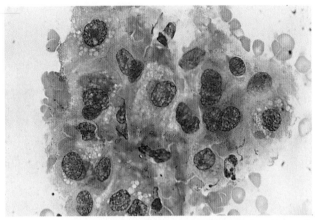

Figure 21-12 Fine-needle aspirate of spleen from a dog with malignant histiocytosis. Lymphoid cells normally present in the spleen have been replaced by pleomorphic cells characterized by marked anisocytosis, indistinct cell margins, cytoplasmic vacuolation, anisokaryosis, and irregular chromatin clumping. (Wright's stain, 1000×.)

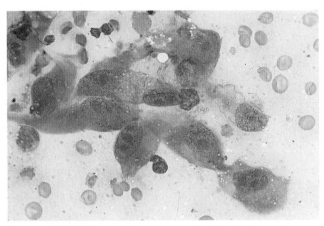

Figure 21-13 Impression smear of splenic tissue from a dog with hemangiosarcoma. The cells have features of connective tissue malignancy, such as anisocytosis, indistinct cell margins, anisokaryosis, and variance in nucleolar size, shape, and number. (Wright's stain, 1000×.)

References

1. Banks WJ: *Histology and Comparative Organology: A Text-Atlas.* Huntington, Krieger, 1980, pp 131-143.
2. Valli KVF, Jubb. In et al: *Pathology of Domestic Animals,* vol 3, ed 3. Orlando, Academic Press, 1985, pp 94-114, 194-200.
3. Feldman and Zinkl. In Ettinger SJ: *Textbook of Veterinary Internal Medicine,* ed 2. Philadelphia, Saunders, 1983, pp 2067-2076.
4. Lipowitz et al. In Slatter D: *Textbook of Small Animal Surgery.* Philadelphia, Saunders, 1985, pp 1204-1218.
5. Christopher MM: Cytology of the spleen. *Vet Clin North Am Small Anim Pract* 33:135-152, 2003.
6. Osborne CA, et al: Needle biopsy of the spleen. *Vet Clin North Am* 4:311-316, 1974.
7. O'Keefe DA, Couto CG: Fine-needle aspiration of the spleen as an aid in the diagnosis of splenomegaly. *J Vet Int Med* 1:102-109, 1987.
8. Lal A, et al: Splenic fine needle aspiration and core biopsy: A review of 49 cases. *Acta Cytol* 47(6):951-959, 2003.
9. Meyer: The management of cytology specimens. *Comp Cont Ed Pract Vet* 9:10-17, 1987.
10. Rebar AH: *Handbook of Veterinary Cytology.* St. Louis, Ralston Purina, 1979.
11. MacWilliams PC: Erythrocytic rickettsiae and protozoa of the dog and cat. *Vet Clin North Am Small Anim Pract* 17:1443-1461, 1987.
12. Spangler WL, Culbertson MR: Prevalence, type, and importance of splenic diseases in dogs: 1,480 cases (1985-1989). *J AM Vet Med Assoc* 200:829-834, 1992.

The Kidneys

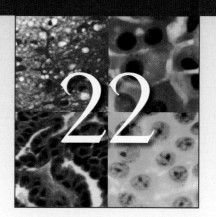

CHAPTER 22

P.J. Ewing, J.H. Meinkoth, R.L. Cowell, and R.D. Tyler

Cytologic examination (e.g., fine-needle biopsy [FNB]) can be a useful tool in diagnosing certain renal lesions, especially neoplasms, in dogs and cats. The advantages and disadvantages of FNB (cytology) as compared with incisional biopsy (histopathology) of the kidney are presented in Table 22-1. Although the examination of cytologic specimens does not provide the cellular architecture necessary to characterize many lesions in which structural relationships are important, it can sometimes provide sufficient diagnostic information to aid in the clinical management of cases and is less invasive and associated with fewer complications than full tissue biopsy. Major complications resulting from FNB of the kidney are uncommon if appropriate procedures are followed.[1]

Disease conditions that are most likely and least likely to yield diagnostic cytologic results are presented in Boxes 22-1 and 22-2. The primary indication for FNB is abnormally sized or shaped kidneys. Cytologic specimens from patients with unilateral or bilateral renomegaly are most likely to yield diagnostic information; small or shrunken kidneys rarely yield positive diagnostic findings. Either fluid or solid tissue lesions may be encountered, and the results of cytologic analysis can help characterize the process as cystic, inflammatory, or neoplastic. Renal cytology is especially useful for the rapid confirmation of renal lymphoma in cats. Although positive cytologic findings are useful in establishing a diagnosis, tentative diagnoses cannot always be excluded based on negative findings because representative material may not have been recovered during collection attempts.

Collecting adequately cellular specimens for evaluation is a limiting factor of renal cytology. FNB of the kidney is easier in cats because their kidneys are more easily palpated and immobilized against the body wall. Using ultrasound to detect optimal sites for specimen collection and to provide additional information about the nature and extent of lesions can significantly increase diagnostic yield. Because of the highly vascular nature of the kidneys, blood contamination is a significant problem during sample collection. Use of a nonaspiration (i.e., capillary action) technique (see Chapter 1) facilitates the collection of cellular specimens that are not heavily contaminated with blood. Highly cellular, solid lesions (e.g., neoplasms) are also more likely to provide cellular samples than many degenerative or inflammatory diseases.

SAMPLING TECHNIQUE

FNB is associated with less tissue trauma than punch biopsies, and there are few contraindications for collecting cytologic specimens from the kidneys. Contraindications for renal FNB are listed in Box 22-3. As with other renal biopsy procedures, the main complication is excessive hemorrhage.[1] Patients should be evaluated for the presence of coagulation defects prior to the procedure; adequate restraint is necessary to prevent unexpected movement during the procedure, and the kidney must be adequately immobilized against the body wall. Seeding of the needle tract with neoplastic cells during fine-needle sampling of malignant lesions has been suggested as a complication; however, clinical experience and results of retrospective studies in humans show such seeding to be uncommon.[2,3]

A blind, percutaneous technique can be used if the lesion appears diffuse (i.e., generalized renomegaly), and the kidney can be immobilized against the wall of the abdomen. The concurrent use of ultrasound to facilitate sample collection is preferred, and tranquilization, sedation, or anesthesia is used as necessary to adequately restrain the patient, preventing unexpected movement during the procedure.

The skin at the site is clipped and prepared as for surgery. The patient is usually restrained in lateral recumbency, and the kidney is manually immobilized against the body wall. As mentioned previously, a nonaspiration technique is preferred to help limit the amount of blood contamination.[4] A 22- or 23-gauge needle attached to a 10- to 12-ml syringe that has been prefilled with air is held at the base of the needle with the thumb and forefinger. Depending on the type of lesion, the needle is directed either into the lesion (focal lesions) or tangentially into the cortex of the kidney (diffuse lesions). Care should be taken to avoid the renal hilus, which contains large vascular structures. The needle is passed through approximately two-thirds the thickness of the lesion about five to seven times with a stabbing motion. The repeated needle punctures should be along a single plane (similar to the action

TABLE 22-1

Advantages and Disadvantages of Renal Cytology as Compared with Incisional Biopsy

Advantages	Disadvantages
Less invasive, fewer complications	Does not allow for assessment of tissue architecture
Less expensive	Does not allow for evaluation of glomeruli
Rapid diagnosis of some conditions such as feline lymphoma	Blood contamination and low cell yield often limit usefulness

---

BOX 22-1

Conditions *Most* Likely to Yield Diagnostic Renal Aspirates

Unilateral renomegaly
Bilateral renomegaly
Solid mass lesions:
  Neoplasms (especially lymphoma)
  Abscesses
  Fungal granulomas

BOX 22-2

Conditions *Least* Likely to Yield Diagnostic Renal Aspirates

Small or shrunken fibrotic kidneys (end-stage kidneys)
Renal tubular degeneration/necrosis
Interstitial nephritis
Glomerulonephritis

BOX 22-3

Contraindications for Renal Aspiration Cytology

Marked thrombocytopenia (platelet count <50,000/μl)
Platelet function disorder (increased buccal mucosal bleeding time)
Coagulopathy (one-stage prothrombin time or activated partial thromboplastin time prolonged >20%)
Patients at high risk for anesthesia/sedation
Obstructive uropathy (severe hydronephrosis or septic pyonephrosis) if risk of abdominal cavity contamination is high

---

of a sewing machine) to minimize blood vessel rupture. Samples may be collected from different portions of the lesion using multiple (two or three) collection attempts. Collection of several slides (at least five) from different areas of the lesion helps increase the chances of obtaining a diagnostic specimen. Whenever blood is visible in the hub of the needle or syringe, collection should be stopped and the material spread onto a glass slide because continued collection attempts usually result in gross blood contamination, rendering the sample worthless.

After collection, the material in the needle (none is usually visible in the syringe) should be carefully dispersed on one end of a glass slide and gently spread out using a slide-over-slide technique (see Chapter 1). If fluid is obtained, direct and line smears should be made, and the remainder of the fluid put into an ethylene-tetra-acetic acid (EDTA) tube. If the fluid is clear (suggesting low cellularity) and there is sufficient sample, concentrated sediment smears, which are similar to urine sediments, are prepared and air-dried.

Impression smears can be made from renal biopsy specimens or kidneys removed at surgery or necropsy before the specimen is fixed in formalin for histologic analysis. Before the impression smears are made, excess blood should be gently blotted from the tissue to increase the number of cells that transfer to the glass slides. Any time there is sufficient tissue for histologic analysis, it should be submitted in case the cytologic preparations are nondiagnostic. Samples for histologic and cytologic examination must be mailed in separate packages because formalin fumes (even from sealed containers) will partially fix the cells on unstained smears, making evaluation impossible.

CYTOLOGIC EVALUATION

Normal and Abnormal Cell Types Encountered

Findings in normal renal aspirates are listed in Table 22-2. Renal tubular epithelial cells are the predominant cell type seen in specimens from normal kidneys. They are rather large, round to polygonal cells that occur singly and in clusters (Figure 22-1). They have a round, centrally placed nucleus and abundant light blue cytoplasm, which, in cats, often contains several distinct, clear vacuoles from the presence of lipid droplets (Figure 22-1, *B*). Clear cytoplasmic vacuoles may also occur in dogs with diabetes mellitus, long-term exposure to corticosteroids, or lysosomal storage disease (Box 22-4). Cells of the distal convoluted tubules and ascending limb of the loop of Henle may contain dark intracytoplasmic granules (Figure 22-1, *C*).[3]

Differentiation of the various epithelial cell types is not practical or of diagnostic importance. The cells and their nuclei should be relatively uniform in size and shape; however, the different types of epithelial cells differ slightly in size. The nuclear-to-cytoplasmic ratio of normal tubular cells is low, and tubular cells that are well spread out often have a single, visible nucleolus (see Figure 22-1). When present, nucleoli should be small and round. Renal tubular cells often remain together as recognizable tubule fragments of various sizes (Figure 22-2). Tubular casts may also be seen in renal aspirates from some animals (Figure 22-3).

TABLE 22-2

Findings in Normal Renal Aspirates

Cell Types or Structures	Appearance	Comments
Renal tubular epithelial cell (see Figure 22-1)	Medium to large, round to polygonal cells that occur singly and in clusters; central round nucleus with single visible nucleolus, light blue cytoplasm, which may have clear vacuoles (cats)	Predominant cell type seen
Intact renal tubules (see Figures 22-2 and 22-3)	Densely packed cells as described above arranged in tubular arrays	Variably present
Glomeruli (see Figure 22-4)	Lobulated clusters of slender, oval to spindle-shaped cells	Infrequently seen
Collagen matrix	Strands of homogeneous, acellular pink material	Absent or present in only small amounts; collagen obtained from renal capsule or interstitium
Peripheral blood	Many erythrocytes with platelet aggregates and leukocytes (neutrophils, lymphocytes, and monocytes)	Marked blood contamination is common; subjective assessment of types and number of leukocytes present is only way to differentiate blood contamination vs. inflammation

Their significance depends on the amount and type of cast present, similar to those in urine sediments. Glomeruli may be seen in cellular samples and appear as somewhat lobulated clusters of slender, spindloid cells (Figure 22-4).[5] Individual cells are difficult to see because they are tightly clustered. Abnormalities of the glomeruli (e.g., glomerulonephritis) are not readily discernible cytologically and require histologic analysis. A few homogeneous strands of acellular pink matrix (collagen) may be seen in normal renal aspirates. The matrix is typically obtained as the needle passes through the fibrous capsule of the kidney.

Some degree (often marked) of peripheral blood contamination is always present in renal aspirates. Various peripheral blood leukocytes (i.e., neutrophils, small mature lymphocytes, monocytes, and possibly eosinophils) and platelets will be present as a result of peripheral blood contamination. A subjective assessment of the number and type of leukocytes present compared with the amount of peripheral blood on the slide is the only way to assess whether the leukocytes most likely represent blood contamination or renal inflammation. Inflammation is suggested by a disproportionate number of leukocytes relative to red blood cells (RBCs) or the presence of cells not associated with peripheral blood (e.g., overt plasma cells, vacuolated/phagocytically active macrophages). Plasma cells are lymphoid cells with eccentric nuclei, increased amounts of deeply basophilic cytoplasm (compared with small lymphocytes), and a perinuclear clear area (Figure 22-5). Macrophages, which must be differentiated from peripheral blood monocytes, have more abundant cytoplasm that may have phagocytized cellular debris or many small vacuoles (see Figure 22-13). Macrophage nuclei are usually round, unlike irregular, pleomorphic monocyte nuclei. Additionally, finding neutrophils with degenerate changes (e.g., swelling of the nuclear lobes) and phagocytized bacteria (see Figure 22-13) is abnormal and indicates septic inflammation.

Small mature lymphocytes, which are approximately 10 μm in diameter (slightly smaller than neutrophils) and have only scant amounts of basophilic cytoplasm, are often present as the result of blood contamination. Their deep purple nuclei are round and slightly indented (see Figure 22-5). The presence of reactive lymphocytes (Figure 22-6) or prolymphocytes, which are slightly larger than small mature lymphocytes, suggests inflammatory infiltrates. Their nuclei are larger, stain a less dense color, and do not have prominent nucleoli. These cells also have moderately increased amounts of blue cytoplasm. Lymphoblasts are usually seen in cases of renal lymphoma. These cells are distinctly larger than the other lymphoid cells (larger than neutrophils) and have prominent nucleoli and less dense nuclear chromatin. Their cytoplasm is more abundant, is deeply basophilic, and often completely encircles the nucleus (Figure 22-7, *B*).

Cytologic Characteristics of Solid Lesions

Cytologic preparations from enlarged or abnormally shaped kidneys or discrete, solid kidney masses are evaluated for the presence of neoplasia or inflammatory responses (Figure 22-8).

Neoplasia: Confirming neoplasia from a patient with renomegaly or a renal mass is a situation in which renal cytology is most likely to be diagnostically rewarding.[1] Renal lymphoma is the most common neoplastic disease affecting feline kidneys and may occur as a single, discrete nodule but more often causes diffuse renal enlargement (typically bilateral).[6] It is not usually limited to the kidneys. Aspirates are of high cellularity and consist almost entirely of lymphoid cells. In most cases, the majority of these cells (>80%) are large lymphoblasts (i.e., lymphoblastic lymphoma) (see Figure 22-7). Lymphoid cells are fragile and slides may contain many ruptured cells. Nearly all cells

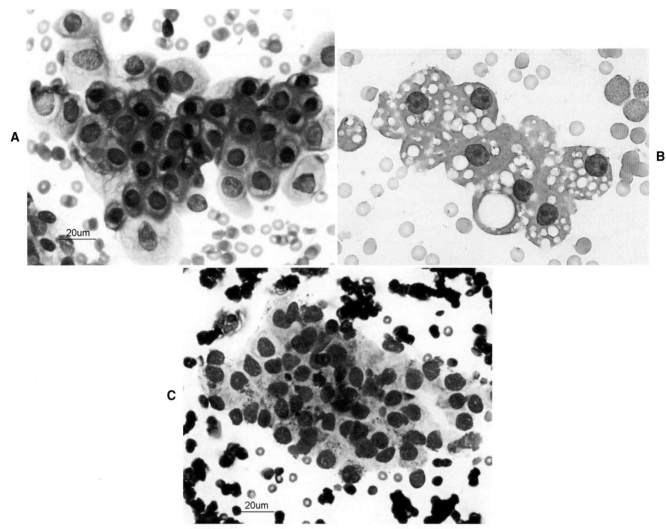

Figure 22-1 A, Renal FNB from a dog. Numerous renal tubular cells showing mature, uniform nuclei with dark, mature chromatin. (Wright-Giemsa stain.) **B**, Renal FNB sample from a cat. Note the cluster of renal tubular epithelial cells with some blood contamination; feline renal tubular cells are often vacuolated. Nucleoli are visible but are small and round. (Wright's stain, original magnification 330×.) **C**, Cluster of renal tubular cells from a renal FNB sample from a cat. The cells are mature and uniform and show cytoplasmic granules. (Wright-Giemsa stain.)

BOX 22-4

Causes of Clear Vacuoles in Renal Tubular Epithelial Cells

Normal cat renal proximal tubular cells (lipid)
Diabetes mellitus in dogs (lipid)
Long-term exposure to corticosteroids in dogs (glycogen)
Lysosomal storage disorders – congenital or drug-induced (lipid or glycogen)

---

may be ruptured if downward pressure is applied to the spreader slide during slide preparation. Depending on the degree to which the tumor has replaced normal tissue in the area sampled, renal tubular cells may be present. Slides made from animals with lymphoma are often very thick, and in many areas the cells are not well spread out. In such

areas, it is difficult to accurately classify the lymphoid cells. Lymphoblasts that are not well spread out appear smaller; their nucleoli are indistinct, and it is difficult to determine the amount of cytoplasm present. Thus it is imperative to find thin areas of the smear where the cells have assumed their normal morphology. Forms of lymphoma in which the neoplastic cell populations cytologically appear as pro-lymphocytes or small lymphocytes occur, but these forms are much less common. In such cases, it may be difficult to differentiate these lesions from severe lymphoid infil-trates resulting from chronic inflammatory conditions. Inflammatory lesions typically result in lower numbers of lymphoid cells admixed with normal renal tubular cells. A mixture of small lymphocytes, prolymphocytes, and some plasma cells may be present. Lymphoma is suggested if there is a dense, monotonous population of lymphoid cells in an extremely cellular smear from an enlarged kid-ney, but histologic confirmation is often warranted.

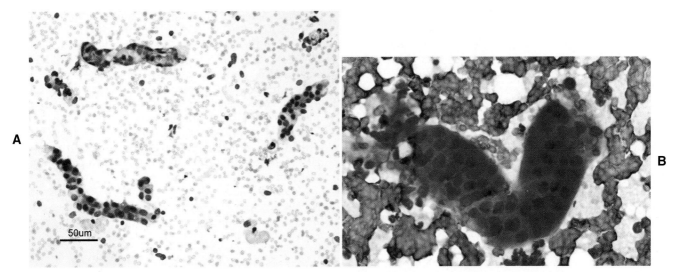

Figure 22-2 A, Small tubular fragments in a renal FNB from a dog. (Wright's stain, original magnification 50×.) **B,** Higher magnification of tubular fragment in a renal FNB from a cat. Dark nuclei of individual tubular cells are visible, but cell margins are difficult to discern. (Wright's stain, original magnification 500×.)

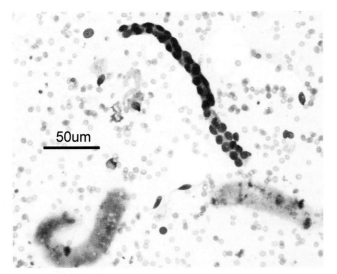

Figure 22-3 A renal tubular fragment and two casts in a renal FNB from a dog. (Wright's stain, original magnification 50×.)

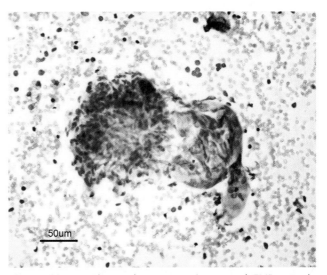

Figure 22-4 A glomerulus present in a renal FNB sample from a dog. (Wright's stain, original magnification 50×.)

Unlike in humans, more than 90% of primary renal tumors in dogs and cats are malignant.[6] Carcinomas (e.g., tubular adenocarcinomas, transitional cell carcinomas) are the most common primary renal neoplasms of dogs and cats, but the overall incidence of renal cancer is fairly low (approximately 1% of all cancers). A diagnosis of carcinoma is made from smears containing a population of epithelial cells that demonstrate adequate criteria of malignancy (see Chapter 2). Aspirates from renal carcinomas are often of much higher cellularity than aspirates from normal kidneys or renal inflammatory diseases and yield a dense population of renal epithelial cells (Figure 22-9, *A*). Some well-differentiated renal carcinomas may yield a majority of cells that are somewhat uniform, and cells demonstrating criteria of malignancy must be found among uniform cells. Poorly differentiated carcinomas may show marked atypia (Figure 22-10). Adrenal carcinomas may be

encountered in animals with masses in the kidney area. If a blind aspirate is performed, these carcinomas are difficult or impossible to differentiate from renal carcinomas. Adrenal cortical cells are larger and have more abundant cytoplasm that often contains many fine vacuoles (Figure 22-11).[5,7] Adrenal carcinomas should be considered if the patient shows clinical evidence of hyperadrenocorticism; diagnostic imaging studies can help identify the location of the tumor in such cases.

Nephroblastoma is an uncommon embryonal tumor that occurs primarily in the kidney and thoracolumbar region of young dogs, but has also been reported to occur as a primary renal tumor of cats.[8,9,10] Nephroblastomas typically present as a solitary unilateral mass at one pole of kidney located primarily in the cortex with possible extension through the capsule. Aspirates or impression smears of nephroblastomas are highly cellular and composed of

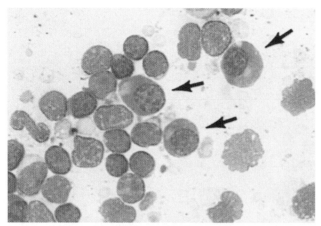

Figure 22-5 Plasma cells *(arrows)* characterized by an eccentric round nucleus with abundant, deep blue cytoplasm and a prominent, clear Golgi apparatus, and small lymphocytes. (Wright's stain, original magnification 250×.)

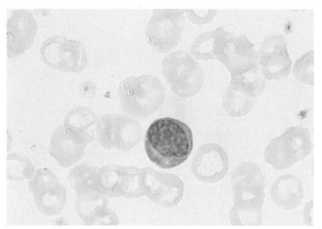

Figure 22-6 A reactive lymphocyte. (Wright's stain, original magnification 250×.)

numerous large (12 to 30 μm in diameter) mononuclear, round to oval cells arranged individually and in clusters of few to many cells. They exhibit mild to moderate anisocytosis and anisokaryosis and a variable but high nuclear-to-cytoplasmic ratio. The cells have eccentrically located round, oval, or pleomorphic nuclei with a finely granular to smudged chromatin, single to multiple small nucleoli, and a scant rim of basophilic and occasionally vacuolated cytoplasm. Nuclear molding and pseudorosette formation may be evident. Small spindloid cells with dark nuclei are frequently intermixed with the round to oval mononuclear cells.[9,10]

Mesenchymal tumors are uncommon, accounting for about 20% of renal malignancies (Figure 22-12).[6] Mesenchymal tumors of the kidney may be primary or metastatic.[8,11,12]

Inflammation: Most inflammatory diseases affecting the kidney (e.g., chronic interstitial nephritis, pyelonephritis, glomerulonephritis) are diagnosed based on history, physical examination findings, and ancillary diagnostic procedure results. Cytologic examination is not usually indicated in such conditions; however, inflammatory responses are occasionally encountered in aspirates from clinical cases or impression smears taken at necropsy. Because kidneys are highly vascular, nearly all renal aspirates contain some inflammatory cells secondary to peripheral blood contamination. A diagnosis of inflammation depends on the presence of cells not typically found in blood (e.g., plasma cells, macrophages) or greater numbers of inflammatory cells than expected from the degree of blood contamination.

Purulent inflammation is denoted by a marked predominance of neutrophils (usually >90%) with only scattered macrophages and suggests inflammation produced by pyogenic bacteria (Figure 22-13) but may also result from noninfectious causes. Many species of pyogenic bacteria, which are usually the result of ascending infection

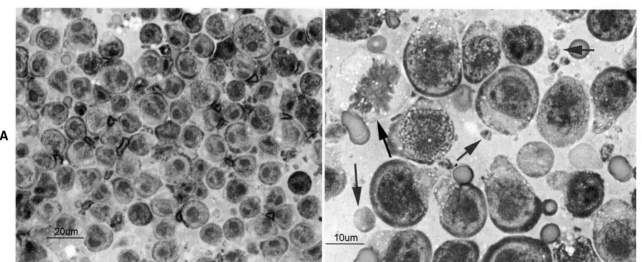

Figure 22-7 FNB samples from a cat with renal lymphoma presenting as bilateral renomegaly. **A,** The specimen is densely cellular with a population of discrete cells. (Wright-Giemsa stain.) **B,** More than 90% of the cells present are lymphoblasts. Numerous lymphoglandular bodies are present *(red arrows)*. One mitotic figure is seen *(black arrow)*. (Wright-Giemsa stain.)

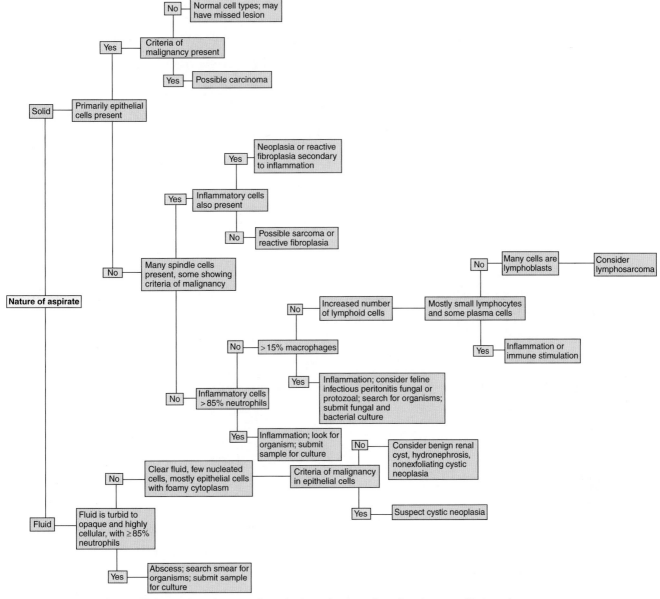

Figure 22-8 An algorithm to aid cytologic evaluation of renal aspirates and impression smears.

from the lower urinary tract, but may also be of hematogenous origin, have been cultured from dogs with acute pyelonephritis. Increased percentages of macrophages (>15%) are seen in cases of pyogranulomatous and granulomatous inflammation. Feline infectious peritonitis is one cause of such lesions that should be considered in cats with appropriate clinical features (Figure 22-14). Slides should also be searched for the presence of fungal organisms. Yeast phases of *Blastomyces dermatitidis, Cryptococcus neoformans, Coccidioides immitis, Histoplasma capsulatum,* and the alga *Prototheca zopfii* (refer to Chapter 3) have all been found in the kidneys of animals with disseminated disease, although such organisms are more commonly encountered in other tissues. Fungal hyphae (Figure 22-15) may occasionally be found in imprints or aspirates, but culture is necessary to further identify the fungus.

Inflammatory infiltrates characterized by a predominance of small, mature lymphocytes and plasma cells are typical of chronic inflammatory lesions and must be differentiated from cases of renal lymphoma, as previously discussed.

Cytologic Characteristics of Fluid Lesions

Fine-needle aspiration can be performed to collect samples for cytologic examination and bacterial culture from animals with fluid lesions (e.g., hydronephrosis or abscesses).

Cysts: In humans, renal cysts are a commonly reported cause of space-occupying kidney lesions and have also been reported in domestic animals. Renal cysts can be

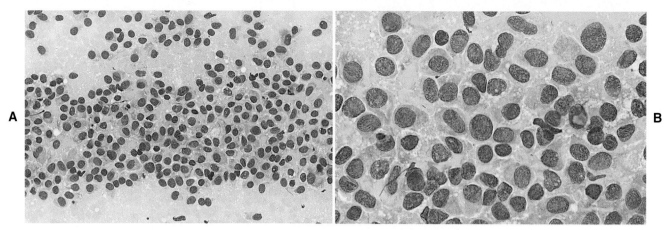

Figure 22-9 FNBs from a mass involving the right kidney of a dog. **A,** The samples are highly cellular, consisting of a single population of epithelial cells. (Wright's stain, original magnification 100×.) **B,** The epithelial cells present show criteria of malignancy, allowing a diagnosis of carcinoma. Histopathologic examination confirmed a renal carcinoma. (Wright's stain, original magnification 250×.)

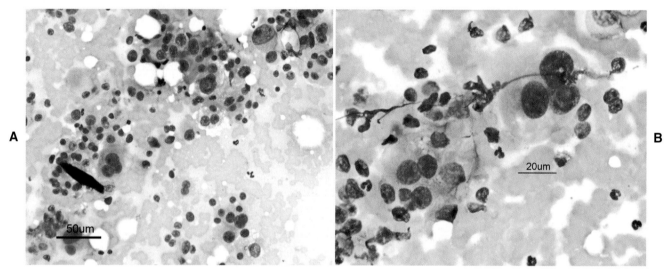

Figure 22-10 FNBs from a German Shepherd with renal cystadenocarcinoma. **A,** Slides are highly cellular and display marked atypia, including marked anisocytosis, marked anisokaryosis, multinucleation, and large prominent nuclei. (Wright-Giemsa stain.) **B,** Higher magnification shows multiple large, irregularly shaped nucleoli. (Wright-Giemsa stain.)

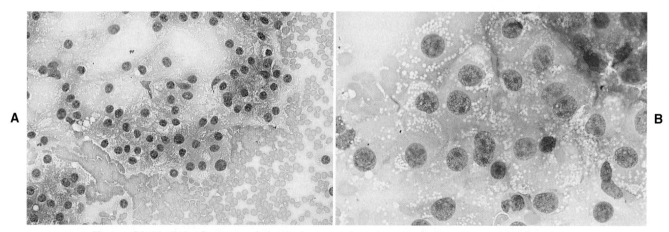

Figure 22-11 FNBs from an abdominal mass of a dog displaying signs of Cushing's syndrome. An ultrasound examination revealed an extremely large right adrenal gland mass. The left adrenal gland could not be seen. **A,** Samples are highly cellular and consist of finely vacuolated epithelial cells. (DipStat, original magnification 100×.) **B,** Cells show moderate variability and prominent nucleoli. Some extremely large cells displaying macronuclei were present in other fields. (DipStat, original magnification 250×.)

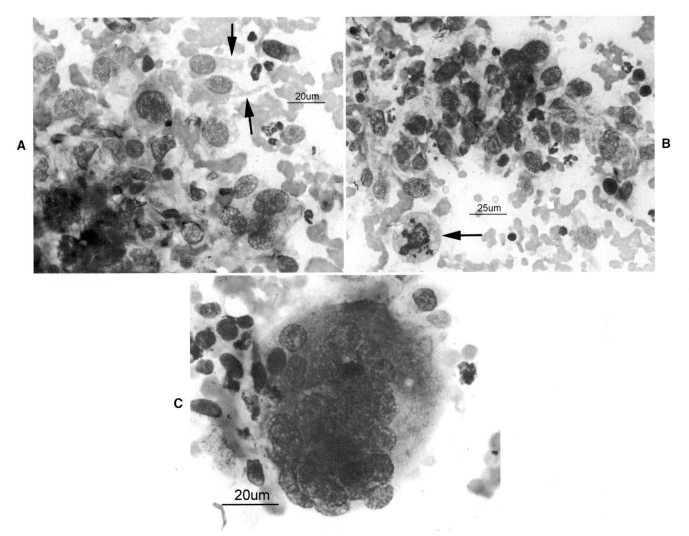

Figure 22-12 FNBs from a renal sarcoma (suspected malignant fibrous histiocytoma) from a cat. **A,** Aspirates are highly cellular and show a pleomorphic population of mesenchymal cells. Tapered cytoplasm is evident in some cells *(arrows)*. Most cells have large, prominent nucleoli. (Wright-Giemsa stain.) **B,** Image showing pleomorphic mesenchymal cells and a bizarre mitotic figure *(arrow)*. (Wright-Giemsa stain.) **C,** Large multinucleated giant cells containing >20 nuclei are common, suggesting malignant fibrous histiocytoma. Further diagnostics were not performed. *(Courtesy Dr. Robin Allison.)*

single or multiple, congenital or acquired, and they frequently do not cause symptomatic disease. They can enlarge and induce a local tissue hypoxia, however, either resulting in overproduction of erythropoietin with resultant polycythemia or causing sufficient loss of parenchyma due to pressure atrophy that renal failure eventually develops. Aspiration of renal cysts may be performed to rule out other causes of renal enlargement and evaluate for secondary bacterial infection. Benign cysts contain a clear, straw-colored fluid that is of low cellularity but may contain a few cuboidal, epithelial lining cells. These cells occur singly and generally have foamy cytoplasm and a low nuclear-to-cytoplasmic ratio with absent or small nucleoli. A few neutrophils and macrophages may also be present.

Some renal carcinomas are cystic and must be differentiated from benign cysts. Exfoliated cells should be evaluated for malignant changes (see Chapter 2), but not all cystic neoplasms exfoliate recognizably malignant cells into the fluid.

Hydronephrosis: Hydronephrosis is the dilation of the renal pelvis and the associated parenchymal atrophy and cystic enlargement of the kidney that result from an obstruction of urine flow. The obstruction can be complete or partial, arise suddenly or progressively, and occur at any level of the urinary tract. A variable amount of clear fluid is recovered from aspiration, and smears of this fluid contain few cells; there may be a few inflammatory cells and epithelial lining cells. High numbers of inflammatory cells are seen with secondary infections. The causes of hydronephrosis, which may be radiographically distinguished from renal cysts, include ectopic ureters, calculi, neoplasia, prostatic hyperplasia, pregnancy, and inadvertent surgical ligation of the ureter.

Abscesses: Renal abscesses occur infrequently in dogs and cats, but may occur secondary to a septic process such as pyelonephritis. The physical appearance of the aspirated material is like that of any other purulent exudate. Cytologically, the smears are very cellular and typically consist of >85% neutrophils with varying numbers

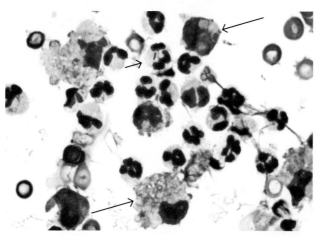

Figure 22-13 FNB from the kidney of a dog with septic pyelonephritis. The smears are highly cellular and contain degenerate neutrophils, some of which contain phagocytized bacterial rods *(short arrow)*. Macrophages containing cytoplasmic vacuoles or phagocytized cellular debris are present in lesser numbers *(long arrows)*. (Diff-Quik, original magnification 1000×.)

of macrophages (see Figure 22-13). A search should be made for infectious agents, and material should be submitted for culture and sensitivity. Identifying bacterial rods or cocci helps in choosing antibiotic therapy while awaiting culture and sensitivity results. With hematologic stains, bacteria (both gram-positive and gram-negative) stain blue-black (see Figure 22-13). If bacterial rods (especially bipolar rods) are seen cytologically, an antimicrobial effective against gram-negative bacteria should be used while culture and sensitivity results are awaited. The pathologic bacterial cocci are generally *Staphylococcus* and *Streptococcus* spp.; therefore when bacterial cocci are seen cytologically, an antimicrobial effective against gram-positive bacteria should be used while culture and sensitivity results are awaited.

Cytologic Characteristics of Crystals

Crystals are rarely encountered in FNB of normal or diseased kidneys. Calcium oxalate monohydrate crystals may be seen in FNB or impression smears of kidneys from dogs or cats with oxalate nephrosis, which occurs most commonly in ethylene glycol–poisoning cases. The calcium oxalate monohydrate crystals may appear as flat, elongate structures with pointed ends that resemble a picket fence or as groupings of crystals that resemble sheaves of wheat (Figure 22-16). The crystals exhibit birefringence when viewed under polarized light (Figure 22-16, *B*).

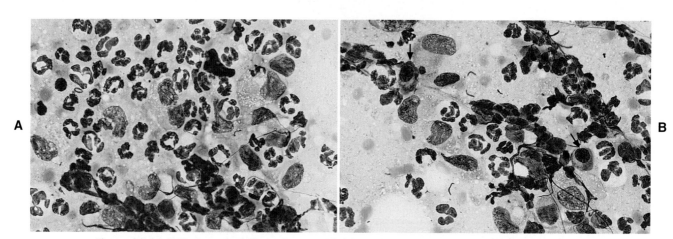

Figure 22-14 FNBs from the kidney of a cat with feline infectious peritonitis. The smears were highly cellular and contained a pyogranulomatous inflammatory response. **A,** Nondegenerate neutrophils and numerous macrophages are shown. In other areas of the smear, macrophages predominate. (Diff-Quik, original magnification 250×.) **B,** Same slide as **A,** similar cell population as **A.** Note the presence of two mature plasma cells *(arrows)*. (Diff-Quik, original magnification 250×.)

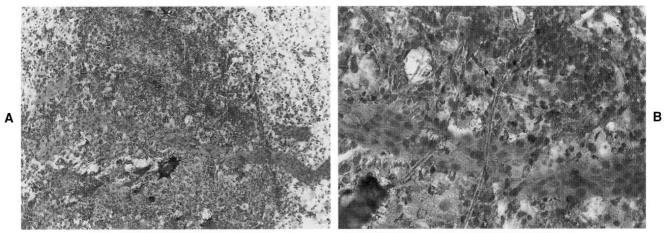

Figure 22-15 Impression smears taken at necropsy from the kidney of a dog. **A,** Highly cellular smear with recognizable tubules and fungal hyphae. (Wright's stain, original magnification 33×.) **B,** Higher magnification of the same area. (Wright's stain, original magnification 200×.)

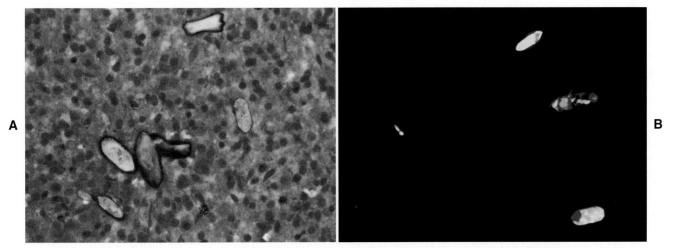

Figure 22-16 Impression smears taken at necropsy from the kidney of a dog. **A,** Highly cellular smear with degenerate tubular epithelial cells and calcium oxalate monohydrate crystals. (Wright's stain, original magnification 500×.) **B,** Lower magnification of crystals as viewed under polarized light demonstrating birefringence. (Wright's stain, original magnification 250×.)

References

1. Bartges, Osborne CA. In Osborne CA, Finco DR: *Canine and Feline Nephrology and Urology.* Philadelphia, Lea & Febiger, 1995, pp 277-303.
2. Leiman G: Audit of fine needle aspiration cytology of 120 renal lesions. *Cytopathology* 1:65-72, 1990.
3. Nguyen GK: Percutaneous fine-needle aspiration biopsy cytology of the kidney and adrenal. *Pathol Annu* 1:163-197, 1987.
4. Menard M, Papageorges M: Technique for ultrasound-guided fine needle biopsies. *Vet Radiol Ultrasound* 36:137-138, 1995.
5. DeMay RM: *The art and science of cytopathology.* Chicago, ASCP Press, 1996, pp 1083-1134.
6. Withrow SJ. In Withrow SJ: MacEwen DM: *Small animal clinical oncology.* Philadelphia, Saunders, 1989, pp 380-385.
7. Barton: Cytology of the endocrine and neuroendocrine tumors. *Vet Can Soc Newsletter* 17:5-9, 1993.
8. Henry CJ, et al: Primary renal tumors in cats: 19 cases (1992-1998). *J Feline Med Surg* 1(3):165-70, 1999.
9. Gasser AM: et al: Extradural spinal, bone marrow, and renal nephroblastoma. *J Am Anim Hosp Assoc* 39(1):80-5, 2003.
10. Neel J, et al: A mass in the spinal column of a dog. *Vet Clin Pathol* 29(3):87-89, 2000.
11. Munday JS, et al: Renal osteosarcoma in a dog. *J Small Anim Pract* 45(12):618-22, 2004.
12. Hahn KA, et al: Bilateral renal metastases of nasal chondrosarcoma in a dog. *Vet Pathol* 34(4):352-326, 1997.

Examination of the Urinary Sediment

J.G. Zinkl

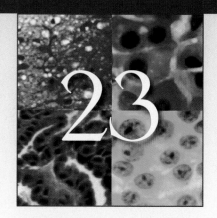

CHAPTER 23

SPECIMEN COLLECTION

Urine must be properly collected to ensure that urinalysis results are reliable. It can be collected in four ways (Table 23-1): catching a sample during urination, expressing the bladder, catheterization, and cystocentesis.[1] Cystocentesis and catheterization are the preferred methods because both provide optimal samples for all aspects of urinalysis by avoiding contamination from the lower genital tract and external genitalia. Although it may be easier to express the bladder or catch a sample during urination, urine collected in these ways may be limited for analysis (particularly for a bacterial culture). Urinalysis is usually performed on preprandial, morning samples, because they tend to be the most concentrated, thus increasing the chance of finding abnormalities.

Fresh urine samples are best for cytologic examination because cell morphology is altered when cells remain in contact with urine for an extended period of time. When applicable, obtaining cells directly from a mass (i.e., traumatic catheterization and ultrasound-assisted fine-needle aspiration biopsy [FNAB]) usually produces a cellular sample with the best morphology for cytologic examination.

Voided Sample

Voided samples, which are collected as an animal urinates, are the simplest samples to obtain. A sample collected in this manner usually is not satisfactory for bacteriologic examination because the sample is often contaminated during urination. Occasionally, the voided samples have increased numbers of white blood cells (WBCs) and epithelial cells due to contamination from inflammatory lesions of the external genitalia or reproductive tract, but other evaluations are unaffected. A voided sample is collected in a clean, although not necessarily sterile, container. Ideally, the vulva or prepuce should be washed to decrease sample contamination. A midurination (i.e., midstream) sample is best because there is less chance of contamination.

Expressing the Bladder

Urine may be collected from small animals by external, manual compression of the bladder. As with collecting voided samples, the external genitalia should be cleaned

before collection. With the animal standing or in lateral recumbency, the bladder is palpated in the caudal abdomen, and urine is expelled by applying gentle, steady pressure. Care must be taken not to exert too much pressure, which could injure or rupture the bladder. This method should never be used on an animal with an obstructed urethra.

Catheterization

Urine may be collected by inserting a catheter of rubber, plastic, or metal into the bladder via the urethra. As in the previous two methods, the external genitalia should be cleaned before the procedure. Sterile catheters are used and sterile gloves worn. Care must be taken to maintain sterility and prevent trauma to the urinary tract. The catheter should pass easily through the urethra. A small amount of sterile, water-soluble lubricating jelly (e.g., K-Y Jelly [Johnson & Johnson Medical Inc, Arlington, Tex.]) should be placed on the tip of the catheter. Because the distal end of many catheters will accept a syringe, urine can be collected with gentle aspiration.

Cystocentesis

Cystocentesis is often used to collect sterile urine samples from dogs and cats. Sometimes as much urine as possible is removed from the bladder to prevent pressure on the bladder wall and urine leakage though the hole created by the needle. Unless the bladder is markedly extended, however, a volume of urine (5 to 10 ml) sufficient to perform urinalysis and culture can be removed without damaging the bladder or causing urine to leak through the bladder wall.

MICROSCOPIC EXAMINATION OF URINE SEDIMENT

Microscopic examination of urine sediment is extremely important, especially for recognizing diseases of the urinary tract. In addition, urine sediment examination is occasionally an aid in diagnosing systemic disease. The best urine samples for sediment examination are morning samples or samples obtained after several hours of water deprivation

TABLE 23-1		
Methods of Urine Collection with Advantages and Disadvantages of Each		
Method	**Advantages**	**Disadvantages**
Voided	Noninvasive, does not require special expertise, can be collected by owner	Contaminated by urethra and prepuce, therefore can have increased RBC and/or WBC due to urethral or prepucial inflammation and is not recommended for culture when cystitis is suspected
Expressing the bladder	Noninvasive, requires only minimal expertise, can be performed at time of examination	Contaminated by urethra and prepuce, therefore can have increased RBC and/or WBC due to urethral or prepucial inflammation and is not recommended for culture when cystitis is suspected
Catheterization	Semi-invasive, requires less expertise than cystocentesis, can be performed at time of examination	Some contamination, but less than voided or expressed urine, can contribute to development of cystitis after catheterization
Cystocentesis	Best for urine culture, less likely to cause cystitis than catheterization, can be performed at time of examination	Invasive but seldom causes cystitis, requires greater expertise than other methods of urine collection

Courtesy R.D. Tyler and R.L. Cowell.

because such samples are more concentrated and the chances of finding formed elements is increased. Urine collected by cystocentesis is the best sample for microscopic examination. The urine sample should be fresh because changes may occur as a sample ages. Samples can be capped and refrigerated for a short time before they are examined, although refrigeration usually increases the numbers of crystals.

Urine obtained from healthy dogs and cats does not contain much sediment. Small numbers of epithelial cells, mucous threads, red blood cells (RBCs), WBCs, hyaline casts, and various types of crystals can be found in the urine of most healthy animals. Bacteria and squamous epithelial cells derived from external genital surfaces may be present in voided and catheterized urine.

In order to semiquantitatively test the formed elements in urine, a standard volume, usually 5 ml, is centrifuged to obtain the sediment on every sample. Then 5 ml of a well-mixed sample is placed in a graduated, conical centrifuge tube and centrifuged for 3 to 5 minutes at approximately 100 G (about 1000 to 2000 rpm depending upon the radius of the centrifuge). The procedure should be standardized for a particular centrifuge to yield uniform results. Some centrifuges such as the Clay-Adams Triac (Becton Dickinson, Parsippany, NJ) are precalibrated to provide the proper force over sufficient time to completely sediment the formed elements in the urine. After centrifugation, the volume of sediment is recorded. The supernatant is gently poured out, leaving about 0.3 ml of urine adhering to the sides of the tube. This urine is allowed to run down the inside of the centrifuge tube, and the sediment is resuspended by gently flicking the bottom of the centrifuge tube.[2]

The sediment may be examined either stained or unstained. When examining unstained sediment, a small drop of the resuspended sediment is placed on a clean glass slide and covered with a coverslip. Microscopic examination should be conducted immediately. For bright field microscopy, subdued light that partially refracts the elements is used to examine unstained urine sediment. Proper lighting is achieved by partially closing the iris diaphragm and moving the substage condenser downward. Properly adjusted phase-contrast microscopy allows for better distinction of elements than reduced illumination with bright field microscopy. However, phase-contrast microscopes are slightly more expensive than bright field microscopes, and they require more precise adjustment in order to properly illuminate objects in urine sediment.

Stained sediment may also be examined. Satisfactory stains include Sternheimer-Malbin stain (Sedi-Stain, Becton Dickinson, Rutherford, NJ) or 0.5% new methylene blue. A drop of stain is added to and mixed with the suspended sediment before a drop of sediment is placed on a slide. When a stained specimen is examined, illumination is less critical than when an unstained specimen is examined; however, reduced illumination further aids visualization of substances by providing contrast.

The specimen is scanned under low power using the 10× objective in order to find the plane where the material has settled, determine the amount of sediment, and find larger elements such as casts or aggregates of cells. The entire area under the coverslip should be examined because casts tend to float to the coverslip's edge. Casts and some crystals are usually identified at low power and are usually reported as the average number seen per low-power field (LPF). A higher-power objective (e.g., 40×) is necessary to detect bacteria, identify some crystals, and differentiate cell types. Epithelial cells, RBCs, and WBCs are reported as the average number seen per high-power field (HPF). Bacteria are reported as few, moderate, or many, and their morphology (i.e., cocci, bacilli, filamentous) is noted.

URINARY SEDIMENT

Cells (Figure 23-1, Table 23-2), microorganisms (Table 23-2), casts (Figure 23-2, Table 23-3), crystals (Figure 23-3, Table 23-4), fat, and contaminating substances may be found in urinary sediment.

Red Blood Cells

Urine sediment normally contains fewer than 2-3 RBCs/HPF. RBCs are small cells that may have several different appearances, depending on the urine concentration (e.g., specific gravity) and the length of time between collection and examination (Figures 23-4 to 23-9). In fresh samples that have intermediate specific gravities, RBCs usually have smooth edges and are yellow to orange. They can be colorless if their hemoglobin diffused while standing. In concentrated urine, RBCs shrink and crenate (see Figures 23-4 and 23-9). Crenated RBCs have ruffled edges and are slightly darker. Extremely crenated RBCs may even appear granular because of membrane irregularities. In dilute or alkaline urine, RBCs swell and may lyse. Swollen RBCs have smooth edges and are pale yellow or orange. Lysed RBCs may be colorless rings (shadow or ghost cells) that vary in size, but, especially when due to marked alkalinity, they usually dissolve and cannot be identified by microscopic examination.

RBCs must be differentiated from WBCs in urine sediments. This is easy on stained sediment smears because RBCs are anucleate, but differences in size and internal structure must be used to differentiate between them on unstained smears. RBCs that maintain their biconcave shape can be easily recognized by their dark central area (see Figure 23-5), but those that shrink or swell in response to urine osmolality may not demonstrate the typical biconcave shape. These RBCs are differentiated from WBCs based on size (approximately half the diameter of a WBC; see Figure 23-6) and lack of internal structure. Although RBCs have no nuclei, they should not be confused with fat globules or yeast. RBCs do not vary much in size, are yellow to orange, and tend to settle onto a slide. Fat globules (Figure 23-10) vary markedly in size and are light green and usually found just under the coverslip. (This last feature causes them to be in a different plane of view from other urine sediment elements.) Yeast organisms are rarely found in fresh urine from dogs and cats, but are typically seen in aged samples with overgrowths of contaminants. When present, yeast organisms are more variable in size than RBCs, and budding can usually be found on some of the organisms.

RBCs in urine usually indicate bleeding somewhere in the urinary or genital tract. Voided samples from females in proestrus, estrus, or postpartum periods often contain RBCs secondary to contamination with secretions from the genital tract. Similar contamination may be present in urine sediments collected by free catch or manual expression of the bladder from animals with any hemorrhagic condition in the genital system. In such cases, RBCs should not be found in urine collected by cystocentesis.

Increased numbers of RBCs along with WBCs are usually found in the urine sediment of animals with inflammatory conditions of the urinary tract. The slight trauma that occurs from catheterization or manual expression, and occasionally with cystocentesis, can increase the number of RBCs in the sediment.

White Blood Cells

Very few WBCs are present in urine from animals without urinary or genital tract disease. WBCs are about twice the size of RBCs and smaller than epithelial cells (see Figures 23-6 to 23-8). They are round and granular and sometimes brownian movement of the cytoplasmic granules in the neutrophils is seen. The polymorphic neutrophil nuclei can usually be seen in stained sediments and with phase-contrast microscopy and may occasionally be seen with reduced illumination bright field microscopy. WBCs are usually in very low numbers in urine (i.e., 0 to 1/HPF); more than 2 to 3 WBCs/HPF indicates inflammation somewhere in the urinary or genital tract. When increased numbers of neutrophils are found in urine sediment, even if bacteria are not found by microscopic examination, the urine sample should be cultured because microscopic examination is much less sensitive than culture to detecting bacteria in urine.

Epithelial Cells

Epithelial cells in urine vary markedly in size depending upon their origin. They are generally larger in the lower portions of the urinary tract than in the ureters, renal pelvis, and renal tubules.

Squamous Epithelial Cells: Squamous epithelial cells, which are derived from the distal urethra, vagina, vulva, or prepuce, are occasionally found in voided samples (Figure 23-11) and are usually not considered significant. They are the largest of the epithelial cells and the largest cells found in urine sediment; they appear flat and often have straight edges and obtuse, angular corners. They usually have a small, round nucleus, although occasionally a nucleus cannot be seen. Squamous epithelial cells are usually not found in samples obtained by cystocentesis. Cells with squamous features can be found in the urine sediment of male dogs with conditions that cause squamous metaplasia of the prostate and occasionally in the sediment of those with urothelial carcinomas (i.e., transitional cell carcinomas) in which there is also squamous metaplasia. In the latter condition, many other features suggestive of epithelial neoplasia, including extreme numbers of epithelial cells with marked pleomorphism, are found.

Urothelial (Transitional) Epithelial Cells: Urothelial, or transitional, epithelial cells come from the proximal urethra, bladder, ureters, renal pelvis, and renal tubules (see Figures 23-8 and 23-9). They vary in size depending upon their origin. Those originating in the proximal urethra and bladder are the largest, are round to elliptical, and have granular cytoplasm and

Red Blood Cells

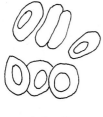

Intact

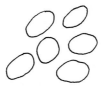

Ghost

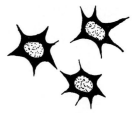

Crenated

Epithelial Cells

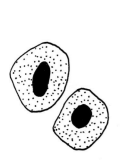

Renal

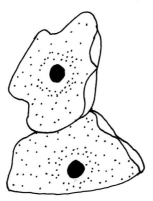

Squamous

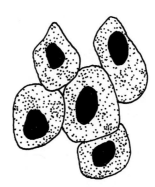

Transitional

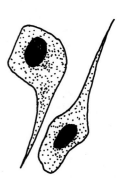

Caudate

Other

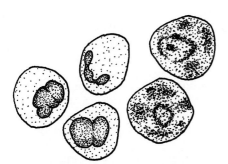

Stained   Unstained

WBC (pus cells)

Fat droplets

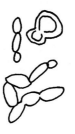

Yeast bodies

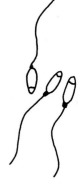

Sperm

Figure 23-1 Cells commonly found in urine sediment smears.

TABLE 23-2

Routine Microscopic Urine Examination: Cells, Cell-like Structures, Microorganisms, Parasites, and Confusing Artifacts

Finding	Normal	Interpretation if Increased	Follow-up
RBCs	≤3/HPF	Bleeding: If voided or expressed, urethra, prepuce, and vagina (e.g., proestrus, estrus, postpartum) must be considered as well as bladder.	Imaging, ultrasound Culture if WBCs are present
WBCs	≤1/HPF	Inflammation: If voided or expressed, urethra, prepuce, and vagina (e.g., proestrus, estrus, postpartum) must be considered as well as bladder.	Culture, imaging, ultrasound
Epithelial cells: Squamous	None in samples collected by Cystocentesis	Presence of squamous epithelial cells in cystocentesis urine samples suggests squamous metaplasia of urinary bladder transitional cells. Consider chronic irritation and/or neoplasia.	Imaging, ultrasound
	Variable in voided, expressed, or catheter-collected samples	None unless cellular abnormalities are noted.	None, unless neoplasia is suspected, then cytology, imaging, and ultrasound should be considered
Urothelial (Transitional)	≤1/HPF	Catheterization, inflammation (WBC should also be present), chronic irritation, neoplasia, chemotherapy.	Cytology, imaging, and ultrasound
Spermatozoa	Occasional in males	None in males. Exposure to male in females.	None
Microorganisms	None	Strongly suggestive of infection if sample collected by cystocentesis or catherization (usually accompanied by WBCs). Voided and expressed samples may be contaminated by organisms from the prepuce, vagina, or vulva.	Culture, look for WBCs in urine, check urine protein and glucose, consider possibility of diabetes mellitus
Parasites	None	Fecal contamination or *Capillaria plica* (bladder worm of dogs and cats) or *Dioctophyma renale* (kidney worm of dogs).	Imaging or ultrasound if bladder or kidney worm suspected
Fat droplets	Cats: Frequent Dogs: Occasional	Increased numbers of fat droplets may be seen with lubricants used for catheterization, obesity, diabetes mellitus, and hypothyroidism.	Physical examination for evidence of hypothyroidism and obesity, urine and serum glucose for diabetes mellitus
Artifacts: Air bubbles, oil droplets, starch granules, material, pollen, fungal spores, yeast, bacteria, ova from intestinal parasites	Variable, depending on method of collection	Associated with contamination or slide preparation.	Beware of contamination

Courtesy R.D. Tyler and R.L. Cowell.

HPF, High-power field (40× objective).

variably sized nuclei. Epithelial cells of the ureters and renal pelvis are smaller, are round to caudate, and have granular cytoplasm. Renal tubular epithelial cells are small, round cells with a distinct, round nucleus. They have granular cytoplasm that may contain a few small to large fat vacuoles. Fatty renal tubular cells are especially common in cat urine. Renal tubular

epithelial cells are only slightly larger than WBCs and are differentiated from WBCs by their round nuclei. A few epithelial cells, especially urothelial cells (i.e., 0 to 1/HPF), are found in sediment from normal animals due to the sloughing of old cells. An increase in epithelial cell numbers may be found in samples obtained by catheterization. Modest to marked increases in epithelial cells are found in inflammatory diseases of the urinary tract because inflammation often causes urothelial hyperplasia. Urine samples from animals with inflammation-induced urothelial hyperplasia also contain increased WBC numbers. Some chemotherapeutic agents (e.g., cyclophosphamide) may induce urothelial hyperplasia with modest pleomorphism. Many epithelial cells are found in sediment from animals with transitional cell carcinomas. Neoplastic urothelial cells usually vary markedly in size. If large numbers of epithelial cells (especially if they vary markedly in size) are found, sediment smears should be made, air-dried, stained with a hematologic stain, and evaluated cytologically.

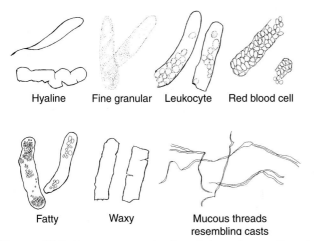

Figure 23-2 Casts commonly found in urine sediment smears.

Spermatozoa

Spermatozoa are occasionally seen in the urine sediment of intact male animals (Figure 23-12). They are easily recognized and have no clinical significance.

TABLE 23-3

Routine microscopic urine examination: Casts and confusing artifacts

Cast Type	Normal	Interpretation if Increased	Follow-up
Hyaline (and cylindroids)	≤1/HPF	Proteinuria (renal or prerenal), mild renal irritation, fever, poor renal perfusion, strenuous exercise, general anesthesia	Urine and serum protein concentration, physical examination, history
Granular	≤1/HPF	Acute to subacute renal tubular injury	Physical examination, history, CBC, serum chemistries
Cellular	None	Acute renal tubular injury	Physical examination, history, CBC, serum chemistries
Waxy	None	Chronic renal injury	Physical examination, history, CBC, serum chemistries
Fatty	≤1/HPF	Excessive numbers suggest renal tubule necrosis/degeneration. They are more commonly seen in cats than dogs. Occasionally they are seen in dogs with diabetes mellitus.	Physical examination, history, CBC, serum chemistries (especially glucose)
Bilirubin	None	Indicate moderate to marked bilirubinuria	Check for hemolysis or hepatic dysfunction
Hemoglobin or myoglobin (red-brown casts)	None	Hemoglobin casts and myglobin casts are both red-brown and cannot be differentiated microscopically. Hemoglobin casts occur with intravascular hemolysis, whereas myoglobin casts occur with severe muscle injury	Check for intravascular hemolysis (CBC) and muscle injury (serum chemistries, especially LDH, CK, and AST)
Casts-like Atifacts (mucous threads)	Occasional	Urethral irritation or contamination with genital secretions	None
Other confusing artifacts: Hair, fecal material, fungal hyphae	None	Associated with contamination or slide preparation	Beware of contamination

Courtesy R.D. Tyler and R.L. Cowell.
HPF, High-power field (40× objective); *CBC,* complete blood count; *LDH,* lactate dehydrogenase; *CK,* creative kinase; *AST,* aspartate aminotransferase.

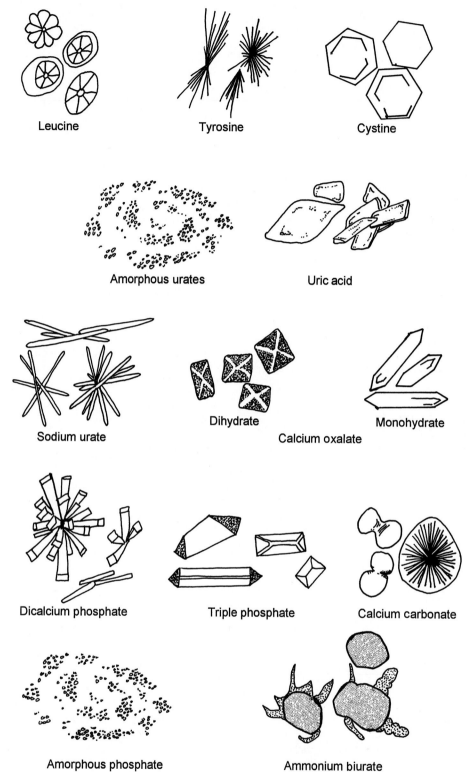

Leucine

Tyrosine

Cystine

Amorphous urates

Uric acid

Sodium urate

Dihydrate

Monohydrate

Calcium oxalate

Dicalcium phosphate

Triple phosphate

Calcium carbonate

Amorphous phosphate

Ammonium biurate

Figure 23-3 Crystals commonly found in urine sediment smears.

Microorganisms

The most common microorganisms found in urine are bacteria (Figures 23-13 and 23-14); fungi and yeast are also found (Figure 23-15), but rarely. Normal urine is free of microorganisms, but it may be contaminated by the vagina, vulva, or prepuce during urination. Normal urine collected by cystocentesis or catheterization does not contain bacteria, but because bacteria proliferate in urine that has been standing at room temperature, it is important to either perform microscopic examination immediately or

TABLE 23-4

Routine Microscopic Urine Examination: Crystals and Confusing Artifacts

Crystal	Normal	Interpretation if Increased	Follow-up
Triple phosphate	Variable	None	None
Amorphous phosphate	Variable	None	None
Calcium carbonate	Variable	None	None
Amorphous urate	Variable	None	None
Bilirubin	None to occasional in highly concentrated urine	High numbers suggest altered bilirubin metabolism (e.g., hemolysis, hepatic disease, biliary disease)	CBC and assessment of hepatobiliary function
Ammonia biurate (also called *ammonia urate*)	Rare	Liver disease. Normal in Dalmations due to difference in purine metabolism for Dalmations.	Check for liver disease, unless patient is a Dalmation
Calcium oxalate (dihydrate or monohydrate)	Uncommon	Increased numbers are found with ethylene glycol intoxication. Dihydrate form may occur idiopathically in dogs. Dihydrate form may occur with ingestion of oxalate-containing plants.	Check history for ingestion of ethylene glycol and check for renal impairment
Sulfonamide	None	May occur in animals treated with sulfonimides.	Beware of sulfonamide-induced nephrosis
Cystine	None	Defect in cystine and other amino acid transport by renal tubules; cystine uroliths may occur and is the only clinical manifestation of the defect.	Check for cystine uroliths
Leucine and tyrosine	None	Associated with severe liver disease in humans, but this has not been commonly found in animals.	Check for liver disease
Crystals: Cholesterol	Uncommon	Unknown, possibly associated with previous urinary tract hemorrhage or degenerative disease of the urinary tract.	Dependant on clinical presentation
Artifacts: Starch granules, fecal material, pollen, fungal spores	Variable, depending on method of collection	Associated with contamination or slide preparation.	Beware of contamination

Courtesy R.D. Tyler and R.L. Cowell.

refrigerate the urine until microscopic examination can be performed. Bacteria are very small and can be identified only at high magnifications. They may be round (cocci), rods (bacilli), or filamentous and usually refract light and quiver because of brownian movement. Amorphous phosphates or urates may also move as the result of brownian movement and can be confused with bacterial cocci. If there is any doubt, an air-dried smear can be made and stained with a cytologic stain for confirmation (Figure 23-16; see Figure 23-40). Bacteria are reported as few, moderate, or many. A large number of bacteria accompanied by a large number of WBCs indicates urinary or genital tract infection with inflammation. Usually when bacteria are found without accompanying WBCs, the sample has been contaminated (e.g., from the external genitalia or nonsterile collection materials) or the observer is mistaking amorphous mineral precipitates for bacteria. Animals with a depressed ability to mount an inflammatory reaction, however, may develop severe urinary tract infections without significant accompanying inflammation. Situations in which urinary tract infection may be present without significant urinary leukocytosis include treatment with high doses of glucocorticoids, Cushing's disease, and diabetes mellitus.

Yeast may be confused with RBCs or lipid droplets, but yeast organisms usually display characteristic budding, often have double refractile walls, and do not dissolve in acetic acid. They are usually contaminants in urine samples, because yeast infections of the urinary tract are rare in domestic animals. Yeast infections of the external genitalia may cause yeast to be present in voided samples.

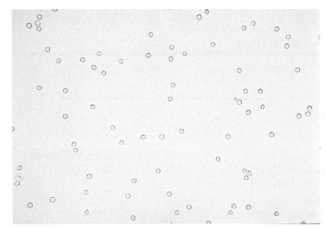

Figure 23-4 RBCs in urine sediment. All the cells are similar in size, but some have irregular borders because they are crenated because of increased urine osmolarity. (Unstained, original magnification 400×.)

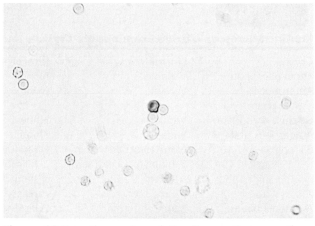

Figure 23-7 In the center of the figure, there are three RBCs and a WBC. The nucleus of the WBC is suggested by the contrast in the center of the cell. (Sedi-Stain, original magnification 560×.)

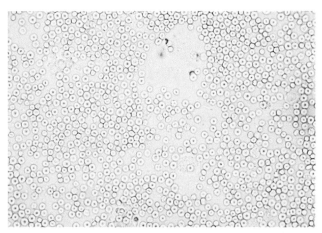

Figure 23-5 Many RBCs in urine sediment. The central dark area in these cells indicates that they have retained their biconcave shape. (Unstained, original magnification 560×.)

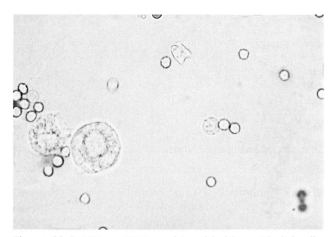

Figure 23-8 RBCs, a WBC, and two bladder epithelial cells. Note the outline of the nucleus in the more distinct epithelial cell. (Unstained, original magnification 1120×.)

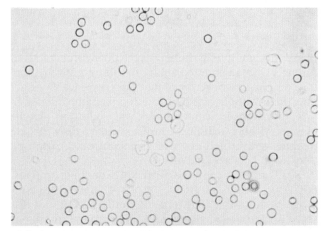

Figure 23-6 RBCs and WBCs in urine sediment. The WBCs, which have uncolored cytoplasm, are approximately twice the diameter of the RBCs. (Unstained, original magnification 560×.)

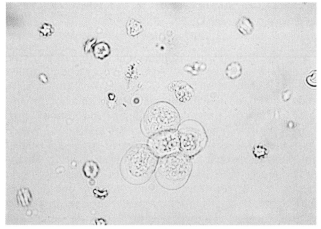

Figure 23-9 A cluster of five bladder epithelial cells and several crenated RBCs. (Unstained, original magnification 1120×.)

Fungal hyphae (see Figure 23-15), which are long, usually branched filaments with septa, are rarely found in urine. Primary fungal infections of the urinary tract are rare, but systemic mycosis may affect the kidneys and lower urinary tract, resulting in fungal elements being found with WBCs and epithelial cells in urine sediment.

When evaluating the importance of potentially infectious agents in the urine (i.e., bacteria and fungi), it is important to consider whether there is clinical and microscopic (i.e., urine sediment) evidence of urinary tract inflammation or the animal has a condition that might inhibit such an inflammatory reaction (e.g., diabetes mellitus). Consideration should also be given to the method of collection and the subsequent handling of the urine sample to assess the likelihood of contamination.

Parasites

Parasite ova in urine sediment are from parasites in the urinary system or fecal contamination of the urine sample. Parasite ova originating in the urinary tract include *Capillaria plica* (bladder worm of dogs and cats; Figure 23-17) and *Dioctophyma renale* (kidney worm of dogs).

Fat Droplets

In urine sediment, fat droplets are lightly tinged green, highly refractile, round bodies of varying sizes (see Figure 23-10). If a sediment sample is allowed to sit for a few moments before it is examined, fat droplets rise to a plane just under the coverslip, and other formed elements settle to the top of the slide. Fat droplets from catheter lubricants or oily surfaces of collecting vials and pipettes frequently contaminate urine. Fat in the urine (i.e., lipiduria) is seen

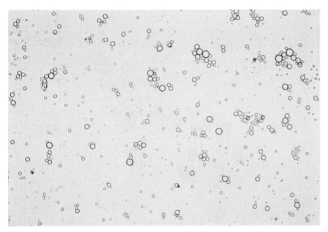

Figure 23-10 There are many fat droplets present in this sample of urine sediment from a cat. The fat droplets are differentiated from RBCs because of the marked variation in size. The fat droplets also settle on a different plain of focus than the cellular elements. (Unstained, original magnification 50×.) *(Courtesy Oklahoma State University, Clinical Pathology Teaching File.)*

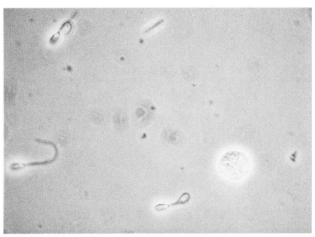

Figure 23-12 A WBC and several spermatozoa as seen with phase-contrast microscopy. (Unstained, original magnification 1600×.)

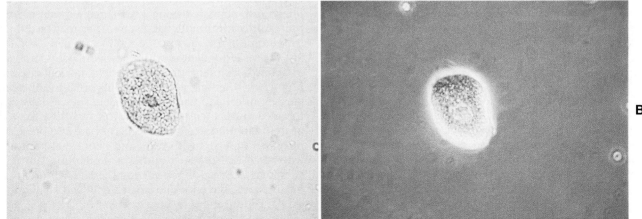

Figure 23-11 A, A squamous epithelial cell from the distal urethra as seen with reduced illumination and bright field microscopy. **B,** The same cell seen with phase-contrast microscopy. (Unstained, original magnification of both figures 880×.)

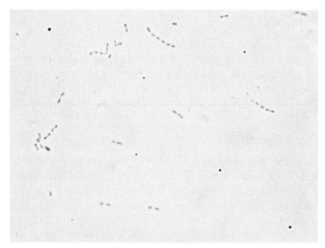

Figure 23-13 Short chains of cocci. (Unstained, original magnification 1600×.)

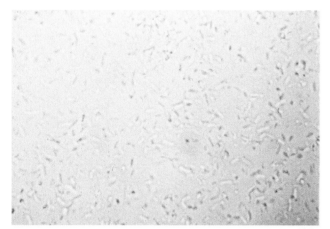

Figure 23-14 Many bacilli rods. (Unstained, original magnification 1600×.)

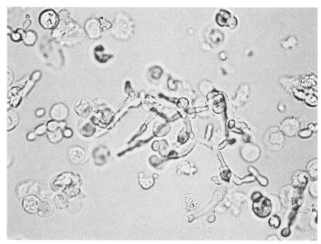

Figure 23-15 WBCs and fungal hyphae. (Unstained, original magnification 1120×.)

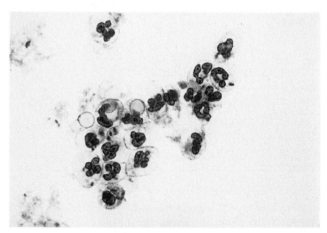

Figure 23-16 Several WBCs, one of which contains a rod-shaped bacterium. (new methylene blue stain, original magnification 1120×.)

to some degree in most cats because the kidneys of cats contain a large amount of lipid. Scattered fat droplets may also be seen with disorders such as obesity, diabetes mellitus, and hypothyroidism. Because fat droplets vary in size and are in a different plane of focus than the rest of the sediment, they can be distinguished from RBCs and yeast.

Casts

Casts (see Table 23-3) are formed in the lumen of the distal and collecting tubules of the kidney. The increased concentration and acidity of urine in the tubules promotes precipitation of the protein secreted in the tubules. Because casts are formed in renal tubules, they are cylindrical with parallel sides. When cells in the tubules exfoliate, the cells are often incorporated into the precipitated protein matrix. Because casts may dissolve in alkaline urine, fresh urine should be evaluated for their presence and quantitation. Also, casts may fracture with high-speed centrifugation, so it is important to use the proper technique when preparing specimens. Very small

numbers of hyaline or granular casts (i.e., 0 to 1/HPF) may be seen in normal urine, but higher numbers of casts indicate a lesion in the renal tubules.

Hyaline Casts: A few hyaline casts, which are clear, colorless, and refractile (Figure 23-18), may be seen in urine from animals without renal disease. They may be difficult to see unless the microscope light is properly adjusted and are easier to identify with phase-contrast microscopy of stained sediment than with bright field microscopy of unstained sediment. Similar to all casts, hyaline casts are cylindrical and have parallel sides. They usually have rounded ends. Increased numbers of hyaline casts may be found in mild renal irritation. They are also present in increased numbers with fever and poor renal perfusion, with renal and prerenal causes of proteinuria, and after strenuous exercise or general anesthesia. Cylindroids are hyaline casts, but with one tapered end, and are found in similar conditions as hyaline casts.

Granular Casts: Granular casts are one of the most common type of casts found in urine sediment (Figure 23-19). The granules originate from tubular epithelial cells and WBCs that degenerated after being incorporated

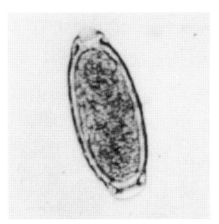

Figure 23-17 An egg of *Capillaria plica*, the bladder worm of dogs and cats. (Unstained, original magnification 400×.)

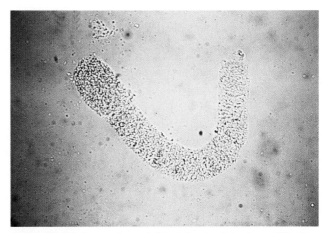

Figure 23-19 A granular cast. (Unstained, original magnification 560×.)

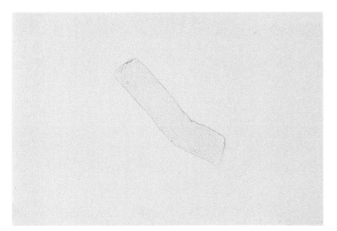

Figure 23-18 A hyaline cast. (Sedi-Stain, original magnification 560×.)

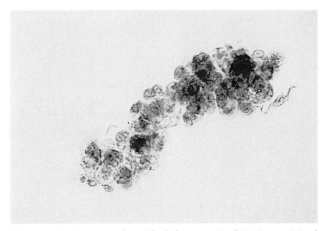

Figure 23-20 A renal epithelial cast. (Sedi-Stain, original magnification 1120×.)

into the protein matrix of the cast. Granular casts are present in large numbers with acute renal diseases and are more specific to renal tubular injury than are hyaline casts.

Cellular Casts: Cellular casts may contain epithelial cells, WBCs, or RBCs (Figure 23-20). Epithelial cell casts are formed when intact epithelial cells are sloughed from the renal tubules and the cast is passed into the urine before the cells degenerate. WBC casts are seen in acute nephritis or toxic conditions that cause degeneration of tubular epithelium. Leukocyte casts are uncommon but can form with inflammation in the tubules (e.g., acute pyelonephritis). RBC casts are also uncommon, but can form with bleeding into the kidneys. These types of casts are usually accompanied by granular casts.

Waxy Casts: Waxy casts, which indicate chronic tubular degeneration, look like hyaline casts but usually are wider, have square instead of round ends, and appear dull, homogenous, and waxy (Figures 23-21 and 23-22). They are more opaque than hyaline casts and may appear to have fissures along their surfaces.

Fatty Casts: Fatty casts contain many small fat droplets, which are round, highly refractile bodies. They are frequently seen in cats, because cats have fat in their

renal parenchyma, but are occasionally seen in dogs with diabetes mellitus. Large numbers of fatty casts suggest renal tubule degeneration.

Other Casts: Casts occasionally incorporate materials such as bilirubin, hemoglobin, or myoglobin into their matrices (Figures 23-23 and 23-24). Bilirubin-stained casts indicate the presence of moderate to marked bilirubinuria. Hemoglobin and myoglobin both impart a red to red-brown color. The presence of hemoglobin casts suggests intravascular hemolysis, but myoglobin staining results from widespread muscle damage.

Castlike Artifacts: Mucous threads are often confused with casts, but they do not have the well-delineated edges of casts. They look more like twisted ribbons than casts. Mucus indicates urethral irritation or contamination of the sample with genital secretions.

Crystals

Crystalluria is usually not clinically significant, but certain types of crystals or great numbers of common crystals may be clinically important (see Table 23-4). Certain crystals form as a consequence of their elements being secreted and

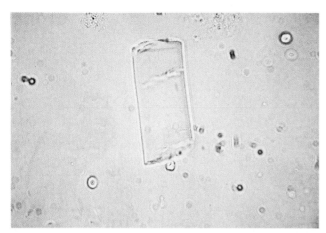

Figure 23-21 A waxy cast. (Unstained, original magnification 560×.)

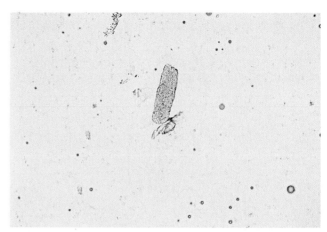

Figure 23-23 A fine, granular cast that has accumulated bilirubin in its matrix. (Unstained, original magnification 280×.)

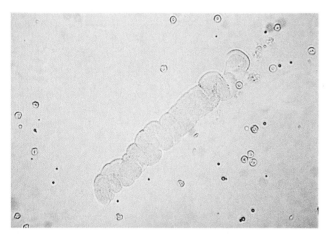

Figure 23-22 A waxy cast. (Unstained, original magnification 280×.)

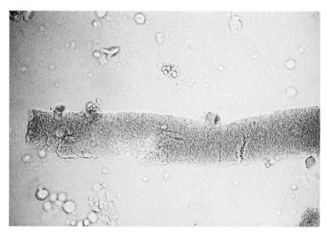

Figure 23-24 A fine, granular cast that has accumulated hemoglobin or myoglobin in its matrix. (Unstained, original magnification 560×.)

concentrated in urine by normal renal activity. Other crystals form because some diseases cause the production of metabolites that are secreted into the urine, forming crystals through precipitation with other elements secreted by the kidneys. Crystals that form in the bladder may lead to the development of urinary calculi. The type of crystals formed depend on urine pH, concentration, and temperature, as well as the solubility of urine elements. If a urine sample is allowed to stand and cool before examination, the number of crystals in the sample increases because the elements that make up crystals are less soluble at lower temperatures. Refrigerated samples often have many more crystals than fresh samples. Crystals are reported as occasional, moderate, or many per LPF (i.e., 10× objective).

Triple Phosphate: Triple phosphate or struvite crystals are found in alkaline to slightly acidic urine. Triple phosphate crystals usually have a coffin-lid appearance but also have other shapes. They are generally prisms with tapering sides and ends (Figure 23-25; see also Figure 23-29) and are found in samples from many normal dogs and cats. Triple phosphate crystals may also be found in animals with struvite uroliths, which are often associated with *Staphylococcus* urinary tract infections. In these cases, there is usually an accompanying inflammatory reaction with increased

numbers of WBCs. Triple phosphate crystals are occasionally shaped like fern leaves (Figure 23-26), especially when the urine contains a high concentration of ammonia.

Amorphous Phosphate: Amorphous phosphate crystals are common in alkaline urine and appear as an amorphous, granular precipitate. They can be present in large amounts but have no clinical significance. They should not be misinterpreted as bacteria.

Calcium Carbonate: Calcium carbonate crystals are commonly seen in the urine of horses but may occasionally be found in the urine of dogs and cats. They are round with many lines radiating from their centers (Figure 23-27) and may also have a short dumbbell shape.

Amorphous Urate: Amorphous urate crystals are similar to amorphous phosphate crystals because they also appear as a granular precipitate, but amorphous urate crystals are usually found in acidic urine, whereas amorphous phosphate crystals are found in alkaline urine. Amorphous urates are also dark green-yellow, whereas amorphous phosphates are a dull brown.

Ammonium Biurate: Ammonium biurate (also called *ammonium urate*) crystals are brown and round with long

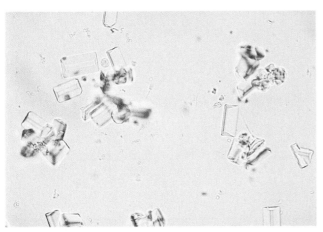

Figure 23-25 Triple phosphate crystals, a WBC (upper left, between two crystals), and spermatozoa. (Unstained, original magnification 560×.)

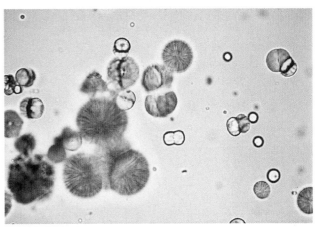

Figure 23-27 Calcium carbonate crystals. (Unstained, original magnification 560×.)

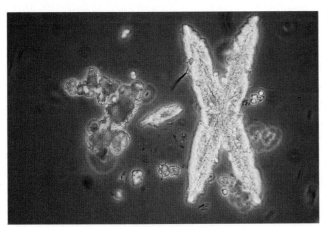

Figure 23-26 A triple phosphate crystal shaped like a fern leaf. (Unstained, original magnification 280×.)

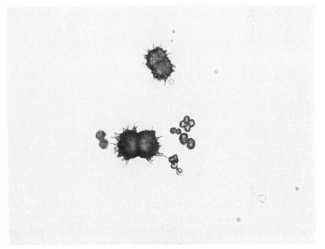

Figure 23-28 An ammonium biurate crystal and a triple phosphate crystal. (Unstained, original magnification 560×.)

spicules (thorn apple shaped) (Figures 23-28 and 23-29). These spicules occasionally break off the main part of the crystal and appear as small brown crystals with fine radiating lines. Ammonium biurate crystals are most common in animals with liver disease, especially in those with portacaval shunts. These crystals are also commonly found in Dalmatians due to altered purine metabolism in this breed.

Calcium Oxalate: Calcium oxalate dihydrate crystals are generally small squares with intersecting, refractile lines that transverse diagonally across the crystal, forming an envelope-like structure (Figure 23-30). These crystals may occasionally take on a cube-like form (Figures 23-31 and 23-32). Calcium oxalate monohydrate crystals are small, flat, elongated structures with pointed ends (Figures 23-33 and 23-34). Calcium oxalate dihydrate crystals are found in acidic and neutral urine and may be seen in small numbers in the urine of healthy dogs. Animals poisoned with ethylene glycol (antifreeze) often have large numbers of calcium oxalate crystals, especially the monohydrate form, in their urine; animals with oxalate urolithiasis may have many calcium oxalate crystals in their urine. Large numbers of calcium oxalate crystals may indicate that an animal is at risk of developing oxalate urolithiasis.

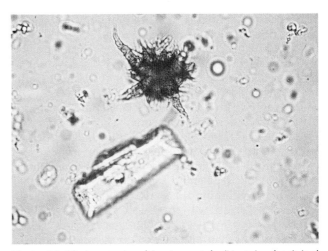

Figure 23-29 Ammonium biurate crystals. (Unstained, original magnification 280×.)

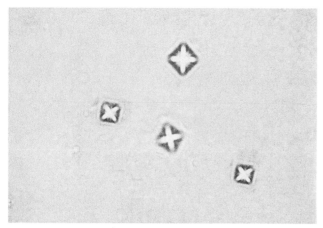

Figure 23-30 Calcium oxalate dihydrate crystals. (Unstained, original magnification 280×.)

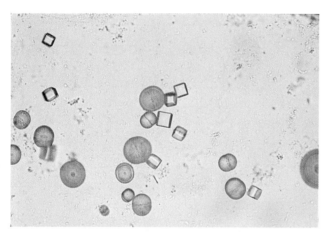

Figure 23-31 Calcium carbonate (large spheres) and cubelike calcium oxalate dihydrate crystals. (Unstained, original magnification 66×.) *(Courtesy Dr. Phillip Clark, Michigan State University.)*

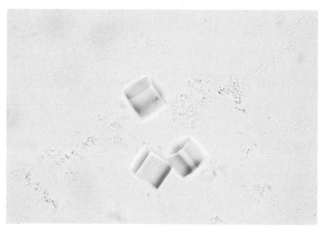

Figure 23-32 Cubelike calcium oxalate monohydrate crystals. (Unstained, original magnification 165×.) *(Courtesy Dr. Phillip Clark, Michigan State University.)*

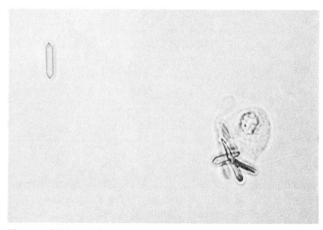

Figure 23-33 Calcium oxalate monohydrate crystals and a bladder epithelial cell. (Unstained, original magnification 560×.)

Figure 23-34 Calcium oxalate monohydrate crystal. (Unstained, original magnification 840×.)

Sulfonamide: Sulfonamide crystals may be seen in animals being treated with sulfonamides. They are less likely to be observed in alkaline urine because they are more soluble in such urine.

Bilirubin: Bilirubin crystals are bundles of elongated, yellow, fine spicules (Figures 23-35 and 23-36). They can be seen in highly concentrated urine of normal dogs, but, if found in large numbers, should arouse suspicion of bilirubin metabolism disorders (e.g., severe hemolytic anemia or severe liver or biliary disease).

Cystine: Cystine crystals are six-sided (hexagonal), flat plates that most commonly form in acidic urine. Cystine crystals are not found in normal animals but in those with cystinuria, a metabolic defect affecting the transport of cystine and other amino acids across the renal tubules (Figure 23-37). These animals are prone to the formation of cystine uroliths, but there are no other clinical manifestations associated with the disease.

Leucine and Tyrosine: Leucine and tyrosine crystals have been associated with severe liver disease in humans, but this has not been commonly found in animals. Their significance in animal urine is not well defined. Tyrosine

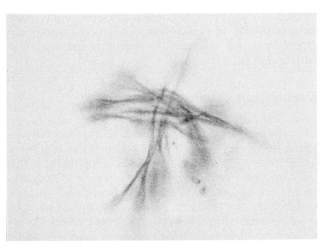

Figure 23-35 Bilirubin crystals. (Unstained, original magnification 840×.)

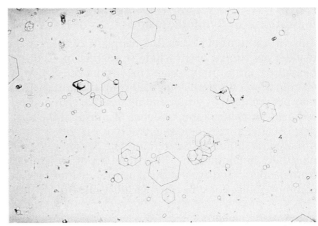

Figure 23-37 Cystine crystals. (Unstained, original magnification 540×.)

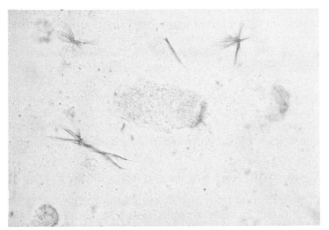

Figure 23-36 Several single bilirubin crystals and a granular cast. (Unstained, original magnification 540×.)

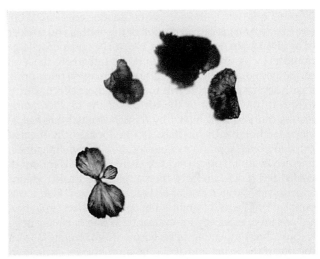

Figure 23-38 Tyrosine crystals. (Unstained, original magnification 540×.)

crystals are dark and needle-like and are often found in small clusters or sheaves (Figure 23-38). Leucine crystals appear as large spheroids with concentric striations.

Cholesterol: Cholesterol crystals are large, flat structures with distinct right angles. They may be rectangular, but usually appear as two or more rectangles joined together. These crystals are not commonly found, and their significance is unknown, but they may be found in the urine of animals with previous urinary tract hemorrhage or degenerative disease (Figure 23-39).

Artifacts: Many substances can contaminate urine during collection, transportation, or examination and be found when urine sediment is examined. Because these contaminants can cause confusion, it is important to recognize them as irrelevant and not a normal part of the sediment.

Air bubbles, oil droplets (usually from lubricated catheters), starch granules (from surgical gloves), hair, fecal material, pollen, fungal spores, yeast, bacteria, and fungi may contaminant urine. Ova of intestinal parasites and many bacteria without an accompanying inflammatory reaction may be found with fecal contamination of the urine sample.

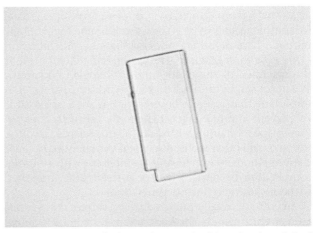

Figure 23-39 A cholesterol crystal. (Unstained, original magnification 540×.)

CYTOLOGY OF THE URINARY TRACT

Indications for Cytologic Examination of Urine

The clinical signs of cystitis and neoplasia of the urinary bladder are similar and include stranguria, pollakiuria, hematuria, urine dribbling, and incontinence.[3] Cytologic examination of material obtained from the urinary tract may be prompted by either finding unusual cells in urine sediment or radiographic evidence of a mass in the bladder. Usually, microscopic evaluation as part of a routine urinalysis is sufficient to determine the presence of a urinary tract inflammation. Differentiation of hyperplasia from neoplasia and evaluation of urinary tract masses are common indications for cytologically evaluating urine.

Obtaining Samples for Cytologic Evaluation

Urine samples collected in a routine manner (e.g., free catch, catheterization, or cytocentesis) may be processed for cytologic purposes. Methods to increase the cell yield from a suspected mass in the bladder or urethra are frequently used. A greater cell yield with fewer contaminating cells can be obtained by traumatic catheterization of the urethra and bladder or by direct aspiration of a mass. Cells can be obtained in large numbers by passing a lubricated urinary catheter to the level of a suspected mass and traumatizing the mass by puncturing it with several quick jabs. This method is most effective with masses in the urethra or the trigone of the bladder. Some masses can also be sampled by transabdominal fine-needle biopsy techniques. If the mass can be localized by manual palpation or is large and its exact location known, unguided, fine-needle aspiration can yield excellent samples. Ultrasound-guided techniques improve the sampling of smaller lesions and provide greater assurance that the desired lesion was sampled.[4] In general, samples obtained by direct aspiration are preferred, especially for evaluating possible malignancies because direct aspiration helps ensure that sampling is from the site of the lesion and avoid the morphologic changes in cells associated with aging and prolonged contact with urine that are commonly seen in smears of urine sediment.

Preparation of Slides from Urine

Although urine collected after a period of time in which an animal has not urinated (e.g., morning samples) is ideal for routine urinalysis, it is the least desirable for cytologic purposes because urine causes exfoliated urothelium and other cells to degenerate. Fresh, unfixed, voided urine is the specimen of choice for initial cytologic evaluations. When a sample cannot be examined immediately, it is important that a smear be prepared as soon as possible to prevent morphologic changes in the cells present. Preservation of urine with acid, formaldehyde, alcohol, freezing, and other methods is not recommended because these methods may lyse cells or interfere with staining. Samples can be refrigerated for a short time, however, without causing cellular degeneration.

Smears are usually prepared from samples concentrated by centrifugation or direct application to a slide using a cytocentrifuge (e.g., Cytospin II, Shandon-Lipshaw, Pittsburgh, Penn.). Cell morphology can be preserved by adding a drop of albumin or autologous serum to the sediment before the smear is made. Cytocentrifugation is especially useful when small volumes of urine are dealt with and cellularity is low.

Normal Urine Cytology

Typically, no or only a few cells are found when urine from normal animals is examined. If very few cells are found on urinalysis, a cytologic examination of urine is usually not performed. A few single urothelial cells that are large and round to oval may be present. Cytoplasm stains pale basophilic to pale acidophilic and is finely vacuolated. Urothelial cell nuclei are usually centrally located and have finely stippled chromatin. Small, tightly molded clusters of urothelial cells are occasionally found and should be interpreted with caution. These cell clusters may indicate neoplasia but may also be found in samples from urinary tract inflammation or urolithiasis. Squamous epithelial cells may also be found in voided urine, and, in males, they are contaminates from the terminal urethra. In females, they come from the vaginal and vulvar squamous epithelium. A few neutrophils and erythrocytes are usually found in cytologic preparations of normal urine. If the smear was made from fresh urine, the neutrophils are usually not degenerate; however, the neutrophils in smears from urine samples that have remained at room temperature for an hour or more may have foamy cytoplasm and mild karyorrhexis, pyknosis, or karyolysis.

Cystitis with Hyperplasia and Metaplasia

Although urine from normal dogs and cats may rarely or occasionally have neutrophils, the presence of many neutrophils indicates inflammation. Often the neutrophils show severe degenerative changes consisting of foamy to vacuolated cytoplasm and karyolysis. Intracellular and extracellular bacteria may accompany the inflammatory cells (Figure 23-40). Even if bacteria are not found in urine with purulent inflammation, the sample should be cultured.

Neutrophils are the predominant cell type in chronic inflammation, but macrophages, lymphocytes, and an occasional plasma cell may also be seen. Macrophage cytoplasm is usually finely vacuolated and contains round, oval, or bean-shaped nuclei that are centric or eccentric. Macrophages may contain phagocytized RBCs, cellular debris, bacteria, or spermatozoa.

Along with high numbers of neutrophils, large numbers of RBCs may be present in urine from patients with cystitis. Hematuria may also be seen with severe glomerular disease (i.e., urinary tract neoplasia) during treatment with chemotherapeutic drugs and with inflammatory and neoplastic disease of the genital tract.

Hyperplasia of the urothelium, which may occasionally be accompanied by squamous metaplasia, often occurs with inflammation of the lower urinary tract and becomes more pronounced as the inflammatory process progresses. Hyperplastic urothelial cells are mildly anaplastic with moderate variation in cell size and increased basophilia. Hyperplasia may also be seen in urolithiasis and with some toxic agents. The finding of atypical urothelial cells

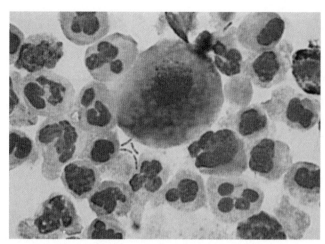

Figure 23-40 Infectious cystitis with many neutrophils, a bladder epithelial cell, and rod-shaped bacilli. (The urine was concentrated by cytospin method.) (Wright-Giemsa stain, original magnification 400×.)

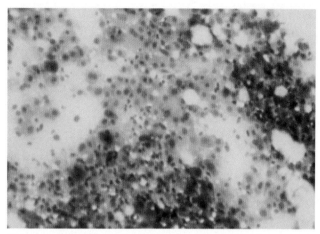

Figure 23-41 A population of moderately pleomorphic epithelial cells from a dog with cyclophosphamide-induced hyperplastic cystitis. The cells vary in size and staining and were concentrated by the cytospin method. (Wright-Giemsa stain, original magnification 40×.) *(Courtesy L. O'Rourke, Louisiana State University.)*

is complicated by the fact that degenerative changes are frequently associated with cells that have been in the urine for some time. When features of anaplasia and degeneration accompany inflammation, their significance should be interpreted conservatively; however, repeating cytologic examination of the urine after the inflammation has subsided is indicated to determine whether the anaplasia was secondary to inflammation or whether it is an indication of urothelial neoplasia.

Squamous metaplasia of the bladder epithelium may be found with chronic inflammation or irritation. Exfoliated squamous-like cells resemble the intermediate or superficial squamous cells found in other locations. That is, they are large cells with abundant, lightly stained cytoplasm. These cells are thin, and their cell membrane may fold back upon itself. Well-differentiated squamous cells have angular outlines and pyknotic or faded nuclei. Squamous-cell carcinomas of the genital or urinary tract may shed well-differentiated squamous cells into the urine, but this is not a common occurrence. Finding large numbers of squamous cells necessitates a search for malignant features and further clinical examination.

Effects of Chemotherapy on the Urinary Bladder

Some chemotherapeutic agents affect the urothelial epithelial cells. The alkylating agents cyclophosphamide and busulfan, which are concentrated in the urine, inhibit DNA replication by binding to nucleic acids. Patients receiving these drugs exfoliate abnormal cells from the urothelium. The cytoplasm is basophilic and often vacuolated; nuclei are large, have a reticulated chromatin pattern, and may have nucleoli. Multinucleated cells may be found. Inflammation and hemorrhage with background cell debris are common findings (Figure 23-41). If the features are sufficiently severe, it may not be possible to differentiate the changes induced from alkylating agents from those of urothelial carcinoma. New malignancies of the urinary bladder have been reported in people receiving cyclophosphamide.[5]

NEOPLASMS OF THE URINARY TRACT

Neoplasms of the bladder may be benign or malignant. Malignant neoplasms arising from the bladder epithelium or urothelium are called *transitional cell carcinomas* or *urothelial carcinomas*.

Papillomas are benign neoplasms composed of urothelium indistinguishable from normal urothelium that grow into the lumen of the bladder.[6] Papillomas may shed moderate numbers of epithelial cells, which are indistinguishable from normal urothelial cells, into the urine. Diagnosis of a papilloma is based on clinical, radiographic, and histologic features, because distinct cytologic features do not occur.

Transitional cell or urothelial carcinomas have papillary, nonpapillary, or invasive growth patterns.[6] Their most common site is the trigonal area of the bladder, but transitional cell carcinomas may also be found in other areas of the bladder and tubular system. Clinical signs and sequelae vary depending on the location of the tumor.

Urothelial carcinomas usually exfoliate large numbers of individual cells and cell clusters. Large clusters of markedly pleomorphic cells with especially marked variation in cellular staining and size are frequently found. Within the clusters, very large cells or individual cells are found, and cell borders are usually not distinct. Some cells have deeply basophilic cytoplasm, but others have lightly basophilic cytoplasm. Cell crowding is evident by cellular and nuclear molding. The nuclear-to-cytoplasmic ratio is distinctly increased in many cells, but there are usually a few very large cells with abundant cytoplasm and a low nuclear-to-cytoplasmic ratio. Some cells have large, relatively light-staining vacuoles, which indicate that they are undergoing hydropic degeneration, possibly induced by the toxic effects of urine. Nuclear chromatin is finely to coarsely reticulated, and large, indistinct nucleoli are occasionally found. Mitotic cells may be present, but are not essential for diagnosis (Figures 23-42 to 23-44).

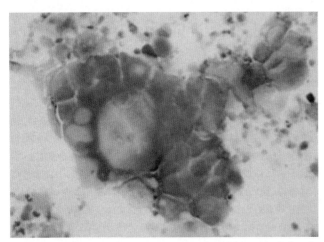

Figure 23-42 A cluster of very pleomorphic epithelial cells from a dog with urothelial carcinoma. The cells vary markedly in size and staining. There is cell crowding, resulting in cellular and nuclear molding. The cells were concentrated by the cytospin method. (Wright-Giemsa stain, original magnification 100×.)

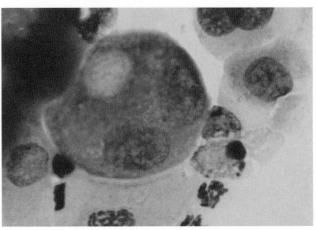

Figure 23-44 A large, basophilic cell containing two nuclei from a urothelial carcinoma. The cells were concentrated by the cytospin method. (Wright-Giemsa stain, original magnification 400×.)

References

1. Ling GV. In Ling GV: *Lower Urinary Tract Diseases of Dogs and Cats*. St. Louis, Mosby, 1995, pp 23-28.
2. Zinkl. In Pratt PW: *Laboratory Procedures for Veterinary Technicians*. St. Louis, Mosby, 1997, pp 259-306.
3. Ling GV. In Ling GV: *Lower Urinary Tract Diseases of Dogs and Cats*. St. Louis, Mosby, 1995, pp 11-16.
4. Nyland and Sammi. In Ling GV: *Lower Urinary Tract Diseases of Dogs and Cats*. St. Louis, Mosby, 1995, pp 61-87.
5. Theilen and Madewell. In Theilen GH, Madewell BR: *Veterinary Cancer Medicine*. Philadelphia, Lea & Febiger, 1987, pp 183-196.
6. Nielsen and Moulton DJ. In Moulton DJ: *Tumors of Domestic Animals*, ed 3. Berkeley, University of California Press, 1990, pp 458-478.
7. Kennedy. In Ling GV: *Lower Urinary Tract Diseases of Dogs and Cats*. St. Louis, Mosby, 1995, pp 107-113.

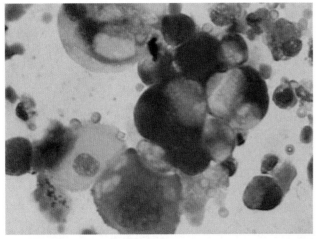

Figure 23-43 A population of pleomorphic, urothelial epithelial cells that vary in size and staining quality, from a dog with urothelial carcinoma. Some of the cells have large vacuoles in their cytoplasm as a result of hydropic change. The cells were concentrated by the cytospin method. (Wright-Giemsa stain, original magnification 160×.)

Some transitional cell carcinomas exfoliate cells with features similar to immature squamous cells. This finding suggests that squamous metaplasia has occurred; however, squamous-cell carcinoma also occurs in the bladder. In addition, adenocarcinomas have also been found in the urinary bladder and may be due to metaplasia of neoplastic transitional epithelial cells.[6,7] Features allowing transitional cell carcinomas to be differentiated from squamous cell carcinomas or adenocarcinomas are difficult to recognize cytologically because they are caused by immaturity and dedifferentiation, resulting in cells that appear similar.

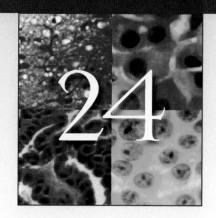

The Male Reproductive Tract: Prostate, Testes, and Semen

J.G. Zinkl

CHAPTER 24

THE PROSTATE GLAND

Collecting and Preparing Samples

Enlargement of the prostate gland is the primary reason for obtaining samples from it. Clinical signs suggesting that the prostate may be enlarged include difficult defecation or micturition, although the latter occurs less frequently. Sometimes urine is tinged red from blood, or blood or pus may drip from the penis. When either of these signs occurs, rectal palpation of the prostate may reveal symmetric or unilateral enlargement, focal bumpiness, or softness.[1,2] Such prostate abnormalities detected by palpation or, occasionally, radiographic examination are the primary indications for obtaining material from the gland for cytologic evaluation.

Material from the prostate can be obtained directly through the urethra or by fine-needle aspiration of the gland. A direct method is to digitally massage the prostate while aspirating through a urinary catheter passed to the level of the gland.[3,4] More prostatic material can be obtained by washing the part of the urethra near the prostate with a small amount of saline through gentle injection and aspiration while gently massaging the prostate. Material may also be obtained from the prostate by ejaculation.[2,4] The prostate is gently massaged during the process to increase the amount of material of prostatic origin because this method may contain contaminants from other parts of the reproductive tract. The first part of the ejaculate contains material primarily derived from the prostate gland.[2,4] The sample size is usually large and has a moderate concentration of cells. In addition to prostatic epithelial cells, ejaculated samples may contain numerous spermatozoa and cells of other reproductive tract and urethral structures. Simultaneously collecting and evaluating urethral wash specimens and urine samples (by antepubic cystocentesis) can alleviate some of the problems of interpreting the cytologic and microbiologic findings of the material collected by ejaculation.

The prostate can be sampled by direct aspiration with a small-gauge needle. Ultrasound-guided aspiration is superior to all other methods for obtaining specimens, especially from focal lesions such as cysts. The patient is sedated and restrained in dorsal recumbency in a padded, V-shaped trough. The inguinal area is anesthetized and the area is prepared as for surgery. Sterile petroleum jelly is applied to the skin to provide an acoustic coupler between the skin and the scanhead, and a small stab incision is made in the skin to facilitate needle passage. While the ultrasound scanhead is held stationary and needle advancement is monitored on the screen, the needle is directed to the prostate or a specific location within the prostate. When the needle has reached the proper site, a small amount of specimen is aspirated into a sterile syringe.[4]

The prostate can be sampled by digital guidance of a needle as well, which may be passed through the posterior abdominal wall or the perineal region, although the latter method has not been widely used in veterinary medicine. At either site, local anesthesia is necessary to prevent discomfort and facilitate needle guidance. When the prostate is so enlarged that it can be palpated through the abdominal wall, the needle can be guided to the prostate while the dog is in either lateral or dorsal recumbency and the prostate is immobilized with one hand. This method is usually effective only when the prostate is markedly enlarged.[4] From the perineal area, a finger is placed in the rectum, and the needle is passed through the skin in the perineal area and guided into the prostate along the finger. With both methods, the gland is gently aspirated while the needle is moved within it.[4] Occasionally, only a small amount of material is obtained by aspiration, but it is usually adequate for making one or two direct smears.

Preparation and staining of slides of prostate material are similar to that of other samples. When samples of low cellularity are obtained (e.g., from cysts), they should be concentrated by centrifugation or with a cytofuge in order to have slides with sufficient material for proper evaluation.

Cytologic Evaluation

When specimens with inadequate numbers of cells are obtained, results are reported as "not diagnostic" and accompanied by a comment indicating the problem and a recommendation that additional sampling be attempted. Fluid from prostatic cysts can be nearly acellular, however, and evaluation of specific gravity and protein concentration may reveal the cystic nature of the lesion.

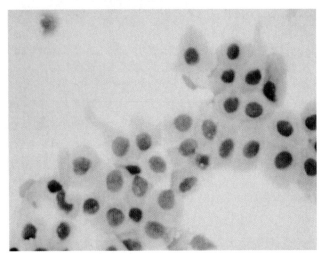

Figure 24-1   Epithelial cells from a normal prostate. The cells are in large clusters and have mildly acidophilic cytoplasm and relatively large nuclei. (Prostatic massage slightly concentrated by centrifugation, Wright-Giemsa stain.)

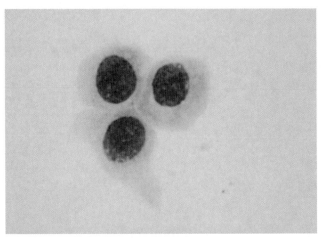

Figure 24-2   Epithelial cells from a normal prostate. The cytoplasm is grainy and acidophilic, and the nuclei are central and have a moderately reticular chromatin network. (Prostatic massage slightly concentrated by centrifugation, Wright-Giemsa stain.)

Normal Prostate

The cytologic features of the normal prostate vary depending upon the method of obtaining materials. Samples obtained by direct aspiration contain fewer contaminating cells and are usually more cellular than samples obtained from ejaculation, massage, or urethral washes. Glandular cells of the normal prostate are found in small to medium clusters and have centric nuclei and a finely stippled or reticular pattern. The cytoplasm stains slightly acidophilic and has a fine, granular appearance due to the very fine, basophilic material coursing through the cytoplasm (Figures 24-1 and 24-2).

Cells and contaminating material from other locations in the urogenital tracts may be found.

Spermatozoa: Sperm heads characteristically stain blue-green with Wright's method. Spermatozoa, which often adhere to other cells, possibly with many attached to a single epithelial cell, are most frequently found in ejaculated material, but can also be found in massage or wash samples (Figure 24-3).

Squamous Cells: Squamous cells are large cells with flattened, floppy appearances. More differentiated squamous cells have pyknotic or karyorrhectic nuclei, and immature squamous cells are difficult to differentiate from urothelial cells and prostatic epithelial cells. Because they originate from the distal urethra or the external genitalia, squamous cells are found in ejaculate, massage, and wash samples, but are also found in prostatic squamous metaplasia. Large, flat and angular or rolled squamous particles may be obtained from the external skin surface as well; these particles do not usually contain even a remnant of a nucleus. Contamination by such particles can be nearly eliminated by cleaning the skin before obtaining a sample.

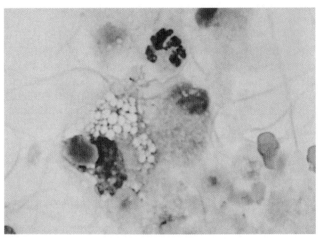

Figure 24-3 A prostatic epithelial cell, neutrophil, macrophage, and many spermatozoa from a dog with mild prostatitis. The background contains proteinaceous material, which is probably the product of prostatic epithelial cells. Spermatozoa characteristically stain aqua with Wright's stain. (Prostatic ejaculate slightly concentrated by centrifugation, Wright-Giemsa stain.)

Urothelial Cells: Urothelial cells (i.e., transitional epithelial cells) usually appear individually but may also be in small clusters. They are larger than prostatic epithelial cells and have homogenous, lightly basophilic cytoplasm and a lower nuclear-to-cytoplasmic ratio than prostatic cells (see Figure 23-1). Urothelial cells originate from the bladder and the tubular structures of the urinary and genital tracts and are most frequently found in samples obtained by ejaculation, massage, and washing.

Other Epithelial Cells: Cells of the ductus deferens and the epididymis are difficult to distinguish from prostatic cells.

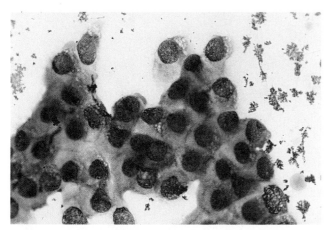

Figure 24-4 A cluster of prostatic epithelial cells from an older dog with benign prostatic hyperplasia. The cells have moderate amounts of basophilic cytoplasm and large nuclei with reticulated chromatin patterns. The azurophilic material found in the noncellular area is ultrasound contact gel. (FNAB, Wright-Giemsa stain.)

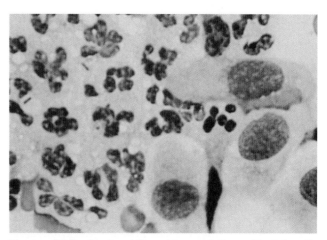

Figure 24-5 Neutrophils and prostatic epithelial cells from a dog with acute prostatitis. Bacilli are in some of the neutrophils, which are mildly degenerated with acidophilic, foamy cytoplasm and minimal nuclear degeneration. (Prostatic massage slightly concentrated by centrifugation, Wright-Giemsa stain.)

Ultrasound-Contact Gel: The gel used to ensure adequate acoustic coupling of the ultrasound scanhead to the body wall may contaminate the material obtained with ultrasound assistance. Small, azurophilic needle-like structures are found individually or in large clusters (Figure 24-4). When there is a large amount of material, the cells may be obscured or not be stained sufficiently for evaluation. The amount of contamination can be minimized by wiping excess gel from the skin before introducing the needle. Enough gel usually remains on the skin and scanhead to ensure sufficient contact for visualization of the prostate and accurate guidance of the needle.

Prostatic Cysts

Prostatic cysts are quite variable cytologically. Some have poorly cellular fluid that, even when concentrated, contains only a few epithelial cells, rare neutrophils, and some debris. Sometimes moderate numbers of normal or slightly hyperplastic (i.e., basophilic) epithelial cells are found. Squamous cells are rarely obtained. The specific gravity and protein concentration of prostatic cysts are usually similar to transudates.

Prostatitis

Purulent inflammation in which neutrophils dominate is the most frequent inflammatory lesion of the prostate. In septic prostatitis, the neutrophils have features, including karyolysis and foamy cytoplasm, that are suggestive of toxic degeneration. There usually are variable numbers of macrophages that typically have abundant, foamy cytoplasm. Bacteria may be found both intracellularly and extracellularly, and when they are found, it is necessary to determine whether they are actually the cause of the inflammation or are contaminants from other locations in the genital or urinary tract.[3] If the sample was obtained by an aspiration technique, the bacteria should be considered

the cause, but if the sample was obtained through the urogenital ductal system, it is necessary to determine if the bacteria are contaminants from the external genitalia or from an inflammatory lesion elsewhere in the urinary or genital system. Intracellular bacteria are certainly a strong indication that the inflammatory process is septic. In addition to inflammatory cells, clusters of various sizes of epithelial cells may be obtained. In aspirates obtained from inflamed prostates, prostatic cells appear to have loose cohesion. Additionally, their cytoplasm usually shows increased basophilia, indicating that the prostatic epithelium is hyperplastic secondary to the inflammation (Figure 24-5).

Prostatic abscesses are focal areas of severe inflammation. Abscesses may be single, large accumulations of pus or multiple, small accumulations. Degenerated neutrophils with karyolysis and foamy cytoplasm with a background of cellular debris are found. Features of prostatic hyperplasia may accompany prostatic abscesses. In addition to hyperplasia, the prostatic epithelium may also develop squamous metaplasia secondary to inflammation (see the discussion of squamous metaplasia later).

Prostatic Hyperplasia

Benign prostatic hyperplasia is a distinct entity that usually occurs in older dogs and is apparently caused by a sex hormone imbalance.[5] Addionally, prostatic hyperplasia usually accompanies inflammatory lesions of the prostate, and the epithelium that lines prostatic cysts is often hyperplastic. The cytologic features of the epithelial cells are similar whatever the cause of the hyperplasia. Moderate cell numbers are usually found; cells are often in variably sized clusters, but many individual cells are also found. In cell clusters, acinar-like arrangements may be found, and cytoplasmic borders are usually indistinct. The cytoplasm is often abundant, basophilic, and slightly granular. Nuclei are

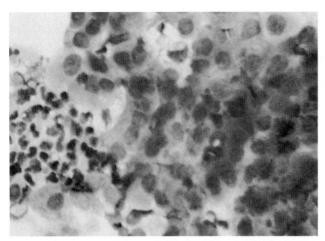

Figure 24-6 Hyperplasia of the prostatic epithelium from a dog with prostatitis. The cells are basophilic and have an increased nuclear-to-cytoplasmic ratio. Pleomorphism is minimal, and differentiation is suggested along the edges of the cell clusters. (Prostate massage slightly concentrated by centrifugation, Wright-Giemsa stain.)

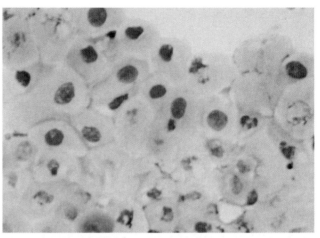

Figure 24-7 Squamous metaplasia of the prostatic epithelium in a dog with a Sertoli cell tumor. The cells are large and light-staining, and some contain karyorrhectic nuclei. (Prostatic massage slightly concentrated by centrifugation, Wright-Giemsa stain.)

round to oval and somewhat large, with finely reticulated or stippled chromatin patterns. Nucleoli are not usually found. The nuclear-to-cytoplasmic ratio is increased compared with that of normal prostatic cells (see Figures 24-4 and 24-6).

When hyperplasia is not accompanied by inflammation, it should be considered a preneoplastic change.[6]

Squamous Metaplasia

Under the influence of the estrogen-like hormone activity that occurs with Sertoli cell tumors, the epithelium of the prostate may undergo metaplasia to become a squamous-like epithelium. Squamous metaplasia may also occur as a sequela to chronic irritation or inflammation, but the most prominent squamous metaplastic changes occur in dogs with Sertoli cell tumors or treated with exogenous estrogens.[3,8] Aspirates are moderately cellular, and large cells (many individual, some in clusters) with slightly basophilic to slightly acidophilic cytoplasm are found. The cells are very large and appear flattened and floppy. Cells occasionally contain an either pyknotic or karyorrhectic nucleus. Inflammatory and hyperplastic cells are occasionally found (Figure 24-7).

Carcinomas

Prostatomegaly and its accompanying signs occur in dogs with prostatic carcinomas. Most prostatic carcinomas arise from the urothelium instead of the glandular prostate.[8] On palpation, the prostate may be very large and have irregular asymmetry.[1,6] Cellularity is moderate to marked, and anisokaryosis, nuclear enlargement and irregularity, and marked increases in the nuclear-to-cytoplasmic ratio are found. Nucleoli are often present and are usually

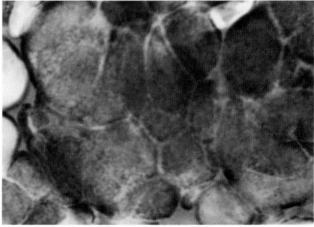

Figure 24-8 Crowded, neoplastic epithelial cells that show cellular and nuclear molding. (Prostatic massage slightly concentrated by centrifugation, Wright-Giemsa stain.)

small, single, and uniform, but sometimes large, irregular nucleoli are found. Cell membranes may be distinct in well-differentiated neoplasms but are indistinct in poorly differentiated tumors. Cell cohesion is often apparent, and acinar-like formation is rarely present within some of the cell clusters (Figures 24-8 and 24-9). It is difficult to distinguish prostatic carcinomas that arise from the urothelium of the genital system from those that arise from the glandular area of the prostate by cytologic examination. However, when acinar-like structures are found, adenocarcinomas are more likely than urothelial carcinomas. Prostatic carcinomas frequently metastasize to the iliac and sublumbar lymph nodes; thus nodular palpation and evaluation are indicated in suspected cases of prostatic neoplasia.[1,6]

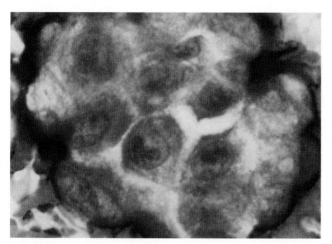

Figure 24-9 A group of neoplastic prostatic epithelial cells, some of which contain distinct nucleoli. Cell borders are indistinct, and modest cell crowding is evident. (Prostatic massage slightly concentrated by centrifugation, Wright-Giemsa stain.)

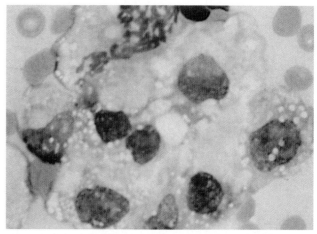

Figure 24-10 A group of vacuolated cells aspirated from a Sertoli cell tumor. The cells have abundant cytoplasm with moderate-sized, clear vacuoles and coarse nuclear chromatin patterns. There is a mitotic figure at the top. (Wright-Giemsa stain.)

TESTES

Obtaining Testicular Samples

Enlargement, either unilateral or bilateral, is the major indication for fine-needle aspiration biopsy and cytologic evaluation of the testes.[8,9] The epididymis may be enlarged and can be aspirated by fine-needle aspiration. Decreased testicular size with increased firmness suggests atrophy. Fine-needle aspiration of atrophic testicles does not usually yield a sample that is adequate for cytologic evaluation, and biopsy and histopathologic evaluation may be required for an informed diagnosis.[9] Semen evaluation may also provide information on testicular lesions, although it is mainly valued for determining sperm quality.

Cytologic Evaluation of Normal Testes

Only a few cells can be obtained from a normal testicle. Spermatozoa or their precursors, round cells such as Sertoli cells, and interstitial cells may occasionally be found, but the material obtained from normal testicles is often contaminated with blood.

Orchitis and Epididymitis

The cytologic findings of orchitis and epididymitis are similar to the cytologic findings of other tissue inflammations. Neutrophils are the predominant cells, but other inflammatory cells (especially macrophages) may be found. The cause of the lesion may occasionally be determined by cytologic or microbiologic methods. In some cases of blastomycosis, *Blastomyces dermatitidis* organisms may be observed in testicular aspirates, but in cases of brucellosis orchitis and epididymitis, *Brucella canis* is rarely seen.[9,10,11] In both blastomycosis and brucellosis of the testes, macrophages including multinucleated phagocytes (i.e., giant cells) may be present.

Neoplasia

The three major tumors of canine testes are Sertoli cell tumors, seminomas, and interstitial cell tumors. These tumors are difficult to differentiate cytologically, but when evaluated with clinical signs and history, a diagnosis is usually possible. The differentiation of testicular neoplasia from inflammation, the other major cause of testicular enlargement, is relatively simple.

Sertoli Cell Tumors: Sertoli cell tumors commonly occur in the testicles of older dogs or the undescended testicles of cryptorchid dogs. Many dogs have feminization syndrome, which along with many other signs, results in atrophy of the contralateral testicle. It is possible to obtain material from intra-abdominal Sertoli cell tumors with ultrasound assistance, and inguinal crypt-orchid testicles are easily aspirated.

Aspirates of Sertoli cell tumors have many cells that vary in size and amount of cytoplasm. Mitotic figures may be found, and small nucleoli may be present; the nuclear chromatin pattern is finely reticulated. The most unique feature is the light-staining, vacuolated cytoplasm in cells with abundant cytoplasm. The vacuoles are small (1 to 2 μm) and very distinct (Figures 24-10 and 24-11). Spindle-shaped cells with abundant cytoplasm are rarely found.

Seminomas: There are few clinical signs in dogs that have seminomas, except when there is a coexisting Sertoli cell tumor, which is a moderately common occurrence. Cryptorchidism is a predisposing factor, and undescended testicles have an increased risk of seminoma development. Some dogs may have feminization syndrome, and prostatitis, prostatic hyperplasia, and perianal adenomas may occur. The major feature of seminomas is testicular enlargement, which is usually unilateral but occasionally may be bilateral. Seminomas may cause multiple enlargements in one or both testicles.

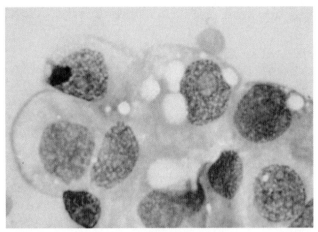

Figure 24-11 A group of cells with abundant cytoplasm that were aspirated from a Sertoli cell tumor. There are several large vacuoles in some cells, the chromatin is coarsely reticular, and a large, somewhat irregular nucleolus is at the top (center). (Wright-Giemsa stain.)

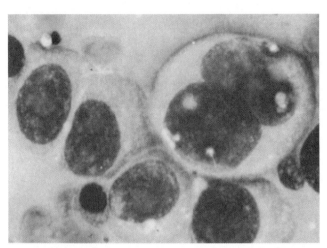

Figure 24-13 A multinucleated cell and several other cells from a seminoma. The cells have a moderate to high nuclear-to-cytoplasmic ratio and a finely reticular chromatin pattern. (Wright-Giemsa stain.)

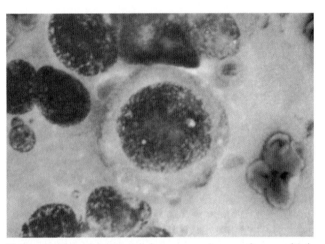

Figure 24-12 A large cell from a seminoma shows a high nuclear-to-cytoplasmic ratio, a finely reticular chromatin pattern, and an irregular nucleolus. (Wright-Giemsa stain.)

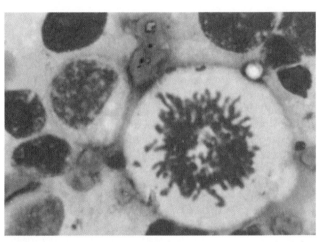

Figure 24-14 A mitotic figure in a seminoma. (Wright-Giemsa stain.)

Aspiration usually yields moderate to large numbers of cells that vary in size and amount of cytoplasm, although the amount of cytoplasm is usually sparse to moderate. The cytoplasm is usually lightly basophilic and homogeneous (Figure 24-12). Nuclei are homogeneous to finely reticular and may be multiple (Figures 24-12 and 24-13). Relatively large nucleoli are found, and mitotic figures are common (Figure 24-14).

Interstitial Cell Tumors: Clinical signs are unusual in dogs with interstitial cell tumors. Aspirates from such tumors are often low in cellularity. Cell clusters frequently surround an endothelial-lined capillary (Figure 24-15). Cells vary in size but usually have abundant cytoplasm that stains basophilic (Figure 24-16). Many cells may contain small vacuoles, but this is not a consistent feature (Figure 24-16). Small, black granules are occasionally seen

in a few cells (Figure 24-17), and the nuclear-to-cytoplasmic ratio is usually low. Nuclei are small to medium, have a fine reticular or homogenous chromatin pattern, and may contain nucleoli.

Canine Transmissible Venereal Tumors: Transmissible venereal tumors (TVTs) usually occur on the external genitalia of dogs, but they may also be found in the nasal cavity, mouth, and pharynx (especially near the tonsils) and on nongenital skin; a TVT may occasionally metastasize to other locations. Impression smears or smears of aspirated material are usually quite cellular, and the tumor cells have distinct characteristics. They are medium-size with a nuclear-to-cytoplasmic ratio that is moderately increased because their nuclei are large and have a moderate amount of cytoplasm. Nuclei are immature with homogenous to finely reticulated chromatin patterns. Large, round nucleoli can be found in a few cells. Cytoplasm stains vary from lightly to heavily basophilic from tumor to tumor. Most cells

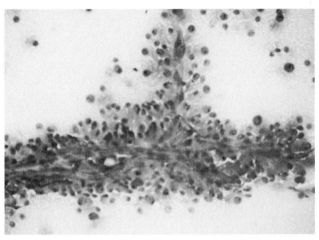

Figure 24-15 An impression smear of an interstitial cell tumor. Note the round to polygonal cells that are free and surrounding an endothelium-lined capillary. (Diff-Quik.)

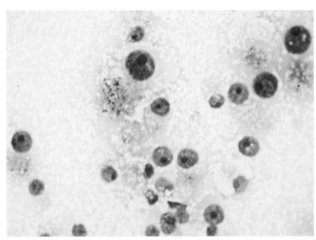

Figure 24-17 Fine-needle aspirate of an interstitial cell tumor. The cells and their nuclei vary in size and show prominent vacuolization. Some cells contain blue-black cytoplasmic granules. (Diff-Quik.)

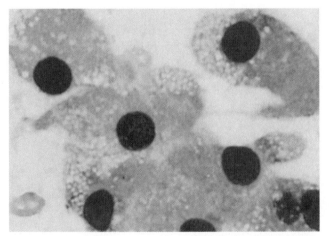

Figure 24-16 Cells in an aspirate of an interstitial cell tumor vary in shape and have moderately basophilic cytoplasm and small, homogenous nuclei. (Wright-Giemsa stain.)

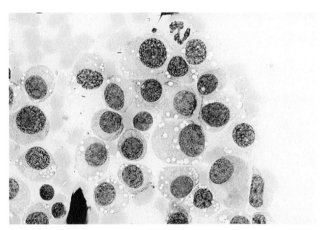

Figure 24-18 Numerous TVT cells with coarse chromatin and smoky gray vacuolated cytoplasm are shown. (Wright's stain.)

contain distinct, small (1 to 2 μm in diameter), punctate vacuoles. Mitotic cells are frequently found (Figure 24-18).

Other cells may be seen in cytologic preparations of TVTs. During the regressive stage, many lymphocytes are present along with a few neutrophils and macrophages. Impression smears made from the surface of ulcerated tumors may contain bacteria, neutrophils, and epithelial cells.

SEMEN

Semen is usually evaluated as part of a routine breeding-soundness examination or to determine its quality in infertile or subfertile males.[12] Semen examination can also provide information on lesions in the genital tract of male dogs, however, because it contains material derived from the testes and also from the remainder of the reproductive tract, including the prostate gland. Thus semen may be examined for breeding purposes, as well as for diagnosis of some inflammatory or neoplastic lesions of the reproductive tract.

Semen Collection

Semen is often collected into an artificial vagina while the penis is manually manipulated in the presence of a teaser bitch. The male's interest can be enhanced by applying a solution of a 1:100 dilution of p-hydroxybenzoate methyl ester to the perineum of the teaser bitch. The technique is more fully described elsewhere.[12,13] Semen may be collected from cats with the use of an artificial vagina or electroejaculation.[14] Dogs produce from 1 to 40 ml of semen ejaculate,[12] and cats produce up to 0.5 ml.[14]

Semen Evaluation

The gross characteristics of the fluid, including color and consistency, should be determined immediately after collection. Normal semen is milky and moderately viscous. A red or pink color indicates that there is blood in the sample, and yellow discoloration suggests the presence

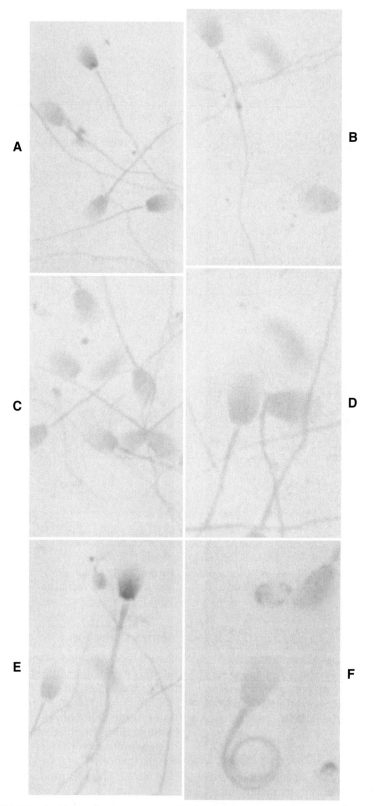

Figure 24-19 **A,** Normal spermatozoa. **B,** Spermatozoa with a protoplasmic droplet. **C,** Detached sperm head. **D,** Spermatozoa with an abnormally attached head. **E,** Spermatozoa with a double tail. **F,** Spermatozoa with a coiled tail. (New methylene blue stain.)

of urine. Serous, greenish or grayish semen indicates inflammation, especially when small flecks of material are present.

The number of spermatozoa per ejaculate is the most important information for evaluating the breeding potential of a male dog.[12] Concentration is determined using a hemacytometer after appropriate dilution. A portion is diluted 1:100 with saline or a red cell Unopette (Becton Dickinson), and the total number of sperm in the central primary square is determined. The total sperm count is calculated by multiplying the count by 10^6 and the volume of the ejaculate. In samples with low numbers of sperm, either the sample is diluted less or a greater area of the hemacytometer should be used for counting. Appropriate adjustments of the multiplication factor are made for calculating the total sperm count.

Sperm motility should be evaluated immediately after collection. The sample should be maintained at body temperature or warmed to body temperature in an incubator. A drop is placed on a warm slide, which is immediately covered with a coverslip. Samples with a high concentration of spermatozoa may be diluted 1:1 with warm physiologic saline or 2.9% sodium citrate.

Progressive, forward motility of individual sperm is estimated at high-dry magnification. Such movement is thought to reflect viability and ability to fertilize the ovum. Spermatozoa may have side-to-side motion without forward progression, move in small circles, or be nonmotile or hypomotile. A normal semen sample should have >70% motility. Decreased motility may be found in semen contaminated with urine or exposed to pus. Overall sperm motility of the first ejaculate after a long period of sexual inactivity is decreased because of the increased percentage of old and dead sperm.[12]

Sperm morphology is assessed by bright field microscopy of a new methylene blue–stained smear or phase-contrast microscopy of an unstained smear. For bright field microscopy, an air-dried smear is mounted in a drop of 0.5% NMB. The following are how 200 sperm are classified: normal sperm, abnormal head, abnormal midpiece, coiled tail, head only, protoplasmic droplet, and abnormal head attachment (Figure 24-19).

In semen of high quality, nearly all sperm should be morphologically normal. Increased percentages of abnormalities indicate poor quality and breeding potential; however, correlations between percentages of sperm abnormalities and conception rate have not been determined in dogs.[12]

Wright-Giemsa–stained semen should be examined after Wright's staining when inflammation or neoplasia is suspected. Neutrophils indicate inflammation in the reproductive tract; however, when abnormal cells are found, contamination from the external surface of the penis and inflammation of the urethra or bladder must be ruled out. Ejaculates, especially the first portion of the ejaculate, occasionally contain cells from the prostate gland, so the diagnosis of prostate gland inflammation or neoplasia may be suggested from such observations. Evaluation of the prostate is indicated with these findings.

References

1. Ling GV, et al: Canine prostatic fluid: Techniques of collection, quantitative bacterial culture, and interpretation of results. *J Am Vet Med Assoc* 183:201-206, 1983.
2. Ling GV: In Ling GV: *Lower Urinary Tract Diseases of Dogs and Cats.* St. Louis, Mosby, 1995, pp 129-141.
3. Thrall DE, et al: Cytologic diagnosis of canine prostatic disease. *J Am Animal Hosp Assoc* 21:95-102, 1985.
4. Ling GV: In Ling GV: *Lower Urinary Tract Diseases of Dogs and Cats.* St. Louis, Mosby, 1995, pp 49-59.
5. Rogers et al: Diagnostic evaluation of the canine prostate. *Compend Contin Educ* 8:799-811, 1986.
6. Madewell BR, Theilen GH: *Veterinary Cancer Medicine,* ed 2. Philadelphia, Lea & Febiger,1987, pp 583-600.
7. Kennedy. In Ling GV: *Lower Urinary Tract Diseases of Dogs and Cats.* St Louis, Mosby, 1995, pp 107-113.
8. DeNicola, et al: *Cytology of the Canine Male Urogenital Tract.* St. Louis, Ralston-Purina, 1980.
9. Larsen RE: Testicular biopsy in the dog. *Vet Clin North Am* 7:747-755, 1977.
10. Barsanti. In Greene CE: *Clinical Microbiology and Infectious Diseases of the Dog and Cat.* Philadelphia, Saunders, 1984, pp 675-686.
11. Greene CE, George: In Green CE: *Clinical Microbiology and Infectious Diseases of the Dog and Cat.* Philadelphia, Saunders, 1984, pp 646-662.
12. Feldman EC: *Canine and Feline Endocrinology and Reproduction.* Philadelphia, Saunders, 1987, pp 481-524.
13. Seager. In Kirk R: *Current Veterinary Therapy VI: Small Animal Practice.* Philadelphia, Saunders, 1977, pp 1245-1251.
14. Seager. In Kirk R: *Current Veterinary Therapy VI: Small Animal Practice.* Philadelphia, Saunders, 1977, pp 1252-1254.

Vaginal Cytology

R.W. Allison, M.A. Thrall, and P.N. Olson

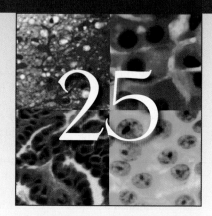

25

CHAPTER

Examination of exfoliated cells from the vagina is a simple technique that is useful to monitor the progression of proestrus and estrus in dogs and cats.[1-3] The vaginal epithelium undergoes a predictable hyperplastic response to increasing plasma estrogen concentrations during proestrus. Starting as only a few cell layers, the epithelium becomes 20 to 30 cell layers thick, eventually exfoliating large numbers of superficial epithelial cells during estrus. Vaginal cytology, often in tandem with hormone analysis, can provide valuable information about the stage of the ovarian cycle.[4] In addition, vaginal cytology has proven useful to detect inflammatory and neoplastic conditions in the female reproductive tract.[5]

THE VAGINA

Collecting Vaginal Samples

Cells are obtained by passing a cotton-tipped swab into the caudal vagina (Figures 25-1 and 25-2). A narrow spreading speculum may be used to allow unimpeded swab passage. If no vaginal discharge is present the swab may be moistened with sterile saline to avoid discomfort. The swab should be directed craniodorsad when entering the vaginal vault in order to avoid the clitoral fossa; keratinized epithelium normally present in the fossa could lead to an inappropriate cytologic interpretation (Figure 25-3).[3] Once cranial to the urethral orifice, the vaginal wall is gently swabbed. The cells are then transferred to a glass slide by gently rolling the swab with minimal pressure to avoid rupturing cells. The smear is allowed to air-dry thoroughly before staining. Romanowsky-type stains typically used for blood films (Wright's or modified Wright-Giemsa stains, including quick-type stains) provide good morphologic detail.

Classifying Vaginal Cells

Vaginal epithelial cells are described beginning with the deepest, most immature layer near the basement membrane and progressing superficially to the most mature layer nearest the vaginal lumen (Figure 25-4).

Basal Cells: Basal cells give rise to all epithelial cell types observed in a vaginal smear. They are small cells with round nuclei and a high nuclar-to-cytoplasmic ratio and are rarely observed in vaginal smears.

Parabasal Cells: Parabasal cells are small round cells with round vesiculated nuclei and a small amount of cytoplasm and are usually quite uniform in size and shape (see Figure 25-4, *A*). Large numbers of parabasal cells may exfoliate when the vagina of a prepubertal animal is swabbed.

Intermediate Cells: Intermediate cells vary in size depending on the amount of cytoplasm present. Although the nuclei of both small and large intermediate cells are similar in size to parabasal cell nuclei, intermediate cells are about twice the size of parabasal cells (see Figure 25-4, *B* and *C*). Intermediate cells still have vesiculated nuclei, but as they increase in size their cytoplasm becomes irregular, folded, and angular, similar to the cytoplasm of superficial cells. Large intermediate cells are sometimes called superficial intermediate or transitional intermediate cells.

Superficial Cells: Superficial cells are the largest epithelial cells seen in vaginal smears (see Figure 25-4, *D*). These are dead cells whose nuclei become pyknotic and then faded, often progressing to anucleate forms (see Figure 25-4, *E*). Their cytoplasm is abundant, angular, and folded. As the cells degenerate, the cytoplasm may contain small vacuoles (Figure 25-5). The degeneration process of stratified squamous epithelial cells into large, flat, dead cells is called cornification; superficial epithelial cells are commonly called cornified cells. Superficial cells with small pyknotic nuclei and anuclear superficial epithelial cells have the same significance.

Other Normal Cytologic Findings: Metestrum cells have been described as vaginal epithelial cells containing neutrophils in their cytoplasm (Figure 25-6).[3,6] They are not specific for any stage of the cycle and may be seen whenever neutrophils are present.

The vagina of dogs and cats contains normal bacterial flora, and bacteria are frequently observed on vaginal cytology slides.[7,8] Unless the bacteria are accompanied by

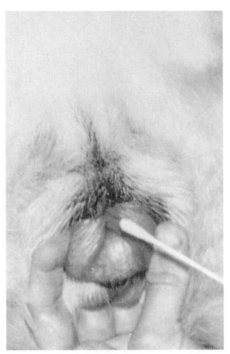

Figure 25-1 The labia are carefully parted to allow unimpeded passage of the swab. *(Courtesy of Kal Kan Forum.)*

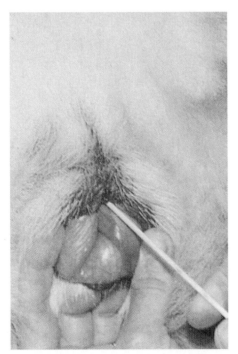

Figure 25-2 The swab is directed craniodorsad to avoid entering the clitoral fossa. *(Courtesy of Kal Kan Forum.)*

large numbers of neutrophils, they are generally considered to be normal flora.

Spermatozoa are sometimes observed in vaginal cytologic preparations from mated bitches (Figure 25-7), but the period during which they are present varies. The presence of spermatozoa confirms a mating, but their absence does not ensure that a bitch was not bred. We have

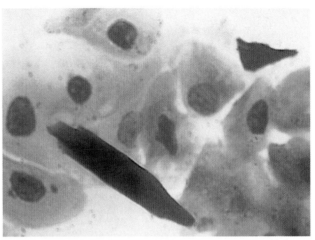

Figure 25-3 Epithelial cells obtained from the clitoral fossa. (Wright's stain, original magnification 400×.)

observed intact spermatozoa or sperm heads in about 65% of vaginal smears made 24 hours after a natural mating and in 50% of smears made 48 hours after mating.

Cells that appear to be placental trophoblast-like syncytia may be occasionally observed in vaginal cytologic preparations, particularly several weeks after whelping in bitches with suspected subinvolution of placental sites (Figure 25-8).[5]

STAGING THE CANINE ESTROUS CYCLE

Figure 25-9 provides an overview of the changes in vaginal cytology related to plasma estrogen levels during the normal canine estrous cycle.

Proestrus

As ovarian follicles mature and serum concentrations of estrogen (estradiol) increase, vaginal epithelium proliferates and erythrocytes pass through uterine capillaries. These changes result in the typical appearance of vaginal cytologic preparations made during proestrus (Figure 25-10). Cytologic specimens obtained in early and mid-proestrus are characterized by a mixture of epithelial cells, including parabasal, small and large intermediates, and superficial cells (Figure 25-11), along with variable numbers of neutrophils and erythrocytes. Basophilic mucous material may be present in the background. As proestrus continues and the vaginal epithelium thickens, neutrophils are no longer able to traverse the vaginal wall, so their numbers decrease. There are progressively higher percentages of large intermediate and superficial cells present with fewer parabasal and small intermediate cells. After serum estrogen levels peak in late proestrus, more than 80% of epithelial cells are superficial, and neutrophils are absent; this is identical to the vaginal cytology during estrus.[9] Erythrocytes may be abundant or absent throughout proestrus. Bacteria, both free and on the surface of epithelial cells, are often present in large numbers (see Figure 25-14). The mean duration of proestrus in mature bitches is 9 days, although a range of 2 to 17 days is seen in normal dogs.[2]

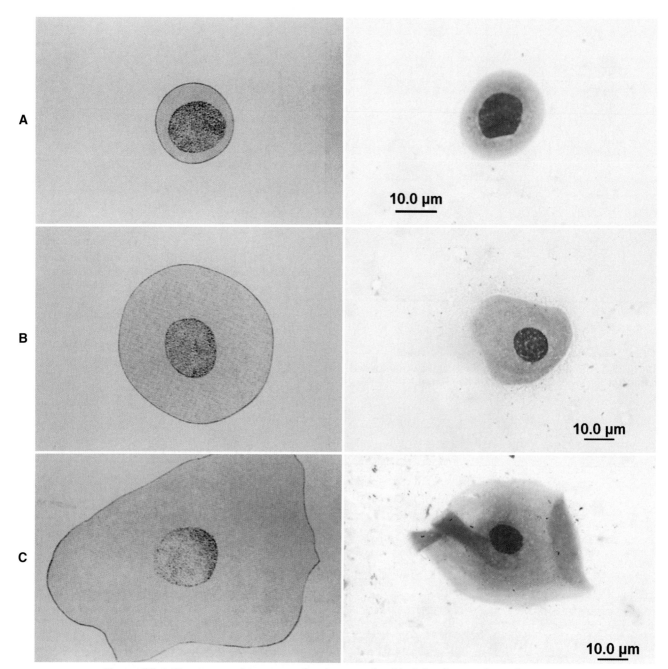

Figure 25-4 Diagrams and corresponding images of epithelial cell types from the canine vagina. **A,** Parabasal epithelial cells. **B,** Small intermediate cells. **C,** Large intermediate cells.

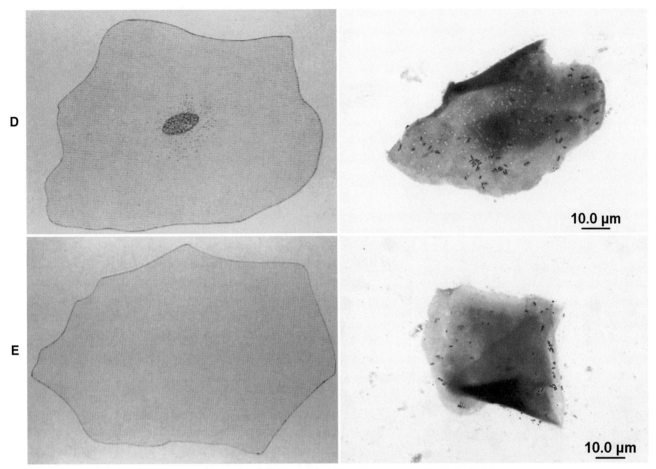

Figure 25-4, cont'd Diagrams and corresponding images of epithelial cell types from the canine vagina. **D,** Superficial cells with pyknotic nuclei (note bacteria adhered to the cell on the right). **E,** Anuclear superficial cells. (All cytology images stained with Wright's stain, original magnification 1000×.) *(All diagrams courtesy of Kal Kan Forum.)*

Estrus

Most (80% to 90%) of the epithelial cells exfoliated during estrus are superficial cells. Typically almost all these superficial cells contain small pyknotic nuclei (Figure 25-12). However, samples from some bitches contain nearly 100% anuclear cells; in other bitches, large intermediate cells are retained. Maximal cornification follows the serum estrogen peak in late proestrus and continues throughout estrus.[1,9] Ovulation usually occurs about 2 days after the luteinizing hormone (LH) surge, following decreases in serum estrogen and increases in serum progesterone (Figure 25-13).[2] Because maximal cornification may occur as much as 6 days before or 3 days after the LH surge, vaginal cytology is an imprecise predictor of ovulation. Cytologic preparations made during estrus usually have a clear background, free of mucus, and may or may not contain erythrocytes. Large numbers of bacteria are commonly observed on and around superficial epithelial cells, but neutrophils are normally absent unless there is inflammation (Figure 25-14).[3] The average duration of estrus is 9 days for mature bitches, but a range of 3 to 21 days has been reported.[2]

Diestrus

Diestrus occurs about 8 days (range 6 to 10 days) after the LH peak in most cycles and is cytologically characterized by an abrupt change in relative numbers of superficial epithelial cells. Over a 24- to 48-hour period, superficial cell numbers dramatically decrease to about 20%, whereas parabasal and intermediate cell numbers

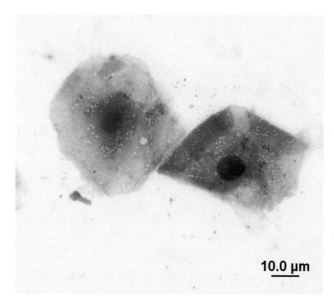

10.0 µm

Figure 25-5 Degenerating superficial vaginal epithelial cells with vacuolated cytoplasm in a canine vaginal smear. (Wright's stain, original magnification 1000×.)

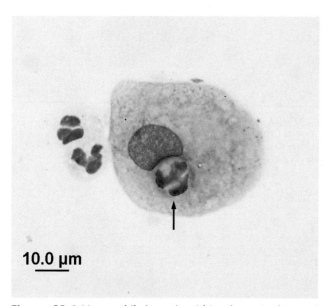

10.0 µm

Figure 25-6 Neutrophil (*arrow*) within the cytoplasm of an epithelial cell. These cells have been termed *metestrum cells* but may be seen at any time neutrophils are present. (Wright's stain, original magnification 400×.)

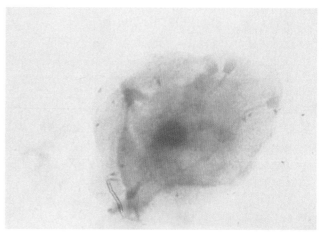

Figure 25-7 Spermatozoa and a superficial epithelial cell in a vaginal smear from a bitch several hours after mating. (Wright's stain, original magnification 400×.)

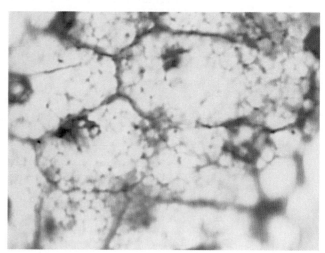

Figure 25-8 Cells that appear to be placental trophoblasts in a vaginal smear from a bitch with subinvolution of placental sites after whelping. (Wright's stain, original magnification 400×.)

increase.[6] Neutrophils appear in variable numbers and usually coincide with increased numbers of parabasal and intermediate cells (Figure 25-15). Some bitches have few or no neutrophils in cytologic preparations made during diestrus (Figure 25-16). Erythrocytes and bacteria may or may not be present. Bacteria engulfed by neutrophils are occasionally seen during diestrus in normal bitches.[5] Behavioral diestrus is defined by the bitch's refusal of the male and usually lags behind cytologic diestrus by several days.[3]

Individual cytologic preparations made during the transition period from late estrus to early diestrus, without benefit of prior preparations, can appear very similar to smears made in early or mid-proestrus. At both times there can be a similar mixture of superficial and nonsuperficial cells, and both erythrocytes and neutrophils may be present. Vaginoscopy, vulvar examination, and the animal's behavior are usually helpful in making differentiations. When in doubt, repeating vaginal cytology in 3 or 4 days should clarify the situation.

Anestrus

Parabasal and intermediate cells predominate during anestrus (Figure 25-17). If present, neutrophils and bacteria are few in number.

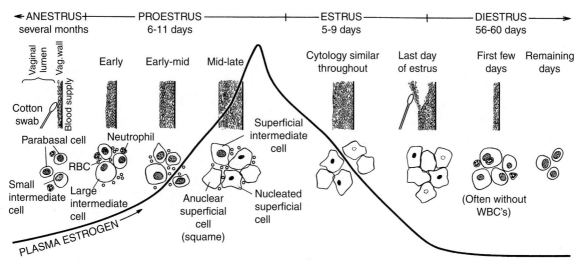

Figure 25-9 Illustration of the changes in vaginal cytology related to plasma estrogen levels: in the average canine estrous cycle. *(From Feldman EC, Nelson RW: Ovarian Cycle and Vaginal Cytology. In Feldman EC, Nelson RW [eds]:* Canine and Feline Endocrinology and Reproduction, *ed 3. Philadelphias, Saunders, 2004, p 755.)*

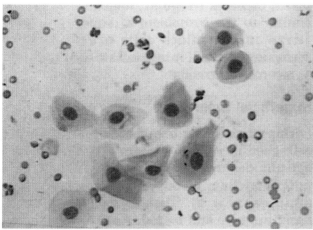

Figure 25-10 Vaginal smear from a dog in proestrus. Intermediate epithelial cells predominate. Note the erythrocytes and a few neutrophils. (Wright's stain, original magnification 100×.)

Figure 25-11 Intermediate cells and neutrophils in a vaginal smear from a dog in proestrus. (Wright's stain, original magnification 400×.)

MANAGEMENT OF BREEDING

There is considerable variation in the duration of proestrus and estrus in normal bitches. Although the average length of time from the onset of proestrus to standing heat (when the bitch will accept a male) is 9 days, it may be as short as 2 or as long as 25 days in normal animals.[6] Some bitches have no discernible behavioral proestrus or estrus, yet they ovulate normally. These variations can cause confusion about the best time to attempt breeding. Vaginal cytology is useful to suggest appropriate breeding times, but cytology alone cannot reliably distinguish between late proestrus and estrus and does not give specific information about the date of ovulation.

Normal, healthy bitches should be bred every 3 to 4 days throughout the period when >90% of vaginal epithelial cells are superficial.[3,9] Because canine spermatozoa can survive for at least 4 to 6 days in the uterus of bitches in estrus, mating may be successful from shortly before the time of ovulation to about 4 days after ovulation. Once diestrus occurs, fertility rapidly declines. Breedings are unlikely to be successful if delayed more than 24 hours after the onset of cytologic diestrus.

Hormone Analysis

Ovulation has been shown to occur about 48 hours (range 24 to 72 hours) after the LH surge.[9,10] Serum LH concentrations can be measured, but stay elevated only

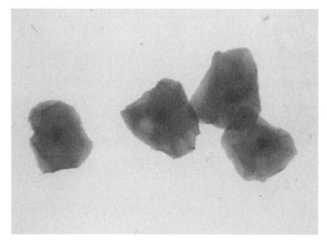

Figure 25-12 Vaginal smear from a dog in estrus. Note superficial epithelial cells with pyknotic nuclei. (Wright's stain, original magnification 100×.)

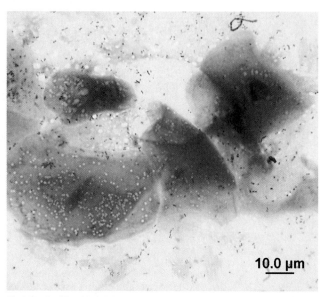

10.0 µm

Figure 25-14 Vaginal smear from a dog in estrus. Superficial cells predominate, and many bacteria are present in the background and adhered to the epithelial cells. (Wright's stain, original magnification 1000×.)

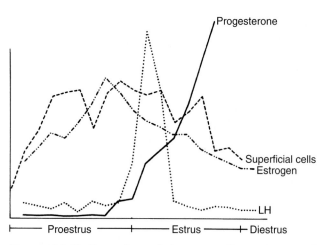

Figure 25-13 Illustration of hormone fluctuations and vaginal cytology during the average canine estrous cycle. *(Modified from Feldman EC, Nelson RW: Ovarian Cycle and Vaginal Cytology. In Feldman EC, Nelson RW [eds]:* Canine and Feline Endocrinology and Reproduction, *ed 3. Philadelphia, Saunders, 2004, p 755.)*

Combining Vaginal Cytology and Hormone Analysis

Determining serial progesterone levels and vaginal cytology during proestrus and estrus will provide the most information about the fertile period and have proven useful in the management of animals with variable estrus cycles.[4] A protocol proposed by Goodman[9] suggests beginning vaginal cytology at the first clinical sign of proestrus (vaginal discharge or vulvar swelling) and following with cytology every few days until cornification reaches 70%. A baseline progesterone level should be performed at the time of the first vaginal cytology. When cornification reaches 70%, serial progesterone assays should be performed every other day until the progesterone level is > 2 ng/ml, at which point breeding should begin and continue every other day for at least two or three breedings. Vaginal cytology should be evaluated concurrently with the progesterone assays to ensure that cornification progresses to 80% to 100%. Following vaginal cytology throughout the breeding period is suggested to identify the onset of diestrus, and at least one additional progesterone assay is suggested to be sure that concentrations continue to rise.

STAGING THE FELINE ESTROUS CYCLE

Female cats (queens) are seasonally polyestrous. Coitus is necessary for ovulation, and successive estrous periods occur in the absence of ovulation. The mean duration of estrus is about 8 days (range 3 to 16 days). The average interval between estrous periods is 9 days (range 4 to 22 days) if ovulation does not occur. Ovulation and the subsequent pseudopregnancy delay the return to estrus for about 45 days. Vaginal smears may be examined to accurately detect estrus in cats.[12-16] Ovulation may be induced while obtaining cells for vaginal cytologic preparations.

12 to 24 hours, making them inconvenient as a marker of ovulation for routine breedings; however, measuring LH levels may be justified in animals experiencing reproductive difficulties or when frozen semen is used for artificial insemination. By contrast, serum progesterone levels rise from basal levels of < 0.5 ng/ml to > 1 ng/ml shortly before the LH surge, 2 to 4 ng/ml during the LH surge, and typically reach > 4 ng/ml by the time ovulation occurs.[4,9,11] Commercial laboratories now offer 24-hour turnaround time on serum progesterone assays, making them a convenient adjunct to vaginal cytology, with the benefit of more precise estimation of the fertile period.

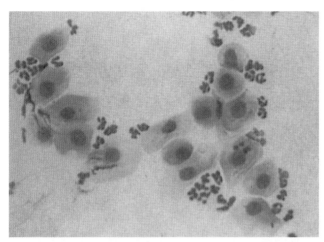

Figure 25-15 Vaginal smear from a dog in diestrus. Note the numerous neutrophils and intermediate cells. (Wright's stain, original magnification 100×.)

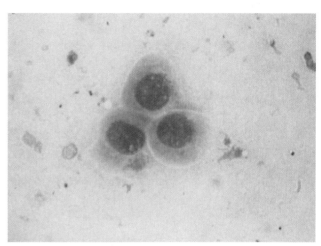

Figure 25-17 Parabasal cells in a vaginal smear from a dog in anestrus. (Wright's stain, original magnification 400×.)

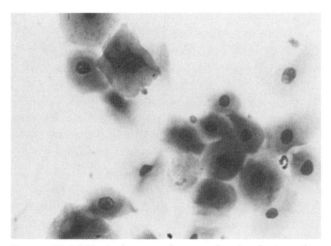

Figure 25-16 Vaginal smear from a dog in diestrus that contains very few neutrophils. (Wright's stain, original magnification 100×.)

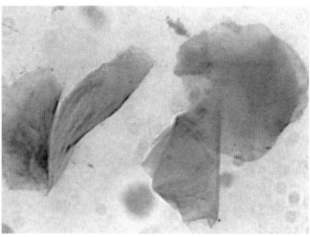

Figure 25-18 Vaginal smear from a cat in estrus. Note the anuclear superficial epithelial cells with folded angular cytoplasm. (Wright's stain, original magnification 400×.)

Vaginal cytologic characteristics of the queen are similar to those of the bitch; differences are outlined subsequently.

Proestrus

Proestrus is usually difficult to detect because queens do not typically have a vaginal discharge as observed in the bitch.[2] Duration of proestrus is short (0.5 to 2 days).[17] Erythrocytes and leukocytes are not usually present on cytologic samples, but there is clearing of the background mucus on vaginal smears due to increasing estrogen levels prior to the onset of estrus. Epithelial cells consist of a mixture of intermediate and nucleated superficial cells, with low numbers of parabasal cells and anuclear superficial cells.[16]

Estrus

Epithelial cells become progressively cornified as serum estrogen levels rise above 20 pg/ml during estrus.[16] The proportion of anuclear superficial cells increases to >10% on the first day of estrus. By the fourth day of estrus, about 40% of the cells are anuclear superficial cells, whereas intermediate cell numbers decrease to <10% (Figure 25-18).[16] Numbers of anuclear superficial cells remain relatively constant during the remainder of estrus, ranging from 40% to 60% of the total. Neutrophils and parabasal cells are absent during estrus. It has been suggested that the pronounced clearing of the background mucus and debris on vaginal smears obtained during estrus may be the most sensitive indicator of estrogen activity in cats.[16]

Interestrous Period and Diestrus

Estrus is followed by the interestrous period (if no ovulation occurs) or diestrus (if ovulation occurs). As estrus ends, background debris and parabasal cells reappear on vaginal smears. Anuclear superficial cell numbers decrease and the majority of cells are a mixture of intermediate and nucleated superficial cells. Low numbers of neutrophils are occasionally present.[16]

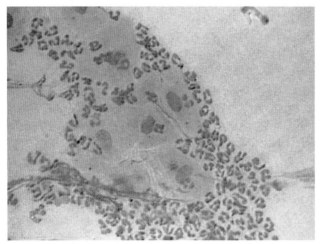

Figure 25-19 Large numbers of neutrophils and intermediate epithelial cells from a puppy with vaginitis. (Wright's stain, original magnification 100×.)

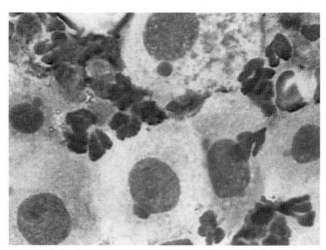

Figure 25-21 Basophilic intracytoplasmic inclusions in epithelial cells in a vaginal smear from a bitch with vaginitis. (Wright's stain, original magnification 400×.)

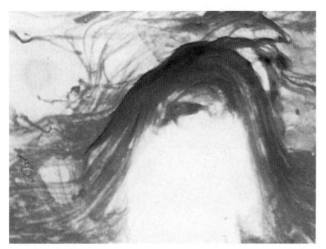

Figure 25-20 Mucus in a vaginal smear from a bitch with a chronic vulvar discharge. (Wright's stain, original magnification 400×.)

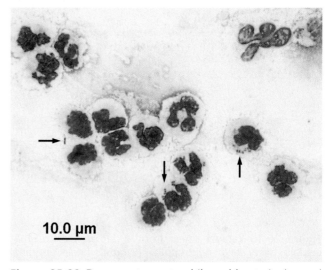

Figure 25-22 Degenerate neutrophils and bacteria *(arrows)* in a vaginal smear from a bitch with metritis. (Wright's stain, original magnification 1000×.)

Anestrus

Vaginal cytology during anestrus is similar to that of the interestrous period. Epithelial cells are predominantly intermediate, with up to 40% nucleated superficial cells and about 10% parabasal cells.[17,18]

CYTOLOGIC CHARACTERISTICS OF VAGINITIS AND METRITIS

Cytologic samples obtained from animals with inflammation of the vagina or uterus are characterized by large numbers of neutrophils (Figure 25-19). If a bacterial infection is the cause, neutrophils often show degenerative changes (swollen, pale nuclei with loss of segmentation) and may contain phagocytized bacteria. Cytologic samples from bitches in early diestrus also contain many neutrophils and may contain bacteria that can occasionally be phagocytized by neutrophils.[5] Thus, vaginal smears from early diestrus can resemble

those from bitches with vaginal or uterine inflammation; however, the number of neutrophils in smears from normal bitches in diestrus markedly decreases by 1 week postestrus. Mucus and a few macrophages and lymphocytes may be seen in cases of chronic vaginitis (Figure 25-20).[5]

Vaginitis is often caused by noninfectious factors, (e.g., vaginal anomalies, clitoral hypertrophy, foreign bodies, or vaginal immaturity), in which case nondegenerate neutrophils will be present. Epithelial intracytoplasmic inclusions that are morphologically similar to *Chlamydia* or *Mycoplasma* spp. have been observed in bitches with vaginitis, but their significance is not known (Figure 25-21). Vaginal smears from animals with pyometra or metritis usually contain large numbers of degenerate neutrophils, and bacteria are frequently observed (Figure 25-22). Muscle fibers from decomposing fetuses may rarely be seen in bitches with metritis secondary to dystocia (Figure 25-23).

CYTOLOGIC CHARACTERISTICS OF NEOPLASIA

Neoplasia of the urinary and reproductive tracts can occasionally be diagnosed by cytologic examination of vaginal smears, although direct aspiration of the mass is often more useful. The most common vaginal tumors in dogs

are of smooth muscle or fibrous tissue origin (leiomyoma, fibroma, and leiomyosarcoma), which do not exfoliate cells readily and so are not generally recognized with routine vaginal cytology.[19,20] If directly aspirated, cytologic samples from benign tumors will contain fairly uniform cells with round to oval nuclei and relatively abundant spindled cytoplasm, present individually or in aggregates. Aspirates from sarcomas will contain similar cells, but with prominent pleomorphism and other criteria of malignancy (Figure 25-24).

Canine transmissible venereal tumors may be diagnosed by vaginal cytology or direct mass aspiration. These contagious tumors are sexually transmitted and occur not only on genitalia but also in other locations (oral and nasal cavity, rectum, skin, subcutaneous tissue).[21] The malignant cells are discrete round cells containing round nuclei with stippled to coarse chromatin and often prominent nucleoli. They have a moderate amount of pale basophilic cytoplasm that usually contains multiple clear, punctate vacuoles (Figure 25-25). Because these tumors are frequently ulcerated and inflamed, variable numbers of neutrophils, macrophages, and lymphocytes may also be present on cytologic samples.[21]

Vaginal carcinomas are less common, but sometimes result from extension of urinary tract carcinomas into the vagina or vestibule (Figures 25-26 and 25-27). These carcinomas may be of transitional cell or squamous cell origin, because the distal portion of the canine urethra is lined by modified squamous epithelium.[22] In one report of seven dogs with urinary tract carcinomas involving the vagina or vestibule, six dogs had vaginal smears performed and neoplastic epithelial cells were identified in all six samples.[23]

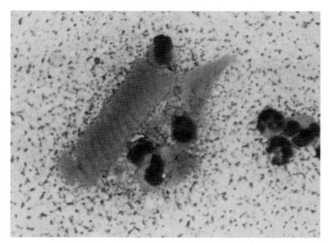

Figure 25-23 Neutrophils and muscle fibers from decomposing puppies in a vaginal smear from a bitch with a herniated uterus and metritis. (Wright's stain, original magnification 400×.)

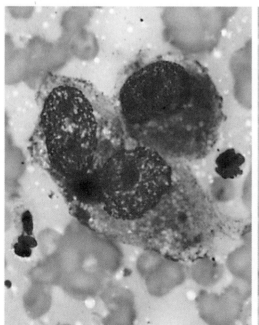
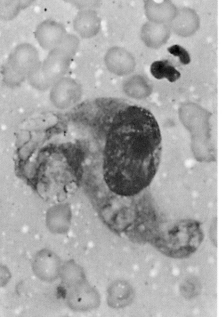

Figure 25-24 Pleomorphic mesenchymal cells from a vaginal sarcoma in a dog. The large vaginal mass was swabbed but not aspirated, resulting in smears of low cellularity. (Wright's stain, original magnification 1000×.)

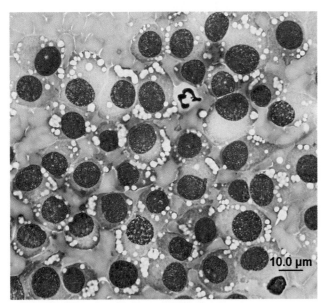

Figure 25-25 Canine transmissible venereal tumor. Direct aspiration of the vaginal mass resulted in highly cellular smears containing the typical vacuolated discrete cells of TVT. (Wright's stain, original magnification 1000×.)

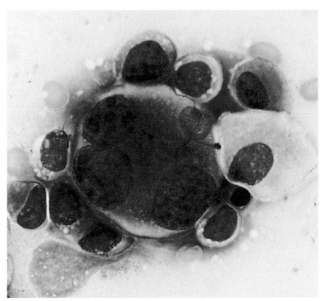

Figure 25-27 These carcinoma cells in a canine vaginal smear exhibit criteria of malignancy including marked anisokaryosis, multinucleation, and multiple prominent nucleoli. (Wright's stain, original magnification 1000×.)

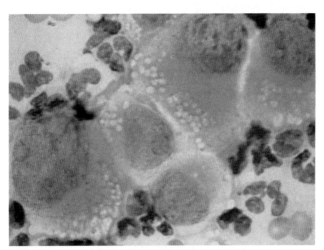

Figure 25-26 Transitional cell carcinoma cells and neutrophils in a vaginal smear from a bitch with transitional cell carcinoma invading the vagina. (Wright's stain, original magnification 1000×.)

Cytologic features of vaginal carcinomas are the same as those occurring in other locations; see discussion of cell types and criteria of malignancy in Chapter 2 and cutaneous carcinomas in Chapter 5.

References

1. Linde C, Karlsson I: The correlation between the cytology of the vaginal smear and the time of ovulation in the bitch. *J Small Anim Pract.* 25:77-82, 1984.
2. Olson PN, et al: Reproductive endocrinology and physiology of the bitch and queen. *Vet Clin North Am Small Anim Pract* 14(4):927-946, 1984.
3. Olson PN, et al: Vaginal cytology. I. A useful tool for staging the canine estrous cycle. *Comp Cont Ed Pract Vet* 6(4):288-297, 1984.
4. Wright PJ: Application of vaginal cytology and plasma progesterone determinations to the management of reproduction in the bitch. *J Small Anim Pract* 31:335-340, 1990.
5. Olson PN, et al: Vaginal cytology. II. Its use in diagnosing canine reproductive disorders. *Comp Cont Ed Pract Vet* 6(5):385-390, 1984.
6. Feldman EC, Nelson RW: Ovarian cycle and vaginal cytology. *Canine and Feline Endocrinology and Reproduction,* ed 3. St. Louis, Saunders, 2004, p 752-774.
7. Clemetson LL, Ward AC: Bacterial flora of the vagina and uterus of healthy cats. *J Am Vet Med Assoc* 196(6):902-906, 1990.
8. Watts JR, Wright PJ, Whithear KC: Uterine, cervical and vaginal microflora of the normal bitch throughout the reproductive cycle. *J Small Anim Pract* 37(2):54-60, 1996.
9. Goodman M: Ovulation timing: Concepts and controversies. *Vet Clin North Am Small Anim Pract* 31(2):219-235, 2001.
10. Hase M, et al: Plasma LH and progesterone levels before and after ovulation and observation of ovarian follicles by ultrasonographic diagnosis system in dogs. *J Vet Med Sci* 62(3):243-248, 2000.
11. Feldman EC, Nelson RW: Breeding, pregnancy, and parturition. In Feldman EC, Nelson RW (eds): *Canine and Feline Endocrinology and Reproduction,* ed 3. St. Louis, Saunders, 2004, p 775-807.
12. Cline EM, Jennings LL, Sojka NJ: Analysis of the feline vaginal epithelial cycle. *Feline Pract* 10(2):47-49, 1980.
13. Herron MA: Feline vaginal cytologic examination. *Feline Pract* 7(2):36-39, 1977.
14. Lofstedt RM: The estrous cycle of the domestic cat. *Compend Cont Ed Pract Vet* 4(1):52-58, 1982.
15. Mowrer RT, Conti PA, Rossow CF: Vaginal cytology an approach of improvement of cat breeding. *Vet Med Small Anim Clin* 70(6):691-696, 1975.

16. Shille VM, Lundstrom KE, Stabenfeldt GH: Follicular function in the domestic cat as determined by estradiol-17 beta concentrations in plasma: Relation to estrous behavior and cornification of exfoliated vaginal epithelium. *Biol Reprod* 21(4):953-963, 1979.

17. Feldman EC, Nelson RW: Feline reproduction. In Feldman EC, Nelson RW (eds): *Canine and Feline Endocrinology and Reproduction*, ed 3. St. Louis, Saunders, 2004, p 1016-1045.

18. Mills JN, Valli VE, Lumsden JH: Cyclical changes of vaginal cytology in the cat. *Can Vet J* 20(4):95-101, 1979.

19. Herron MA: Tumors of the canine genital system. *J Am Anim Hosp Assoc* 19(6):981-994, 1983.

20. Thacher C, Bradley RL: Vulvar and vaginal tumors in the dog: A retrospective study. *J Am Vet Med Assoc* 183(6): 690-692, 1983.

21. Rogers KS: Transmissible venereal tumor. *Compend Cont Ed Pract Vet* 19(9):1036-1045, 1997.

22. MacLachlan NJ, Kennedy PC: Tumors of the genital systems. In Meuten DJ, (ed): *Tumors of Domestic Animals*, ed 4. Ames, Iowa, Iowa State Press, 2002, pp 547-573.

23. Magne ML, et al: Urinary tract carcinomas involving the canine vagina and vestibule. *J Am Anim Hosp Assoc* 21(6):767-772, 1985.

Peripheral Blood Smears

D. Walker

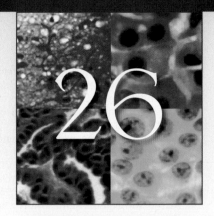

CHAPTER 26

Blood smear evaluation as part of the complete hematology profile (complete blood count [CBC]) is a fundamental step in overall patient health assessment. Blood smear examination can yield a broad range of diagnostic information well beyond obtaining a differential leukocyte count. For example, altered red cell morphology can suggest chronic blood loss, exposure to exogenous toxins, disease involving select organs, or primary immune-mediated condition. Changes in leukocyte morphology may be the earliest laboratory finding suggestive of acute inflammation, leukemia, or certain inherited conditions. In some cases, specific organisms, pathognomonic inclusions, or particular neoplastic cell types on blood films yield an immediate definitive diagnosis. In addition, monitoring cytologic changes found in peripheral blood can help determine a patient's response to treatment, short- and long-term prognoses, and future treatment plan.

Blood smear evaluation can be performed as supplement to an automated CBC whether the latter is obtained in-house or from an outside laboratory. The evaluation provides a synopsis of essentially all other hematologic parameter values and an assurance of the accuracy of values obtained from other methods and sources. The greatest amount of information is generally obtained when the white blood cell (WBC) differential count is not a primary objective, and the person evaluating the smear has access to the patient's current and previous laboratory findings, current clinical condition, and medical history.

Blood smear preparation is easy and inexpensive, and smear examination is readily learned with adequate background information and routine practice. This chapter describes techniques of preparation and interpretation of canine and feline blood smears and addresses integrating findings from blood smears with other parameters in CBCs. Supplementary information on interpreting routine hematologic parameter values is available in several well-written reviews and texts.[1-5]

EQUIPMENT AND SUPPLIES

The only major equipment for blood smear evaluation is a well-maintained binocular microscope with high-quality 10, 20, 40, or 50 (ideally, oil-immersion), and 100×

(oil-immersion) objectives. Other items, such as Coplin jars and staining racks, are convenient for preparing smears. Standard plain or frosted glass slides can be used directly from the package without special treatment or cleaning. Slides with frosted ends facilitate labeling with patient information. Slide surfaces should be free of dust, fingerprints, and residue from detergent, alcohol, or tap water. The use of special cytologic adhesives can result in background staining and is not recommended. An ample supply of slides facilitates preparation of multiple smears per sample, avoiding the frustration of interpreting any poorly made smears. Any additional smears can also be reserved for alternative types of staining or, if indicated, a specialist's review.

SAMPLE COLLECTION

Ideally, blood samples should be collected on the first attempt from a medium to large vein of a calm patient. Ethylene-tetra-acetic acid (EDTA) is the preferred anticoagulant for blood used in cytologic preparations. The liquid form of EDTA (usually K_3EDTA) disperses more rapidly in samples than the powder form (usually K_2EDTA) and may be preferable to help prevent platelet aggregates with feline blood or for viscous or difficult-to-collect samples. However, powdered K_2EDTA provides better erythrocyte preservation for automated counts and lacks dilutional effect on low-volume samples. Both forms of EDTA preserve general cellular morphology in refrigerated samples for up to 4 hours, although the fresher the sample, the more reliable the morphology.

Alternatively (particularly if sample volume is limited), blood without an anticoagulant can be placed directly from the collection needle onto the slide. Samples collected from superficial skin-puncture wounds or clipped toenails (due to excessive contamination with tissue procoagulants) and blood anticoagulated with heparin (a relatively poor preservative of cellular morphology and staining characteristics) are less acceptable. Blood anticoagulated with citrate can be used to evaluate cell morphology on blood smears and may be particularly useful to avoid anticoagulant-associated pseudothrombocytopenia; however, the required 10% sample dilution interferes with cell count estimates.

Collection of blood in proper proportion to anticoagulant helps avoid certain artifacts of cell morphology and may be facilitated by the use of commercial Vacutainers.

HEMATOLOGIC REFERENCE RANGES

Hematologic reference ranges must be established by individual diagnostic laboratories; however, published reference ranges can be used as a general guide for in-clinic laboratories. Typical values for dogs and cats are listed in Table 26-1. Certain physiologic factors occasionally cause a healthy patient's hematologic values to deviate from reference ranges. Because they are rapidly expanding their vascular space, very young animals tend to have relatively low hematocrits. Because they are also actively replacing fetal with adult red blood cells (RBCs), animals in early growth periods have greater RBC anisocytosis, polychromasia, and incidence of nucleated RBCs when compared with mature animals.

Relatively high lymphocyte counts are also common in young animals, and lymphopenia is suggested if lymphocyte counts drop below 2000 cells/μl in puppies and kittens under 6 months of age.[3] Transient elevations above the reference range for lymphocyte counts are common in excited or vigorously exercised patients, especially if they are immature. This epinephrine-induced response can also result in temporarily increased counts of other WBC types in the peripheral blood of healthy patients. At least one canine breed, the Greyhound, has hematologic reference ranges reported to fall slightly outside of reference ranges commonly used for the species.[6,7] Although these normal physiologic conditions should be considered, they generally explain less than 5% of the patient values that fall outside reference ranges for any single hematologic parameter.

SMEAR PREPARATION

Well-made smears are required for reliable identification and evaluation of peripheral blood cells. Smears can be prepared on glass slides or coverslips. The glass slide

TABLE 26-1

Reference range for Hematologic Values in Dogs and Cats

Erythrocytes

	Canine Values	Feline Values
Hematocrit (%)	37.0-55.0	24.0-45.0
Hemoglobin (g/dl)	12.0-18.0	8.0-15.0
Erythrocyte count (×10⁶/μl)	5.5-8.5	5.0-10.0
Reticulocytes (%)	≤1.0	≤1.0
MCV (fl)	60.6-77.0	39.0-55.0
MCH (pg)	19.5-24.5	12.5-17.5
MCHC (g/dl)	32.0-36.0	30.0-36.0

Leukocytes

	CANINE VALUES		FELINE VALUES	
Cell Types	Distribution Range (%)	Absolute Range (cells/μl)	Distribution Range (%)	Absolute Range (cells/μl)
Total leukocytes	-	6,000-17,000	-	5,500-19,500
Neutrophils segmented	60-77	3,000-11,000	35-75	2,500-12,500
band	0-3	0-500	0-3	0-500
Lymphocytes	12-30	1,000-4,800	20-55	1,500-7,000
Monocytes	3-10	150-1,350	1-4	0-850
Eosinophils	2-10	100-1,250	2-12	0-1,500
Basophils	Rare	Rare	Rare	Rare

Platelets

	Canine Values	Feline Values
Platelets count (×10³/μl)	200-500	300-800
Mean platelet volume (fl)	5.4-9.2	12.1-15.1

Proteins

	Canine Values	Feline Values
Plasma protein (refractometry; g/dl)	5.7-7.0	6.1-7.4
Albumin (g/dl)	2.4-3.6	2.5-3.3
Globulins (g/dl)	2.1-4.6	2.6-4.9

MCV, Mean corpuscular volume; *MCH,* mean corpuscular hemoglobin; *MCHC,* mean corpuscular hemoglobin concentration.

technique is generally easier and more reliable than preparing smears on coverslips. Glass slides can also be processed through automatic stainers and so may be most suitable for laboratories using such equipment. However, the coverslip method generally results in more uniform WBC distribution and less trauma to fragile blood components, such as large or neoplastic cells, within the sample. For both methods, blood samples should be fresh and well-mixed at smear preparation time, and smears should be completely air-dried before staining.

Glass Slides

Smears are prepared on glass slides by placing a drop of blood (2 to 3 mm in diameter) on the broad face of the slide about 1.0 to 1.5 cm from the frosted border (or edge of a nonfrosted slide). Another clean, dry slide (i.e., spreader slide) is held loosely against the surface of the first slide at a 30-degree angle and drawn smoothly toward the blood drop, as illustrated in Figure 1-16. The spreader slide should be brought to a position where it just meets, but is not drawn into, the blood drop. When the spreader slide makes contact with the blood, capillary action immediately distributes the blood between the two slides. Then, with no downward pressure, the spreader slide is quickly and smoothly swept across the remaining length of the underlying slide.

Ideally, blood smears have a smooth transition from the thick region to the feathered edge and cover an area half the length and slightly less than the width of the slide (see Figure 1-16, *D*). If the edge is blunt instead of feathered, the second slide was probably raised off the first before the blood was spread completely. Unequal smear thickness usually results from the spreader slide being held at too obtuse an angle or placing too much pressure on the first slide while spreading the blood. Too much pressure on the second slide can also result in WBC clumping along the smear's feathered edge. Too little pressure can result in short, thick smears. Smear thickness can also be affected by the viscosity of the blood sample. Adjusting the angle at which the second slide is held against the first can help compensate for very viscous (e.g., hemoconcentrated) or watery (i.e., anemic) blood samples. A more obtuse, 40- to 45-degree angle between the two slides makes thicker smears for very anemic samples, and an angle less than 30 degrees may be necessary for preparing smears of severely hemoconcentrated blood. Smears need to be thoroughly air-dried before staining; those that are thick may require additional drying time. Use (at the low setting) of a heat block or a blow dryer may shorten the drying time.

Glass Coverslips

The first step in creating coverslip smears is to place a small drop of blood drawn from a capillary tube in the center of a 22- × 22-mm glass coverslip and a second coverslip on top. The corners of the two coverslips should point in opposite directions. Then, without downward pressure, the top coverslip is quickly and smoothly drawn horizontally off the underlying one. The smears created on both coverslips are air-dried, stained (see the following discussion of stains), and placed face down on a drop of immersion oil or mounting medium on the same or separate glass slide(s) for evaluation.

Coverslip smears can also be made using both sides of a single coverslip to spread blood in two separate regions of a glass slide surface, resulting in two adjacent smears with fairly uniform WBC distribution on a single slide. This method provides the benefits of coverslip smears but avoids the problems inherent to handling delicate glass coverslips during manual staining. This method also allows smears to be processed with an automatic stainer.

STAINS

As with cytologic preparations, Romanowsky-type stains are good general stains for microscopically evaluating blood smears. Quick Romanowsky-type stains are advantageous because they are less sensitive to solution pH and staining time and less susceptible to precipitate formation than Wright's stains. However, many quick stains are also less effective at demonstrating polychromasia of immature erythrocytes.

Wright's staining is achieved by flooding the air-dried blood smear with, or dipping it into Coplin jars containing, filtered Wright's stain. After 2 to 4 minutes of incubation with the stain, the smear is flooded with a volume of phosphate buffer solution roughly equal to the amount of stain. To mix the buffer with the stain, gently rock or blow on the slide, or dip it into another Coplin jar containing the buffer. The slides are incubated for another 3 to 6 minutes with the buffer. A metallic sheen will begin to appear on the fluid surface of flooded smears. The slide is then rinsed with tap water (or a 50:50 mixture of tap and distilled water to achieve a pH around 7.0) and blotted with bibulous paper or placed upright on an absorptive surface to hasten drying. A blow dryer set on low power and held 8 to 10 inches from the slide also shortens drying time.

Quick stain methods vary somewhat and should be used according to manufacturer's recommendations. The two-step Prodiff is unique among quick stains in differentially staining polychromatophilic and mature RBCs. Most quick stains such as Diff-Quik, Hemacolor, and Quick III lack good distinction of polychromatophilic erythrocytes, but provide particularly consistent staining between smear preparations. The quick stains generally require slowly dipping the smear first in an alcohol fixative, then a methylene blue dye mixture, and lastly, an eosin-containing solution. One edge of the slide is briefly blotted between solutions. Tap or distilled water can be used to rinse the slide after the last solution and before air-drying.

TROUBLESHOOTING

Artifacts of Cell Morphology and Staining

Most artifactual changes in cell morphology and staining can be readily recognized by their appearance and/or distribution within a smear. Examining multiple smears of the same blood sample is also helpful, because alterations that are inconstant from smear to smear are likely to be artifactual.

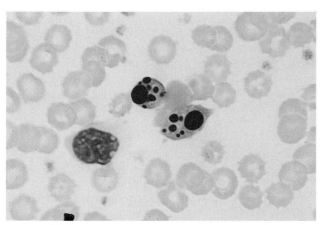

Figure 26-1 Degenerating cells resulting from prolonged storage of blood before smears were made. (Diff-Quik stain, original magnification 330×.)

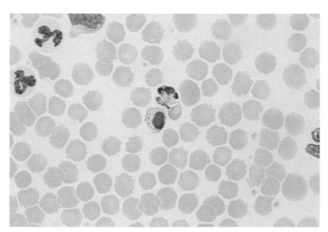

Figure 26-2 Aging artifact in blood stored at room temperature for more than 1 hour. One cell has a densely stained, fragmented nucleus and cytoplasmic blebbing, and the adjacent cell has a condensed, rounded nucleus with a homogeneous chromatin pattern. (Wright's stain, original magnification 250×.)

Crenated Erythrocytes: Crenated erythrocytes (see Figure 26-33), artifacts especially common in feline blood samples, have a thorn-apple shape with many short, uniformly spaced, blunt or pointed spicules that protrude from the cell membrane. Crenated RBCs can result from drying the smear too slowly or a relative excess of anticoagulant in the sample. Prolonged storage time of the blood (e.g., more than 2 hours at either 4° C or room temperature), particularly with an EDTA anticoagulant, can also result in RBC crenation. Differences in surface tension between the cell membrane and the glass slide may be an unpredictable cause of the artifact.

In Vitro Aging Artifacts: These are common in smears made from blood samples left at room temperature for more than 2 to 4 hours or refrigerated for longer than 12 hours. Neutrophils, monocytes, and immature and neoplastic WBCs degenerate slightly earlier than other cell types. The nuclei of affected cells initially become

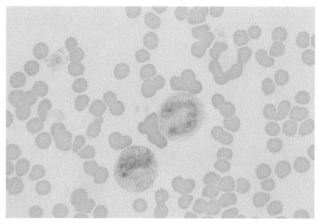

Figure 26-3 Inadequate incubation of this blood smear resulted in poorly stained WBCs despite adequate RBC staining. (Wright's stain, original magnification 250×.)

condensed and homogeneous-staining, and segmentation of granulocyte nuclei becomes more prominent, with only thin stands of chromatin separating lobules (e.g., hypersegmented neutrophils). Basophilia and vacuolation may be evident in the cytoplasm of neutrophils, and nuclei later become pyknotic and fragmented (Figure 26-1). The cytoplasmic borders of degenerating cells often show blebbing (Figure 26-2), and the cytoplasm of lymphocytes and monocytes may become vacuolated. These changes interfere with accurate identification of cell type and invalidate differential WBC counts if more than 10% of the cells in the smear are affected. Platelet aggregation/agglutination is also prevalent in aged samples. Avoiding aging artifacts is one reason to include fresh well-made smears with a sample submitted for hematology analysis to an outside laboratory.

Pale or Unstained Nuclei: Pale or unstained nuclei (Figure 26-3) on smears suggest that there has been inadequate staining time, or the stain has aged. Of the three-step quick stain solutions, the methylene blue mixture is usually that which has begun to degrade and may require longer incubation time with the smear or replacement. On Wright's-stained preparations, pale nuclei with bright orange-red RBCs can result from overzealous washing or low pH of the buffer. Conversely, Wright's-stained smears with pale nuclei and RBCs that stain slightly brown to green may occur when preparations are thick, inadequately washed, or stained with too little or too alkaline a buffer. A neutral buffer (i.e., pH 6.4 to 7.0) is most effective for Wright's staining. The pH of the distilled or tap water wash solution can occasionally interfere with the intensity of the nuclear staining with both Wright's and quick stains. Additional causes of inadequate nuclear staining are noted in Table 1-3.

Drying Artifact: Drying artifact (Figures 26-4 and 26-5) results if a smear is insufficiently air-dried before it is stained. The artifact is recognized in RBCs as round to crescent-shaped, punched-out regions or refractile vacuole-like structures. Stain condensations may border these pale cell areas or precipitate in the background between cells.

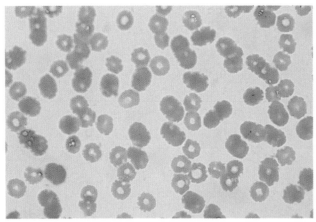

Figure 26-4 This blood film was inadequately dried before staining. The punched out, unstained regions in the RBCs are a result of moisture interfering with the contact between cells and stain. (Diff-Quik stain, original magnification 250×.)

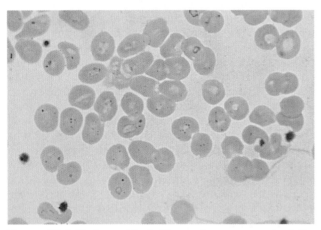

Figure 26-5 Drying artifact. The eosin component of the Diff-Quik stain has precipitated around RBC areas that were inadequately dried. This artifact could be mistaken for erythroparasites, cytoplasmic inclusions, or basophilic stippling. (Diff-Quik stain, original magnification 330×.)

Overall Blue Tint: This may be seen on blood smears stained after prolonged storage, prepared from heparin-anticoagulated blood, or exposed to formalin or formalin fumes before staining. Even indirect exposure to formalin fumes (as may occur when slides are packaged with fixed tissues for shipment) may result in an overall pale, hazy smear.

Stain Precipitate: Stain precipitate is more often a problem with Wright's stains than with quick stains. Wright's stain will precipitate in storage, if incubated on a slide too long, or if insufficiently washed from a slide after incubation. Precipitate formed during storage and from insufficient washing occurs as random aggregates of spherical and dumbbell-shaped granules that appear both in and out of the smear's plane of focus (Figure 26-6). With prolonged incubation time, stain precipitate appears throughout the smear as uniformly dispersed, irregular globules of stain. Precipitate formed during storage can be removed by filtering the stain through Whatman filter paper into clean vials.

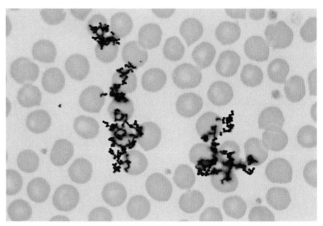

Figure 26-6 The granular stain precipitate appears in and out of the plane of focus for the smear. This precipitate formed as a result of insufficient washing of Wright's stain after buffer application. The granular precipitate that forms in the stain during storage can also be deposited on blood smears. The latter can be prevented by filtering the stain before use. (Wright's stain, original magnification 330×.)

BLOOD SMEAR EVALUATION

Smears should be initially examined from the thickest region to the feathered edge using the 10 or 20× objective. At this low magnification, blood films can be checked for staining, overall thickness, smooth transitions in thickness, cell distribution, and adequacy of the monolayer area. The monolayer is generally found within the distal half of the smear adjacent to the feathered edge and is luminescent when the unstained slide is held under indirect light. The monolayer represents the limited region where cell morphology is most reliably evaluated. WBCs should be fairly uniformly distributed within this region and only mildly clustered along the feathered edge. Examination of the borders and especially the feathered edge of the smear under low magnification may demonstrate the presence of platelet aggregates, microfilaria, large atypical cells, or cells with phagocytosed organisms.

A patient's hematocrit can be roughly approximated by examining a blood smear at low magnification. Blood films from nonanemic animals generally have RBCs that are closely apposed in the monolayer as well as several RBC layers at the thick end of the smear that obstruct penetrance of most condenser light. In contrast, smears from animals that are moderately to markedly anemic usually have RBCs that are widely separated from one another in the monolayer and only one or two RBC layers in the thick end of the smear that allow considerable condenser light to penetrate. Unless the angle between slides was adjusted during smear preparation of hemoconcentrated samples, the monolayer occupies a relatively reduced area. Estimates should ultimately be checked against the patient's measured hematocrit or packed-cell volume.

The WBC count can also be roughly estimated or simply classified as low, normal, or high by examining the smear under low magnification. Accurate identification of the different WBC types and their relative proportions is more easily performed using the 40× or 50× objective. Cell morphology is typically evaluated under magnifications of 40× to 100×; platelet number and morphology are assessed at the highest of these magnification levels.

NORMAL CELL COMPONENTS OF BLOOD

Red Blood Cells

RBC morphology is primarily evaluated within the monolayer where artifactual distortion induced during preparation and differences in smear thickness are less apt to influence cell appearance. Nearly all significant morphologic abnormalities of RBCs can be detected at 40× or 50× magnification, although some alterations may require additional examination at higher magnification. Initial examination of RBC morphology with the 100× objective, however, often results in overdiagnosis of aberrations.

Mature RBCs in healthy adult dogs are about 7 μm in diameter (slightly larger than the 5.5- to 6.0-μm diameter of feline RBCs). As is apparent in the monolayer of blood smears, canine RBCs are biconcave with an area of central pallor occupying about one third of the cell's diameter. Feline RBCs do not consistently have discernible central pallor and tend to vary slightly more in shape than canine RBCs. Both species have mild RBC anisocytosis and may show an occasional immature polychromatophilic cell on peripheral blood smears.

White Blood Cells

Neutrophils: Canine and feline neutrophils have similar appearance on blood films (Figure 26-7). The neutrophil nucleus is elongate and separated into multiple lobules by invaginations of the nuclear border. Demarcations between lobules are seldom distinct enough to be considered filamentous. Chromatin is organized into dense clumps of dark purple to black staining heterochromatin separated by narrow areas of less condensed euchromatin. Cytoplasm is clear, pale eosinophilic to faintly basophilic with a fine grainy texture, and rarely, contains one or two small vacuoles. Neutrophil granules range from indiscernible to faintly eosinophilic but are pale and much smaller than the prominent granules of mature eosinophils.

Band Neutrophils: Band neutrophils, low numbers of which occur in the peripheral blood of healthy dogs and cats, have an elongate, U- or J-shaped to slightly twisted nucleus with less chromatin condensation than mature neutrophils (Figure 26-8). Nuclear lobulation is absent or poorly defined. Constrictions of canine band neutrophil nuclei are less than half the width of the remainder (nonconstricted sections) of the nucleus; feline band neutrophils lack nuclear constrictions entirely. Cytoplasm is similar in granule content and staining to that of mature neutrophils.

Monocytes: Canine and feline monocytes are larger than neutrophils and similar in size to eosinophils and basophils. Nuclei vary greatly in morphology, ranging from elongate U shapes that resemble band neutrophils to irregular multilobulated forms. The nuclear chromatin of monocytes is generally distinct from that of both mature and immature granulocytes and is characteristically lacy to ropy with only a few small isolated clumps of heterochromatin (Figure 26-9). The moderate to abundant gray-blue cytoplasm of monocytes has a ground-glass texture, is often sparsely dusted with minute eosinophilic granules, and occasionally contains vacuoles. Cytoplasmic borders are usually irregular, sometimes with fine, filamentous, pseudopodia-like extensions. Because of their relatively large size, monocytes may be concentrated along the feathered edge, and their proportion underestimated in blood smear differential WBC counts.

Lymphocytes: Lymphocytes vary in size in the peripheral blood of dogs and cats, with small cells predominating. Small lymphocytes have densely staining, round to oval nuclei that are sometimes slightly indented and usually have large, well-defined chromatin clumps (Figure 26-10). Alternatively, nuclear chromatin may appear smudged, especially when stained with a quick stain. The moderately blue cytoplasm of small lymphocytes is scant, and cytoplasmic borders are partially obscured by the nuclei, particularly with feline lymphocytes. Larger lymphocytes in peripheral blood have less densely staining, but still clearly clumped, nuclear chromatin. Cytoplasm of the larger cells is more abundant and ranges from light to moderately basophilic. Some lymphocytes have a few variably sized eosinophilic cytoplasmic granules that are usually concentrated within a single perinuclear cell area (Figure 26-11).

Eosinophils: Eosinophils, which are slightly larger than neutrophils, can usually be found in very low numbers on blood smears of healthy dogs and cats. Nuclei are less lobulated (often being divided into only two distinct lobules) with less condensed chromatin (Figure 26-12) than those of mature neutrohils. Cytoplasm is clear to faintly basophilic and contains prominent pink granules, which are abundant, small, and rod-shaped in cats (Figure 26-13) but vary widely in number and size in dogs. Canine eosinophils occasionally contain a single, large granule that may be mistaken for an inclusion body or unusual organism (Figure 26-14). Eosinophils of Greyhounds are peculiar in that they may appear vacuolated on smears—a breed difference that has been attributed to differential staining properties of the specific granules.[8] Eosinophil granules that are ruptured in vitro are also sometimes freely scattered in the background of canine and feline blood smears.

Basophils: Basophils are the largest of the mature granulocytic cell types and rare in peripheral blood of healthy dogs and cats. Nuclei are less densely staining and have fewer lobulations and a more elongated, ribbon-like appearance than the nuclei of other granulocytic cell types (Figure 26-15). Cytoplasm is moderately blue-gray to slightly purple and usually contains granules. In dogs, basophil granules are usually low in number and stain dark blue to metachromatic. Canine basophils also occasionally lack obvious granules but are recognizable by their size, nuclear morphology, and cytoplasmic staining (Figure 26-16). In cats, basophils contain abundant oval, pale lavender to gray specific granules (Figure 26-17), although immature basophils may also contain a few primary, dark purple granules.

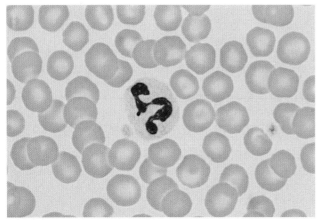

Figure 26-7 A canine neutrophil with pale, eosinophilic cytoplasm and a lobulated nucleus containing mostly dense heterochromatin. (Wright's stain, original magnification 330×.)

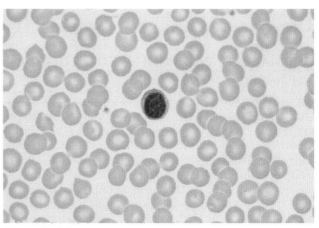

Figure 26-10 A canine lymphocyte with densely clumped nuclear chromatin and scant basophilic cytoplasm. (Wright's stain, original magnification 250×.)

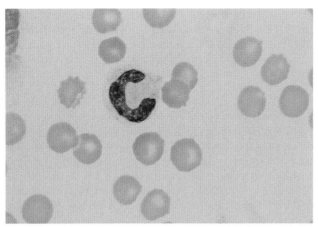

Figure 26-8 A canine band neutrophil with pale eosinophilic cytoplasm that is similar to a mature cell and a U-shaped nucleus lacking distinct segmentation. (Wright's stain, original magnification 330×.)

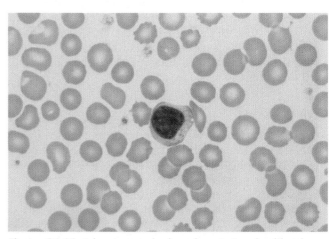

Figure 26-11 A large granular lymphocyte in a healthy dog. Both canine and feline lymphocytes occasionally contain a few eosinophilic granules in a moderate amount of homogeneous basophilic cytoplasm. (Wright's stain, original magnification 250×.)

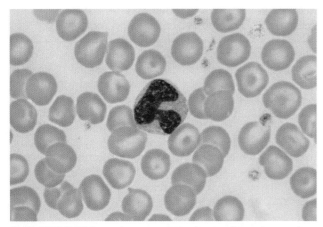

Figure 26-9 This canine monocyte has an irregular nucleus with a ropey chromatin pattern and grainy basophilic cytoplasm. (Wright's stain, original magnification 330×.)

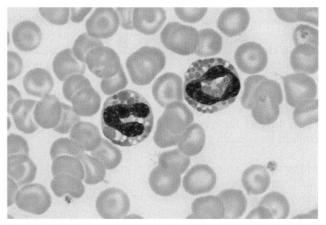

Figure 26-12 Two canine eosinophils, one of which has partially degranulated cytoplasm. Eosinophil nuclei are less condensed and lobulated than those of neutrophils. (Wright's stain, original magnification 330×.)

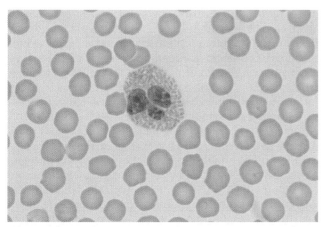

Figure 26-13 A feline eosinophil with small, rod-shaped, eosinophilic granules filling the cytoplasm and partially obscuring the nucleus. (Wright's stain, original magnification 250×.)

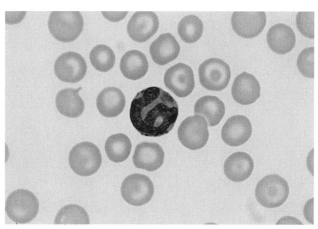

Figure 26-16 A poorly granulated canine basophil, which can be identified as such by its size, ribbon-like nuclear shape, and cytoplasmic staining, despite the near absence of cytoplasmic granules. (Wright's stain, original magnification 330×.)

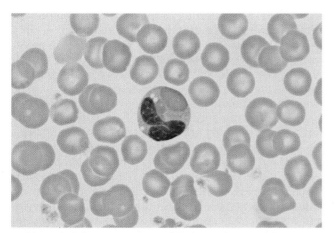

Figure 26-14 A canine eosinophil with only two large cytoplasmic granules. (Wright's stain, original magnification 330×.)

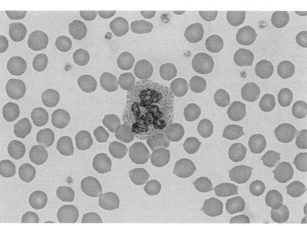

Figure 26-17 A feline basophil with a segmented nucleus and abundant oval to polygonal, lavender-gray, cytoplasmic granules. (Wright's stain, original magnification 250×.)

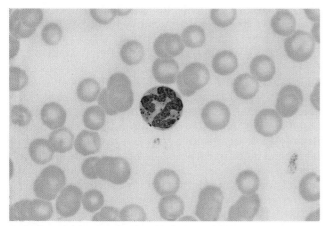

Figure 26-15 A canine basophil with metachromatic granules scattered in the cytoplasm. (Wright's stain, original magnification 250×.)

Platelets

Canine and feline platelets appear oval, round, or rod-shaped on peripheral blood smears. Their clear to pale gray cytoplasm usually contains a central cluster of eosinophilic to metachromatic granules. Platelets normally vary in size from about one fourth to two thirds of the diameter of RBCs in canine blood, and occasionally are even larger than the RBCs in feline blood. Partially activated platelets have a spider-like appearance with thin cytoplasmic processes extending from a small spherical cell body. Platelets may also appear aggregated (Figure 26-18) or agglutinated into an amorphous mass on blood smears, a finding particularly common in feline blood smears. Aggregated and agglutinated platelets are usually pushed to the feathered edge, which may result in the false impression of thrombocytopenia if only the monolayer of the smear is evaluated.

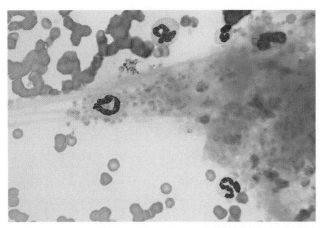

Figure 26-18 A large mass of aggregated platelets, fibrin, and a few enmeshed leukocytes. Platelet aggregation or agglutination sometimes results in artifactually low platelet counts. (Wright's stain, original magnification 200×.)

ALTERATIONS OF RBCs IN DISEASE

Alterations in RBC Numbers

Alterations in RBC density on a smear may reflect polycythemia or anemia. The most common cause of polycythemia is hemoconcentration with dehydration, resulting in a relative increase in RBC numbers and plasma protein concentration. Alternatively, relative polycythemia may occur secondary to splenic contraction, a condition that is more likely to occur in dogs than cats, and can be supported by the animal's recent history, lack of a corresponding increase in plasma proteins, and transient nature of the finding. Absolute polycythemia is less common, but when observed is usually the result of an appropriate erythropoietic response to chronic hypoxia. The hypoxia may be generalized, as with respiratory or cardiovascular conditions, or localized to the kidney; both conditions can lead to low renal tissue oxygenation and increased circulating erythropoietin.

Absolute polycythemia secondary to inappropriate erythropoietin production, and primary polycythemia, or polycythemia vera, which is independent of erythropoietin levels, are both rare in dogs and cats. These two conditions are tentatively diagnosed by excluding the more common causes of erythrocytosis. Polycythemia associated with tumor erythropoietin production has been reported in dogs with renal and nonrenal tumor types, with the latter including cecal leiomyoma, nasal fibrosarcoma, and extradural schwannoma.[9-11] Inappropriate administration of recombinant erythropoietin or androgens may also be a cause of absolute secondary polycythemia in dogs or cats as in other species, although treatment with human erythropoietin can also lead to red cell aplasia in both species.[12] The algorithm of Figure 26-19 may further help in determining the cause of polycythemia in dogs and cats.

Anemia is an especially common finding in dogs and cats and can be secondary to almost any type of illness. Anemia is often suspected before blood samples are collected based on a patient's clinical signs and physical examination. Evidence to support the condition as being acute or chronic can be derived from the clinical

presentation and history. An animal with peracute to acute blood loss is often anxious and tachypneic and may have mucous membranes that are paler than expected for the degree of anemia as a result of transient peripheral vasoconstriction. With chronic blood loss, through upregulation of RBC 2,3-diphosphoglycerate in dogs and likely by an alternative mechanism in cats, oxygen is more readily released from hemoglobin to the tissues. Animals with chronic anemia are apt to be relatively inactive and show distress and dyspnea only if further stressed by physical exertion or an additional medical condition or if the blood loss is severe. A dog or cat presenting with a packed cell volume (PCV) of 12% or less typically has some degree of chronic anemia, because acute or subacute blood loss to this magnitude is generally not life-supporting. Blood smear examination, as described in the following section and Figure 26-20, may further aid in determining the cause of anemia in dogs and cats.

Blood Smear Examination in the Evaluation of Anemia

Cytologic examination of peripheral blood is important in determining the cause, treatment, and prognosis of a patient's anemia. The procedure is also valuable in monitoring anemic conditions over time. Alterations of red cell morphology are usually most indicative of the primary cause of the anemia. For example, anisocytosis may be detected in animals with regenerative erythropoietic response or immune-mediated hemolysis with spherocytic RBC, and is especially profound when the two conditions are concurrent (see Figure 26-26). An increasing proportion of large, immature RBCs over time without a change in absolute red cell count suggests that an animal has persistent blood loss (or hemolysis) and a responsive marrow. Other components of the smear, including leukocytes and platelets, may also provide clues about the cause of anemia. Increased numbers of normal or enlarged platelets may been seen in association with acute or persistent blood loss. Low platelet numbers support platelet consumption or destruction, with anemia secondary to hemorrhage or immune-mediated hemolysis. Leukocytosis is usually also seen with immune-mediated red cell destruction, whereas leukopenia (especially neutropenia) and thrombocytopenia occur concomitant with anemia with impaired bone marrow hematopoiesis.

Evaluating smears for the extent of erythropoietic response can provide critical information on the cause of an anemia. Responding anemia, as suggested by an orderly shift to a greater than normal proportion of large, variably basophilic, immature RBCs on an anemic patient's blood smears, indicates RBC loss from hemorrhage or hemolysis. A regenerative response may be detected in peripheral blood as early as 2 to 4 days after initial blood loss in dogs and cats, depending upon the cause, magnitude of anemia, and the animal's concurrent conditions. The response is typically rapid and profound in dogs and cats with hemolytic conditions, and more variable in onset and magnitude in patients with only mild blood loss. In all cases, if the regenerative response appears less than adequate for the degree of anemia (assuming adequate

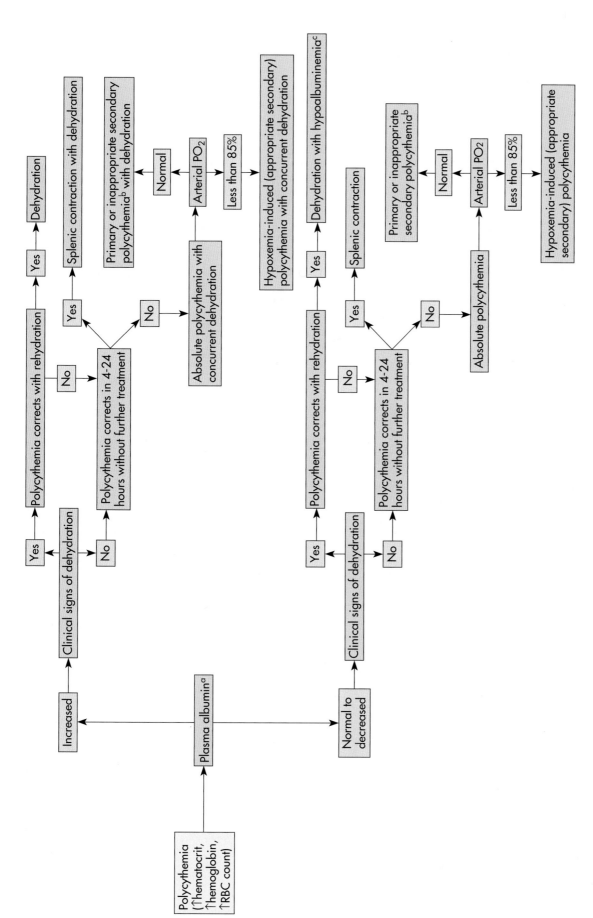

Figure 26-19 An algorithm to aid in the diagnosis of polycythemia.

[a]Total protein can be substituted in most cases if serum albumin value is unavailable and serum globulins are unlikely to be markedly elevated.
[b]Inappropriate secondary polycythemia may be caused by renal lesions or selective neoplastic conditions (presumably associated with tumor production of erythropoietin-like factors) including, but not limited to, primary renal tumors (see text).
[c]Albumin loss may be due to plasma protein loss, insufficient dietary protein, hepatic protein synthesis, or a combination of these.

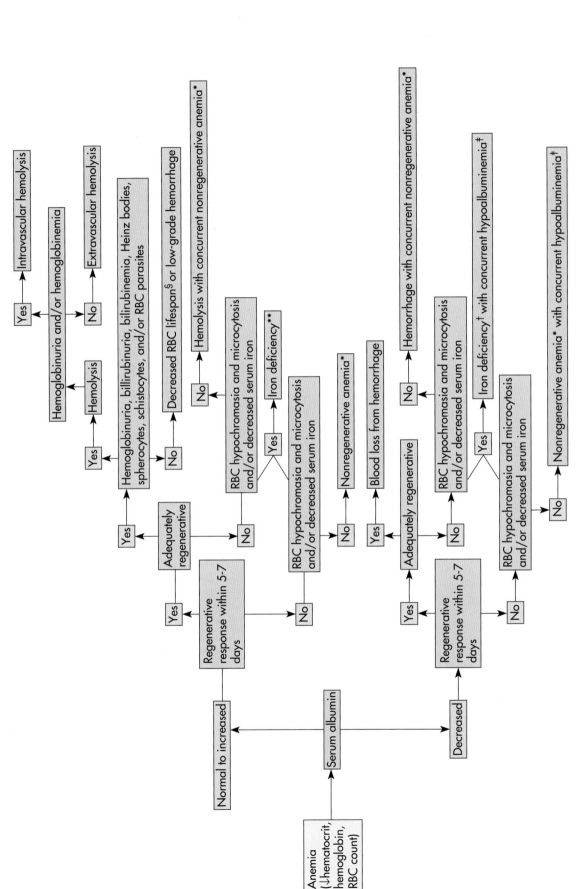

Figure 26-20 An algorithm to aid in the diagnosis of anemia.

*Refers to anemia of chronic systemic disease or the underlying condition of the bone marrow impairing RBC production. The former includes anemia of chronic inflammation, certain endocrinopathies, and major organ (e.g., kidney, liver) diseases, neoplasia, and malnutrition. The latter includes toxin-induced and immune-mediated conditions affecting RBC precursor cells.

† Copper deficiency may also be a consideration in these cases.

‡ Hypoalbuminemia may be a result of plasma protein loss (including plasma protein loss through hemorrhage), insufficient hepatic synthesis, or insufficient dietary protein.

§ Includes chronic low-grade hemolysis. The presence of abnormally high polychromasia/reticulocyte count in mildly anemic or nonanemic animals suggests chronic lead toxicity or an intrinsic RBC abnormality.

** Portosystemic shunt, copper, and/or vitamin B_6 deficiency may also be considerations in these cases.

time has elapsed for the marrow to maximally respond), a reticulocyte count, which allows anemia to be classified as adequately regenerative, inadequately regenerative, or nonregenerative, is indicated. Inadequately regenerative or nonregenerative anemias indicate some degree of impaired erythropoiesis for which evaluation of the patient's bone marrow may provide further diagnostic information.

Reticulocyte Evaluation and Quantitation

One of a few vital stains that can be used to distinguish immature from mature erythrocytes on blood films is new methylene blue (NMB). The stain combines with polyribosomes retained in immature RBCs (reticulocytes), which are then recognized as dark blue granules or "reticulum" within the RBC cytoplasm. Mature RBCs lack cytoplasmic ribosomes and stain uniformly pale blue with NMB.

Method: One part blood is mixed with 1 to 1.5 parts NMB (0.5% in saline) in either a test or capillary tube (rolling the latter to mix well). This mixture is then allowed to

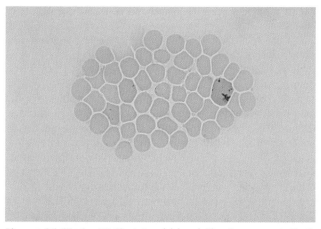

Figure 26-21 An NMB-stained blood film from a cat. Both aggregate and sparsely stippled punctate reticulocytes are seen in this field. (NMB stain, original magnification 250×.)

stand at room temperature for either 10 (canine blood) or 15 to 20 (feline blood) minutes. The blood/stain combination is mixed again, and a small drop is used to make a thin smear, which is then air-dried and examined under the 100× oil-immersion objective. For manual reticulocyte quantitation, at least 1000 total RBCs are quantified, and the number of reticulocytes is expressed as a percentage (i.e., number of reticulocytes among 1000 total RBCs/10). An eyepiece etched with a Miller disk (available through retailers of microscope accessories) may facilitate counting.

Canine reticulocytes are of the aggregate type, recognized by their dark blue, interlacing network of cytoplasmic precipitate. Feline reticulocytes are of two readily recognizable types, aggregate reticulocytes (as in dogs) and punctate reticulocytes (Figure 26-21). Punctate reticulocytes lack the reticular pattern of cytoplasmic staining but contain a few scattered, variably sized, dark blue cytoplasmic granules. These two reticulocyte types are counted separately in feline blood because their kinetics during a regenerative response differ. Note that epierythrocytic *Hemobartonella felis* organisms, basophilic stippling, and drying artifacts on RBCs can appear similar to and may need to be differentiated from punctate reticulocytes on NMB-stained feline blood smears.

Interpretation: A maximal erythropoietic response from the bone marrow is expected within 7 days of the onset of anemia. At this time, a reticulocyte percentage that is at least equal to the average expected value for the species and the corresponding level of anemia (Table 26-2) represents an adequate marrow response, which is indicative of blood loss from hemorrhage or hemolysis. A reticulocyte count greater than 50% of the expected response but less than that considered adequate for the species and the severity of anemia represents an inadequately regenerative marrow response. Inadequately regenerative anemias occur in animals with hemorrhage or hemolysis concomitant with impaired marrow erythropoiesis. Animals whose marrow has had time to respond (about 7 days) but who have <50% of the expected reticulocyte response for their corresponding hematocrit should be considered to have a nonregenerative anemia. Note that erythropoietic

TABLE 26-2

Expected Reticulocyte Count Relative to Hematocrit value in Dogs and Cats with Adequately Regenerative Anemias*

CANINE[†]		FELINE		
PCV (%)	Reticulocyte (%)	PCV (%)	Aggregate Reticulocyte (%)	Punctuate Reticulocyte (%)
45	<1.0	45	-	-
35	≥1.0	35	≤0.5	≤10
25	≥4.0	25	0.5-2.0	>10
20	≥6.0	20	2.0-4.0	>10
10	≥10.0	10	>4.0	>10

*Adapted from material from Oklahoma State University, Department of Anatomy, Pathology, and Pharmacology.
[†]Findings further based on corrected reticulocyte count and reticulocyte production index calculations.

responses are highly variable and less readily classified in dogs with only mild anemia (i.e., PCV >25%).

When based solely on the aggregate reticulocyte percentage, an adequate erythropoietic response to anemia in cats is about half of that expected in dogs; however, punctate reticulocyte numbers should also be considered because this may be the only reticulocyte type to increase in cats with mild blood loss. Furthermore, feline punctate reticulocytes remain elevated longer (up to 2 weeks after resolution of anemia) than aggregate reticulocytes in the peripheral blood. Thus an increase in punctate (without a detectable increase in aggregate) reticulocytes can represent an adequate marrow response in cats with either mild acute or recently resolved anemia.

If a patient's total RBC count is available, some veterinarians prefer to interpret the response to anemia based on absolute reticulocyte counts (i.e., total RBC count × reticulocyte percentage). Counts greater than 50,000 aggregate reticulocytes/μl in cats and 60,000 aggregate reticulocytes/μl in dogs are considered indicative of at least a mild regenerative response. Classification of anemia in dogs can also be based on calculation of the corrected reticulocyte count as is described in most comprehensive hematology texts.[1-3]

Alterations of RBC Shape or Size

Although occasional alterations of RBC shape or size can be seen on virtually all smears, such changes that occur in high proportion (i.e., greater than 5% of RBC) or that are prominent in their appearance should be carefully evaluated for their potential diagnostic significance. Common RBC shape changes that can be detected on peripheral blood smears of dogs and cats and have diagnostic significance can be grouped into five major categories: (1) RBC fragmentation, (2) oxidative injury, (3) immune-mediated damage, (4) altered diameter, and (5) shape distortion or poikilocytosis. Table 26-3 may serve as a quick aid in the diagnosis of the major red cell shape changes.

Fragmentation: RBC fragmentation on blood smears represents RBCs that have lost a portion of their cell membrane generally with some associated cytoplasm. RBC fragmentation is most often a result of excessive blood turbulence from altered blood flow or extensive deposition of fibrin within microvascular lumina. The former is likely the primary mechanism of RBC fragmentation associated with cardiac valvular stenosis and caval syndrome of heartworm disease. The latter mechanism is responsible for the fragmentation hemolysis that is frequently seen in animals with disseminated intravascular coagulation or extensive inflammation of highly vascular tissues (i.e., spleen, liver, pulmonary parenchyma, bone marrow, and renal cortex). Both mechanisms may be active in cases of fragmentation hemolysis associated with large, highly vascular tumors (especially hemangiosarcomas). RBC fragmentation can also result from intrinsic abnormalities of the RBCs themselves, as with RBC oxidative injury or moderate to severe iron deficiency. Fragmented RBCs are usually recognized on blood smears as one of three morphologic forms: schistocytes, keratocytes, or blister cells.

Schistocytes (or schizocytes) are irregularly shaped RBC fragments that typically have ragged asymmetrical borders and sharp, pointed projections (Figure 26-22). Keratocytes are RBC fragments with two adjacent horn-like projections as a result of one-sided loss of cell membrane and cytoplasm. Keratocytes are sometimes referred to as bite or helmet cells because of their two-dimensional shape on blood smears (see Figure 26-22). Blister cells are RBCs with a single, eccentric, vacuole-like structure thought to be created when the cell encounters fibrin strands bridging a vessel lumen. Blister cells are usually found with other forms of fragmented RBCs and probably represent the transitional form between intact erythrocytes and keratocytes (see Figure 26-27). If >1% of these abnormal RBCs are present in peripheral blood, significant RBC fragmentation is suggested. When 10% or more of the RBCs on a blood film appear fragmented, clinical and other laboratory findings are likely to further support the presence of intravascular hemolytic anemia in the patient.

Increased red cell distribution width (RDW) with a shoulder on the left side of the RBC histogram tracing may be seen with automated analysis of blood samples with larger numbers of fragmented red cells; this finding is supportive but not diagnostic of the condition because it can also be seen with other red cell and even platelet alterations.

Oxidative Injury: Oxidative injury of red cells can lead to denaturation of the hemoglobin protein that, when pronounced, can appear as Heinz bodies and/or eccentrocytes on patient blood films. Heinz bodies appear as single, rounded protrusions of the RBC membrane (Figure 26-23), often with a pale staining collar of cytoplasm around the base of the projection. They may also be seen as eccentric, round, pale-staining areas within, or refractile bodies overlying, RBCs. The presence and percentage of RBCs containing Heinz bodies can be most accurately determined by preparing wet or dry blood smears stained with 0.5% NMB. Heinz bodies occasionally fragment from the cell during sample processing and are seen as small, spherical, pink or refractile (or NMB-stained) bodies in the background of a smear. Heinz bodies vary in size depending upon the severity of oxidative injury. Cats, whose hemoglobin molecules are particularly susceptible to oxidative injury, may have very small Heinz bodies in varying percentages (generally <10%) of their circulating RBCs when healthy. Many small and, occasionally, large Heinz bodies may be found in the RBCs of cats with certain chronic conditions (e.g., diabetes mellitus, lymphoma, hyperthyroidism, chronic renal disease). Canine Heinz bodies and numerous or large feline Heinz bodies in RBCs suggest a potential hemolytic crisis. Eccentrocytes, which may also be detected in blood smears of dogs and cats exposed to exogenous oxidative toxins, have an eccentric, ghosted region of cytoplasm with the remaining cytoplasm being slightly condensed (see Figure 26-23). Several exogenous toxins associated with oxidative RBC injury and Heinz bodies and/or eccentrocytes in dogs or cats are listed in Table 26-3.

TABLE 26-3

Major Changes in Peripheral Blood Smear Red Cell Morphology as Indicators of the Cause of Anemia

Prominent Morphology	Expected Associated Red Cell Morphologic Findings	Additional Morphology/ Other Findings Often Seen	Causes to Consider
Hypochromatic erythrocytes	Hypochromic RBCs often appear as acanthocytes, codocytes, or fragmented cells	Insufficient erythropoietic response (polychromatophilic cells) relative to degree of anemia	Iron deficiency: consider dietary deficiency or chronic blood loss (e.g., through GI or urinary tract, repeated blood collection, chronic parasitemia); portosystemic shunt
Fragmented erythrocytes (schistocytes)	Keratocytes (helmet cells), blister cells, possibly occasional spherocytes	Sufficient polychromatophilic cells to indicate a regenerative erythropoietic response	Microangiopathic hemolytic anemia secondary to disseminated intravascular coagulation, inflammation of a highly vascular organ (e.g., liver, spleen, lung, renal glomeruli), turbulent blood flow (e.g., caval syndrome, hemangiosarcoma), severe burns, advanced neoplasia, lymphosarcoma[13,14]
Eccentrocytes and/or Heinz bodies	Sufficient polychromatophilic cells to indicate a regenerative erythropoietic response	Pyknocytes (small, dense, irregularly shaped RBCs), ghosted erythrocytes	Hemolytic anemia secondary to oxidative injury: consider ingestion of onion garlic, zinc, copper, or naphthalene; drug toxicity (e.g., acetaminophen, benzocaine products, propofol, d-L methionine, vitamin K_3, or phenazopyridine)[15-17]
Anisocytosis	Due to polychromatophilic macrocytes indicative of a regenerative response	Codocytes and stomatocytes (among polychromatophilic cells) and a few nRBC may be seen with a regenerative response	If erythropoietic regenerative response is adequate relative to degree of anemia, consider blood loss from hemolysis or hemorrhage (see Table 26-2); if less than adequate regenerative response, consider nonregenerative cause in addition to hemolysis and/ or hemorrhage
	Or due to combined polychromatophilic macrocytes and spherocytes or microcytes	Erythrocyte agglutination, thrombocytopenia, red cell parasites, nRBC	Immune-mediated hemolytic anemia; infection with erythroparasites, especially hemotropic *Mycoplasma* spp.; crotalid snake or bee envenomation[18,19]; may also be seen with Heinz body formation (presumed reformed erythrocyte following removal of membrane protrusion)
	Or due primarily to normocytic macrocytes with few/no polychromatophilic cells	nRBC, other immature erythroid, or abnormal nucleated cells	Myelodysplastic or myeloproliferative disorder (myeloid, erythroid, or lymphoid)

GI, Gastrointestinal; *nRBC,* nucleated red blood cell.

Continued

TABLE 26-3

Major Changes in Peripheral Blood Smear Red Cell Morphology as Indicators of the Cause of Anemia—cont'd

Prominent Morphology	Expected Associated Red Cell Morphologic Findings	Additional Morphology/ Other Findings Often Seen	Causes to Consider
Acanthocytes, echinocytes	Few to no polychromatophilic erythrocytes	If >1% fragmented cells (e.g., schistocytes, keratocytes) – see this section on previous page	Artifact of collection/preparation (see text), disorders of lipid metabolism, liver disease, glomerulonephritis, lymphosarcoma, doxorubicin administration and elapid or crotalid snake envenomation, myeloproliferative disorders, myelofibrosis, uremia, and possibly electrolyte abnormality[14,18-25]
Nucleated erythrocytes	Sufficient polychromatophilic cells to indicate a regenerative erythropoietic response	nRBC with normal morphology; Howell-Jolly bodies	Low numbers of nRBCs sometimes accompany a robust regenerative erythropoietic response
	Few or no polychromatophilic macrocytes indicative of a nonregenerative or poorly regenerative erythropoietic response	nRBC with normal morphology; Howell-Jolly bodies	Splenic or bone marrow dysfunction (e.g., secondary to hypoxia, neoplasia, trauma), persistent glucocorticoid treatment, hyperadrenocorticism, severe physiologic stress, hemangiosarcoma, reported as occasional in some breeds (generally without anemia)
	Few or no polychromatophilic macrocytes indicative of a nonregenerative or poorly regenerative erythropoietic response	Abnormal nRBC (e.g., asynchronous nuclear-to-cytoplasmic ratio), other immature or abnormal nucleated cells	Dyserythropoietic, myelodysplastic, or myeloproliferative (myeloid, erythroid, or lymphoid) disorders; bone marrow dyscrasia in Poodles (with macrocytosis, and usually without anemia)

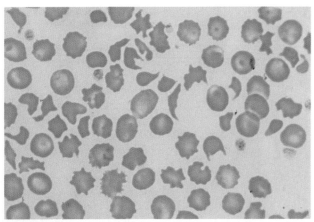

Figure 26-22 Many fragmented RBCs are seen in this blood smear from a dog with stenosis of the pulmonic valve. Numerous schistocytes and a helmet-shaped cell can be seen. (Wright's stain, original magnification 250×.)

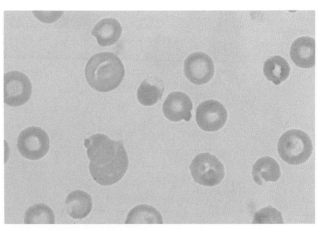

Figure 26-23 Three canine erythrocytes with large Heinz bodies and an eccentrocyte (center) can be seen in this field. (Wright's stain, original magnification 330×.)

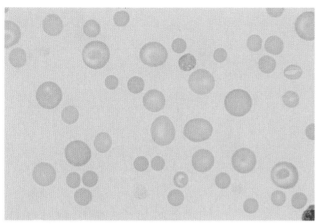

Figure 26-24 A blood smear from a dog with immune-mediated hemolytic anemia. Note the marked anisocytosis resulting from a mixed population of small spherocytes and large, immature, and normal RBCs. The spherocytes are dense staining and lack central pallor. A few poly-chromatophils are in the shape of codocytes. (Wright's stain, original magnification 250×.)

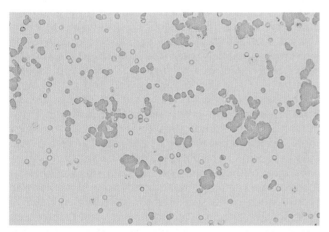

Figure 26-25 RBC agglutination is seen in this blood film from a dog with immune-mediated hemolytic anemia. The cells remained agglutinated after saline dilution of the blood. (Wright's stain, original magnification 100×.)

Immune-Mediated RBC Damage: Immune-mediated RBC damage is suggested by the presence of spherocytes and/or agglutinated RBCs on smears of peripheral blood. Spherocytes are densely staining, small (less than two thirds of the normal diameter) RBCs that lack central pallor (Figure 26-24). They predominantly occur as a result of immune opsonization and piecemeal removal of the RBC membrane by phagocytic cells of the vascular system. This membrane damage weakens the cell and decreases its deformability, leading to RBC loss through cell rupture. In some cases, complement may directly lyse opsonized cells. Significant spherocytosis (>1%) is usually accompanied by overt extravascular or combined extravascular and intravascular hemolytic anemia. Spherocytosis can be reliably detected only in species whose RBCs have distinct central pallor (e.g., dogs) and then only in the monolayer of blood smears. Both dogs and cats with

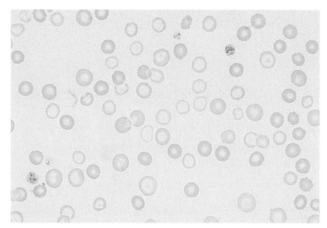

Figure 26-26 Blood from a dog with chronic blood loss and severe iron deficiency. Iron-deficient RBCs have a broad area of central pallor and a thin rim of stained cytoplasm. Anisocytosis is also apparent. (Diff-Quik stain, original magnification 132×.)

immune-mediated hemolytic anemia, however, may have pronounced anisocytosis on blood films (due to a mixture of spherocytic, normal, and—in cases with regenerative responses—large immature RBCs). Note that spherocyte-like particles may also be seen in a few cases of traumatic RBC injury, along with more typical morphologic forms of fragmented RBCs, and may also be seen on smears from animals with recent blood transfusions.

RBC agglutination (Figure 26-25) represents a particularly severe form of immune-mediated hemolytic anemia and may be detected grossly in samples within the collection vial or on unstained blood films. A saline dilution test is suggested for all suspect samples to aid in distinguishing immune-mediated agglutination from nonspecific RBC aggregation or rouleaux. Mixing 2 or 3 drops of saline with a drop of blood on a glass slide or tube causes cells that are simply aggregated or in rouleaux to disperse. Unstained, coverslipped preparations should be evaluated under 40× magnification with the substage condenser lowered.

Alterations in RBC Diameter: RBCs with smaller or larger diameter than average can be classified as microcytes or macrocytes, respectively. Blood smear evaluation is a sensitive means of detecting these alterations if RBC diameter in peripheral blood is mixed. Uniform microcytosis or macrocytosis is not easily recognized in peripheral smears, but can be indicated by the mean cell volume (MCV) value generated with automated hematology analysis of the sample. In smears containing mixed red cell diameters, or anisocytosis, determining which cells represent the abnormal population may be difficult. Adjacent leukocytes on the smear can be helpful for size comparisons. Anisocytosis with microcytosis and poorly regenerative anemia can be seen in dogs and cats with pronounced iron-deficiency anemia (Figure 26-26). The decrease in cell diameter is a result of additional mitoses during erythropoiesis in association with delayed hemoglobin synthesis. Measurable microcytosis generally occurs slightly earlier than RBC hypochromasia in animals with iron deficiency, but hyopchromasia is usually the

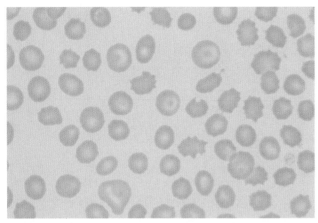

Figure 26-27 Irregularly spiculated codocytes, echinocytes, and ovalocytes in the blood of a dog with multicentric lymphoma. The blister cell near the center of the field indicates that RBC trauma may be at least partially responsible for the acanthocytic RBCs. (Wright's stain, original magnification 250×.)

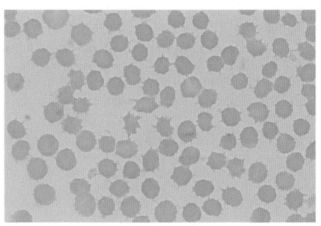

Figure 26-28 Acanthocytes demonstrating irregularly sized spicules in a blood smear from a dog with cholestatic liver disease. (Wright's stain, original magnification 132×.)

more prominent blood smear finding. Microcytic and normochromic to hypochromic RBCs can also be seen in dogs with congenital portosystemic shunt (likely in association with abnormal iron metabolism[26]), and generalized microcytosis of normochromic RBCs occurs as a nonpathologic breed characteristic in Shibas, Akitas, and possibly Chow Chows.[27]

Macrocytosis occurs most commonly in animals with regenerative anemias, reflecting the relatively large size of immature polychromatophilic RBCs. The polychromatophilic staining of these cells is less apparent with some quick stains, so the cells may appear as normochromic macrocytes on blood films. True normochromic macrocytosis can result from impaired mitosis of RBC precursors and may be seen with myelodysplastic and myeloproliferative diseases and feline leukemia virus (FELV) infections. Macrocytosis in association with familial bone marrow dysplasia has also been reported in some poodles, including Miniature and Toy Poodles.[28] Macrocytosis that is attributed to these erythroid dysplastic or neoplastic conditions is usually accompanied by additional findings of increased erythrocyte anisocytosis and circulating nucleated erythroid cells (sometimes with asynchronized nuclear to cytoplasm development).

Macrocytosis has been rarely associated in dogs and/or cats with alterations of red cell fluid balance or cytoskeletal or membrane properties. Any of these causes may contribute to the familial macrocytosis with stomatocytosis (central fold resulting in a linear central pale region) that is uncommonly seen in Miniature or Standard Schnauzers. In affected Schnauzers, the RBC shape change may be associated with other blood smear red cell alterations (anisocytosis, polychromasia) as well as increased RBC fragility and slight anemia.[29,30] Rare familial macrocytosis has been reported with other breeds (e.g., Giant Schnauzer, Alaskan Malamute, and Drentse Patrijshond) in association with pronounced clinical manifestations.[31,32]

Poikilocytosis: Poikilocytosis is the presence of striking shape variation in a significant number (generally 10% or more) of peripheral blood RBCs. Poikilocytosis is a nonspecific term and may refer to acanthocytes, echinocytes, elliptocytes/ovalocytes, codocytes, and less often, other red cell shape changes (Figures 26-27 and 26-28). Poikilocytosis has been linked to altered RBC membrane lipid content and lipid metabolism in humans; this may also be a contributing mechanism for the association of poikilocytosis in animals with hepatic disease, including cats with hepatic lipidosis, cholangiohepatitis, hepatitis/hepatopathy, systemic histoplasmosis, and portocaval shunt, and dogs with chronic hepatic or renal glomerular disease, lymphosarcoma or hypothyroidism.[15,23,24] However, it is as likely that the poikilocytosis in these cases is also multifactorial because abnormalities of the microvasculature and blood viscosity, hypertension, and inflammation accompany most of these conditions and can alter the physical stress on circulating erythrocytes. Poikilocytosis has also been reported in both species administered doxorubicin.[21,22] Poikilocytes may be the most frequent shape change seen in animals with RBC fragmentation injury as well, but the latter is generally the more diagnostic finding.

Acanthocytes are poikilocytes with one or more irregularly spaced and shaped membrane projections that may be slightly knobbed at the tip (see Figure 26-28), whereas echinocytes have more numerous and uniformly spaced membrane projections. Acanthocytes or echinocytes can resemble, but are usually distinguishable from, in vitro crenated cells or preparation artifacts by their random distribution within blood smears (whereas the in vitro effects are generally seen in broad regions of the smear). Elliptocytes, or ovalocytes, are oval RBCs with smooth or scalloped borders that (along with acanthocytes) have been particularly reported in cats with hepatic lipidosis.

Codocytes, or target cells are poikilocytes with three-dimensional hat-like shapes that appear on blood smears as RBCs with pale to unstained rings separating peripheral and central-stained cytoplasmic regions (see Figure 26-24). Codocytes represent RBCs with relative excess of membrane compared with volume of cytoplasm. In dogs, relatively high numbers of codocytes have been associated with the hypercholesterolemia of hypothyroidism.

However, immature RBCs, which similarly have an excess of membrane to cytoplasm, can also be commonly seen as large, slightly polychromatophilic codocytes on smears.

With samples that show pronounced poikilocytosis on smears, increased RDW may be seen on histograms with automated analysis. However, this may also reflect the additional occurrence of fragmented or immature RBCs and is not specifically supportive of the morphologic findings.

Alterations in RBC Staining

Polychromatophils: Polychromatophils are immature RBCs that are usually larger and more basophilic than mature cells (see Figure 26-26). Polychromatophils occur in up to 0.5% and 1% of the circulating RBC pool of healthy cats and dogs, respectively. Higher proportions of polychromatophils suggest increased erythropoiesis.

Hypochromasia: Hypochromasia characterizes the RBCs of pronounced iron deficiency (see Figure 26-26). These cells are recognized by their prominent central pallor and a relatively thin, peripheral ring of stained cytoplasm. Hypochromic RBCs are generally more variable in shape than normochromic RBCs, often occurring as poikilocytes, folded cells, and codocytes on blood smears. The hypochromic cells in iron deficiency may also appear microcytic, although this is often more subtle on blood smears than the change in tinctorial properties. Polychromatophilic RBCs are considered hypochromic in reference to their hemoglobin content but do not appear hypochromic on routinely stained blood films. Table 26-3 may further aid in determining the cause of hypochromatic erythrocytes in dogs and cats.

Howell-Jolly Bodies: Howell-Jolly bodies are dark blue to black spherical inclusions that usually occur individually within RBC cytoplasm. These discrete structures represent nuclear remnants that are not appropriately extruded from the cell during maturation. Howell-Jolly bodies are occasionally seen as an insignificant finding in the RBCs of healthy dogs and cats. Higher numbers of cells may contain the inclusions in animals with regenerative anemia, with decreased splenic function, or in association with abnormal erythropoiesis. It is particularly important not to confuse Howell-Jolly bodies with other cellular inclusions or erythroparasites.

Basophilic Stippling: Basophilic stippling appears as a faint dusting of the RBC cytoplasm with fine, gray to dark blue granules. This finding is an indication of interference with, or incomplete utilization of, polyribosomes for hemoglobin synthesis and is most often a nonspecific finding in dogs and cats with profound regenerative responses to anemia. Basophilic stippling has classically been linked to lead toxicity in dogs, but is generally limited to cases with severe lead exposure and associated with no, or only mild, anemia.[33]

Nucleated RBCs: Nucleated RBCs, or normoblasts, are occasionally seen in the blood of healthy dogs and cats. Higher numbers of nucleated RBCs (but generally less than 5 RBCs/100 WBCs) are expected on blood smears from animals with regenerative anemias or splenic dysfunction/asplenia. Normoblastemia with the latter condition can occur transiently with splenic trauma and inconsistently with splenic neoplasia, inflammation, and extramedullary hematopoiesis. Hyperadrenocorticism, severe physiologic stress, and corticosteroid treatment are also associated with reduced splenic trapping of the nucleated cells and possible mild normoblastosis. Variable numbers of circulating normoblasts may be seen in animals with hemangiosarcoma of the spleen or other organs and inflammatory liver conditions. Certain dog breeds (e.g., Miniature Schnauzer, Dachshund), when healthy, have also been reported to have increased numbers of nucleated RBCs.[34]

If there are >5 nucleated RBCs/100 WBCs in peripheral blood, bone marrow alterations are particularly suggested. Hypoxia of the bone marrow, as occurs with hypovolemic shock, and marked or peracute anemia can transiently impair marrow sinusoidal integrity and result in mild to moderate normoblastemia. Marrow hypoxia may be a reason that circulating, nucleated RBCs are commonly associated with—but are not an indication of—a regenerative response to anemia. In cases with 15 or more nucleated RBCs/100 WBCs on blood smears, bone marrow severe injury or disruption of architecture, or lead poisoning is more likely. Erythremic myelosis, a myeloproliferative disorder predominantly occurring in cats, is characterized by severe peripheral blood normoblastosis that includes erythroid progenitor cells of multiple stages (e.g., metarubricytes, rubricytes, and rubriblasts) (see Figure 26-52). Table 26-3 may further aid in determining the cause of increased numbers of circulating nucleated erythrocytes in dogs and cats.

Parasitic Organisms of RBCs

Dogs and cats can be infected with several species and variants of RBC-associated parasitic organisms. A complete list of the known organisms is too large to adequately review here; hence, only those that have been reported on blood films from dogs and cats in North America are described. Notably, the taxonomy of erythrocyte-associated parasitic organisms has been evolving in the last few years with advancements in molecular-based classification. For this reason and because new variants and new hosts of the organisms are increasingly being discovered in other global regions, it is prudent to keep in mind that this list may not be comprehensive in the near future.

Hemotropic Mycoplasmosis: Infection with *Mycoplasma haemofelis* and *Mycoplasma haemominutum* (previously classified as *Hemobartonella felis*, large and small forms, or *H. felis* Ohio and California variants) has been reported for cats in most areas of the United States, although regional differences in prevalence, and greater incidence in older, male and/or outdoor cats have been noted.[35-37] Infection with either organism can be asymptomatic or associated with a mild anemia. Infection with *M. haemofelis* can also cause a moderate to severe acute extravascular hemolytic anemia in cats.

In Wright's-stained smears of peripheral blood, *M. haemofelis* appears as basophilic cocci, short rods (that may represent chains of cocci), or faint rings on the RBC

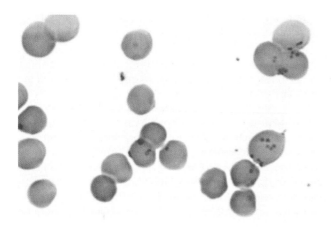

Figure 26-29 This blood smear from a domestic cat shows a high proportion of the RBCs with single scattered or short chains of basophilic cocci or faint rings on the cell membrane that are characteristic of *Mycoplasma haemofelis* organisms. (Diff-Quik stain, original magnification 400×.)

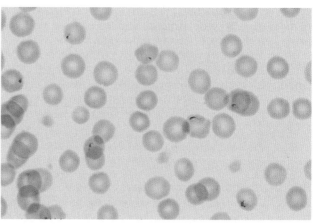

Figure 26-30 In this smear from a domestic cat, signet ring-shaped *Cytauxzoon felis* organisms are apparent in several RBCs. (Diff-Quik stain, original magnification 330×.)

membrane, and are most reliably identifiable if found in chains that extend across the face of an RBC (Figure 26-29). *M. haemominutum* appear similar in staining and shape in smears, but cocci are about half the diameter and generally not found as rings or in chains. With both organisms, few to a majority of red cells can appear infected on smears. However, the number of infected red cells seen does not necessarily correlate with the occurrence or severity of anemia. Fresh blood (without use of anticoagulants) seems to be the most reliable for detecting the bacteria; organisms are apt to detach from the RBC membrane in shaken or stored samples, especially those containing a calcium-chelating anticoagulant. Organisms also need to be differentiated on blood smears from artifacts of preparation and staining (e.g., membrane blebs in crenated RBCs or granular stain precipitate). In suspected infections, repeat sampling may be useful to detect either organism on blood smears. However, more sensitive molecular diagnostic methods are commercially available to confirm infection. Molecular methods have also shown that cats can be infected with both organisms.

In dogs, two mycoplasma epierythrocytic parasites have also been reported. Distinction between these has been by molecular procedures rather than blood smear evaluation because infections appear to be mostly occult. However, circulating infected red cells may rarely be seen in asplenic or immunosuppressed dogs. On Wright's-stained smears, these organisms appear as basophilic epierythrocytic cocci, with *Mycoplasma haemocanis* being larger than the more recently described variant. Although infection is most commonly asymptomatic, a variety of symptoms with or without anemia have been reported with acute, or resurgence of latent infection in some dogs, and rare cases of severe symptoms or pronounced anemia have been described in association with *M. haemocanis*.[38,39] For suspected active cases of *M. haemocanis*, a polymerase chain reaction–based method of detection with whole blood is also available through some university laboratories.

Cytauxzoon felis: *Cytauxzoon felis* has been reported in North American cats primarily from midwestern, southeastern, and mid-Atlantic regions of the United States. Organisms occur within RBCs as signet rings and occasionally matchstick, safety pin, and maltese cross forms (Figure 26-30). Typically <1% of feline RBCs appear infected unless a cat is in the terminal stages of infection. Schizogonous forms in swollen macrophages are readily detected in aspirates of the lymph nodes, spleen, liver, lungs, and bone marrow of clinically ill cats. Cytauxzoonosis is commonly acutely fatal in cats as a result of vascular obstruction from schizogony within phagocytic cells (particularly endothelial macrophages) throughout the body. The anemia that develops is usually only mild to moderate, partially masked by dehydration, and minimally regenerative at the time of the animal's death. Leukopenia and thrombocytopenia are also common during terminal stages.[40]

Babesia spp.: *Babesia* spp. have been detected in dogs but not, at the time of this writing, in cats in North America. *B. canis* is the largest of these organisms that infect canine RBCs. Pyriform to amoeboid shapes of *B. canis* can extend across most of the RBC diameter (Figure 26-31), whereas rod and fusiform shapes, which are usually present concomitantly, are much smaller and more difficult to detect. Intraerythrocytic forms of the other two species identified in dogs, *B. gibsoni* and *Babesia conradae*, are also relatively small compared with *B. canis* pyriforms and particularly pleomorphic, occurring within RBCs as rings, rods, pyriform, band-like, and coccoid-like forms. Multiple organisms per RBC may be seen in acute infections with any of these species; however, only rare parasites are detected with chronic babesiosis. Detection may be facilitated by examining capillary blood smears (e.g., collected from an ear vein) and the RBCs located immediately below the buffy coat of a spun hematocrit tube. Infected cells are also most likely to be located along the periphery and feathered edge of a smear.

Additional supportive findings with acute *B. canis* infections include intravascular hemolysis with hemoglobinuria,

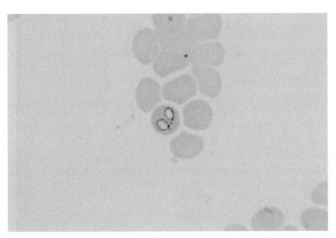

Figure 26-31 Peripheral blood from a dog with a *Babesia canis* infection. Two piroplasms are seen in a single RBC in this field. (Wright's stain, original magnification 330×.)

bilirubinuria, and bilirubinemia. Extravascular hemolysis with anemia, as well as thrombocytopenia and neutropenia, can be found in dogs with acute infections of any of these *Babesia* species. Chronic infection can result in an undulating pattern of variably regenerative anemia with clinical and laboratory evidence of chronic immune stimulation. An indirect fluorescent antibody test (IFA) can also support diagnosis, although false-negative results can occur in acutely infected animals, and antibody cross-reactivity is considerable between *Babesia* spp. Molecular methods (polymerase chain reaction [PCR]) for detection of the different species in whole blood is offered by some university laboratories.

ALTERATIONS IN PLATELET NUMBERS AND MORPHOLOGY

A patient's platelet count can be roughly estimated from the monolayer of a blood smear, if there are no platelet clumps along the feathered edge. Under 100× oil-immersion magnification, the platelets in each of 10 microscopic fields are counted, averaged, and multiplied by 15,000 to arrive at the estimated number per μl. Alternatively, 7 to 35 platelets per oil-immersion 100× field can be used as a reference for adequate platelet numbers (i.e., ≥100,000 platelets/μl).[3] Platelet clumps suggest that numbers are at least adequate for hemostasis (i.e., ≥50,000 platelets/μl).[3] When abnormal platelet numbers are detected on dog or cat blood smears, thrombocytopenia is found more often than thrombocytosis. A wide variety of conditions, with inflammatory states and neoplasia being the two most commonly associated with the finding in both species, have been associated with thrombocytopenia in dogs and cats.[41,42] However, marked thrombocytopenia can usually be attributed to one of the four primary causes listed with examples in Box 26-1. Conditions associated with thrombocytosis are also listed in Box 26-1.

The diameter of most platelets in healthy dogs range from 2 to 4 μm, or about a fourth to half the size of the erythrocytes. Platelets in cats are more variable in size, larger on average than those in dogs, and about a fourth

to almost the same size of the erythrocytes. Enlarged platelets in both species are considered to be those with approximately the same diameter as RBCs. Platelets this size are uncommon in normal canine blood and constitute a minor percentage in normal feline blood. Giant platelets (i.e., "stress platelets," "shift platelets," or megathrombocytes; Figure 26-32) are larger than RBCs and unusual in blood smears from healthy dogs and cats. Giant or increased numbers of enlarged platelets on routinely prepared blood films suggest active thrombopoiesis or, less often, abnormal thrombopoiesis associated with myelodysplastic or myeloproliferative conditions or myelofibrosis. Irregularly shaped and/or atypically granulated platelets may also be seen in the peripheral blood of animals with bone marrow disorders, especially those animals with myeloproliferative conditions and cats with FeLV infections.

Increased incidence of small platelets has been reported as a finding on blood smears from dogs with immune-mediated thrombocytopenia or with various chronic conditions; however, because small platelets overlap into the normal range, this is a more difficult determination on blood smears alone without supportive mean platelet volume (MPV) data from automated analysis of the blood. Overall, increased platelet variation in size and granulation, cytoplasmic polychromasia or vacuolation, and filamentous extensions suggestive of activation can be observed more often on smears from dogs and cats with clinical illness than healthy animals,[43] although these findings generally have little to no specific diagnostic value. A rare reason for abnormal platelet morphology is the appearance of a single large granule (sometimes vacuolated) in a canine platelet, which represents the morula of *Anaplasma (Ehrlichia) platys*; infected dogs usually present with mild to moderate thrombocytopenia or cyclic thrombocytopenia.

Familial and other genetic defects that affect platelets are usually not associated abnormal platelet morphology that can be detected by routine blood smear evaluation. One exception recently reported is an asymptomatic familial disorder in Cavalier King Charles Spaniels characterized by slight thrombocytopenia and enlarged platelets that have normal ultrastructure.[44]

ALTERATIONS OF WBCs IN DISEASE

Alterations of WBC Numbers

The WBC count can be roughly classified as high, normal, or low by scanning the blood smear monolayer and the feathered edge with the 10 or 20× objective. The percentages of each WBC type can be estimated by scanning the smear or determined by a 100-differential nucleated cell count. Mature neutrophils are the most common WBC type in peripheral blood of healthy adult cats and dogs, respectively averaging 60% and 70% of the differential cell count, although cats have a slightly wider reference range than dogs. Lymphocytes, the second most common nucleated cell type, average 20% of the differential count in adult dogs and slightly more than 30% in cats. Monocytes constitute about 5% and eosinophils are usually less than 5% of canine and feline peripheral blood WBCs. There are six major patterns of alterations in the WBC-differential count commonly seen in animals; these are listed with the general

BOX 26-1

Causes and Conditions Associated with Clinically Significant Alteration in Peripheral Blood-Platelet Count

Thrombocytopenia

Increased Destruction
Immune-mediated thrombocytopenia
Drug induced (usually an immune-mediated process
    [e.g., certain antibiotics or heparin therapy])
Accelerated Utilization
Disseminated intravascular coagulation
Major vessel thrombosis
Acute severe hemorrhage (e.g., some cases of brodi-
    facoum toxicity)
Increased Storage Site Sequestration
Splenic disease (e.g., splenomegaly, splenic torsion, severe
    splenic congestion, and splenic neoplasia)
Anaphylaxis, endotoxemia (sequestration in microvascu-
    lature)
Certain drugs (e.g., barbiturates)
Addison's disease
Decreased Production
Pancytopenic syndrome (e.g., chronic *Ehrlichia* spp. infec-
    tion, Fanconi's syndrome, estrogen toxicity)
Marrow infiltration (leukemia, myelofibrosis, myelophthisic
    conditions)
Cyclic hematopoiesis
Chemotherapeutic cytotoxic and cytostatic drugs
    Severe nutritional deficiencies
Mixed or Idiosyncratic Causes
Certain infections, especially those involving the bone
    marrow (e.g., FeLV or histoplasmosis), acute pathologic
    viral infections, *Babesia* spp., and rickettsial infections
Nonleukemic neoplasia
Bacterial septicemia or endotoxemia
Pronounced inflammation or necrosis (especially of highly
    vascular organs)
Uremia

Thrombocytosis

Reactive
Acute hemorrhage/hemolysis
Increased granulopoiesis (especially when associated with
    chronic inflammation)
Increased erythropoiesis
Storage Site Release (Transient Thrombocytosis)
Splenic contraction (fear, pain, trauma, physical exertion,
    postoperative)
Certain drugs (e.g., corticosteroids or epinephrine)
Canine Cushing's disease
Post-splenectomy
Increased Production
Certain drugs (e.g., vincristine)
Myeloproliferative syndromes (*eg,* myelogenous leukemia
    and erythremic myelosis)
Mixed or Idiosyncratic Causes
Various neoplasias (e.g., squamous cell carcinoma, mast
    cell sarcoma)
Iron deficiency

---

mechanism of their induction in Box 26-2. Conditions associated with changes in the number of each specific WBC type have been published in several veterinary texts.[1-3]

Alterations of WBC Morphology

Neutrophilic Toxic Changes: Neutrophilic toxic changes are probably the most common morphologic WBC alterations detected on blood films. These cellular changes are an outcome of aberrant granulopoiesis and indicate a systemic inflammatory effect on the bone marrow. The most severe changes are primarily seen in animals with sepsis, endotoxemia, or tissue necrosis. Toxic changes represent qualitative abnormalities of neutrophils, with the severity, or degree of alteration, considered at least as significant as the actual proportion of cells involved.

Döhle bodies are the mildest form of toxic neutrophilic change. These irregular gray patches in neutrophil cytoplasm (Figure 26-33) represent aberrant aggregations of endoplasmic reticulum. Döhle bodies always indicate a systemic effect of inflammation in dogs but are occasionally seen without significant inflammation in cats with increased granulopoiesis.

Cytoplasmic basophilia is a more severe form of toxic change that appears as pale, homogeneous, blue to patchy blue-purple cytoplasm in affected cells. As with Döhle bodies, cytoplasmic basophilia may occur in band, as well as mature, neutrophils.

Foamy cytoplasmic vacuolization is an indication of severe systemic toxicity and considered a result of abnormal lysosome formation and intracellular release of the autolyzing enzymes. This toxic change appears as many vaguely defined vacuoles throughout the cytoplasm, giving it a soap bubbles–like appearance (Figure 26-34).

Toxic granulation is an uncommon finding that occurs with severely aberrant granulopoiesis. The small, scattered, red-pink cytoplasmic granules (Figure 26-35)

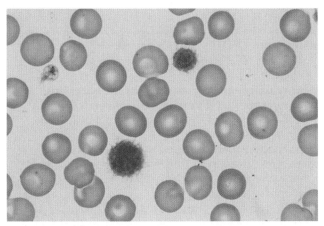

Figure 26-32 A giant and a slightly enlarged platelet in a dog with hemorrhagic pancreatitis and a markedly inflammatory leukogram. Enlarged platelets are consistent with increased thrombopoiesis, which may be a reactive response associated with acute hemorrhage and increased granulocytopoiesis in this dog. (Wright's stain, original magnification 330×.)

represent the retained primary granule mucopolysaccharide that is normally lost during neutrophil maturation.

Giant neutrophils represent skipped mitotic divisions of rapidly developing neutrophil precursor cells. Giant neutrophils are similar in appearance to, but about twice the size of, band or mature neutrophils and are generally found more often in cats with toxic neutropoiesis than dogs (Figure 26-36).

Ring-shaped nuclei in neutrophils are a sign of extreme systemic toxicity and are typically associated with sepsis (Figure 26-37). When evaluating blood smears for toxic changes, it is important not to mistake neutrophil nuclei with overlapping ends as toxic ring-shaped nuclei.

Immature Granulocytes: Increased immature granulocytes in the peripheral blood of dogs and cats usually indicates an inflammatory process. During inflammation, as in health, granulocytes exit the bone marrow in an orderly manner dependent upon their stage of maturation. For each granulocyte line, cells of the most mature stages available to an animal are found in the highest proportion in peripheral blood. Cells of sequentially less mature stages are expected to occur in blood in numbers directly proportional to their level of development. A particularly guarded prognosis is indicated when the total number of immature neutrophils, including band cells, on an inflammatory leukogram is greater than that of mature segmented neutrophils. A similar prognosis is indicated when 10% or more of the circulating neutrophils are immature in an animal with neutropenia. Both of these conditions are called degenerative left shifts. In addition, accurately staging immature granulocytes may be difficult because of asynchronous cellular development in particularly pronounced inflammatory responses. This is often recognized as a delay in nuclear shape change relative to the degree of chromatin condensation and cytoplasmic development (Figure 26-38).

Band cells of granulocytes contain cytoplasmic granules specific to cell type and nuclei generally similar to those of mature neutrophils, but lack distinct segmentation and have less condensed chromatin.

Metamyelocytes have nuclei shaped like kidney beans or broad hourglasses with fewer, smaller, and more widely spaced clumps of heterochromatin compared with band and segmented granulocyte nuclei (Figure 26-39). The cytoplasm of neutrophilic metamyelocytes ranges from pale pink to variably basophilic, depending upon the degree of immaturity and toxic change. Cytoplasmic granules specific to cell type are present and are usually prominent in eosinophil and basophil metamyelocytes.

Myelocytes have round to oval, slightly eccentric nuclei that are sometimes slightly flattened on one side; they have coarse, ropy chromatin separating a few small chromatin clumps. Myelocytes are larger with a considerably higher nuclear-to-cytoplasmic ratio than more mature WBCs. The cytoplasm is slightly basophilic and contains granules specific to the cell type.

Pelger-Huët Anomaly: Pelger-Huët anomaly is an idiosyncratic finding reported in several dog breeds, canine mongrels, and domestic short-haired cats. It is generally considered a familial disorder in which all or most granulocyte and monocyte nuclei fail to undergo segmentation. The defect is presumed to originate at the stem cell level because bone marrow megakaryocytes are also affected.[45] Nuclei of affected circulating cells may be round or kidney bean shaped, whereas chromatin condensation and cytoplasmic development resemble that of normal mature cells (Figure 26-40). The granulocytes of animals with Pelger-Huët anomaly can usually be distinguished from the immature cells of an inflammatory response based on their uniform appearance and absence of toxic changes. Animals with Pelger-Huët anomaly lack overt functional immune system alterations; however, at least one study of an affected family of Foxhounds has shown impaired neutrophil and lymphocyte functions.[46] A prolonged acquired Pelger-Huët–like anomaly has also been reported in a dog as a presumed idiosyncratic reaction to chemotherapeutic treatment.[47]

Hypersegmented Neutrophils: Hypersegmented neutrophils in peripheral blood represent neutrophils that have remained in circulation for an extended period instead of migrating into the tissues. These cells, which are recognized as neutrophils with five or more distinct separations between nuclear lobes (Figure 26-41), can be seen in peripheral blood of patients with increases in the circulating levels of exogenous or endogenous corticosteroids. Hypersegmented neutrophils are also occasionally seen in the peripheral blood of animals with marked neutrophilia associated with chronic inflammatory states and for a brief period after treatment or elimination of the source of inflammation. Hypersegmented neutrophils may be distinguished from partially pyknotic cells that have aged in vitro by evaluating other WBCs in the smear for evidence of in vitro aging changes.

Chediak-Higashi Syndrome: Chediak-Higashi syndrome is a genetic disorder that affects intracellular protein transport in a wide variety of tissue types and is associated

BOX 26-2

Common Patterns of Alterations in the Leukocyte Differential Count

Leukocytosis

Physiologic (Epinephrine-Mediated) Responses (e.g., with fear, excitement, pain, and trauma)
Neutrophils: mildly increased
Lymphocytes: increased
Monocytes: normal to mildly increased
Eosinophils: normal to increased
Basophils: usually absent

Stress-Related (Corticosteroid-Mediated) Responses
Neutrophils: increased
Lymphocytes: decreased
Monocytes: increased (in dogs) or variable (in cats)
Eosinophils: decreased
Basophils: absent

Acute Inflammatory Conditions
Neutrophils: increased, usually with a shift toward immature stages
Lymphocytes: normal to decreased
Monocytes: normal to increased
Eosinophils: normal to decreased
Basophils: usually absent

Chronic Inflammatory Conditions
Neutrophils: increased, with or without a shift toward immature stages
Lymphocytes: usually increased, especially with chronic infectious diseases
Monocytes: usually increased
Eosinophils: variable; may be increased
Basophils: variable; may be increased

Leukopenia

Acute Cutopenias (e.g., acute systemic infections, viral infections, endotoxemia, anaphylaxis)
Neutrophils: decreased (may have a left shift with acute inflammatory disease)
Lymphocytes: often decreased
Monocytes: variable (e.g., often increased with acute immune-mediated cytopenias)
Eosinophils: decreased
Basophils: absent

Chronic sutopenias (e.g., bone marrow infiltration and/or infections involving the marrow, aplastic anemia, or estrogen toxicity)
Neutrophils: decreased (often without a left shift)
Lymphocytes: usually normal to increased (increased with chronic immune stimulation)
Monocytes: usually normal to increased (may be partly compensatory to neutropenia)
Eosinophils: variable
Basophils: variable

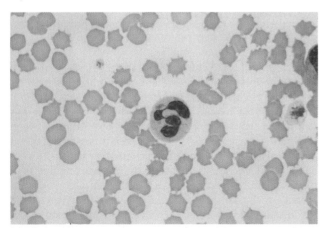

Figure 26-33 Cytoplasmic basophilia and a large Döhle body in this neutrophil from a cat with pyothorax indicate systemic toxicity affecting marrow granulocytopoiesis. The RBCs in the background are crenated as a result of excess EDTA in the collected blood sample. (Wright's stain, original magnification 250×.)

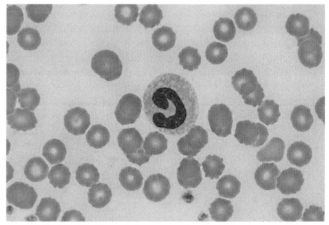

Figure 26-34 A canine neutrophil showing changes associated with inflammation and marked systemic toxicity. The cytoplasm appears slightly basophilic and foamy. (Wright's stain, original magnification 250×.)

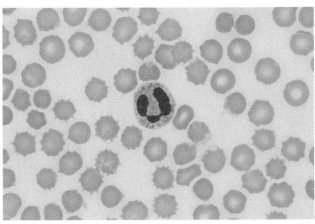

Figure 26-35 Toxic granulation, as noted by the scattered, small, round, eosinophilic to metachromatic cytoplasmic granules, in a canine neutrophil. The cell also shows cytoplasmic basophilia and foaminess. (Wright's stain, original magnification 250×.)

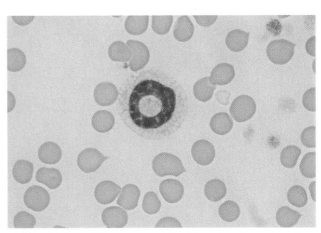

Figure 26-37 A feline neutrophil with a ring-shaped nucleus indicating severe systemic toxicity. The cell also has highly vacuolated or foamy cytoplasm. (Wright's stain, original magnification 250×.)

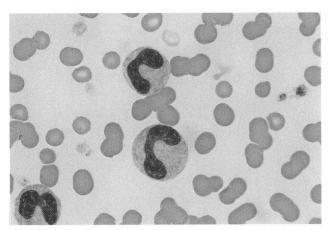

Figure 26-36 A giant neutrophil adjacent to a normally proportioned neutrophil in a feline blood smear. The basophilic cytoplasm and Döhle bodies in both neutrophils indicate systemic toxicity. (Wright's stain, original magnification 250×.)

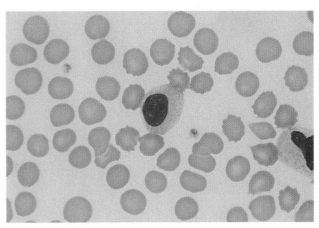

Figure 26-38 Asynchronous development of nuclear shape (compared with cytoplasmic maturation and chromatin condensation) is seen in this canine neutrophilic myelocyte. (Wright's stain, original magnification 250×.)

with abnormally large cytoplasmic granules in peripheral blood leukocytes. The condition has been described in Persian cats with blue smoke–colored hair coats, as well as other species, but not in dogs. In peripheral blood smears, the abnormal granules may be seen in neutrophils, eosinophils, monocytes, and an occasional lymphocyte. With Romanowsky-type stains, the granules in affected leukocytes are usually eosinophilic and often irregular in shape. In neutrophils, the granules are considered to represent fused primary (i.e., azurophilic) granules, which have properties of lysosomes. Cats with Chediak-Higashi syndrome often have low neutrophil counts as well as functionally impaired leukocyte bacteriocidal activity and mild bleeding tendency due to platelet defects.[48-50]

Altered Staining of Neutrophil Granules: Neutrophils with prominent magenta granules scattered throughout the cytoplasm have been reported in peripheral blood

smears of some Birman cats as an inherited condition. Granules in affected cells have similar shape and size as that of the normally barely discernible granules in neutrophils of unaffected cats. Affected cats appear clinically healthy, and no ultrastructural or functional abnormalities of their neutrophils have been found.[51] The finding is thought to reflect a benign genetic difference in neutrophil lysosomal contents, which affects affinity for acidic dyes.

Other familial canine or feline conditions in cats or dogs can be associated with altered neutrophil granules. In mucopolysaccharidosis type VI and type VII, and GM2-gangliosidosis, reddish-purple granules may be present within the cytoplasm of circulating neutrophils and monocytes.[52,53] Eosinophil granules may be unstained or more brighly eosinoplic and abnormally shaped in affected animals. However, gross dysmorphic features and, sometimes, neurologic deficits are generally far more prominent in dogs and cats with these conditions.

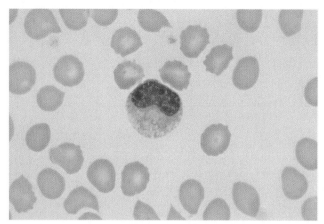

Figure 26-39 A metamyelocyte in the blood of a dog with an inflammatory leukogram and left shift. The cell's cytoplasm is more deeply basophilic than expected as a result of systemic toxicity. (Wright's stain, original magnification 330×.)

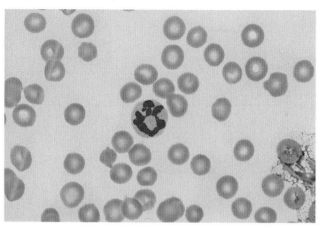

Figure 26-41 A neutrophil with a hypersegmented nucleus in the blood of a dog 1 day after an ovariohysterectomy for pyometra. (Wright's stain, original magnification 250×.)

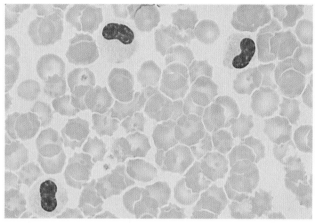

Figure 26-40 Pelger-Huët anomaly. The nuclei of granulocyte cells retain immature shapes despite a condensed, mature, chromatin pattern. (Wright's stain, original magnification 250×.)

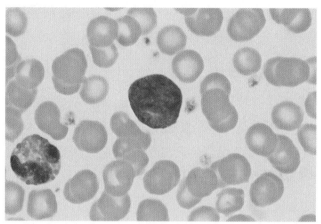

Figure 26-42 A large, reactive lymphocyte in a cat with histoplasmosis. The cell's nuclear chromatin is less densely clumped compared with that of small mature lymphocytes. The cytoplasm is abundant, is deeply basophilic, and shows a prominent, pale perinuclear Golgi region. (Wright's stain, original magnification 330×.)

Reactive Lymphocytes: Reactive lymphocytes are generally regarded as immune-stimulated T- or B-cells with upregulated synthesis of inflammatory mediators and/or immunoglobulins (B-cells). The cells are generally large-sized, with abundant cytoplasm and less-condensed nuclear chromatin than the more common small, mature lymphocytes. The gray to deeply basophilic cytoplasm represents an abundance of polyribosomes associated with the increased protein synthesis and often shows a contrasting pale, perinuclear Golgi region (Figure 26-42). Reactive lymphocytes in peripheral blood suggest active immune stimulation but are etiologically nonspecific.

Mast Cells: Mast cells have been observed in peripheral blood of dogs and cats with systemic mastocytosis (Figure 26-43) and in very low numbers on blood smears from dogs with pronounced inflammatory conditions, regenerative anemia, trauma, or non–mast cell neoplasia.[54,55]

Mitotic Figures: Mitotic figures are rarely seen on blood films. When present, they are most often found at the feathered edges of smears and are part of a leukemic cell population (Figure 26-44). Mitotic figures are rarely seen in peripheral blood of nonleukemic animals, but in these cases, the most common association has been with reactive lymphocytosis.

WBC Inclusions: WBC inclusions on blood smears usually represent phagocytosed material, including other cells, cell debris, and infectious organisms. Phagocytosed RBCs, hematoidin, or hemosiderin (with the last two appearing as light brown or black cytoplasmic material) are seen only rarely in the circulating monocytes or neutrophils of animals, generally in association with marked inflammatory responses or hemolytic anemias.

Inclusions of canine distemper virus can occur in either WBCs (i.e., lymphocytes, neutrophils, monocytes) or RBCs. The inclusions are pathognomonic for the infection

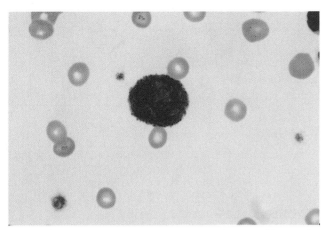

Figure 26-43 A well-granulated mast cell in the blood of a cat with splenic mast-cell neoplasm. (Wright's stain, original magnification 250×.)

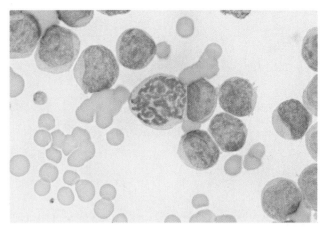

Figure 26-44 A large, mitotic figure among other leukemic cells in the blood of a cat with large cell lymphoid leukemia. (Wright's stain, original magnification 250×.)

and usually appear as one or two variably sized, discrete, eosinophilic, round to oval bodies in the cytoplasm of lymphocytes and monocytes, and as smaller, eosinophilic to basophilic bodies in neutrophils. In addition to, or in lieu of, their appearance in WBCs, viral inclusions may also be observed in RBCs. When seen in RBCs, the inclusions are found in a relatively high percentage of the cells and appear as pale blue, pink, or red-brown, round to irregular structures (Figure 22-45). The occurrence of the inclusions in peripheral blood cells of infected dogs is highly variable, even within the same individual at different stages of the disease. They are reported to be found most often in the early stages of the infection but can rarely be found during the neurologic phase of the disease.

Intracellular morulae of *Ehrlichia canis, Erlichia ewingii,* or *Anaplasma phagocytophilum* may be seen in canine WBCs, especially those with clinical signs of illness (e.g., fever, thrombocytopenia, leukopenia, anemia, lymphadenopathy, splenomegaly, weight loss, and/or lameness; dogs with chronic *E. canis* infections can also show severe pancytopenia). Morulae of all three species (in the bacterial order Rickettsiales) are similar in appearance as round to oval, eosinophilic to basophilic bodies in the cytoplasm of affected cells. With good microscopic resolution, morulae can be seen to be composed of varying numbers of minute cocci (Figure 26-46). Morulae of *E. ewingii* and *A. phagocytophilum* can be readily seen in peripheral blood neutrophils of affected dogs. In contrast, *E. canis* morulae occur in canine lymphocytes and monocytes and are detected only rarely in peripheral blood, and then only during the very early stages of infection. Diagnosis and patient monitoring of *E. canis* infection in dogs can be supplemented by testing serum with a commercial in-house or diagnostic laboratory indirect fluorescent antibody (IFA) assay. However, these tests do not completely differentiate among rickettsial organisms, and false negatives based on low IFA titers can occur. Molecular (PCR) analysis is the most reliable way to distinguish between infections with the different *Ehrlichia* or *Anaplasma* species. However, due to the low numbers of circulating organisms, cases of monocytic ehrlichiosis, false negatives

with whole blood samples from dogs with *E. canis* infection may still occur with this method.

Hepatozoon americanum gamonts are rarely found in peripheral blood leukocytes of dogs infected with the organism. The majority of infections have been in the Gulf Coast region, but the range appears to be expanding to include Southeastern and South Central areas of the United States.[56,57] Despite the pronounced leukocytosis accompanying the disease (e.g., 20,000 to 200,000 WBCs/μl), the organism is usually found in very few circulating nucleated cells (probable monocytes). Examination of buffy coat preparations may aid detection of the intracellular parasite. *H. americanum* gamonts in Wright's-stained blood films appear as aqua-staining ovoid bodies with a single eosinophilic to basophilic patch; these are large enough to displace cell nuclei and distort cytoplasmic borders (Figure 22-47). Sometimes the ovoid structure remains unstained but is discretely outlined by the displaced host cell cytoplasm and nucleus. In addition to the high WBC count (attributed to a mostly mature neutrophilic leukocytosis), clinical infection is primarily associated with fever, muscular hyperesthesia and atrophy, and long bone and/or vertebral periosteal proliferation. Definitive diagnosis can usually be made with skeletal muscle biopsy. Serology for detection of antibodies to *H. americanum* sporozoites or PCR with whole blood are also commercially available.

Very rarely, yeast, fungal, or other types of bacterial organisms are seen within leukocytes on blood smears from dogs or cats. If these are seen in fresh samples, however, they are diagnostic of the systemic infections. Special stains may aid in further characterizing the organism.

Table 26-4 may serve as a quick reference for interpretation of morphologic alterations in leukocytes in peripheral blood smears and conditions to consider in association with these findings.

LEUKEMIAS

Atypical or bizarre cells or a disordered collection of immature cells on peripheral blood smears suggest leukemia. A persistent, unexplained increase of a specific cell

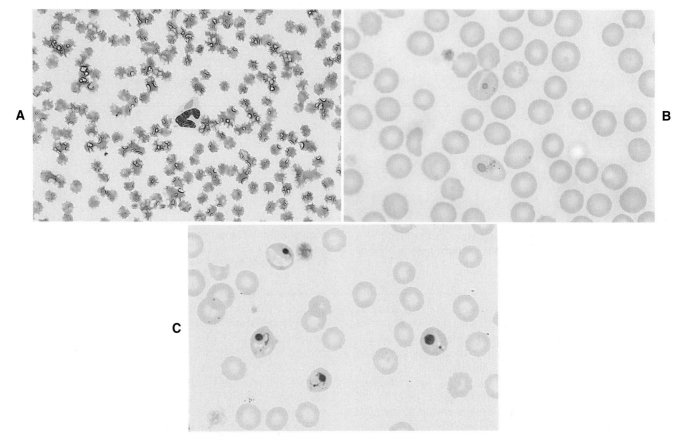

Figure 26-45 A, A canine distemper virus (CDV) inclusion in this neutrophil stains red-orange. (Wright's stain, original magnification 200×.) **B,** CDV inclusions in two RBCs stain pale sky blue with Diff-Quik. (Original magnification 330×.) **C,** CDV inclusions in three RBCs stained with Wright's stain. Wright's stained inclusions are bright pink-purple to reddish-brown inclusions. (Original magnification 330×.)

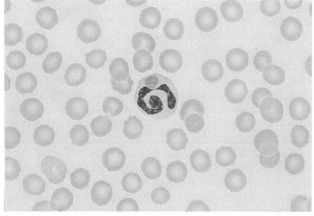

Figure 26-46 A canine neutrophil containing an *Ehrlichia ewingii* morula. (Wright's stain, original magnification 250×.)

type in peripheral blood can also suggest leukemia, as exemplified by chronic lymphocytic leukemia. The majority of dogs and cats with leukemia have a moderate to marked leukocytosis (i.e., >50,000 WBCs/µl in dogs and >35,000 WBCs/µl in cats), consisting predominantly of the neoplastic cell population. Exceptions are common,

however, and some patients even present with leukopenia. Peripheral blood RBC and platelet counts are usually altered (i.e., most often decreased) in leukemic dogs and cats. Concomitantly, macrocytic RBCs and mega-thrombocytes, abnormally shaped or granulated platelets, and/or increases in nucleated RBCs may be evident on blood films, supporting bone marrow involvement. Monocytosis is also common and, in some cases, eosinophilia or basophilia are seen in addition to the neoplastic nucleated cells in peripheral blood. Numbers of neutrophils and lymphocytes in blood from dogs and cats with leukemias are highly variable, although a shift toward immature cell stages and/or toxic changes is uncommon unless secondary systemic inflammation or tissue necrosis is present. Hypersegmented neutrophils may also be seen in some cases.

Because of immaturity and anaplasia, recognition of the cell line from which the leukemic cells originated is often difficult to impossible by evaluating only routinely stained peripheral blood films. Examination of marrow aspirates may be important for confirmation and prognostication of leukemia; but, because leukemic cells within the bone marrow are typically more immature than those in the peripheral blood, the procedure may not aid in specifically identifying the neoplastic cell type unless special cytochemical staining or immunophenotyping is employed. A few of the more common leukemias in dogs and cats may be suggested by a combination of leukemic cell morphology, patient history, and associated hematologic abnormalities, as discussed in the following sections.

Lymphoid Leukemias

Lymphoid leukemias of two major clinical forms are recognized in dogs and cats: acute lymphoblastic leukemia (ALL) and chronic lymphocytic leukemia (CLL). ALL most often affects young adult to middle-aged animals,

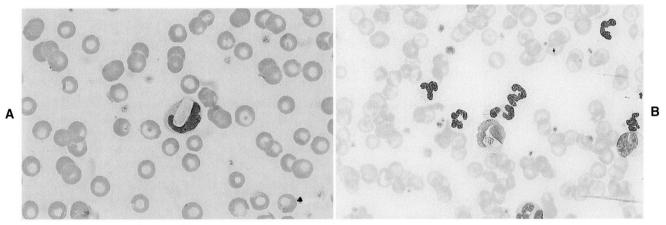

Figure 26-47 A, A nonstaining *Hepatozoon canis* capsule distorts this neutrophil's cytoplasmic and nuclear shape. (Diff-Quik, original magnification 250×.) **B,** Stained with Wright-Giemsa stain, the nuclear material of the organism can be seen in the large WBC in the center of the field. Giemsa stains the organism better than Wright's or Diff-Quik. (Original magnification 132×.)

TABLE 26-4

Changes in Peripheral Blood Smear Leukocyte Morphology as Indicators of the Cause of Disease

Prominent Change	Specific Morphologic Findings	Other Criteria/ Considerations	Causes to Consider
Neutrophil toxic changes	Döhle bodies, cytoplasmic basophilia, cytoplasmic vacuolization, giant neutrophils, ring-shaped nuclei (listed in order of significance [see text])	Döhle bodies occasionally seen without significant inflammation in cats with increased granulopoiesis	Tissue necrosis, sepsis, endotoxemia
Regenerative left shift	Increase in proportion of immature neutrophils, with orderly progression of developmental stages	Normal to increased neutrophil count, or <10% of cells are bands or more immature stages if neutropenia	Tissue necrosis, sepsis, endotoxemia
Degenerative left shift	Pronounced increase in proportion of immature neutrophils, with orderly progression of developmental stages; may also see asynchronous maturation (e.g., nuclear shape more immature relative to chromatin and cytoplasmic features)	Immature neutrophil stages comprise >50% of total neutrophil count with normal to increased neutrophil count, or >10% of count if neutropenia	Severe sepsis, endotoxemia
Leukocyte dysplasia	Increase in proportion of immature or bizarre leukocytes on blood smears, with discontinuous or disordered leukocyte maturation stages	Changes may involve one or multiple cell lines	Myelodysplastic or myeloproliferative disorder; Pelger-Huët anomaly; recovery from chemotherapy or severe leukocytopenia

Continued

TABLE 26-4

Changes in Peripheral Blood Smear Leukocyte Morphology as Indicators of the Cause of Disease—cont'd

Prominent Change	Specific Morphologic Findings	Other Criteria/ Considerations	Causes to Consider
Cytoplasmic inclusions	Morphology consistent with specific infectious organism or viral inclusion (see text)	Usually with inflammatory leukogram, cytopenia, and/or thrombopenia (depending on the organism and disease stage); consider species, cell type (s) affected, age, regional factors	*Ehrlichia* spp., *Hepatozoon* spp., CDV, *Histoplasma* spp., *Mycobacteria* spp.
	Cytoplasmic granules appear abnormally stained and/or shaped, and are often surrounded by a vacuole	If familial or genetic abnormality, multiple cell types may be similarly affected and cell counts may be unaffected or decreased	Chediak-Higashi anomaly, neutrophil granulation anomaly in Birman cats, mucopolysaccharidosis types VI and VII, or GM2-gangliosidosis
	Cytoplasmic granules appear abnormally stained and/or shaped	Transient condition	Postchemotherapy, recovery from severe leukocytopenia
	Phagocytosed cells, cell debris, RBCs, hematoidin, or hemosiderin	Affected cells may be neutrophils, monocytes/macrophages or neoplastic cells	May accompany marked inflammatory responses, hemolytic anemias, significant hemorrhage into tissues, blood transfusion, or neoplastic, especially myeloproliferative conditions
Neutrophil hypersegmentation	Multilobed nuclei with typically hypercondensed chromatin and mature cytoplasm staining	Rule out in vitro aging artifact	Recovery from severe chronic inflammation, corticosteroid excess (hyperadrenocorticism and iatrogenic), myelodysplastic or myeloproliferative disorder, chemotherapy, or megaloblastic anemia (e.g., Poodles)[28]
Smudged cells, or "basket cells"	Numerous ruptured cells, often found at feathered edge and periphery of smear	Repeatable and not attributable to smear technique or in vitro aging artifact	Circulating blast cells–especially leukemic lymphoblasts or myeloblasts
Basophilia and/or eosinophila	Increased counts of eosinophils and/or basophils with normal morphology		Helminthiasis (especially with *Dirofilaria immitis*), eosinophil-associated pulmonary disease, chronic inflammation with immune stimulation (e.g., infections of epithelial surfaces), hypoadrenocorticism, snake bite toxicosis, neoplastic (especially myeloproliferative) conditions

CDV, Canine distemper virus.

and CLL is more common in dogs over 7 years of age and cats of a wide range of ages. Circulating blast cells of ALL usually occur in high numbers and have oval or bizarre clover leaf–shaped nuclei with coarse, reticulated chromatin and moderate amounts of basophilic cytoplasm (Figure 26-48). These cells may also have one or more variably sized, dark, nucleolar rings (Figure 26-49). Neoplastic cells of CLL always occur in high numbers in peripheral blood and appear as typical mature lymphocytes, although they tend to vary more in size and have especially dark-staining cytoplasm and a few cytoplasmic vacuoles. As with other leukemic cell types, these cells may also show cytophagia and erythrophagia (Figure 26-50). About half of all canine CLL cases further exhibit monoclonal gammopathy.[1] In addition, about 10% of canine solid lymphomas, especially the multicentric

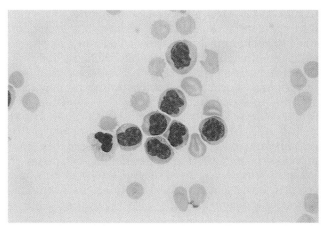

Figure 26-48 Canine leukemic lymphocytes displaying a variety of convoluted nuclear shapes that can resemble the nuclei of monocytes or immature granulocytes. The chromatin of these cells is partially clumped into blocks of heterochromatin. (Wright's stain, original magnification 250×.)

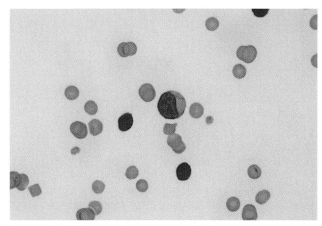

Figure 26-50 A neoplastic lymphoid cell containing a single phagocytosed RBC in this blood smear from a cat. (Wright's stain, original magnification 132×.)

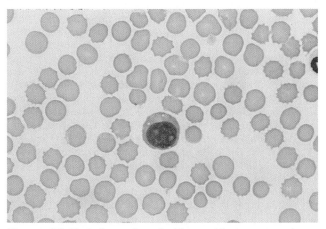

Figure 26-49 A large lymphoblast with two prominent nucleolar rings in the peripheral blood of a cat with lymphoid leukemia. (Wright's stain, original magnification 250×.)

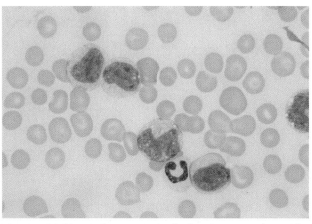

Figure 26-51 Myelomonocytic leukemia in a dog. The neoplastic cells have irregular nuclei with minimally clumped chromatin and abundant, grainy, basophilic cytoplasm. (Wright's stain, original magnification 250×.)

forms and those in the advanced stages, have detectable neoplastic lymphoid cells in circulation, although these cells generally occur in much lower numbers than the leukemic cells of dogs with ALL and CLL. Feline lymphoma is rarely associated with circulating neoplastic cells.

Myeloid Leukemias

In both dogs and cats, myeloid leukemia of every major lineage has been reported, including malignant (systemic) mastocytosis and eosinophilic, basophilic, and megakaryocytic leukemias. Acute myeloid and myelomonocytic leukemias (Figure 26-51) are especially common in dogs.

Acute myelogenous (granulocytic) leukemia in dogs occurs predominantly in young animals, including dogs under 2 years of age. Leukocytosis tends to be extreme and composed of a disordered mixture of immature cells that resemble myeloblasts, giant band neutrophils, and neutrophilic metamyelocytes with a separate, smaller

population of seemingly normal mature to hypersegmented granulocytes. Immature myeloid cells have finely stippled, lacy or ropy chromatin and, occasionally, prominent nucleolar rings. Their cytoplasm is relatively abundant and blue-gray with a ground-glass consistency and is occasionally scattered with fine eosinophilic granules.

Acute myelomonocytic leukemia is considered if some of the more differentiated circulating neoplastic cells have monocytoid appearances while others resemble immature granulocytic cells (based on nuclear shape, chromatin pattern, and cytoplasmic features). Immunophenotyping methods have been developed to differentiate between these two forms of myeloid leukemia,[58] although the progression of the condition in dogs is generally similar.

Chronic myelogenous leukemia is much less common in dogs and cats, and without age predilection. Cases have presented with fluctuating moderate to marked leukocytosis of predominantly mature leukocytes, with a lower proportion of immature and dysplastic cells. However,

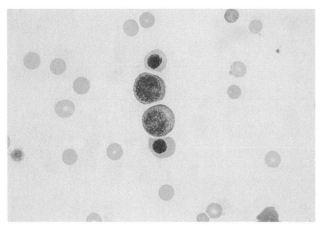

Figure 26-52 Erythremic myelosis in a cat, characterized by erythroblasts of varying maturity in the peripheral blood. Note the macrocytosis of at least one of the metarubricytes on either end of this row of nucleated cells. The other two cells are basophilic rubricytes with centrally located nuclei, coarsely clumped chromatin, and deeply basophilic cytoplasm. (Wright's stain, original magnification 250×.)

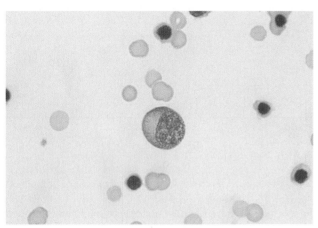

Figure 26-53 A large plasmacytoid-like erythroblast in the blood of a cat with erythremic myelosis. (Wright's stain, original magnification 250×.)

normal total leukocyte counts can also occur. Animals may survive up to 2 years with this condition, which is usually accompanied by persistent anemia and sometimes altered platelet counts. Chronic myeloid leukemias are differentiated from a leukemoid response, in part, by the lack of orderly progression of developmental stages among the leukocytes in peripheral blood and absence of a corresponding pyogenic condition. Chronic myelogenous leukemia can also be associated with a subsequent showering of immature forms in the peripheral blood or a blast crisis.

Erythremic Myelosis

Erythremic myelosis is relatively common in cats and extremely rare in dogs. Affected cats usually have severe, nonregenerative anemia and high numbers of circulating nucleated RBCs in various stages of development

(Figure 22-52). Over a few weeks to months, the leukemic population usually shifts toward higher proportions of more immature stages of RBCs and sometimes to an erythroleukemic population involving both erythroid and granulocytic cell lines. There is often atypical morphology—particularly macrocytosis of the nucleated and nonnucleated erythroid cells. Very immature erythroid cells can usually be differentiated from immature cells of other blood cell lines by their centric nuclei that contain dark, coarsely clumped chromatin and their scant to moderate amount of deeply basophilic cytoplasm. In some cases, however, the neoplastic erythroid cells have eccentric nuclei and prominent Golgi regions, resembling plasma cells (Figure 22-53).

References

1. Feldman BF, et al: *Schalm's Veterinary Hematology*, ed 5. Philadelphia, Lea & Febiger, 2000.
2. Latimer KS, Rakich PM: Clinical interpretation of leukocyte responses. *Vet Clin North Am Small Anim Prac* 19:637-668, 1989.
3. Duncan JR, et al: Veterinary Laboratory Medicine. In *Clinical Pathology*, ed 3. Ames, Iowa, Iowa State University Press, 1994.
4. Wyrick-Glatzel, Gwaltney-Krause. In Harmening DM: *Clinical Hematology and Fundamentals of Hemostasis*, ed 2. Philadelphia, FA Davis, 1992, pp 523-617.
5. Shafer, et al. In Hoffman R: *Hematology Basic Principles and Practice*. New York, Churchill Livingstone, 1991, pp 1790-1801.
6. Sullivan, et al: Platelet concentration and hemoglobin function in greyhounds. *J Am Vet Med Assoc* 205:838-841, 1994.
7. Lording. In Post-graduate Committee in Veterinary Science: Proceedings No. 122, University of Sydney, 1989, pp 369-392.
8. Iazbik MC, Couto CG: Morphologic characterization of specific granules in Greyhound eosinophils. *Vet Clin Pathol* 34:140-143, 2005.
9. Yamauchi A, et al: Secondary erythrocytosis associated with schwannoma in a dog. *J Vet Med Sci* 66:1605-1608, 2004.
10. Sato K, et al: Secondary erythrocytosis associated with high plasma erythropoietin concentrations in a dog with cecal leiomyosarcoma. *J Am Vet Med Assoc* 220:486-490, 2002.
11. Couto CG, et al: Tumor-associated erythrocytosis in a dog with nasal fibrosarcoma. *J Vet Intern Med* 3:183-185, 1989.
12. Cowgill LD, et al: Use of recombinant human erythropoietin for management of anemia in dogs and cats with renal failure. *J Am Vet Med Assoc* 212:521-528, 1998.
13. Rebar AH, et al: Red cell fragmentation in the dog: An editorial review. *Vet Pathol* 18:415-426, 1981.
14. Weiss DJ, et al: Quantitative evaluation of irregulary spiculated red-blood cells in the dog. *Vet Clin Pathol* 22:117-121, 1993.
15. Lee KW, et al: Hematologic changes associated with the appearance of eccentrocytes after intragastric administration of garlic extract to dogs. *Am J Vet Res* 61:1446-1450, 2000.
16. Caldin M, et al: A retrospective study of 60 cases of eccentrocytosis in the dog. *Vet Clin Pathol* 34:224-231, 2005.
17. Andress JL, et al: The effects of consecutive day propofol anesthesia on feline red blood cells. *Vet Surg* 24:277-282, 1995.
18. Walton RM: et al: Mechanisms of echinocytosis induced by *Crotalus atrox* venom. *Vet Pathol* 34:442-449, 1997.
19. Wysoke JM, et al: Bee sting-induced haemolysis, spherocytosis and neural dysfunction in three dogs. *J South Afr Vet Assoc* 61:29-32, 1990.
20. Weiss DJ, et al: Quantitative evaluation of echinocytes in the dog. *Vet Clin Pathol* 19:114-118, 1990.

21. Badylak SF, et al: Poikilocytosis in dogs with chronic doxorubicin toxicosis. *Am J Vet Res* 46:505-508, 1985.

22. O'Keefe DA, Schaeffer DJ: Hematologic toxicosis associated with doxorubicin administration in cats. *J Vet Intern Med* 6:276-282, 1992.

23. Cooper RA, et al: Red cell cholesterol enrichment and spur cell anemia in dogs fed a cholesterol-enriched atherogenic diet. *J Lipid Res* 21:1082-1089, 1980.

24. Christopher MM, Lee SE: Red cell morphologic alterations in cats with hepatic disease. *Vet Clin Pathol* 23:7-12, 1994.

25. Ogilivie GK, et al: Alterations in lipoprotein profiles in dogs with lymphoma. *J Vet Intern Med* 8:62-22, 1994.

26. Simpson KW, et al: Iron status and erythrocyte volume in dogs with congenital portosystemic vascular anomalies. *J Vet Intern Med* 11:14-19, 1997.

27. Gookin JL: Evaluation of microcytosis in 18 Shibas. *J Am Vet Med Assoc* 212:1258-1259, 1998.

28. Canfield PJ, Watson AD: Investigations of bone marrow dyscrasia in a Poodle with macrocytosis. *J Comp Pathol* 101:269-278, 1989.

29. Bonfanti U, et al: Stomatocytosis in 7 related standard Schnauzers. *Vet Clin Pathol* 33:234-239, 2004.

30. Brown DE, et al: Erythrocyte indices and volume distribution in a dog with stomatocytosis. *Vet Pathol* 31:247-250, 1994.

31. Pinkerton PH, et al: Hereditary stomatocytosis with hemolytic anemia in the dog. *Blood* 44:557-567, 1974.

32. Slappendel RJ, et al: Familial stomatocytosis–hypertrophic gastritis (FSHG), a newly recognised disease in the dog (Drentse patrijshond). *Vet Q* 13:30-40, 1991.

33. Berny PJ, et al: Low blood lead concentration associated with various biomarkers in household pets. *Am J Vet Res* 55:55-62, 1994.

34. Meyers, et al: *Veterinary Laboratory Medicine*. Philadelphia, Saunders, 1992, pp 21.

35. Willi B, et al: prevalence, risk factor analysis, and follow-up of infections caused by three feline *Hemoplasma* species in cats in Switzerland. *J Clin Microbiol* 44:961-969, 2006.

36. Lappin MR, et al: Prevalence of *Bartonella* species, *Haemoplasma* species, *Ehrlichia* species, *Anaplasma phagocytophilum*, and *Neorickettsia risticii* DNA in the blood of cats and their fleas in the United States. *J Feline Med Surg* 8:85-90, 2006.

37. Jensen WA, et al: Use of a polymerase chain reaction assay to detect and differentiate two strains of *Haemobartonella felis* in naturally infected cats. *Am J Vet Res* 62:604-608, 2001.

38. Benjamin MM, Lumb WV: *Haemobartonella canis* infection in a dog. *J Am Vet Med Assoc* 135:388-390, 1959.

39. Kemming G, et al: Can we continue research in splenectomized dogs? *Mycoplasma haemocanis*: old problem–new insight. *Eur Surg Res* 36:198-205, 2004.

40. Hoover JP, et al: Cytauxzoonosis in domestic cats: 8 cases (1985-1992). *J Am Vet Med Assoc* 205:455-460, 1994.

41. Grindem CB, et al: Epidemiologic survey of thrombocytopenia in dogs: A report on 987 cases. *Vet Clin Pathol* 20:43, 1992.

42. Jordan HJ: et al: Thrombocytopenia in cats: A retrospective study of 41 cases. *J Vet Intern Med* 7:261-265, 1993.

43. Halmay D, et al: Morphological evaluation of canine platelets on Giemsa- and PAS-stained blood smears. *Acta Veterinaria Hungarica* 53:337-350, 2005.

44. Cowan SM, et al: Giant platelet disorder in the Cavalier King Charles Spaniel. *Exp Hematol* 32:344-350, 2004.

45. Latimer KS, et al: Nuclear segmentation, ultrastructure, and cytochemistry of blood cells from dogs with Pelger-Huët anomaly. *J Comp Pathol* 97:61-72, 1987.

46. Bowles CA, et al: Studies of the Pelger-Huët anomaly in foxhounds. *Am J Pathol* 96:237-247, 1979.

47. Shull RM, Powell D: Acquired hyposegmentation of granulocytes (pseudo-Pelger-Huët anomaly) in a dog. *Cornell Vet* 69:241-247, 1979.

48. Colgan SP, et al: Platelet aggregation and ATP secretion in whole blood of normal cats and cats homozygous and heterozygous for Chediak-Higashi syndrome. *Blood Cells* 15:585-595, 1989.

49. Colgan SP, et al: Defective in vitro motility of polymorphonuclear leukocytes of homozygote and heterozygote Chediak-Higashi cats. *Vet Immunol Immunopathol* 31:205-227, 1992.

50. Prieur DJ, Collier LL: Neutropenia in cats with the Chediak-Higashi syndrome. *Can J Vet Res* 51:407-408, 1987.

51. Hirsch VM, Cunningham TA: Hereditary anomaly of neutrophil granulation in Birman cats. *Am J Vet Res* 45:2170-2174, 1984.

52. Alroy J, et al: Morphology of leukocytes from cats affected with alpha-mannosidosis and mucopolysaccharidosis VI (MPS VI). *Vet Pathol* 26:294-302, 1989.

53. Gitzelmann R, et al: Feline mucopolysaccharidosis VII due to beta-glucuronidase deficiency. *Vet Pathol* 31:435-443, 1994.

54. Stockham SL, et al: Idiopathic mastocythemia in dogs. *Vet Clin Pathol* 15:16-21, 1986.

55. McManus PM: Frequency and severity of mastocytemia in dogs with and without mast cell tumors: 120 cases (1995-1997). *J Am Vet Med Assoc* 215:355-357, 1999.

56. Ewing SA, et al: American canine hepatozoonosis: An emerging disease in the New World. *Ann NY Acad Sci* 916:81-92, 2000.

57. Cummings CA, et al: Characterization of stages of *Hepatozoon americanum* and of parasitized canine host cells. *Vet Pathol* 42:788-796, 2005.

58. Weiss DJ: Evaluation of proliferative disorders in canine bone marrow by use of flow cytometric scatter plots and monoclonal antibodies. *Vet Pathol* 38:512-518, 2001.

The Bone Marrow

C.B. Grindem, R.D. Tyler, and R.L. Cowell

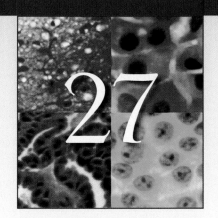

CHAPTER 27

Bone marrow is the major hematopoietic organ of the body. In young animals, active hematopoietic tissue is found throughout both flat and long bones. As growth ceases, hematopoietic activity in the central areas of long bones regresses. In adults, most active hematopoiesis occurs in the flat bones and the extremities of long bones. The central area of long bones contains mostly fat, with very little active hematopoietic tissue.

Active hematopoietic tissue is highly vascular and consists of islands of hematopoietic tissue surrounded by vascular sinuses. The islands of hematopoietic tissue are composed of the following: erythroid, granulocytic, monocytic and thrombocytic series cells; marrow structural cells (adventitial cells); fat cells; and a few macrophages, lymphocytes, plasma cells, and mast cells. The hematopoietic tissue islands are bounded by the endothelium lining the vascular sinuses.

INDICATIONS

The most common indication for bone marrow cytologic examination is recognition of hematologic abnormalities not readily explained by a good history, physical examination, chemistry profile, and/or other clinical procedures. Bone marrow examination is often rewarding in evaluating animals with nonregenerative anemia, persistent neutropenia, or persistent thrombocytopenia.[1-3]

Bone marrow cytologic evaluation can also be used to assess the marrow's involvement in some neoplastic conditions, such as lymphoid neoplasia and mast cell neoplasia; to identify suspected infectious agents, such as *Histoplasma capsulatum*, *Leishmania donovani*, *Ehrlichia* spp., *Cytauxzoon felis*, and *Toxoplasma gondii*; and to evaluate patients with evidence of hyperglobulinemic conditions (e.g., multiple myeloma, lymphoma, ehrlichiosis/anaplasmosis, leishmaniasis, and disseminated histoplasmosis) (Box 27-1).[4-8]

CONTRAINDICATIONS

Contraindications of bone marrow biopsies are few, and complications are uncommon. Restraint, sedation, and anesthesia usually pose a greater risk to the patient than the biopsy procedure. Bone marrow aspiration biopsies can often be collected without sedation; general anesthesia is seldom necessary. Hemorrhage is a theoretical concern in thrombocytopenic animals, but significant bleeding rarely occurs, even in severely thrombocytopenic animals. Bleeding complications can be controlled with fresh whole blood or appropriate component therapy.[4,9,10] Iatrogenic marrow infection is possible, but the risk is miniscule, especially if the area of skin through which the aspirate is collected has been properly prepared. The main contraindication for bone marrow biopsy is performing an unnecessary biopsy. Evaluation of a current blood smear and a thorough clinical workup are mandatory before performing a bone marrow biopsy.

SAMPLE COLLECTION AND PREPARATION

Proper collection and preparation of marrow are necessary for maximal diagnostic usefulness.[4,5,7,11-13] Bone marrow degenerates rapidly after collection or the animal's death; therefore bone marrow samples from dead animals should be collected immediately (within 30 minutes) after the animal's death. Regardless of whether the animal is alive or dead, bone marrow cytologic preparations should be prepared immediately after collection. Interestingly, granulocytes appear to be the first cells to undergo significant morphologic distortion after marrow sample collection or the animal's death. Granulocytic nuclei swell and, losing their contorted lobulated pattern, become large and round to ovoid. The nuclear chromatin pattern loses its dense clumped areas and stains less intensely and more uniformly. As a result, neutrophils that have undergone this alteration may be mistaken for blast cells. This error can lead to misdiagnosis of neoplasia. Extreme caution must be used when examining samples from animals dead for 30 minutes or more before slide preparation. These samples can be examined for cellularity, organisms, mast cell infiltration, erythrophagocytosis, plasmacytosis, and accumulation of iron-containing pigments, but examination for evidence of neoplasia can result in misdiagnosis. The same requirements and limitations apply for bone marrow samples submitted for histopathologic examination.

Bone Marrow Cytologic Evaluation

Historical or Physical Findings

Fever of unknown origin or occult disease

Diagnosing, staging, or monitoring neoplasia (lymphoma, leukemia, mast cell tumor, multiple myeloma, histiocytic sarcoma, metastatic neoplasia)

Drug toxicity (estrogens, phenylbutazone, various antibiotics)

Abnormal CBC Findings

Unexplained cytopenias (leukopenia, anemia, thrombocytopenia)

Unexplained cytosis (leukocytosis, polycythemia, thrombocytosis)

Abnormal cell morphology

WBC: myeloblasts, lymphoblasts, monoblasts, giant neutrophils, doughnut-shaped nuclei, pseudo-Pelger-Huët cells

RBC: dacrocytes, sideroblasts, unexplained macrocytosis or microcytosis

Atypical cellular reactions

Excessive nucleated red cells

Neutrophilia with an inappropriate or disorderly left shift

Abnormal Serum Chemistry Findings

Hypercalcemia

Hyperglobulinemia (monoclonal and polyclonal)

Decreased serum iron

CBC, Complete blood count; *WBC*, white blood cell; *RBC*, red blood cell.

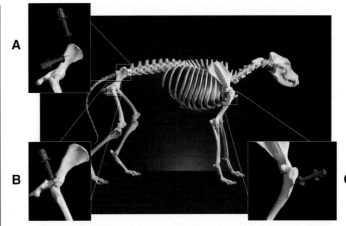

Figure 27-1 Dog skeleton showing common sites for bone marrow collection. In large dogs, the dorsal approach to the iliac crest **(A)** is an excellent site for aspiration and core biopsies. In small dogs and cats the lateral approach to the wing of the ilium **(A)** is a good site for core biopsies, and the trochanter fossa of proximal femur **(B)** is a good site for aspiration biopsies. For all small animals, the proximal humerus **(C)** is an excellent site for both aspiration and core biopsies. *(Reprinted with permission from Grindem CB, Neel JA, Juopperi TA: Cytology of bone marrow. Vet Clin Small Anim 32[6]:1316, 2002.)*

After bone marrow preparations are air-dried, they should be stained as soon as possible. When submitting bone marrow cytologic preparations for consultation, several air-dried unfixed preparations and air-dried stained preparations should be submitted.

Some techniques for collecting, preparing, and staining bone marrow cytologic preparations are discussed subsequently.

Instruments and Supplies

A 15- to 18-gauge, 1- to 2-inch bone marrow aspiration biopsy needle, clear Petri dish or watch glass, 10- to 12-ml syringe, several clean microscope slides and coverslips, the supplies for a surgical prep and, optionally, ethylene-tetra-acetic acid (EDTA) and isotonic fluid solution are required for collecting and preparing bone marrow aspirate biopsies. These instruments and supplies should be located on a clean work counter in close proximity to the work area where the sample is to be collected. If anticoagulant is not used, smears must be prepared from the aspirate immediately (within 30 seconds of collection). Some acceptable bone marrow biopsy needles are the Rosenthal (Popper and Sons, New Hyde Park, NY), Illinois sternal, and Jamshidi needles (Tyco Healthcare-Kendall, Mansfield, MA 02048).

A sterile 2% to 3% EDTA/isotonic saline solution can be prepared using commercially available EDTA blood collection tubes, which contain about 1.5 mg of EDTA (as a freeze-dried powder or liquid solution) per milliliter of blood to be added. Injecting 0.35 ml of sterile isotonic saline into a 7-ml EDTA tube produces about 0.35 ml of 3% EDTA or 0.42 ml of 2.5% EDTA, depending on whether the tube originally contained powdered or liquid EDTA.

Aspiration Biopsy

Site: Bone marrow aspiration biopsies may be collected from the proximal humerus, iliac crest, trochanteric fossa of the femur, and sternebrae of dogs and cats (Figure 27-1).[4,5,7,11-13] The proximal humerus and iliac crest in large dogs and the proximal humerus and trochanteric fossa in small dogs and cats are the most accessible. As a result, they are the most commonly used sites. Because of the danger of penetrating the thoracic cavity, the sternebrae should be avoided in cats and small dogs. For the same reason, the ribs should be used only when incisional biopsies are performed. The trochanteric fossa may not be approachable in large, well-muscled, or very obese patients. Also, the cortical bone of the trochanteric fossa may be so dense in older dogs that it prevents easy penetration of the marrow cavity. Because of the small diameter of the bones of cats and small dogs, the trochanteric fossa often supersedes the iliac crest as a site for bone marrow aspiration in these animals.

Collection: To aspirate bone marrow via the humerus or trochanteric fossa of the femur, the animal is placed in lateral recumbency. If the iliac crest is used, the animal can be standing, sitting, or in sternal recumbency. Regardless of the site used, the hair is clipped from the skin several inches around the area where needle puncture is anticipated. The skin is then prepared as for surgery, and a local anesthetic is injected into the skin and under the periosteum at the puncture site.

A small stab incision is made at the biopsy site with a sterile scalpel blade (number 11). The greater trochanter of the proximal femur is located by palpation, and the biopsy needle is passed medial to the trochanter, with its long axis parallel to the long axis of the femur, until the needle reaches the trochanteric fossa. When bone is contacted, moderate pressure is applied and the needle is rotated in an alternating clockwise-counterclockwise motion. The operator usually feels the resistance decrease when the needle enters the bone marrow in the trochanteric fossa or humerus, but this sensation may not be as obvious for the iliac crest. To aspirate the humerus, palpate the greater tubercle and insert the needle into the flat area on the craniolateral surface of the proximal humerus distal to the greater tubercle, avoiding the articular cartilage. For the iliac crest, palpate the greatest prominence of the crest and, once the needle is firmly in bone, it is probably in the marrow cavity. With core biopsies of the iliac crest it is important to keep the needle parallel to the long axis of the wing of the ilium.

When the marrow cavity has been entered, the stylet is removed and a 10- to 20-ml syringe containing 0.3 to 0.5 ml of sterile 2% to 3% EDTA/isotonic saline solution is attached to the needle. Strong negative pressure is applied by rapidly pulling the plunger back as far as possible (usually two thirds to three fourths of the volume of the syringe). Most animals show evidence of pain when bone marrow aspiration begins, and this is good evidence that the needle is in the marrow cavity. After a few drops of marrow are collected, the negative pressure is released. If EDTA is used, the volume of marrow collected should not exceed the volume of EDTA/isotonic saline solution in the syringe. Continued negative pressure contaminates the marrow sample with blood. Whether a marrow sample appears in the syringe or not, negative pressure should not be applied to the syringe twice in the same area. This causes aspiration of excessive amounts of blood.

If marrow is not collected at the first site, the syringe is removed, the stylet is replaced in the biopsy needle, the needle is repositioned by slight advancement and rotation, and negative pressure is reapplied. If marrow is still not collected, the negative pressure is maintained and the needle is slowly withdrawn until marrow is obtained or the needle exits the bone. If this fails to collect an adequate sample, aspiration can be attempted from another site in the same bone or from another bone. If a sample cannot be collected by aspiration, a core biopsy or incisional biopsy is necessary.

Smear Preparation without EDTA: If EDTA/isotonic saline is not used, as soon as a few drops of marrow sample appear in the syringe, the plunger is released, the syringe is detached from the needle, and the stylet is replaced in the needle. The needle remains embedded in the bone.

Then the sample is immediately expelled directly onto a glass microscope slide. Direct smears similar to blood smears can be made and squash preps should also be prepared by tilting a slide 45 to 70 degrees, allowing the blood to drain from the slide into a watch glass or Petri dish (Figure 27-2). Marrow flecks tend to adhere to the glass microscope slide. A second glass microscope slide is placed perpendicularly across the marrow flecks adhered to the first slide, causing the marrow flecks to spread. The two slides are then smoothly pulled apart in a horizontal plane, dispersing the flecks.

In Romanowsky-stained smears, the marrow flecks appear as blue-purple streaks. If the sample does not contain marrow flecks, the needle can be repositioned by slight advancement and rotation. The stylet is removed, another syringe is attached, and the aspiration procedure is repeated. After two or three aspiration attempts or when marrow flecks are recovered, the needle is removed.

Smear Preparation with EDTA: If EDTA/isotonic saline is used, once the marrow sample is collected, the plunger is released to relieve the negative pressure, and the needle is detached from the syringe. The stylet is replaced in the needle and the needle remains embedded in the bone. The contents of the syringe are thoroughly mixed, and the anticoagulated marrow sample is expelled into a watch glass or clear Petri dish. If the sample does not contain marrow flecks, the needle can be repositioned by slight advancement and rotation. The stylet is removed, another syringe containing EDTA/saline solution is attached, and the aspiration procedure is repeated. After two or three aspiration attempts, or when marrow flecks are recovered, the needle is removed.

Marrow samples collected in EDTA/isotonic saline solution and expelled into a Petri dish are prepared as follows. The Petri dish is tilted and/or rotated under a soft light so that the marrow flecks can be seen and distinguished from fat droplets. Marrow flecks are clear to slightly opaque and light gray; fat droplets are clear and glistening. Marrow flecks may be slightly irregular in shape; fat droplets are spherical. Generally, marrow flecks are easily located if an adequate sample has been collected.

Flecks are transferred from the sample in the Petri dish to glass microscope slides by tilting the Petri dish, causing the sample to drain to one side of the dish. Some flecks cling to the bottom of the Petri dish, and the fluid portion of the sample drains away from them. These flecks are harvested with a microhematocrit capillary tube, one end of which is touched to the side of the fleck. Often the fleck is partially aspirated into the capillary tube and can be transferred to the glass microscope slide. If the fleck does not partially aspirate into the capillary tube, the tube is gently advanced, forcing the fleck into it. The marrow fleck is then transferred onto the glass microscope slide by tapping the capillary tube end containing the fleck on the slide. Any excessive fluid transferred can be removed by touching the fluid with a piece of absorbent paper or cloth.

After the fleck is transferred to the glass microscope slide, a 22- × 22-mm coverslip is placed over the fleck at a 45-degree angle to the glass microscope slide, allowing one corner of the coverslip to hang over the edge of the microscope slide (Figure 27-3). When the coverslip is placed over the fleck, the fleck spreads to about twice its previous size. Some smears should be made without any pressure other than that caused by the coverslip, and others should be made with gentle thumb pressure sufficient to cause the smears to spread to about twice the diameter caused by coverslip pressure alone. This ensures that some of the flecks are optimally spread.

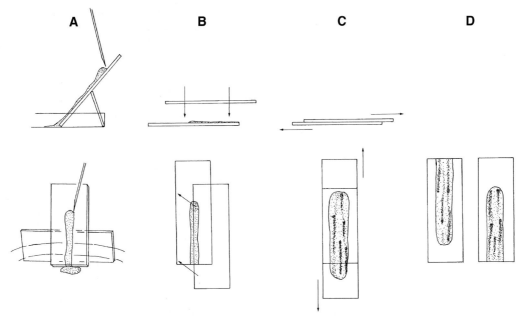

Figure 27-2 Smear preparation for bone marrow aspirates not collected in EDTA/ isotonic saline solution. **A,** Some of the aspirate is expelled onto a tilted glass microscope slide. The slide can be propped up with another glass slide braced against the side of a Petri dish. Marrow flecks tend to adhere to the slide as the marrow runs down it. **B,** Another glass slide is placed over the slide containing the aspirate, which spreads the aspirate. **C,** The two slides are slid apart. **D,** This produces two preparations.

Excessive pressure, which causes cell rupture, is the most common error when preparing cytologic smears of marrow flecks. When making smears from marrow samples in EDTA/isotonic saline solution, using another glass microscope slide instead of a coverslip to spread the fleck may cause excessive pressure and result in rupture of nucleated cells.

Core Biopsy

Core biopsies can be collected with a Jamshidi infant (cats and small dogs) or pediatric (large dogs) marrow biopsy needle. The same procedure is used for collecting core biopsies as described for collecting marrow aspirate biopsies, except after the point of the needle has penetrated the cortex of the bone and entered the marrow cavity, the stylet is removed from the needle and the needle is advanced about 3 mm with a rotating motion.[4,5,7,8,11-13] This cuts and collects a core of bone marrow. The needle is removed from the animal, and the core of marrow is forced onto a glass microscope slide by passing the stylet through the barrel of the needle from the hub end or retrograde from the needle end if the biopsy needle is tapered.

Using the point of the needle, the core of marrow is gently rolled the length of the microscope slide. After making one or two slide preparations in this manner, the core of marrow is placed in a container filled with 10% neutral buffered formalin. If the cytologic preparations are to be sent to an outside laboratory, they should not be mailed with the formalin-filled container because formalin vapors alter the cells' staining qualities.

COLLECTING MARROW SAMPLES FROM DEAD ANIMALS

Bone marrow samples are occasionally collected from dead animals. If a complete evaluation of the marrow is expected, the samples must be collected and the cytologic preparations made immediately (within 30 minutes) after the animal's death. When collection and/or preparation is delayed, the preparations can be evaluated for cellularity, organisms, mast cell infiltration, plasmacytosis, erythrophagocytosis, and iron-containing pigments, but should not be evaluated for myeloid or lymphoid neoplasia. Delay in sample preparation can result in rupture of all of the cells.

Although samples can be collected from most flat bones and the extremities of most long bones of dead animals, it is advisable to collect marrow samples from the same location(s) used in live animals (see Figure 27-1). Remember that in adults, the central areas of long bones contain mostly fat. Access to the marrow can be gained by sawing the bone, cutting it with rongeurs, or fracturing it. If the bone is sawed, heat generated at the saw line can damage adjacent cells; therefore samples from sawed bones should be collected well away from the saw line. Marrow is dug from between bony trabeculae, trying to avoid collecting bone spicules. The marrow is placed on one end of a glass microscope slide and gently rolled (by lifting upward with a needle or other instrument at the back of the sample) the length of the slide. Several slides are prepared from samples collected from several different areas of the bone marrow. The slides are air-dried and stained as described later.

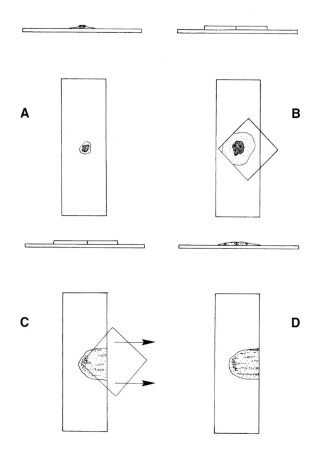

Figure 27-3 Smear preparation for bone marrow aspirates collected in EDTA/isotonic saline solution. **A,** A fleck, collected from the Petri dish containing the sample, is placed on a glass microscope slide. **B,** A microscope slide coverslip is placed over the fleck at a 45-degree angle to the slide. This spreads the fleck and accompanying fluid. **C,** The coverslip is slid horizontally and smoothly off the glass slide. **D,** Both the glass microscope slide preparation and coverslip preparation can be used. However, the coverslip preparation is usually hard to handle during staining and is often discarded. Multiple preparations can be made on a glass slide, and multiple slides can be prepared.

STAINING MARROW PREPARATIONS

After fleck smears or core biopsy or necropsy imprints are made, they are air-dried. The general Romanowsky-type staining procedures for staining blood smears are followed, except the stains and buffers are left in contact with the cells for a longer time. The extent to which the times must be lengthened depends on the thickness and cell density of the smears, but staining times must usually be increased two times or more. Macroscopically, the marrow fleck streaks in the smear appear blue-purple to purple when the smear is properly stained.

CELLS IN MARROW

To evaluate cytologic preparations of bone marrow, one must be able to recognize the normal cells that occur in bone marrow, the neoplastic cells that have a propensity for infiltrating bone marrow, the organisms that can infect the marrow, and the processes (e.g., erythrophagia) that occur in some pathologic conditions.[4-9,13,14]

Erythroid Series

During proliferation and maturation, erythroid progenitor cells undergo 4 to 5 mitoses, producing 16 to 32 daughter cells. As they mature, erythroid cells decrease in size, their nuclei condense, and their cytoplasm changes from dark blue to red-orange. The general characteristics of the different cell stages of erythroid production are described later. Table 27-1 lists the different stages of erythroid development and provides an estimate of the relative proportions and a brief description and a generalized schematic of the classic morphology of each stage.

Rubriblasts: The rubriblast is the most immature identifiable erythroid cell. Its nucleus is round with a smooth nuclear border, a fine granular chromatin pattern, and one or two pale to medium blue nucleoli (Figures 27-4 and 27-5). Its cytoplasm is intensely basophilic and forms a narrow rim around the nucleus. The rubriblast has the highest nuclear-to-cytoplasmic ratio of the erythroid series.

Prorubricytes: The next maturation stage of the erythroid series is the prorubricyte. Its nucleus is round with a smooth nuclear border and a nuclear chromatin pattern that is slightly coarser than that of the rubriblast. Nucleoli are usually not visible in the prorubricyte stage. Cytoplasm is slightly less intensely blue and forms a thicker rim around the nucleus. The nuclear-to-cytoplasmic ratio is less than that of the rubriblast but greater than that of the rubricyte (the next stage of maturation).

Rubricytes: The next stage of erythroid maturation is the rubricyte. This stage is divided into basophilic and polychromatophilic rubricytes or sometimes divided into basophilic, polychromatophilic, and orthochromic rubricytes. The rubricyte and its nucleus are smaller than the prorubricyte and its nucleus. The rubricyte nucleus has an extremely coarse chromatin pattern that may resemble the spokes of a wheel. Cytoplasm is blue (basophilic) to bluish-red-orange (polychromic or polychromatophilic) to red-orange (orthochromic) (Figures 27-6 and 27-7; see Figure 27-4). The nuclear-to-cytoplasmic ratio is less than that of prorubricytes but greater than that of metarubricytes (the next stage of maturation). Mitosis occurs in the early rubricyte stage but ceases by the later rubricyte stages.

Metarubricytes: The next stage of erythroid development is the metarubricyte. Its nucleus is extremely pyknotic and appears black, without a distinguishable chromatin pattern (see Figure 27-4). Cytoplasm may be polychromatophilic or orthochromic.

Polychromatophilic Erythrocytes: The next stage of development is the polychromatophilic erythrocyte. In blood smears stained with Romanowsky-type stains, polychromatophilic erythrocytes are nonnucleated, larger than

TABLE 27-1

Nucleated Erythroid Cell Developmental Stages and Their Relative Percentage, Description, and Schematic Morphology

Developmental Stage	APPROXIMATE PERCENTAGE OF CLASSIFIABLE NUCLEATED ERYTHROID CELLS OF MARROW*		Description	Schematic Morphology
	Dogs	Cats		
Rubriblast	0.5	0.5	*Cell:* large; small to moderate amount of dark blue cytoplasm *Nucleus:* large; 1-2 nucleoli; dense granular chromatin	
Prorubricyte	2.0	3.5	*Cell:* medium to large; moderate amount of medium to dark blue cytoplasm *Nucleus:* medium to large; nucleoli usually not visible; coarse chromatin pattern	
Rubricyte	65	75	*Cell:* medium to small; small to moderate amount of medium blue (basophilic) to blue-pink (polychromatophilic) to orange (orthochromic) cytoplasm *Nucleus:* medium to small; no visible nucleoli; coarse, clumped chromatin pattern with clear spaces	
Metarubruicyte	32.5	21	*Cell:* small, small amount of blue-pink (polychromatophilic) to orange (orthochromic) cytoplasm *Nucleus:* small and pyknotic; no nucleoli visible; chromatin is densely clumped with few or no clear spaces	

*Broad variations may occur in normal animals because of the influence of things such as the subjectivity of cell classification and normal variation among individuals.

TABLE 27-2

Developmental Stages of Neutrophils and Their Relative Percentage, Description, and Schematic Morphology

Developmental Stage	APPROXIMATE PERCENTAGE OF CLASSIFIABLE NEUTROPHILIC GRANULOCYTES OF MARROW*		Description	Schematic Morphology
	Dogs	Cats		
Myeloblast	1	1	*Cytoplasm:* light to medium blue without granules *Nucleus:* round with prominent nucleoli *Chromatin pattern:* fine, lacy	
Progranulocyte (promyelocyte)	3	3	*Cytoplasm:* light blue with scattered, small, red/purple,(azurophilic) nonspecific (primary) granules *Nucleus:* round to oval; nucleoli indistinct or not visible *Chromatin pattern:* becoming coarse	
Myelocyte	12	10	*Cytoplasm:* nonspecific (primary) granules no longer visible, so clear to slightly granular *Nucleus:* round to oval with slight indentation *Chromatin pattern:* coarse	
Metamyelocyte	20	20	*Cytoplasm:* clear to slightly granular *Nucleus:* kidney bean shaped *Chromatin pattern:* coarse with clumps	
Band neutrophil	26	30	*Cytoplasm:* clear to slightly granular *Nucleus:* curved rod or band shaped, with smooth borders *Chromatin pattern:* coarse with dense clumps	
Segmented neutrophil	38	36	*Cytoplasm:* clear to slightly granular *Nucleus:* has marked indentations *Chromatin pattern:* coarse with dense clumps	

*Broad variations may occur in normal animals because of the influence of things such as the subjectivity of cell classification and normal variation among individuals.

mature erythrocytes (orthochromic erythrocytes), and bluish-pink (polychromatophilic). Polychromatophilic erythrocytes stain as reticulocytes with supravital stains (e.g., new methylene blue [NMB]).

Reticulocytes are nonnucleated erythrocytes that develop one or more granules or a network of granules when stained with supravital stains. More mature reticulocytes may be orthochromic (red-orange), and as a result, all polychromatophilic cells are reticulocytes, but some reticulocytes are not polychromatophilic; instead, they are orthochromic.

The cytoplasm of some cells matures before the nucleus is extruded. These cells skip the polychromatophilic erythrocyte stage.

Mature Erythrocytes: The last stage of erythroid development is the mature erythrocyte, which stains red-orange (orthochromic) with Romanowsky-type stains. Mature erythrocytes do not stain nor form granules (reticulocyte formation) with NMB.

Granulocyte Series

Myeloid progenitor cells usually undergo four mitoses; however, depending on circumstances, a mitosis may be skipped or additional mitoses may occur. The developmental stages, immature to mature, of the granulocyte series are myeloblast, progranulocyte (promyelocyte), myelocyte, metamyelocyte, band cell, and segmented granulocyte (mature neutrophil, eosinophil, and basophil). The myeloblast, myelocyte, and metamyelocyte stages of neutrophilic granulocytes cannot be reliably differentiated from monocytes. Table 27-2 lists the different stages of development of the granulocyte series and gives the relative proportions and a brief description of the classic morphology of each stage.

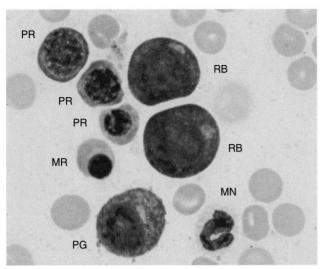

Figure 27-4 Bone marrow aspirate. Rubriblasts *(RB)*, polychromatophilic rubricytes *(PR)*, metarubricyte *(MR)*, progranulocyte *(PG)*, and mature neutrophil *(MN)* are indicated. (Wright-Giemsa stain, original magnification 250×.)

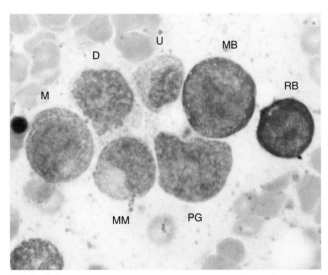

Figure 27-5 Bone marrow aspirate. Rubriblast *(RB)*, myeloblast *(MB)*, progranulocyte *(PG)*, early myelocyte *(M)*, metamyelocyte *(MM)*, damaged cell nucleus *(D)*, and an unidentified late stage granulocyte *(U)*, most likely distorted band neutrophil, are indicated. (Wright-Giemsa stain, original magnification 250×.)

Myeloblasts: The myeloblast is large and may be round or irregular in shape. It has a large nucleus with a fine to finely stippled chromatin pattern and one or more visible nucleoli (see Figure 27-5). The cytoplasm is blue to blue-gray and does not contain visible granules. The myeloblast has the highest nuclear-to-cytoplasmic ratio of any of the granulocytic developmental stages.

Progranulocytes (Promyelocytes): The next stage of granulocyte development is the progranulocyte or pro-myelocyte. Often, the progranulocyte is slightly larger than the myeloblast due to increased cytoplasm. The

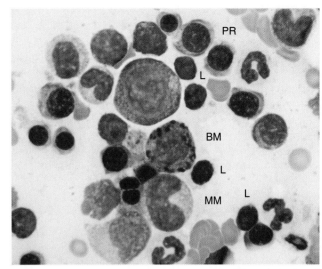

Figure 27-6 Bone marrow from a healthy cat. Small lymphocytes *(L)* are usually <10% of nucleated cells in the bone marrow of healthy cats. Basophilic myelocyte *(BM)*, neutrophilic metamyelocyte *(MM)*, polychromatophilic rubricytes *(PR)*, and lymphocytes are indicated. Basophil precursors have prominent magenta to blue-black granules. Also notice that metamyelocytes can be difficult to impossible to distinguish from monocytes in the bone marrow. (Wright-Giemsa stain, original magnification 250×.)

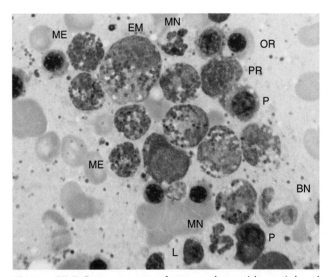

Figure 27-7 Bone marrow from a dog with peripheral eosinophilia (>50,000/μl). The bone marrow was hyper-cellular with an increased myeroid-to-erythroid ratio, but eosinophils were the predominant granulocyte. Maturation appears orderly, but definitive cell stages can be difficult to determine because the eosinophilic granules cover the nucleus. Mature eosinophils *(ME)* outnumber earlier precursors such as eosinophilic myelocytes *(EM)*. Mature neutrophils *(MN)*, band neutrophils *(BN)*, polychromatophilic rubricytes *(PR)*, orthochromic rubricyte *(OR)*, plasma cells *(P)*, and a lymphocyte *(L)* are also present. Hypereosinophilic disorders include hypersensitivity reactions (often GI), parasites, fungi, paraneoplasia, and very rarely eosinophilic leukemia. This dog was treated for heartworm disease, and the eosinophilia resolved. (Wright-Giemsa stain, original magnification 250×.)

BOX 27-2

Some Diseases that Can Cause Nonregenerative Anemia, Neutropenia, and/or Thrombocytopenia in Dogs and Cats, Classified by the Overall Marrow Cellularity with which They Can Be Associated

Hypocellular Marrow	Normocellular Marrow	Hypercellular Marrow
FeLV suppression (cat)–A	FeLV suppression (cat)–A, d	Histoplasmosis–A
Ehrlichiosis (dog)–A	Ehrlichiosis (dog)–A, d	Ehrlichiosis (dog)–TP, e
Renal insufficiency–NA	Histoplasmosis–A, d	Myeloproliferative disease–A
Marrow necrosis–A, a	Myeloproliferative disease–A, d	Lymphosarcoma–A
Radiation, cytotoxic drugs, etc–A, a	Lymphosarcoma–A, d	Anemia of inflammatory disease (i.e., anemia of chronic disease)–NA
Myelofibrosis (sclerosis)–A, b		
Pure red cell aplasia–NA, c		
Immune-mediated		
idiopatic		

FeLV, Feline leukemia virus; *A,* one to all of the marrow cell lines may be affected; *NA,* nonregenerative anemia; *NP,* neutropenia; *TP,* thrombocytopenia; *a,* anemia may not be present in the acute phase; *b,* flecks, if any are collected, may appear small but hypercellular because fibrous tissue has replaced most of the marrow elements, but a few pockets of hypercellular marrow may remain; *c,* rarely, thrombocytopenia and/or neutropenia may also be present; *d,* usually associated with hypocellular marrow; *e,* ehrlichiosis can be associated with hypocellular marrow, but then it is usually in the acute to subacute phase of infection and is associated with thrombocytopenia alone—clinical signs are often unapparent.

major differentiating feature of the progranulocyte is the presence of scattered, small, azurophilic (red-purple) primary granules throughout the cytoplasm (Figure 27-8; see Figure 27-5). Primary granules are also called *nonspecific granules*. Nuclei are the same size to slightly smaller than nuclei of myeloblasts, have lacy to coarse chromatin patterns, and may contain visible nucleoli (which are usually fewer and less prominent than those of myeloblasts) or nucleolar rings. Nucleolar rings are rings of densely staining chromatin that demark obscured nucleoli. The nuclear-to-cytoplasmic ratio of promyelocytes is less than that of myeloblasts. The presence of primary granules allows progranulocytes to be recognized as members of the granulocyte series and differentiates them from the monocyte series. Therefore progranulocytes can be identified more specifically than myeloblasts, neutrophil myelocytes, and neutrophil metamyelocytes, which lack visible primary granules. As a result, the term *progranulocyte,* instead of *promyelocyte,* can be used to identify members of this developmental stage.

Myelocytes: The next developmental stage of the granulocyte series is the myelocyte. The disappearance of the primary granules (seen in the progranulocyte stage) aids differentiation of the myelocyte from the progranulocyte. Also, myelocytes are smaller than progranulocytes, and their nuclear chromatin is more dense, giving a coarser pattern (Figure 27-9; see Figures 27-5 to 27-8). Nuclei are round to oval, and nucleoli are not visible. Cytoplasm is light blue to clear and contains secondary (specific) granules, which are poorly visualized in the neutrophil series but give eosinophils and basophils their characteristic appearance.

The granules of feline eosinophils are rod shaped, and the granules of canine eosinophils are pleomorphic (but typically round) and variable in size (see Figures 27-7 and 27-8). Feline basophils contain granules that are oval, tend to stain lavender, and fill the cytoplasm. The oval granules may appear round when viewed end-on. Immature feline basophils contain many red-purple granules (see Figures 27-6 and 27-9). Canine basophils contain a few to many round, variably sized, red-purple (metachromatic) granules. The myelocyte is the last stage capable of mitosis.

Metamyelocytes: The next stage of granulocyte development is the metamyelocyte. Its nucleus is classically described as kidney bean shaped. Generally, cells with nuclei having indentations extending less than 25% of the way into the nucleus are classified as myelocytes, whereas those with nuclei having indentations extending 25% to 75% of the way into the nucleus are classified as metamyelocytes (see Figure 27-6). The cytoplasmic characteristics of metamyelocytes are similar to those of myelocytes, with the neutrophil myelocyte cytoplasm being clear. This stage and subsequent stages do not undergo mitosis.

Band Cells: The next stage of granulocyte development is the band cell. It has a nucleus with a curved band or rod shape and smooth, parallel sides (see Figures 27-7 and 27-8). Some chromatin clumps are present. No area of the nucleus has a diameter less than one-half the diameter of any other area of the nucleus. Membrane irregularity and excessive narrowing of the nucleus warrant classifying of the cell as a mature neutrophil. The cytoplasmic characteristics of band cells are similar to those of metamyelocytes.

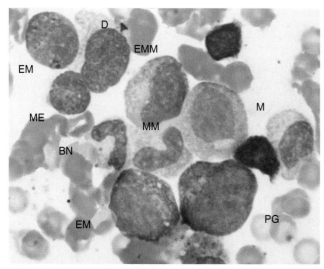

Figure 27-8 Bone marrow aspirate. Progranulocyte *(PG)*, neutrophilic myelocyte *(M)*, eosinophilic myelocyte *(EM)*, early metamyelocyte *(EMM)*, metamyelocyte *(MM)*, band neutrophil *(BN)*, mature eosinophil *(ME)*, and damaged cell nucleus *(D)* are indicated. (Wright-Giemsa stain, original magnification 250×.)

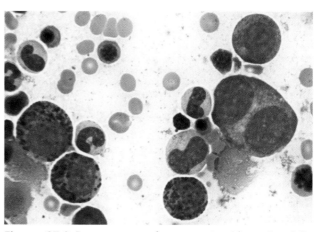

Figure 27-9 Bone marrow from a cat with eosinophilia and basophilia. Note three basophilic myelocytes, a progranulocyte, and a binucleated promegakaryocyte. (Wright-Giemsa stain, original magnification 250×.)

Segmented Granulocytes: The final stage of granulocyte development is the segmented granulocyte (mature neutrophil, eosinophil, or basophil). Its nucleus is lobate or has areas of marked constriction (see Figure 27-7). The nuclear border is often irregular with large, dense chromatin clumps. Its cytoplasmic characteristics are similar to those of myelocytes, metamyelocytes, and band cells.

Monocyte Series

Cells of the monocyte series account for only a small percentage of the total marrow cells. As mentioned earlier, monoblasts cannot be differentiated from myeloblasts by light microscopy. Also, promonocytes are morphologically similar to neutrophilic myelocytes and metamyelocytes in bone marrow cytologic preparations stained with Romanowsky-type stains. Mature monocytes in bone marrow smears have the same appearance as monocytes in peripheral blood.

Thrombocyte (Megakaryocyte) Series

Megakaryoblasts: The most immature developmental stage of the megakaryocyte series recognizable by light microscopy is the megakaryoblast. It is not commonly identified in marrow aspirates, however, because it usually occurs in small numbers and is difficult to differentiate from other blast cells.

Promegakaryocytes: The promegakaryocyte is the next recognizable stage. It has deep blue cytoplasm and contains two to four nuclei that may appear separate but are linked by thin strands of nuclear material (see Figure 27-9). Promegakaryocytes are much larger than WBC and RBC precursors.

Megakaryocytes: The megakaryocyte is the next developmental stage. Megakaryocytes are gigantic (50 to 200 microns in diameter) and contain more than four nuclei that are joined and form a lobulated mass (Figures 27-10 and 27-11). The larger the cell, the greater the nuclear ploidy (number). Megakaryocytes with deeply basophilic cytoplasm are less mature than those with light blue cytoplasm containing eosinophilic granules. Immature megakaryocytes are sometimes called *basophilic megakaryocytes*, and mature megakaryocytes are sometimes called *eosinophilic* or *granular megakaryocytes*. Bare nuclei of megakaryocytes may be seen in bone marrow cytologic preparations. They may represent nuclei of megakaryocytes that have shed their cytoplasm as platelets into the peripheral blood or megakaryocytes whose cytoplasm has been torn from their nuclei during smear preparation.

Lymphocytes and Plasma Cells

Small lymphocytes (Figure 27-12; see Figure 27-6) are recognizably smaller than neutrophils and have a scanty amount of light to medium blue cytoplasm and an indented but otherwise round nucleus with a dense smudged chromatin pattern without visible nucleoli. Intermediate-sized lymphocytes (often referred to as prolymphocytes) are about the same size as neutrophils and have a little more medium to light blue cytoplasm than small lymphocytes. Their nuclei are round, other than an indentation in one area of the nucleus where the cytoplasm is most visible. The nuclear chromatin pattern appears smudged and nucleoli are rarely visible. Large lymphocytes, frequently called lymphoblasts when their nucleoli are prominent (Figure 27-13), are larger than neutrophils and have a small to moderate amount of light to dark blue cytoplasm. Their nuclei may be indented or irregular and have a fine reticular or lacy chromatin pattern. Multiple prominent nucleoli often are present.

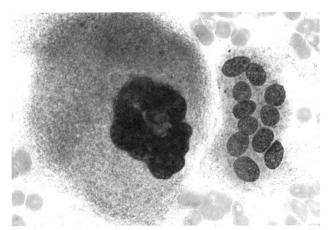

Figure 27-10 Bone marrow aspirate. Mature megakaryocyte with a condensed multilobulated nucleus and eosinophilic, granular cytoplasm on the left and a multinucleated osteoclast on the right. Osteoclasts are uncommonly seen in bone marrow aspirates and are associated with bone remodeling such as in young animals or animals with renal disease, metabolic bone disease, or neoplasia. (Wright-Giemsa stain, original magnification 240×). *(Reprinted with permission from Grindem CB: Bone marrow biopsy and evaluation.* Vet Clin Small Anim *19[4]:680, 1989.)*

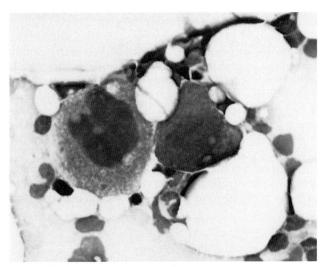

Figure 27-11 Bone marrow aspirate. A mature megakaryocyte with eosinophilic cytoplasm is on the left, and an immature basophilic megakaryocyte is on the right. (Wright-Giemsa stain, original magnification 250×.)

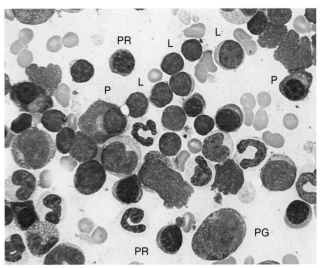

Figure 27-12 Bone marrow from a healthy cat. A focal area of numerous small lymphocytes is present. Small lymphocytes *(L)* can easily be confused with nucleated red cells, but small lymphocytes have scant to almost no visible cytoplasm and often a less coarsely clumped nuclear chromatin pattern. Small lymphocytes usually comprise < 5% of nucleated bone marrow cells in healthy dogs and <10% in cats. Progranulocyte *(PG)*, polychromatophilic rubricytes *(PR)*, plasma cell *(P)*, and lymphocytes are indicated. (Wright-Giemsa stain, original magnification 250×.)

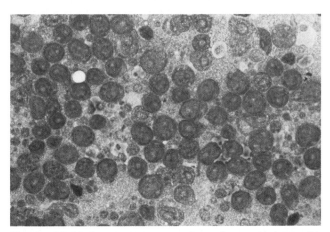

Figure 27-13 Bone marrow aspirate from a dog with lymphoma. Numerous lymphoblasts are on a basophilic background that contains lymphoglandular bodies. Although lymphoglandular bodies (cytoplasmic fragments) can be seen with any rapidly dividing cell population, they are most often associated with lymphoma. (Wright-Giemsa stain, original magnification 250×.)

Plasma cells are about the same size as or slightly larger than neutrophils (see Figures 27-7 and 27-12). They have a round, eccentric nucleus and a moderate to abundant amount of deep blue cytoplasm. The Golgi apparatus can be recognized as a clear area in the cytoplasm adjacent to the nucleus where the cytoplasm is most abundant. Sometimes the cytoplasm contains round structures called Russell bodies, which are areas of rough endoplasmic reticulum that are markedly dilated by immunoglobulin. Plasma cells packed with Russell bodies are called *Mott cells.*

The bone marrow of normal dogs and cats usually contains <5% and <10%, respectively, lymphocytes and <2% (both dogs and cats) plasma cells.[5-7,13-15] However, higher lymphocyte ranges have been reported (<15% in dogs and <20% in cats).[5,7,15] Lymphocytes and plasma cells are not uniformly distributed throughout the bone marrow; therefore their proportions vary from area to area and fleck to fleck.

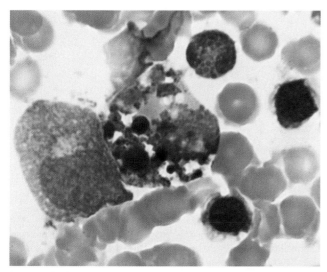

Figure 27-14 Bone marrow aspirate. The large macrophage in the center of the field contains pyknotic debris, red cell fragments, and golden-brown hemosiderin pigment. (Wright-Giemsa stain, original magnification 250×.)

Macrophages

Usually <2% of the cells in normal canine and feline marrow are macrophages. Marrow macrophages are large, but often not as large as early myeloid precursor cells (Figure 27-14). Their nuclei are usually eccentric, and their cytoplasm is abundant and light blue-staining with indistinct boundaries. The cytoplasm is often vacuolated and may contain phagocytized material, such as pyknotic nuclear debris, WBCs, RBCs, and/or their breakdown products, or organisms (e.g., *Histoplasma capsulatum* or *Leishmania donovani*).

Osteoclasts and Osteoblasts

Osteoclasts and osteoblasts are occasionally encountered in bone marrow aspirates. Osteoclasts are giant multinucleated cells that phagocytize bone and can be confused with megakaryocytes (see Figure 27-10). Osteoclast nuclei are discernibly separate, whereas megakaryocyte nuclei are fused. The cytoplasm of osteoclasts stains blue and often contains azurophilic granular material. Osteoclasts are more common in aspirates from young animals than from old animals.

Osteoblasts are relatively large cells that somewhat resemble plasma cells. They have eccentric nuclei and basophilic, sometimes foamy, cytoplasm. The Golgi apparatus may be visible as a clear area adjacent to the nucleus. Osteoblasts are larger and have less condensed nuclear chromatin than plasma cells. Their nuclei are round to oval with a reticular chromatin pattern and one or two nucleoli. As with osteoclasts, they are more common in bone marrow aspirates from young, growing animals than from older animals.

Miscellaneous Cells

Fat cells (adipocytes, lipocytes), endothelial cells (Figure 27-15), a few fibrocytes/fibroblasts, a few mast cells (Figure 27-16), unidentifiable blast cells, and free nuclei may be

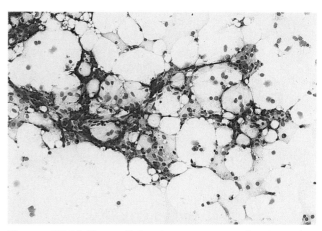

Figure 27-15 Hypocellular bone marrow from a dog with chronic ehrlichiosis. Marrow flecks are extrememly hypocellular and nearly devoid of developing hematopoietic cells. The flecks contain mostly fat cells, capillaries, and stromal cells. (Wright's stain, original magnification 50×.)

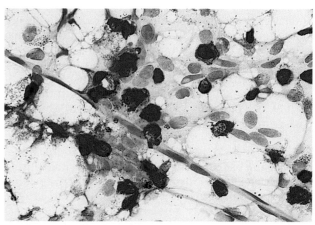

Figure 27-16 Hypocelluar bone marrow from a pancytopenic dog with chronic ehrlichiosis. Numerous well-differentiated mast cells are present along with capillaries and stromal cells. Prolonged treatment with doxycycline resulted in recovery of the marrow and resolution of the pancytopenia, although increased numbers of mast cells were still present in the marrow. (Wright's stain, original magnification 160×.)

found in aspirates from normal animals. The free nuclei may be hematogones (small, round, condensed nuclei shed from metarubricytes) or basket cells (large, free nuclei with dispersed lace-like chromatin from ruptured cells).

ORGANISMS IN MARROW

Although bacterial infections may involve bone marrow, the organisms usually sought on bone marrow cytologic preparations are *H. capsulatum* (Figure 27-17), *L. donovani* (Figure 27-18), *Mycobacterium* spp. (Figure 27-19), *Cytauxzoon felis* (Figure 27-20), *Babesia* spp. (Figure 27-21), *Mycoplasma* spp. (Figure 27-22), *Toxoplasma gondii*, and *Ehrlichia/Anaplasma* spp.[16] *H. capsulatum* (see Figure 27-17) is one of the most common organisms identified in bone marrow cytologic preparations from dogs

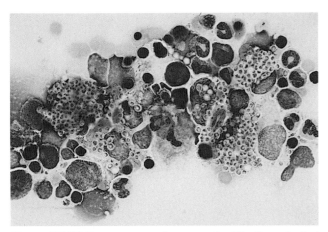

Figure 27-17 Bone marrow from a cat with disseminated histoplasmosis. Several large macrophages are present, each containing numerous *Histoplasma* organisms. Note the half-moon appearance of the organisms. (Wright's stain, original magnification 250×.)

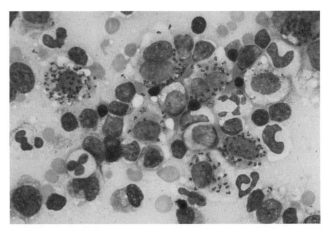

Figure 27-18 Bone marrow from a dog with disseminated leishmaniasis. Round to oval amastigotes of *Leishmania* with the "parachute men" appearance of small dark-staining rodshaped kinetoplasts and paler round nuclei are seen within macrophages and in the background. A few nucleated red cells, neutrophils, lymphocytes, and a plasma cell are also present. Amastigotes are approximately 2.5 to 5.0 μm long and 1.5 to 2.0 μm wide. (Wright-Giemsa stain, original magnification 250×.)

and cats. Systemic histoplasmosis often causes nonregenerative anemia, thrombocytopenia, and/or neutropenia. In a very high proportion of systemic histoplasmosis cases, the organism can be identified in bone marrow cytologic preparations. Macrophages containing amastigotes of leishmania are frequently observed in the bone marrow of dogs with visceral leishmaniasis. The small dark-staining kinetoplast and nucleus distinguish leishmania "parachute men" from histoplasma "half-moons" (see Figures 27-17 and 27-18). Although *Ehrlichia* spp. morulae can be found in the bone marrow of dogs during the early stages of ehrlichial infection, they are seldom identified during chronic ehrlichiosis. Because chronic ehrlichiosis is the most common stage in which clinical disease is recognized, bone marrow evaluation seldom results in ehrlichial organisms being found. Care must be taken not to mistake platelets overlying monocytes, macrophages, and/or neutrophils for *Ehrlichia* morulae. In cytauxzoonosis, schizogony occurs within cells of the mononuclear-phagocytic system that primarily line veins in vascular organs such as spleen, lung, liver, kidney, lymph node, and bone marrow (see Figure 27-20). Bone marrow should be scanned at low power to identify these large structures. Remember to look for piroplasms within the mature red cells in the background blood using high magnification (100×). Babesial and mycoplasmal infections do not have developmental stages in organs. Therefore, to diagnose these diseases from bone marrow cytology, the organisms must be found in the background mature red cells (see Figures 27-21 and 27-22).

BONE MARROW EVALUATION

Evaluation of bone marrow cytologic preparations must be made in light of available historic information, the animal's clinical signs, physical examination and laboratory findings, and the hematologic findings from a peripheral blood sample collected within hours of the

bone marrow cytologic sample.[4-9] Care should be taken not to overinterpret results. When an interpretation cannot be made with certainty, the bone marrow cytologic preparations along with a concurrent complete blood count (CBC) and blood smear should be referred for interpretation.

MARROW SAMPLE EVALUATION

Bone marrow evaluation begins with aspiration. Easy collection of numerous flecks suggests normocellular or hypercellular marrow. On the other hand, if the marrow collection technique is adequate, difficult aspiration or failure to aspirate flecks from several sites suggests hypocellular, fibrotic, or very densely packed marrow.

Aspirate samples containing only a few or no flecks and very little fat suggest fibrotic marrow. Those containing a few or no flecks and many fat globules suggest fatty hypoplastic marrow. Those containing many flecks suggest normocellular or hypercellular marrow. These subjective impressions should be confirmed by microscopic examination.

Core biopsies that yield red-gray marrow suggest normocellular or hypercellular marrow, and white or yellow-white marrow suggests hypocellular or fibrotic marrow. Core biopsies of fibrotic marrow may be recognizably firm.

Bone marrow flecks normally vary in cellularity and cell composition; therefore several flecks should be evaluated. Macroscopically, hypercellular marrow tends to have large flecks that yield large, densely staining smears, and hypocellular marrow has small flecks that yield small smears with a reticular network of stain material outlining small to large unstained areas. Macroscopically, well-stained bone marrow preparations should be dark blue-purple. Reddish areas usually indicate clots.

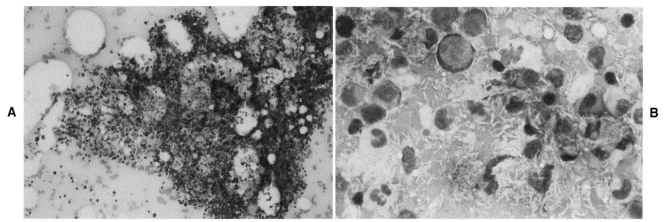

Figure 27-19 Bone marrow from an anemic feline immunodeficiency virus–positive cat with mycobacteriosis. **A,** Lower-power image of bone marrow granuloma. The "unit particle" has a pale-staining vacuolated appearance of foamy macrophages and distorted, almost necrotic, appearing cells and lacks the normal mixed population of discrete round hemic cells. (Wright-Giemsa stain, original magnification 40×.) **B,** Examination at higher power reveals numerous intracellular and extracellular linear nonstaining rods (0.2 to 0.5 µm wide, 1.0 to 3.0 µm long). Organisms are most often observed in macrophages but only occasionally in granulocytes. Reexamination of the peripheral blood smear revealed rare mycobacterial organisms in neutrophils. Acid-fast staining for mycobacteriosis was positive. Culture and classification or polymerase chain reaction are necessary for determination of *Mycobacterium* species. (Wright-Giemsa stain, original magnification 250×.)

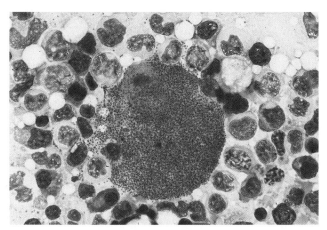

Figure 27-20 Necropsy bone marrow from a cat with cytauxzoonosis. A large macrophage containing a schizont of *Cytauxzoon felis* is surrounded by slightly degenerative-appearing myeloid cells and a few nucleated red cells, lymphocytes, and plasma cells. *Cytauxzoon* piroplasms were seen in the peripheral blood of this cat prior to death. Scanning bone marrow smears at low power are helpful in identifying the large schizonts. (Wright-Giemsa stain, original magnification 250×.) *(Case courtesy Dr. Jaime Tarigo.)*

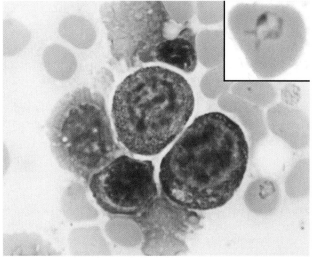

Figure 27-21 Bone marrow from a pancytopenic dog with babesiosis. Erythroid hyperplasia with pleomorphic large intracellular *Babesia* organisms in the red cells in the background. Organisms occurred singly or in doublets, but most organisms were irregular in shape; however, a few classic tear drop-shaped *Babesia* were seen. The large size is consistent with *B. canis* (2.4 to 5 µm) in contrast to the smaller *B. gibsoni* (1 to 3.2 µm). (Wright-Giemsa stain, original magnification 250×.)

Microscopic evaluation of bone marrow cytologic preparations should be methodical and thorough. A systematic approach is outlined later and in Box 27-3. Thick and thin areas of flecks on several well-stained smears should be examined.

Adequacy of Preparation: At low magnification (4× to 10× objective) the smear is quickly scanned to ensure that there are well-stained areas where flecks have been sufficiently spread (without excessive rupturing of cells) to form a cell monolayer with good cell morphology. If the flecks are insufficiently spread or excessive numbers of cells are ruptured, new preparations can be made if the sample was collected in EDTA. If the fleck smears are adequate but not sufficiently stained, they can be restained. If they are overstained, they can be destained in methanol and restained.

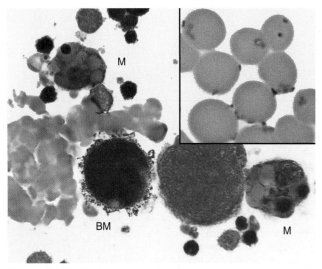

Figure 27-22 Bone marrow from a severely anemic cat with immune-mediated hemolytic anemia. Red cell agglutination and erythrophagocytosis are prominent features of this bone marrow. Macrophages *(M)* have engulfed numerous erythrocytes. A basophilic megakaryocyte *(BM)* and a nucleus from a damaged megakaryocyte are present. Background red cells in bone marrow taken from any severely anemic cat should be scrutinized for *Mycoplasma* spp. *(inset).* (Wright-Giemsa stain, original magnification 250×.)

Low-Power Observations (4× to 10×): Adequate smears should be examined at low power for estimation of cellularity; number, morphology, and maturation of megakaryocytes; quantitation of iron stores; and identification of atypical cell clusters or background. Well-stained monolayer areas are selected for examination at higher powers (Table 27-3 and Box 27-4; also see Box 27-3).

Evaluation of Marrow Cellularity

Bone marrow cellularity is estimated on low magnification (4× to 10× objective) by comparing the proportion of fat and cells in the fleck smear (Figures 27-23 through 27-25). Normal marrow cellularity varies, depending on the age of the animal (see Figure 27-23). Marrow flecks of very young animals contain very little fat, and flecks from juvenile animals contain about 25% fat and 75% cells. Flecks from young adult animals contain about 50% fat and 50% cells, and flecks from older animals contain about 75% fat and 25% cells. Cellularity also varies from fleck to fleck; therefore multiple flecks should be evaluated to form an estimate of overall marrow cellularity. Hypocellular marrow (see Figures 27-15, 27-16, and 27-25) usually yields only a few flecks or, on some occasions, may not yield any flecks (dry tap). The flecks collected have a low cell-to-fat ratio (age must be considered). Hypocellular marrow can result from suppressive conditions (e.g., feline leukemia virus marrow suppression), hypoplastic conditions (e.g., renal insufficiency), infectious diseases (e.g., chronic ehrlichiosis, parvovirus infection), toxic conditions (e.g., estrogen toxicity), and idiopathic hypoplastic diseases. The cell lines affected, as

well as clinical, historical, and/or clinicopathologic information, often suggest the cause of hypocellular marrow.

Normocellular marrow usually yields many marrow flecks with a normal (considering the animal's age) cell-to-fat ratio. Normocellular marrow may be normal or contain dysplastic and/or dyscrasic changes or organisms indicating pathologic changes. Dysplastic changes are alterations in cell morphology caused by a pathologic process. Dyscrasic changes are abnormal proportions of developmental stages of a cell series or abnormal proportions of different cell series. For example, excessive numbers of rubriblasts constitute a dyscrasia or dyscrasic change, whereas the presence of rubriblasts with abnormal cellular morphology (e.g., abundant cytoplasm, very coarse chromatin, and eccentric nuclear location) is a dysplasia or dysplastic change (see Figure 27-26 and Table 27-4). Also, normal cellular marrow preparations may contain organisms, macrophages demonstrating erythrophagocytosis, excessive numbers of mast cells, or metastatic tumor cells (e.g., metastatic carcinoma cells, Figures 27-27 and 27-28).

Hypercellular marrow usually yields an abundance of marrow flecks, but, occasionally, tightly packed neoplastically hypercellular marrow may yield only a few or no flecks. Hypercellular marrow has an increased cell-to-fat ratio (the animal's age must be considered) and can be caused by erythroid hyperplasia (Figure 27-29), myeloid or granulocytic hyperplasia, myeloproliferative diseases including leukemias (Figures 27-30 and 27-31), or infiltration of neoplastic cells (e.g., lymphoma or metastatic neoplasia) (see Figures 27-13, 27-27, and 27-28), plasma cell tumors (multiple myelomas) (Figure 27-32), and mast cell tumors (Figures 27-33 and 27-34). Dysplastic cellular changes can also be seen in hyperplastic marrow specimens (see Figure 27-30). The hemogram (including RBC morphology and platelet count), clinical signs, historical information, and duration of the animal's illness help differentiate the causes of different types of hypercellular marrow.

Ultimately, a core biopsy is the best specimen for estimation of bone marrow cellularity. Core biopsies are especially valuable in determining whether hypocellular aspiration biopsies are due to poor technique, are hypercellular marrows that will not aspirate ("dry taps"), or are truly hypocellular marrows.

Evaluation of the Megakaryocytic Series

The abundance and maturation of megakaryocytes are estimated at low magnification (4× to 10× objectives). Megakaryocytes are not uniformly distributed in the bone marrow or on smears. They are usually associated with unit particles or at the edges of the smear. Therefore, it is imperative to examine multiple smears and preferably a core biopsy before diagnosing megakaryocytic hypoplasia. Reported guidelines for estimating megkaryocytes numbers vary widely.[5,7,8,13,17] However, in general, each fleck normally contains several megakaryocytes, and less than three megakaryocytes per large fleck or less than three to five per slide suggests megakaryocytic hypoplasia. More than 10 to 20 megakaryocytes per cellular 10× field or smear suggests hyperplasia (Figures 27-35 and 27-36).[5,7,13,17] Usually, ≥70% of the

BOX 27-3

Systematic Approach to the Microscopic Evaluation of Bone Marrow

Low-Power Observations (4× to 10×)

Assess adequacy of specimen
   Presence of unit particles to determine cellularity
   Adequate, increased, decreased cellularity
   Thick and thin areas to evaluate cell morphology
   Assess staining quality of specimen
   Acceptable, unacceptable
Determine number, morphology, and maturity of megakaryocytes
   Adequate, increased, decreased megakaryocytes
   Unremarkable, dysplastic, or neoplastic appearance of megakaryocytes
   Orderly, arrested, left or right shifted, disorderly maturation
Quantitate iron stores (Prussian blue stain used to confirm iron)*
   Adequate, increased, decreased
Identify atypical cell clusters, cells, or background
Identify good areas to examine at higher power

High-Power Observations (40× or 50× to 100×)

Evaluate erythroid and myeloid morphology and maturation
   Unremarkable, dysplastic, or neoplastic morphology
   Orderly, arrested, left or right-shifted, dysplastic or neoplastic maturation
Determine myeloid-to-erythroid ratio
   Unremarkable (approximately 1:1)
   Increased (>3:1, myeloid hyperplasia and/or erythroid hypoplasia)
   Decreased (<1:3, myeloid hypoplasia, and/or erythroid hyperplasia)
Estimate the percentage of blast cells present
   Unremarkable (< 2% to 5%)
   Increased—(5% to 20%) hyperplasia or early neoplasia, (>30%) neoplasia (leukemia)
   Lymphoblasts and lymphoglandular bodies—lymphoma
Identify erythrophagocytosis (for iron stores see Box 27-6)
   Increased—ineffective erythropoiesis, extravascular hemolytic anemia (immune-mediated, hemic parasites), post-transfusion, histiocytic neoplasia, hemophagic histiocytosis
Calculate percentage of plasma cells
   Unremarkable (< 2%)
   Increased (> 3%)—immune-mediated disease, chronic (rickettsial) infections, multiple myeloma (usually > 15%)
Calculate percentage of small lymphocytes
   Unremarkable (< 5% dogs, <10% cats)
   Increased—lymphoid follicle, lymphoid hyperplasia, lymphoma
Identify other cell types
   Mast cells (unremarkable <2%), increased—systemic mastocytosis, reactive process, myelofibrosis, marrow hypoplasia or aplasia
   Osteoblasts, osteoclasts—young animal, active bone remodeling (do not confuse with megakaryocytes)
   Fibroblasts—myelofibrosis, marrow hypoplasia or aplasia, bone fibrosarcoma
   Smudge cells—fragile cells (young, old, dying, neoplastic), tramatic specimen handling
   Histiocytes—Reactive (IMHA, granulomatous disease, storage diseases, hemophagic histiocytosis), neoplastic (systemic histiocytosis, histiocytic sarcoma including MH, malignant fibrous histiocytoma)†
Evaluate stromal cell reactions†
   Myelofibrosis, necrosis, osteosclerosis, inflammatory reactions, vascular lesions (amyloidosis, atherosclerosis), or serous atrophy of fat
Identify pathologic agents
   Histoplasma *spp.*, Leishmania *spp.*, Mycobacterium *spp.*, Cytauxzoon *spp.*, Babesia *spp.*, Mycoplasma *spp.*, Ehrlichia/Anaplasma *spp.*, Dirofilaria *spp.*, Blastomyces *spp.*, Cryptococcus *spp.*, Coccidioides *spp.*
Identify neoplasia
   Leukemia (acute and chronic myeloid, acute and chronic lymphoid), lymphoma, multiple myeloma, systemic mastocytosis, sarcoma, metastatic neoplasia

---

*Iron stores are usually not observed in cat bone marrow specimens.
†Core biopsy is necessary to definitively identify stromal cell reactions.
IMHA, Immune-mediated hemolytic anemia; *MH,* malignant histiocytosis.

TABLE 27-3

Interpretation of Myeloid and Erythroid Maturation Patterns

Maturation Pattern	Characteristics	Disorders/Conditions/Diseases
Orderly	All stages of maturation are present in normal proportions. Blast cells are uncommon (< 5%), the majority of the erythroid cells are in the proliferative pool (rubricytes – approximately 65%-75%) and the majority of the myeloid cells are in the maturation pool (metamyelocytes, bands, and segmented neutrophils – approximately 80%-85%).	Healthy animals Hyperplasia
Left-shifted	All stages of maturation are present and orderly except early stages are overrepresented.	Early hyperplasia Chronic myeloid leukemia
Right-shifted	All stages of maturation are present and orderly except late stages are overrepresented.	Late hyperplasia Early hypoplasia
Arrested	Virtually all cells are in the blast and/or proliferative pool with lack of maturation past this stage.	Early bone marrow recovery Myeloproliferative disorders Immune-mediated destruction of later stages
Dyscrasic/dysplastic	Inappropriate increase in blast cells and/or morphologically atypical cells.	Myeloproliferative disorders Myelodysplastic syndrome Toxicity Drugs/chemotherapy Early neoplasia (leukemia)
Neoplastic	Marked increase in blast (>30%) and early precursors with minimal maturation, presence of foreign cells (lymphoma or metastatic neoplasia).	Leukemia Lymphoma Metastatic neoplasia

BOX 27-4

Normal Myeloid and Erythroid Maturation

Myeloid Series	Maturation Pyramid	Erythroid Series
Myeloblasts (< 5% of AMC) Progranulocytes, myelocytes (~15% of AMC) Metamyelocytes, bands, segmented neutrophils (~80%-85% AMC)	Blasts / Proliferative pool / Maturation & storage pool	Rubriblasts (< 5% AEC) Prorubricytes, rubricytes (~65%-75% AEC) Metarubricytes (~20%-30% AEC)

AMC, All myeloid cells; *AEC*, all erythroid cells (nucleated).

megakaryocytes are mature (see the discussion of mega-karyocytic stages earlier in this chapter).[13] When <50% of the megakaryocytes are mature, a regenerative response in the megakaryocytic series is indicated (see Figures 27-35 and 27-36). If many promegakaryocytes (four or fewer nuclei) are present, a maturation defect or early regenerative response is suspected. Box 27-5 lists mega-karyocytic disorders.

Thrombocytopenia can be caused by platelet destruction (e.g., immune-mediated thrombocytopenia) (see Figures 27-35 and 27-36), increased utilization (disseminated intra-vascular coagulation), sequestration (often in the spleen), or suppression of platelet production (e.g., estrogen tox-icity). In thrombocytopenic animals, megakaryocytic hyperplasia indicates platelet destruction or utilization, whereas megakaryocytic hypoplasia indicates suppression

of platelet production. Platelet sequestration is usually transient and associated with normal megakaryopoiesis.

Bone marrow aspiration is seldom indicated in evalu-ation of patients with thrombocytosis, but it may be helpful in evaluation of patients with suspected essential thrombocythemia, polycythemia vera, or megakaryocytic leukemia (Figure 27-37). These can cause thrombocytosis but are very rare.

Evaluation of the Erythrocytic Series

The abundance, proportions, and morphology of the eryth-rocytic series should be assessed using the 10×, 20×, 40× or 50×, and 100× (oil-immersion) objectives. Determining the abundance of erythroid cells (erythroid hypoplasia/hyperplasia) requires consideration of the overall marrow

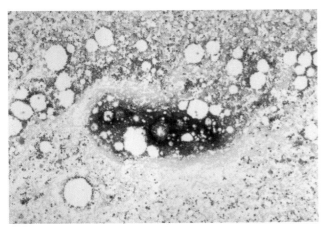

Figure 27-23 Bone marrow aspirate. Normocellular marrow for an adult but mildly hypocelluar for a young dog or cat younger than 1 year. (Wright-Giemsa stain, original magnification 20×.)

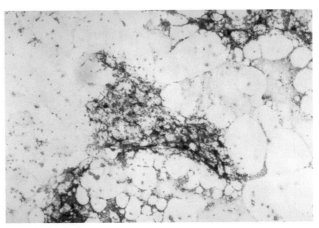

Figure 27-25 Bone marrow aspirate. Hypocellular marrow from a dog with half-body irradiation therapy. (Wright-Giemsa stain, original magnification 20×.)

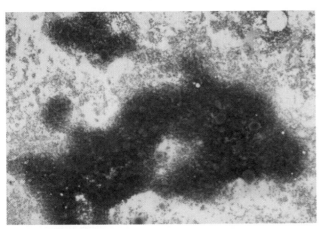

Figure 27-24 Bone marrow from a dog with immune-mediated hemolytic anemia and immune-mediated thrombocytopenia. Marrow is hypercellular with virtually no fat in the unit particle. Note the increased numbers of paler-staining megakaryocytes imbedded in the unit particle. (Wright-Giemsa stain, original magnification 40×.)

cellularity and the marrow cell proportion of the erythroid series (see Figures 27-29 and 27-36). Tables 27-1 and 27-3 and Box 27-4 give the relative proportions and maturation patterns of the erythroid series. The morphology of the erythroid cells can be evaluated for abnormalities, such as megaloblastic change, karyolysis, pyknosis of immature cells, and cytoplasmic and/or nuclear vacuolation (see Table 27-4). Megaloblastic changes include excessively coarse chromatin patterns, increased cytoplasm, macrocytic orthochromic erythrocytes, and increased hemoglobin content (causing polychromasia or orthochromia) in immature rubricytic cells (see Figures 27-26 and 27-30). Megaloblastic change is most commonly seen in cats with feline leukemia virus–induced erythroid dysplasia (Table 27-5). Karyolysis, pyknosis, and cytoplasmic and nuclear vacuolation can be caused by conditions such as marrow necrosis due to toxins (e.g., drugs), infectious agents (bacterial or viral), and irradiation.

Nonregenerative anemia is a common indication for cytologic examination of bone marrow. Some causes of nonregenerative anemia in dogs and cats are listed in Table 27-5. Associated bone marrow findings and procedures that can help differentiate the causes are also listed. Frequently with nonregenerative anemias the bone marrow is hypocellular to normocellular with increased myeloid-to-erythroid. In the dog, iron stores should be critically evaluated (Box 27-6; see Figure 27-36). Iron stores are usually not visible in cat marrow. Adequate to increased iron stores differentiate anemia of chronic inflammatory disease from nutritional iron deficiency or chronic blood loss. Increased iron stores with erythrophagocytosis suggest extravascular hemolytic anemia, ineffective erythropoiesis, or previous blood transfusions. Bone marrow cytologic examination is seldom of diagnostic value in evaluating secondary polycythemia but may be helpful in evaluating patients with suspected polycythemia vera, which is an extremely rare neoplasia.

Evaluation of the Granulocytic Series

The abundance, proportions, and morphology of the granulocytic series are assessed using the 10×, 20×, 40× or 50×, and 100× (oil-immersion) objectives. Normal proportions for the different granulocytic maturation stages are given in Tables 27-2 and 27-3 and Box 27-4. To determine whether there is an overall increase in the granulocytic series, marrow cellularity and the proportion of the marrow cells that are granulocytes must be considered. The presence of excessive numbers of one or more developmental stages, in comparison with the other developmental stages of the series, is referred to as dyscrasia. Dyscrasias can be caused by neoplasia (see Figure 27-30), regenerative response, and/or maturation arrest (with or without neoplasia). See Table 27-3 for the different maturation patterns. Acute myeloid leukemia is indicated by finding a high number of blast cells (>30% of the cell population) (see Figures 27-30 and 27-31). Some causes of abnormal morphology (dysplasia) are chemicals, nutritional imbalances (e.g., folic acid/B$_{12}$ deficiency), hereditary disorders (e.g., macrocytosis of Poodles), neoplasia,

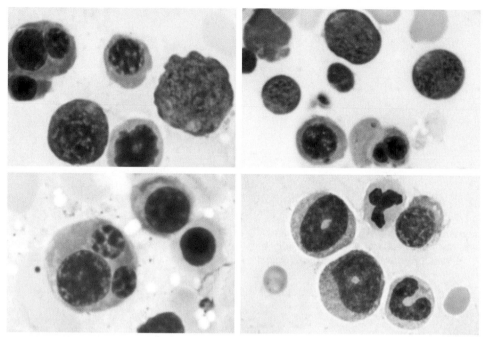

Figure 27-26 Bone marrow from a pancytopenic dog with suspected drug toxicity. Dysplastic changes include giant-sized red cell precursors, binucleated and multinucleated red cells, nuclear fragments, nuclear-cytoplasmic asynchrony, irregular cytoplasmic outlines, and doughnut-shaped myeloid cells.

TABLE 27-4

Characteristics of Bone Marrow Dysplasia

Cell Type	Morphologic Features	Causes
Erythroid	Scant, ragged cytoplasm	Iron deficiency
	Ringed sideroblasts	MPD
	Megalocytosis/macrocytosis	FeLV, B_{12}/folic acid deficiency, Poodle macrocytosis, drugs
Myeloid	Binucleation and multinucleation, nuclear fragmentation	MPD, drugs, virus (parvovirus)
	Hypersegmentation	MPD
	Hyposegmentation (pseudo-Pelger-Huët)	MPD, toxicity, or drugs
	Doughnut-shaped nucleus	MPD, toxicity, or drugs
	Abnormal cytoplasmic granulation	MPD, toxicity, glycogen storage disorders
Megakaryocyte	Dwarf forms	MPD
	Multinucleation	MPD, B_{12} or folic acid deficiency
General features – All cell lines	Cytoplasmic vacuolation	Toxicity, drugs, MPD
	Asynchronous N:C maturation	MPD, BM recovery, toxicity
	Giant forms	Skipped maturation divisions and/or MPD

MPD, Myeloproliferative disorders including myeloid leukemias and myelodysplastic disorders; *FeLV*, feline leukemia virus; *N:C*, nuclear-to-cytoplasmic ratio.

feline leukemia virus infection, marrow necrosis, and marrow infection (e.g., parvovirus infection).

Occasionally, bone marrow is examined to evaluate animals with persistent neutropenia. Some causes of persistent neutropenia are canine ehrlichiosis, feline leukemia virus suppression, myeloproliferative disease, lymphoma, myelofibrosis (sclerosis), estrogen toxicity, marrow necrosis, histoplasmosis, and cyclic hematopoiesis (cyclic neutropenia). These conditions, except cyclic hematopoiesis, can also cause severe nonregenerative anemia and/or thrombocytopenia. Cyclic hematopoiesis is associated with periodic marrow hypoplasia that is synchronous with the cycle of neutropenia. The bone marrow changes usually associated with these diseases, except cyclic hematopoiesis, and some procedures that may help diagnose them are given in Table 27-5. Bone marrow cytologic examination may aid in the diagnosis of extreme neutrophilia and/or abnormal neutrophil morphology; however, leukemoid inflammatory responses (nonneoplastic extreme neutrophilia with or without

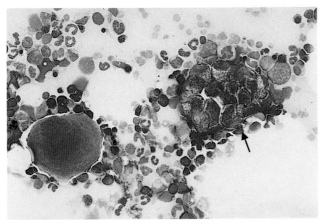

Figure 27-27 Bone marrow from a dog with a metastatic bronchiolar-alveolar carcinoma. A cluster of cohesive, vacuolated epithelial cells is present among the hematopoietic precursors *(arrow)*. A mature megakaryocyte is present to the left. (Wright's stain, original magnification 250×.)

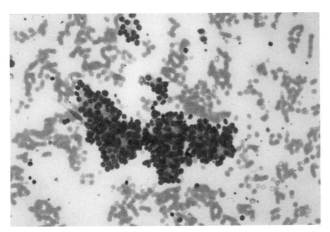

Figure 27-28 Bone marrow from a dog with metastatic carcinoma. Aggregates of a homogeneous population of epithelial cells are forming acinar-like structures, which can be seen at low power. The bone marrow has been virtually replaced by these neoplastic cells. The dog had diffuse metastatic gastrointestinal carcinoma. (Wright-Giemsa stain, original magnification 80×). *(Courtesy Dr. Jennifer Neel.)*

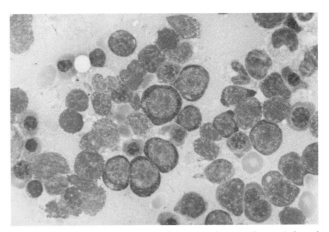

Figure 27-29 Bone marrow from a dog with peripheral nonregenerative anemia but an early bone marrow regenerative response. Marked erythroid hyperplasia (decreased M:E ratio) with an excessive number of rubriblasts compared with late-stage precursors (polychromatophilic and orthochromic rubricytes) indicating a severe left shift in maturation. A binucleated polychromatophilic rubricyte in the lower right corner is a dysplastic change. Often, in a very hyperplastic marrow, a few dysplastic cells can be identified. If increased dysplastic cells are observed and polychromasia is not observed in the peripheral blood within several days, ineffective erythropoiesis with some form of dyscrasia should be suspected. (Wright-Giemsa stain, original magnification 250×.)

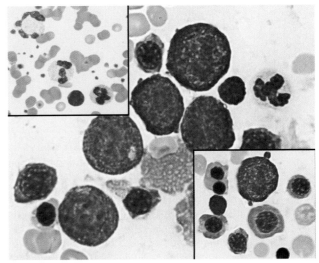

Figure 27-30 Bone marrow from an FeLV-positive cat with erythroleukemia with erythroid predominance. Erythroleukemia can be difficult to differentiate from myelodysplastic syndrome. The distinguishing features in this cat are that more than 50% of nucleated, cells in the bone marrow are erythroid and blast cells, including rubriblasts comprising >30% of nonerythroid cells. Dysplastic cells are prominent in the blood and bone marrow of this cat. Giant hypersegmented neutrophils are present in the peripheral blood *(upper left inset)*. Erythroid changes in the bone marrow include megaloblastic changes (large cell size, increased cytoplasm, excessively coarse chromatin in immature cell, nuclear-cytoplasmic aynchrony), binucleated red cells, and cytoplasmic blebbing *(lower right inset)*. (Wright-Giemsa stain, original magnification 250×.)

an extreme left shift) can cause severe marrow dyscrasia. If a diagnosis of chronic granulocytic leukemia cannot be made from the peripheral blood and history, it often cannot be made from bone marrow cytologic evaluation until the terminal blast crisis develops. Cytochemistry stains and cytogenetics may be helpful to differentiate chronic granulocytic neoplasia from a leukemoid response. Distinguishing chronic myeloid neoplasia from nonneoplastic proliferations, including reactive or paraneoplastic causes, is extremely challenging. Chronic myeloid leukemias (CML) are relatively uncommon compared with reactive or paraneoplastic causes.

Evaluation of the Myeloid-to-Erythroid Ratio

The myeloid-to-erythroid (M:E) ratio is the ratio of myeloid cells to nucleated erythroid cells. Quantitative M:E ratios are determined by appropriately classifying

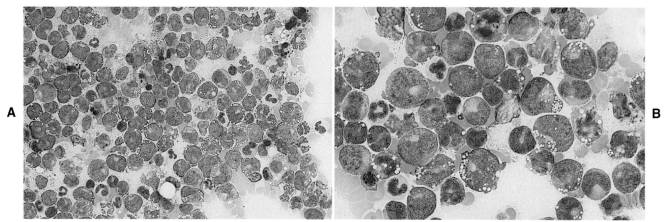

Figure 27-31 Bone marrow from a dog with monocytic leukemia. The dog had a peripheral WBC count of 60,000 cells/μl. **A,** The marrow flecks are hypercellular, and there is a marked increase in the number of blast cells present. Mature neutrophils are markedly reduced in number. (Wright's stain, original magnification 132×.) **B,** Higher magnification of bone marrow sample in **A.** The cells have many features typical of monocytes, including irregular, lobulated nuclei; diffusely basophilic cytoplasm; and clear cytosplasmic granules. Cytochemical stains of bone marrow smears confirmed the monocytic nature of the cells. (Wright's stain, original magnification 330×.)

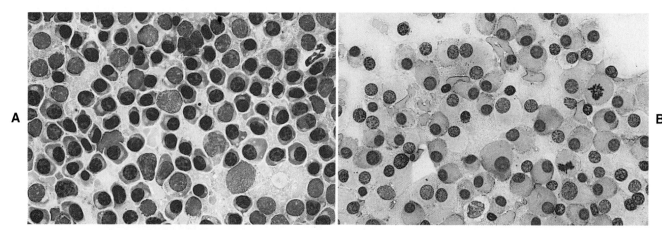

Figure 27-32 Cytologic features of a plasma cell myeloma (multiple myeloma). **A,** Bone marrow from a dog with a plasma cell myeloma containing sheets of well-differentiated plasma cells. The marrow flecks were all extremely hypercellular. Plasma cells were diffusely present in increased numbers throughout the flecks. The high cellularity of the flecks and the monotonous pattern of plasma cells, which in some areas are crowding out all other hematopoietic cells, differentiated this from immune stimulation. (Wright's stain, original magnification 160×.) **B,** Bone marrow from a cat with plasma cell myeloma. This marrow shows features similar to those in **A,** except that the cells display greater cellular variability and atypia and lack the perinuclear clear zone seen in the cells in **A.** Mitotic figures are numerous. (Wright's stain, original magnification 160×.)

500 nucleated cells as myeloid or erythroid using the 100× (oil-immersion) objective. Cells should be classified from several fields of several different flecks. Harvey[9] suggests 50% of the cells be classified from areas of the marrow flecks and 50% be classified from inter-fleck areas. Alternatively, a subjective M:E ratio can be estimated from the proportions of myeloid and erythroid cells seen while the marrow cytologic preparations are evaluated.

Accurate quantitative M:E ratios require classification of all myeloid and nucleated erythroid cells encountered in the fields viewed. This requires considerable experience and can be very frustrating. Although M:E ratios for normal dogs and cats are usually between 0.75:1 and 2.0:1, the range of M:E ratios for normal dogs and cats is very broad and can extend from 0.6:1 to 4.4:1.[4-8] Because some cells are difficult to classify, the broad range of M:E ratios encountered in normal dogs and cats, and the ease with which most diagnostically significant changes in the M:E ratio can be perceived subjectively, the use of quantitative M:E ratios are usually more masochistic than diagnostic.

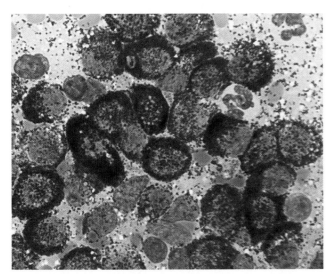

Figure 27-33 Bone marrow metastasis of a mast cell tumor in a dog. A solitary cutaneous mast cell tumor was removed 6 months previously. The dog had acute onset of vomiting and abdominal pain. There was no evidence of local recurrence of the original tumor or of any other masses. All marrow flecks had numerous mast cells; some flecks, like this one, contain almost exclusively mast cells. The markedly cellular mast cell infiltration differentiates this from mast cell hyperplasia, as depicted in Figure 27-16. (Wright-Giemsa stain, original magnification 250×.)

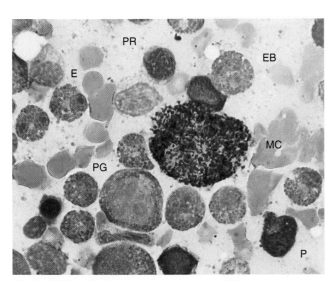

Figure 27-34 Bone marrow from a dog with systemic mastocytosis. Atypical, giant mast cells even in low numbers are indicative of mast cell neoplasia. Eosinophilic hyperplasia is often associated with mast cell tumors. Progranulocyte *(PG)*, eosinophilic bands *(EB)*, eosinophils *(E)*, plasma cells *(P)*, and polychromatophilic rubricytes *(PR)* surround an atypical mast cell *(MC)*. (Wright-Giemsa stain, original magnification 250×.)

In general, subjective evaluation of the proportions of myeloid and erythroid cells (subjective M:E ratio) is sufficient for diagnostic purposes, but quantitative ratios may be necessary in research studies and are an excellent way to learn hematopoietic cell morphology.

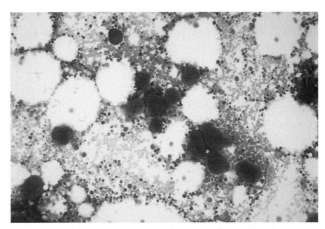

Figure 27-35 Bone marrow from a dog with immune-mediated thrombocytopenia. Increased numbers of megakaryocytes with basophilic cytoplasm indicate an appropriate regenerative response to platelet destruction. Megakaryocytes often are associated with unit particles or edges of the marrow smears and can best be located at low power. (Wright-Giemsa stain, original magnification 40×.)

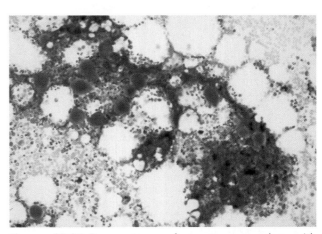

Figure 27-36 Bone marrow from a young dog with immune-mediated hemolytic anemia and immune-mediated thrombocytopenia. Hypercellular bone marrow with increased megakaryocytes and increased iron stores (brown-black pigment in unit particle) from a young dog with a diagnosis of increased iron turnover usually associated with hemolytic anemias or blood transfusions. This amount of iron could be acceptable for an old dog. Iron stores are not normally visible in cat bone marrow. (Wright-Giemsa stain, original magnification 40×.)

The M:E ratio is interpreted in relation to marrow cellularity and peripheral blood (hemogram) values. Table 27-6 gives several examples of how to interpret M:E ratios.

Examination for Erythrophagocytosis, Iron-Containing Pigments, Plasmacytosis/Lymphocytosis, Mast Cell Disorders, and Myelofibrosis

The marrow is examined for these conditions at all magnifications, and their presence is confirmed on the higher magnifications (40× or 50× and 100× objectives).

Interpretation of Megakaryocytes

Increased Megakaryocytes and/or Immature Forms	Decreased Megakaryocytes	Abnormal Megakaryocytes
Platelet consumption/destruction	Immune-mediated thrombocytopenia	Myeloproliferative disease
Immune-mediated thrombocytopenia	Infections (e.g., parovirus)	Megakaryocytic leukemia
Chronic anemia	Drug toxicities or idiosyncratic reactions (e.g., estrogen, chemotherapy, antibiotics)	B_{12} and/or folic acid deficiency
Inflammation	Aplastic anemia	
Essential thrombocythemia		
Megakaryocytic leukemia		

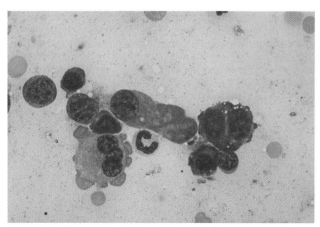

Figure 27-37 Bone marrow from a cat with megakaryocytic leukemia. The large basophilic binucleated cell is a promegakaryocyte. The multinucleated cell and the mononuclear cell with abundant trailing cytoplasm are atypical megkaryocytes. Megakaryocytic leukemia is rare and can be associated with either thrombocytopenia as in this case or thrombocytosis. (Wright-Giemsa stain, original magnification 250×.)

Erythrophagocytosis is rarely seen in marrow samples from normal animals. When erythrophagocytosis is a prominent feature of the marrow sample, ineffective erythropoiesis and/or extravascular hemolysis is suggested (see Figure 27-22). Ineffective erythropoiesis is the destruction of erythroid cells before they leave the marrow. Mild ineffective erythropoiesis may occur in some strongly regenerative anemias; however, marrow samples are seldom collected from animals with regenerative anemia. Additionally, erythrophagocytosis can be seen with hemic parasites (e.g., *Babesia* spp. and *Mycoplasma* spp.), post blood transfusions, histiocytic neoplasia and hemophagocytic histiocytosis.[18]

Evaluation of the marrow for iron pigments may require special stains, such as Prussian blue. However, black-brown aggregates of iron can frequently be observed in canine unit particles at low power (4× to10×) (see Figure 27-36). Hemosiderin can usually be seen as blue-black particulate material in macrophages when iron stores are plentiful in dogs. However, recognizable iron pigments may not be present in Romanowsky-type–stained marrow preparations from normal cats. Iron stores vary with age. Young dogs have little to no iron stores, whereas older dogs should have visible iron stores. Recognizable marrow iron associated with low serum iron and ferritin levels can result from anemia of inflammatory disease. Depleted marrow iron stores associated with low serum iron and ferritin levels are associated with iron deficiency. Box 27-6 lists causes for increased and decreased iron stores.

In dogs and cats, usually <2% of nucleated marrow cells are plasma cells. When >3% are plasma cells, immune stimulation should be suspected. Sometimes, chronic immune stimulation results in development of Mott cells (plasma cells stuffed with Russell bodies). Marrow plasmacytosis is often associated with myeloid hyperplasia. Plasmacytosis is sometimes associated with myeloid hypoplasia or a normal myeloid component in canine ehrlichiosis.

Plasmacytosis secondary to inflammatory conditions (e.g., chronic ehrlichiosis, immune-mediated hemolytic anemia, and/or thrombocytopenia) must be differentiated from multiple myeloma (plasma cell myeloma), which is a neoplastic proliferation (Figure 27-38). With multiple myeloma, there is usually a markedly hypercellular marrow with a diffuse increase in the concentration of plasma cells throughout the marrow and the plasma cells may exhibit atypical morphology. Dense sheets of plasma cells are usually present (see Figure 27-32).

Rickettsial titers, electrophoretic patterns, Bence Jones urine protein, and radiographs are diagnostic tools to distinguish multiple myeloma from a reactive plasmacytosis. Multiple myeloma is characterized by plasmacytosis, monoclonal gammopathy, Bence Jones proteinuria, and punched-out lytic bone lesions. Remember that ehrlichiosis and lymphoma occasionally have a monoclonal gammopathy.

Cytologically, mast cells are easily recognized in bone marrow smears. A few mast cells may be present normally; however, when mast cells are abundant, infiltration by mast cell neoplasia should be considered (see Figure 27-33). Mast cell hyperplasia associated with anemia (regenerative, nonregenerative, aplastic, and iron deficiency), myelofibrosis, lymphoma, and marrow hypocellularity has been reported.[19] In these cases, the low cellularity of the marrow accentuates the presence of the mast cells

TABLE 27-5

Some Causes of Nonregenerative Anemia in Dogs and Cats

Disease	Prominent marrow features	Helpful diagnostic procedures
Anemia of chronic disease	Erythroid hypoplasia and granulocytic hyperplasia with increased marrow iron and plasma cells	History, physical examination, clinical signs, marrow iron, serum ferritin
Renal insufficiency	Erythroid hypoplasia	History, physical examination, clinical signs, BUN and/or serum creatinine concentration, urinalysis
Nutritional iron deficiency or chronic blood loss	Erythroid hypoplasia; absent or decreased iron stores; small RBC precursors with scant, ragged cytoplasm	History, physical examination, clinical signs, marrow iron, serum ferritin
FeLV marrow suppression (in cats)	Erythroid hypoplasia with or without maturation arrest and/or abnormal morphology (e.g., megaloblastic erythroid cells); granulocytic hypoplasia may also be present.	Increased MCV on hemogram and/or the presence of megaloblastic erythrocytes in peripheral blood smears; ELISA, IFA, PCR, or virus isolation testing for FeLV
Ehrlichiosis (in dogs)	Early: Variable findings often hypercellular Late: Erythroid hypoplasia, usually granulocytic and megakaryocytic hypoplasia, increased plasma cells, rarely cytoplasmic morulae	*Ehrlichia* spp. titer or PCR and/or response to therapy
Estrogen toxicity (in dogs)	Erythroid, granulocytic, and megakaryocytic hypoplasia/aplasia; increase in lymphocytes, mast cells, and plasma cells.	History and physical examination
Drug toxicity (e.g., trimethoprim/sulfadiazine, chemotherapy drugs)	Usually granulocytic and megakaryocytic hypoplasia but erythroid hypoplasia or aplasia may be observed	History
Marrow necrosis	Erythroid, granulocytic, and megakaryocytic hypoplasia with pink homogeneous strands of necrotic nuclear material; early changes include cytoplasmic and nuclear vacuolation	History, core biopsy
Myelofibrosis (sclerosis)	Erythroid hypoplasia: flecks are sparse, collected flecks may be normocellular or hypercellular	Core biopsy is necessary to confirm myelofibrosis
Histoplasmosis	Organisms present: variable findings, but most commonly erythroid hypoplasia and granulocytic hyperplasia	Refer slide for identification, culture, titers
Hypothyroidism	Erythroid hypoplasia, variable iron stores	Thyroid panel, physical examination, clinical signs, hypercholesterolemia
Nonerythroid neoplasia (e.g., granulocytic leukemia, lymphocytic leukemia, lymphoma)	Erythroid hypoplasia with marked increase in cells of the neoplastic cell line; blast cell make up >30% of the cell population	Cytochemistry and/or flow cytometry or immunohistochemistry (core biopsy) to specifically identify the type of neoplasia, PCR for lymphoma
Erythoid neoplasia (in cats, extremely rare in dogs)	Increased erythroid cells often with a maturation arrest and/or abnormal morphology; may need to repeat aspirate to separate from early regenerative response	Refer bone marrow cytologic sample and peripheral blood smear for interpretation; ELISA, IFA, PCR, or virus isolation testing for FeLV

BUN, Blood urea nitrogen; *RBC,* red blood cell; *FeLV,* feline leukemia virus; *MCV,* mean cell volume; *ELISA,* enzyme-linked imunosorbent assay; *IFA,* indiret fluorescent antibody; *PCR,* polymerase chain reaction.

BOX 27-6

Interpretation of Bone Marrow Iron Stores

Increased Iron Stores
Hemolytic anemia
Anemia of chronic disease
Multiple blood transfusions
Old age
Hemochromatosis/hemosiderosis
Parenteral administration of iron

Decreased Iron Stores
Newborn or young animal
Nutritional iron deficiency
Chronic blood loss
Chronic phlebotomies

TABLE 27-6

Calculation and Interpretation of M:E ratio

BM Cellularity	Normal M:E*	Increased M:E*	Decreased M:E*
Normal	Normal	Myeloid hyperplasia and erythroid hypoplasia	Erythroid hyperplasia and myeloid hypoplasia
Increased	Myeloid and erythroid hyperplasia	Myeloid hyperplasia[†]	Erythroid hyperplasia[‡]
Decreased	Myeloid and erythroid hypoplasia	Erythroid hypoplasia	Myeloid hypoplasia

Example 1
BM cellularity—increased
Increased M:E ratio (6:1)
PCV 20%, nonregenerative anemia
WBC 25,000/μl, neutrophilia with a left shift
Interpretation: Myeloid hyperplasia and erythroid hypoplasia

Example 2
BM cellularity—increased
Decreased M:E ratio (1:6)
PCV 20%, regenerative anemia
WBC 10,000/μl with normal differential
Interpretation: Erythroid hyperplasia

$$\text{M:E ratio} = \frac{\text{Total myeloid cells}}{\text{Total nucleated erythroid cells}}$$

*Normal M:E ratio is slightly greater than 1:1; a range of 0.75-2.5 is often used when a 200-500 cell differential is performed. A ratio of 1:3 to 3:1 can be used as a crude normal range when M:E ratios are estimated.
[†]Evaluate CBC taken at time of BM biopsy to determine whether erythroid hypoplasia is also present.
[‡]Evaluate CBC taken at time of BM biopsy to determine whether myeloid hypoplasia is also present.

(see Figure 27-16). The overall marrow cellularity plus the absolute number and morphology of mast cells is used to differentiate mast cell hyperplasia from mast cell neoplasia (see Figure 27-34).

Myelofibrosis is the displacement of normal marrow elements (myelophthisis) by fibrous tissue. A few pockets of marrow usually persist within the fibrous tissue and undergo compensatory hyperplasia. Aspiration usually does not yield any marrow flecks, but occasionally a few small flecks may be recovered. These flecks usually contain very little fat and therefore appear hypercellular. Bone marrow core biopsy is necessary to definitively diagnose myelofibrosis.

Examinations of Bone Marrow for Organisms

Bone marrow cytologic preparations can be examined for organisms, such as *H. capsulatum* (see Figure 27-17), *L. donovani* (see Figure 27-18), *Mycobacterium* spp. (see Figure 27-19), *C. felis* (see Figure 27-20), *Babesia* spp. (see Figure 27-21), *Mycoplasma* spp. (see Figure 27-22), *T. gondii*, *Ehrlichia* spp. and *Anaplasma* spp., using the 40× or 50× and 100× (oil-immersion) objectives.[16] Usually, the areas of the

smear adjacent to the fleck and the edges of the fleck are the most rewarding because they tend to contain a greater concentration of marrow macrophages than other areas. When organisms are suspected, a short search should be performed. If they are not found quickly, the cytologic preparations should be sent to a consultant with more experience in identifying organisms and time to search for them. However, the examiner who has the time and enjoys bone marrow perusal should not be dissuaded from performing longer searches.

Diagnosis of Leukemia, Lymphoma, and Metastatic Neoplasia

The differentiation of neoplastic and myelodysplastic proliferative bone marrow disorders can be difficult (Box 27-7) (see Figure 27-30).[4-8,18-20] Primary bone marrow neoplasia can be subdivided into myeloproliferative, meaning myeloid, erythroid, or megakaryocytic (see Figures 27-30, 27-31, and 27-37); lymphoid (Figure 27-39; see Figure 27-13); histiocytic (Figure 27-40); and undifferentiated (Figure 27-41). The diagnosis of neoplasia can be especially challenging when the marrow has not been totally effaced by tumor cells. Early bone marrow recovery (e.g., repopulation after parvovirus infection) or an early regenerative response may look neoplastic with increased blast cells approaching 30% (see Figure 27-29). Therefore, it is imperative to scrutinize all available information and if still in doubt, re-evaluate the CBC and, if necessary, the marrow in 3 to 5 days. By that time an early regenerative marrow will exhibit orderly maturation, whereas neoplasia will have the same or increased blast population. A good guideline for diagnosing neoplasia is finding ≥ 30% blast cells (leukemia), ≥ 30% lymphoblasts/lymphocytes (lymphoma), ≥ 15% plasma cells (multiple myeloma), and sheets or large clusters of cells (metastatic mast cell tumor, histiocytic sarcoma, metastatic carcinoma, or sarcoma).

In addition to numbers, cellular atypia can also suggest neoplasia even in the face of relatively few neoplastic-appearing cells (e.g., atypical plasma cells or mast cells) (see Figure 27-34). Suspected myelodysplastic syndromes, chronic leukemias, and specific classification of leukemia need to be referred to an experienced clinical pathologist.

Lymphoid neoplasia often infiltrates bone marrow (see Figures 27-13 and 27-39). However, it is important to remember that although uncommon, normal dog and cat marrow can contain up to 15% and 20% lymphocytes, respectively.[4-8,13-15] Increased small lymphocytes can occasionally occur in reactive processes often associated with increased plasma cells. But, whenever lymphocytes are increased in the bone marrow, Stage V

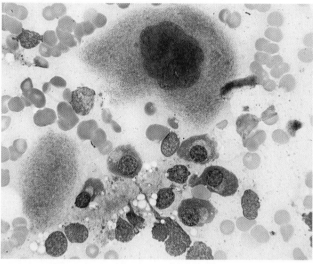

Figure 27-38 Bone marrow from a dog with immune-mediated hemolytic anemia. A small cluster of well-differentiated plasma cells is adjacent to a mature megakaryocyte. Immune-mediated hemolytic anemia and ehrlichiosis are common causes of reactive plasmacytosis. (Wright-Giemsa stain, original magnification 250×.)

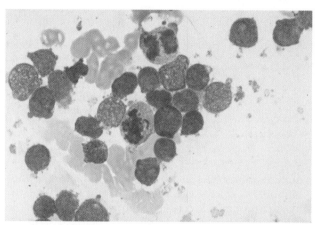

Figure 27-39 Bone marrow from a dog with hypercalcemia and Stage V lymphoma. Note the homogeneous appearance of these rounds cells and the scant amount of cytoplasm. Two mitotic figures are present. Lymphoma may have many different morphologic appearances and sometimes requires special staining techniques to prove that the cells are lymphoid and not another round cell population. Immunophenotyping confirmed T-cell lymphoma. (Wright-Giemsa stain, original magnification 250×.)

BOX 27-7

Classification of Nonneoplastic and Neoplastic Proliferative Bone Marrow Disorders

Myeloproliferative*	Lymphoproliferative	Histiocytic
Acute myeloid leukemias	Acute lymphocytic leukemia	Histiocytic sarcoma‡
Chronic myeloid leukemia	Lymphoma stage V	Systemic histiocytosis
First- and second-degree polycythemia	Chronic lymphocytic leukemia	Malignant fibrous histiocytoma
Essential thrombocythemia	Plasma cell neoplasia	Hemophagic histiocytosis
Mast cell leukemia	Plasmacytosis†	Storage diseases
Myelodysplastic syndrome		IMHA
Inflammatory disease		
Regenerative anemia		

*Includes myeloid, erythroid, and megakaryocytic cell lines.
†Ehrlichiosis, IMHA, etc.
‡Includes malignant histiocytosis (MH).
IMHA, Immune-mediated hemolytic anemia.

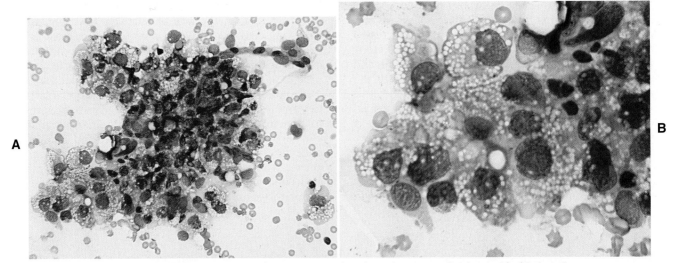

Figure 27-40 Bone marrow from an anemic, thrombocytopenic dog with histiocytic sarcoma (malignant histiocytosis). **A,** Cohesive clusters of large histiocytic cells with abundant pale blue vacuolated cytoplasm have displaced normal bone marrow hemic cells. (Wright-Giemsa stain, original magnification 80×.) **B,** Higher magnification of bone marrow sample in **A** reinforces the large cell size (compare with red cell size), abundant cytoplasm, moderate to marked anisocytosis and anisokaryosis, and erythrophagia. (Wright-Giemsa stain, original magnification 250×.)

lymphoma must be ruled out. Neoplastic lymphocytes/lymphoblasts can be confused with other blasts in the bone marrow and special techniques (flow cytometry, immunohistochemical staining, cytochemical staining) may be necessary for definitive identification. When ≥30% of the nucleated cells in marrow can be definitely recognized as lymphoblasts, lymphoid neoplasia is indicated. Lymphoglandular bodies (basophilic cytoplasmic fragments) are frequently associated with lymphoma in the bone marrow. Bone marrow evaluation for staging of lymphoma can be challenging because the early infiltration is focal or multifocal and identification of the scattered neoplastic lymphocyte population can easily be overlooked. Also, acute lymphocytic leukemia (lymphoid neoplasia arising first in the blood and bone marrow as compared with lymphoma that initially develops in primary lymphoid tissue and secondarily infiltrates the bone marrow) can be cytologically indistinguishable from acute myeloid leukemia. For these reasons, it is best to send these samples to a diagnostic laboratory. Core biopsy with immunohistochemical lymphocyte markers, flow cytometric analysis, polymerase chain reaction (PCR), and cytochemical staining are helpful diagnostic tools to detect lymphoma or lymphoid leukemia in the bone marrow. Bone marrow examination from patients with chronic lymphocytic leukemia can be unrewarding, and evaluation of spleen is recommended in these cases.

Metastatic neoplasia is uncommon in dog and cat bone marrow especially as compared to humans. Rarely, neoplasms such as carcinomas may metastasize to bone marrow (see Figures 27-27 and 27-28). Carcinomas tend to form cohesive cell clusters, which distinguish them from hematopoietic cells even at low power. Multiple smears should be examined because the lesion(s) may be

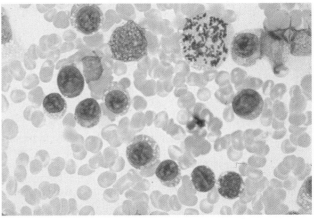

Figure 27-41 Bone marrow from a cat with round cell neoplasia. A relatively uniform population of discrete round cells with round nuclei and scant, often finely vacuolated cytoplasm has replaced the normal marrow population. A large mitotic figure is at the top of the field. These cells did not mark for any of the standard leukemia, lymphoma, or histiocytic markers, indicating their undifferentiated status. (Wright-Giemsa stain, original magnification 250×.)

focal or multifocal. Thorough scanning of marrow smears at low power is essential to identify suspicious areas of homogeneous cell populations or cohesive cell clusters to examine at higher magnification (see Figures 27-27 and 27-28). Neoplastic mast cell tumors and plasma cell tumors present a unique problem because mast cells and plasma cells can normally be in the bone marrow in low numbers and can be increased in nonneoplastic disease process.[19] Therefore it is important to evaluate both numbers and morphology of mast cells and plasma cells to determine wheather neoplasia is present.

BOX 27-8

Some Causes of Bone Marrow Dysfunction

Bone Marrow Damage

Infections*
- Viral
  - FeLV
  - FIV
  - Parvovirus
  - Canine distemper
- Rickettsial
  - Ehrlichiosis
  - Anaplasmosis
- Bacterial
  - Mycobacteriosis
  - Any septicemia
- Mycoplasma-like
  - *M. haemofelis*
  - *M. haemominutum*
  - *M. haemocanis*
- Protozoal
  - Cytauxzoonosis
  - Babesiosis
  - Leishmaniasis
- Fungal/Yeast
  - Histoplasmosis
  - Any systemic fungi

Toxic drugs
- Chemotherapy drugs
- Estrogen*
- Trimethoprim/sulfadiazine
- Phenylbutazone
- Medicated skin creams
- Thiacetarsamide
- Griseofulvin
- Meclofenamic acid
- Quinidine
- Fenbendazole

Radiation

Immunologic mechanism
- Pure red cell aplasia
- Anti-rhEPO antibodies

Bone Marrow Replacement

Leukemia
Lymphoma
Myelofibrosis
Myelonecrosis
Osteosclerosis
Metastatic neoplasia
Infectious granulomas

Microenvironment or Hereditary Factors

Acquired deficiencies/defects
- Inflammation
  - Iron utilization defect
- Erythropoietin
  - Renal disease
  - Liver disease?
- Nutritional deficiencies
  - Iron deficiency
  - Starvation (protein)
  - Vitamin B_{12}/folic acid
- Toxins
  - Lead
  - Uremic toxins
- Hypothyroidism

Hereditary or congenital
- Pyruvate kinase deficiency
- Canine cyclic hematopoiesis
- Leukocyte adhesion deficiency
- Chediak-Higashi syndrome
- Pelger-Huët syndrome[†]
- Poodle macrocytosis
- Vitamin B_{12} malabsorption - Giant Schnauzers
- Congenital dyserythropoiesis— English Springer Spaniels

*Cellularity varies with stage of disease.
[†]Hyposegmented granulocytes (neutrophils and eosinophils) without clinical disease effects.
FeLV, Feline leukemia virus; *FIV*, feline immunodeficiency virus.

SUMMARY OF BONE MARROW EVALUATION AND INTERPRETATION

Bone marrow examination is a valuable diagnostic and prognostic tool for the evaluation of hematopoietic disorders. A primary goal of the practitioner is taking quality bone marrow samples and preparing good smears. A good sample is mandatory for accurate assessment of the bone marrow. After a thorough, methodical examination of the marrow (see Box 27-3), a brief but complete report should be generated that includes all observations. Final conclusions and interpretations must incorporate signalment, history, physical findings, laboratory results including concurrent blood smear examination, and bone marrow findings. See Figure 27-42 for an interpretation algorithm and Tables 27-5 and Box 27-8 for some causes of bone marrow dysfunction.

A core biopsy is necessary to document myelofibrosis/myelonecrosis, confirm hypocellularity, and help identify focal metastatic neoplasia. To refer bone marrow cytology samples, submit both stained and unstained smears and liquid bone marrow in EDTA. Avoid shipping smears with formalin specimens as formalin vapors fix the smears

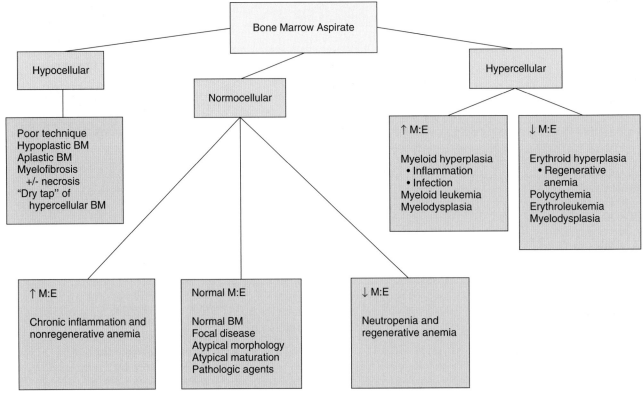

Figure 27-42 Algorithm for bone marrow *(BM)* interpretation. *M:E,* Myeloid-to-erythroid ratio.

and alter staining quality. For special procedures such as flow cytometry, immunohistochemistry, cytochemistry, electron microscopy, and PCR that help identify or characterize neoplastic cell populations or etiologic agents, contact the reference laboratory regarding specific instructions for sample submission.

References

1. Kearns SH, Ewing P: Causes of canine and feline pancytopenia. *Comp Cont Ed Pract Vet* 28:122, 2006.
2. Neel JA, Birkenheuer AJ, Grindem CB: Immune mediated and infectious thrombocytopenia in dogs and cats. In Bonagura J (ed): *Kirk's Current Veterinary Therapy XIV*, St. Louis, Saunders, In press.
3. Weiss DJ: A retrospective study of the incidence and the classification of bone marrow disorders in the dog at a veterinary teaching hospital (1996-2004). *J Vet Intern Med* 20:955, 2006.
4. Grindem CB, Neel JA, Juopperi TA: Cytology of bone marrow. *Vet Clin Small Anim* 32:1313, 2002.
5. Harvey JW: *Atlas of Veterinary Hematology.* Philadelphia, Saunders, 2001.
6. Jain NC: Examination of the blood and bone marrow. In Jain NC (ed): *Essentials of Veterinary Hematology*, Philadelphia, Lea & Febiger, 1993.
7. Thrall MA, Weiser G, Jain N: Laboratory evaluation of bone marrow. In Thrall MA (ed): *Veterinary hematology and clinical chemistry.* Baltimore, Lippincott Williams & Wilkins, 2004.
8. Wellman ML, Radin MJ: *Bone Marrow Evaluation in Dogs and Cats.* Wimington, Del, The Gloyd Group, 1999.
9. Harvey JW: Canine bone marrow: Normal hematopoiesis, biopsy techniques and cell identification and evaluation. *Comp Cont Ed Pract Vet* 6:909, 1984.
10. Hoff B, Lumsden JH, Valli VEO: An appraisal of bone marrow biopsy in assessment of sick dogs. *Can J Comp Med* 49:34-42, 1985.
11. Friedrichs KR, Young KM: How to collect diagnostic bone marrow samples. *Vet Med* 100:578, 2005.
12. Relford RL: The steps in performing a bone marrow aspiration and core biopsy. *Vet Med* 86:670, 1991.
13. Grindem CB: Bone marrow biopsy and evaluation. *Vet Clin North Am Small Anim Pract* 19:669, 1989.
14. Mischke R, Busse L: Reference values for the bone marrow aspirates in adult dogs. *J Vet Med Assoc* 49:499, 2002.
15. Weiss DJ: Differentiating benign and malignant causes of lymphocytosis in feline bone marrow. *J Vet Intern Med* 19:855, 2005.
16. Greene CE: *Infectious Diseases of the Dog and Cat*, ed 3. St. Louis, Saunders, 2006.
17. Mischke R, et al: Quantification of thrombopoietic activity in bone marrow aspirates of dogs. *Vet J* 164:269, 2002.
18. DeHeer HL, Grindem CB: Histiocytic disorders. In Feldman BF, Zinkl JG, Jain NC (eds): *Schalm's Veterinary Hematology*, ed 5. Philadelphia, Lippincott Williams & Wilkins, 2000.
19. Plier ML, MacWilliams PS: Systemic mastocytosis and mast cell leukemia. In Feldman BF, Zinkl JG, Jain NC (eds): *Schalm's Veterinary Hematology*, ed 5. Philadelphia, Lippincott Williams & Wilkins, 2000.
20. Blue JT: Myelodysplastic syndromes and myelofibrosis. In Feldman BF, Zinkl JG, Jain NC, (eds): *Schalm's Veterinary Hematology*, ed 5. Philadelphia, Lippincott Williams & Wilkins, 2000.

Index

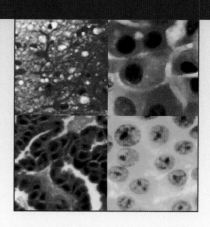

Note: Page numbers followed by *f* indicate figures; *t*, tables; and *b*, boxes.